RESEARCH METHODS IN THE SOCIAL AND HEALTH SCIENCES

For Anne-Marie and Jodi

RESEARCH METHODS IN THE SOCIAL AND HEALTH SCIENCES

Making Research Decisions

Ted Palys
Simon Fraser University

Chris Atchison
University of British Columbia

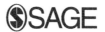

Los Angeles | London | New Delhi
Singapore | Washington DC | Melbourne

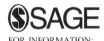

FOR INFORMATION:

SAGE Publications, Inc.
2455 Teller Road
Thousand Oaks, California 91320
E-mail: order@sagepub.com

SAGE Publications Ltd.
1 Oliver's Yard
55 City Road
London EC1Y 1SP
United Kingdom

SAGE Publications India Pvt. Ltd.
B 1/I 1 Mohan Cooperative Industrial Area
Mathura Road, New Delhi 110 044
India

SAGE Publications Asia-Pacific Pte. Ltd.
3 Church Street
#10-04 Samsung Hub
Singapore 049483

Printed in the United States of America

ISBN 978-1-5443-5767-6

This book is printed on acid-free paper.

Acquisitions Editor: Leah Fargotstein
Editorial Assistant: Sam Diaz
Production Editor: TNQ
Copy Editor: TNQ
Typesetter: TNQ
Proofreader: TNQ
Cover Designer: Gail Buschman

21 22 23 24 25 10 9 8 7 6 5 4 3 2 1

BRIEF CONTENTS

DETAILED CONTENTS

PREFACE

We have to begin by expressing our great pleasure at joining the SAGE family with the publication of *Research Methods in the Social and Health Sciences: Making Research Decisions*, and we are honored by the opportunity this gives us to explain research methods in the contemporary world to students, the next generation of researchers. Our title pays homage to one of the first contemporary texts to offer advice on how to design and implement a broad range of research methods used in the social and behavioral sciences—*Research Methods in the Behavioral Sciences* by Leon Festinger and Daniel Katz (1953). Looking back to their book and the context in which it was written reveals much about how the world and thinking about research methods have changed in those intervening years as well as providing a backdrop against which to highlight the principles that frame this book.

One obvious change from the world that Festinger and Katz wrote in is the assortment of technology that has become integral to the conduct of research in the 21st century. Computers first had an impact on the range of and ease with which analyses could be done; nowadays anyone with no more than a laptop can engage in complex analyses of qualitative, quantitative, and mixed data with a mouse click. Then came the internet. For researchers this brought the creation of digital libraries accessible from anywhere; access to other resource materials including myriad sources of data; access to communities that otherwise could never have been reached in any significant number; and the creation of means of ongoing communication between researchers and research participants that have made the world a much smaller and more connected place. Clearly any book about research methods for the 21st century needs to incorporate discussion about all these advances, both in terms of the many doors that have opened and opportunities created via the digital revolution, but also with appropriate cautions about what this might mean for researchers given how digital surveillance has emerged thus far as the digital world's driving economic principle.

The students who come to us to learn about research also are very different from those who were going to universities and colleges when Festinger and Katz's book came out. For one thing, many of the students who take our courses these days are the first never to have known a world without digital and information technology. But the demographic changes are dramatic as well. Chris tells a story in Chapter 12 about his days in the doctoral program at the University of Toronto, seeing pictures of graduating classes in the corridors of buildings that have been part of the U of T campus for almost 150 years. He notes it was only in the years following World War II where nonmale and nonwhite faces start to appear in the pictures with any regularity. Although access to postsecondary education still has a long way to go to achieve anything even mildly approximating equity and universality, those who come now are most certainly far more diverse than was the case in the 1950s. The upshot of these developments is that research methods texts need to be able to speak to people who are undaunted by and eager to embrace technology and are collectively connected to far more diverse communities than was the case for Festinger and Katz.

There is also far less we can assume about our students' aspirations than was the case for Festinger and Katz. If you wanted to be a researcher in their day, odds are that you would be pursuing graduate degrees and looking for an academic appointment. These days lucrative research opportunities exist throughout society with government, corporations, and the nonprofit sector all looking for people who know how to put together a survey, conduct an interview, analyze a data set, or are able simply to critically analyze a report based on such data. Clearly a methods text for the 21st century needs to include not only theory-driven research that still fuels the academy but also has useful guidance for those who will be marketing and applying their research skills in nonacademic environments where people are looking to understand their markets, get a handle on consumer sentiment, and evaluate programs and policies in terms of everything from their broader impact down to the simple question of whether they accomplish what they set out to do.

The academy has changed as well. The faculty are far more diverse than they were in the 1950s, which has brought a whole new dimension of courses, programs, and lines of inquiry. First came greater diversity of courses as Women's studies, Indigenous programs, and African-American studies programs came into existence in the 1960s. The 1970s and 1980s also brought with them a new interest in interdisciplinarity, which saw the creation of new transdisciplinary disciplines such as communications, health studies, sexology, human ecology, criminology, environmental studies, and kinesiology. We see a similar cross-fertilization these days where multidisciplinary and often multiinstitutional research teams come together with a large research grant that brings broad focus to the study of important social and health issues. It surprises us how many research books are still written as if the researcher will be working alone or perhaps with a student or two. Certainly such researchers still exist; Ted is an example of someone who more typically works that way. But researchers like Chris, who these days more commonly works with teams of researchers from different disciplines where data gathering and data management strategies are integral to ensuring that everyone stays on the same page, exemplify a growingly common scenario.

All of these changes have had further implications for the types of research that is done and the methods that are implemented. We see far greater sensitivity to cultural issues and acknowledgment of the harm that can be done to communities when researchers execute hit-and-run research without regard to the community that will be impacted by their work. We also see a more participant-centered consideration of research ethics. The transition of calling those who take part in our research "research participants" instead of "research subjects," as Festinger and Katz knew them, speaks volumes about our changing relationship with communities—more egalitarian, more collaborative, less exploitative, more respectful. Methodological models based on a more collaborative relationship with the community—as you see in participatory action research and critical ethnography to give but two examples—help ensure that cooperation will be realized.

Further exemplifying this trend, one of the biggest transitions in academe in the last decade has been growing attention to the idea of "knowledge transfer"—encouraging researchers to figure out ways their research can get exposure beyond the twenty other experts in the field who will read their journal article. Social media now helps researchers both respond to and build the communities they will work with through a career. Any research methods text for the 21st century needs to discuss this broader presence and greater connectedness that many researchers seek and that their institutions and funders encourage.

Accompanying the greater diversity and more team-based and interdisciplinary research we describe above has also been more tolerance about embracing a wider array of methodological models. When Ted published his first book on research methods in 1992, it was the first one we know of that actually included both qualitative and quantitative methods under one cover (Palys, 1992). That combination has now become commonplace, with the bulk of the academy now embracing the utility and wisdom of mixed-methods approaches and the more comprehensive understanding such approaches bring.

We mention all these changes not only to highlight how much things have changed since Festinger and Katz (1953) published their monograph but also to introduce you to the content and perspective of *Research Methods in the Social and Health Sciences: Making Research Decisions*. All of these shifts have implications for what gets included in a research methods text and how they are discussed, and they set the backdrop for the themes that have found fertile ground in this book.

Chapter by Chapter

Chapter 1 lays out the broad organizing scheme for the book. After outlining some of the key characteristics of qualitative and quantitative traditions in research, we discuss and give examples of how the introduction of mixed-methods approaches have allowed social and health researchers to conduct research that leverages the strengths of each tradition to ask and answer more complex research questions and thereby to generate more comprehensive descriptions, understandings, or explanations. This theme appears throughout the book.

Chapter 2 on "Getting Started" distinguishes deductive, inductive, and abductive approaches while noting their complementarity; introduces the notion of operationalization; discusses reliability and validity; encourages using our "sociological imagination" to identify the bigger issues that are reflected in our research questions; and reaffirms the empirical commitment to both theory and data. Our discussion of the literature includes attention to the bourgeoning creation of virtual libraries and other internet-based sources and how software developed for the analysis of talk, text, image, and video—such as NVivo—can be used with electronic libraries as an information management tool at every stage of the research process.

With greater emphasis on the ability to secure funding in order to be able to conduct research, coupled with more onerous process requirements that must be met prior to getting approval to do your research, proposal writing has become a requisite skill, and we are aware of more and more courses that require students to write a proposal as their term project rather than undertaking an actual piece of research. Accordingly, **Chapter 3** outlines those elements would-be researchers need to address that speak to the concerns of those who evaluate such proposals—including research methods professors!

Chapter 4 begins with a broad discussion of some of the main ethical principles to consider when undertaking any research project—informed consent, confidentiality, conflicts of interest and roles—but also encourages readers to connect with ethical issues that Institutional Review Boards often pay less attention to, such as questions of voice and privilege, the general nature of the relationship we have with participants before and after a project, and so on. Attention is also devoted to some of the new ethical issues that have arisen because of the wide array of internet-based sources and computer-assisted means of gathering data, such as the more ambiguous boundaries that exist between "public" and "private" forums and the question of whether data that are transmitted over the internet can be considered secure and confidential. The government-created regulatory systems that academic institutions have implemented in the US, Canada, Australia, New Zealand and the UK are also discussed. Although we focus on the Common Rule in the US, Canadian readers can find a Canadian-focused version among the book's supplementary materials on the Sage website.

Chapter 5 focuses on both sampling and recruitment, that is, the latter recognizing that finding people who might participate in your research is one thing, but actually convincing them to agree to participate is another. As an example, the chapter includes an extensive discussion of Chris's research with sex workers and their clients—two groups that have been notoriously difficult to engage in research and hence about whom little has been known—and his pioneering work that allowed him to engage samples of thousands of individuals who have completed his surveys and agreed to be interviewed.

Chapters 6–8 then deal with different aspects of causal inference and data analysis, each of which emphasizes the idea that the challenge of research design is typically one of gathering information to enhance our understanding of phenomena while at the same time eliminating as many rival plausible explanations for their occurrence as possible. Chapter 6 does so within the context of classic experimental design where students learn a vocabulary (thanks to Donald T. Campbell) that can be applied to any research design, and where the logic of eliminating rival plausible explanations is clear. This is followed in Chapter 7 with discussions of quasi-experimental design and evaluation research in a manner that extends the rival plausible explanations theme to incorporate notions of analytic control, which is further developed in Chapter 8 on case study analysis.

In **Chapters 9–12** we present some of the main techniques that are used by social and health science researchers to gather data—including surveys, interviews, oral histories, observation, ethnography, participant observation, content analysis, and archival data including official statistics and secondary data sources. We discuss in each the many data-gathering opportunities that are now available via the internet and intranets, new ways that digital technologies can facilitate and enhance the data-gathering process, and ways that the various techniques can be combined with one another to gain the benefits of mixed-method inquiry.

Chapters 13 and 14 focus more exclusively on analysis. Chapter 13 pays considerable attention to the impacts that the digital revolution is having on the research process. This is evident both in the range of nonnumerical sources that are available to researchers via the internet—where the predominantly textual sources of yesteryear are being expanded through virtual libraries and extensive archives that exist and/or can be created from videos, audio sources, Twitter feeds, Facebook entries, and so on—and in the availability of qualitative data analysis (QDA) software that can be used to both manage and analyze these diverse sources. We introduce readers to an array of qualitative data analysis software but focus most on the program that suits our research best—NVivo—to illustrate just what can be accomplished if you take the digital plunge. While important to discuss, we also were aware that many universities and colleges have yet to make QDA software available to their faculty and students, and hence have sought at this time mostly to whet your appetite for what such programs can accomplish in the hope that we will be further along when and if another edition of this book is contemplated in the future. In the interim, we encourage students and faculty to download free trial versions of the programs that will give you an opportunity to try out the software firsthand, preferably with data you have gathered, and to take advantage of the many tutorials and webinars that are available online to help new users get started and those who are already familiar with the software to expand their proficiency.

Chapter 14 offers a conceptual introduction to the analysis of numerical data that keeps to more basic and foundational conceptual tools for describing data (e.g., standard deviation, variance, degrees of freedom, central tendency and skew) and very basic statistical techniques (e.g., z-scores, chi-square, correlation, t-test). We made this choice for two reasons. First is that we presume this text will not be used in a statistics class. Accordingly, we decided to keep with very basic techniques that are foundational for more advanced statistics and to leave those more advanced statistical techniques for the professor in students' next statistics course. Secondly, we are always astonished to find how many people who can execute various razzle-dazzle statistical procedures nonetheless really do not understand very basic statistical concepts. Thus, we felt that the best service we could do for our readers was to provide the very foundational conceptual introduction you see here, and thereby to prepare students for advanced techniques that for the most part are simply more complicated and generalized versions of the techniques we talk about in this book.

We close the book with **Chapter 15**, which we have entitled "Disseminating Your Research." In previous years this would have been strictly a "writing" chapter, but for all the reasons we cite at the beginning of this preface, we believe it important that any research methods text for the 21st century needs to recognize that even though writing journal articles and books remains an important thing we do, being a 21st-century researcher calls for a broader range of skills. First of all, we talk about presentations and all that you can do not only to avoid "death by PowerPoint" but also to create a powerful presentation that engages and "speaks to" the diverse audiences you are likely to be addressing in your classes, at conferences, and in community meetings. We conclude with a discussion of some of the ways you can mobilize social media both to build a community around your research interests and to remain connected with and continue to inform them even after your project has ended.

Pedagogical Features

Research Methods in the Social and Health Sciences: Making Research Decisions includes several pedagogical features to help professors, teaching assistants, and students work through and benefit from the material contained in the book:

- We direct students' attention to key material and concepts throughout the book by highlighting key concepts and compiling them at the end of each chapter.

- We provide opportunities for independent practice by providing study questions at the end of each chapter. The questions and definitions of key concepts help students focus their studying (either individually or as part of a study group) and provide a learning check on key concepts discussed in each chapter.

- Instructors will find the study questions and lists of key concepts a useful source for exam questions that reflect the main themes and ideas of each chapter. Problems also are included that can be used to promote critical discussion in a class, lab, or tutorial group; suggested activities are included that can be a basis for student essays and term projects.

- Liberal use of citations provides numerous literature sources—both classic and contemporary—for professors and more advanced students who wish to examine the issues discussed in this book in more detail.

- Each chapter ends with a section entitled "Summing up and looking ahead" that summarizes each chapter's main themes and provides a segue to the chapters that follow.

- A series of appendices provides supplementary information that negates the need for other sources with respect to tests of significance.

The most important pedagogical feature we include, however, from our perspective, is that this book has been written by two people who love doing research, love talking about research, and love explaining research to anyone interested in hearing about it.

We typically find when we read other research methods texts that every research methods book has one great chapter—which usually involves the method in which the author has expertise—while the rest of the book sounds more distant and as if it were based largely on secondary sources. In contrast, the two of us have several decades of collective experience using virtually every method we talk about in this book in a wide array of social and health research settings, which allows us not only to articulate research methods at a conceptual level but also to share stories about our work to give readers a feel for how those concepts play out in the course of actually doing research. We feel that this, accompanied by our narrative writing style, makes the book very accessible and the sometimes complex material much more understandable.

Personal Notes

We are indebted to many for their collegiality and feedback along the way. At the top of the list are our fine colleagues and friends who understand how much we appreciate their trenchant criticism and the unconditional affection and encouragement in which it is always wrapped. The list is a lengthy one, but we especially wish to thank Howie Becker, Patrick John Burnett, the late Donald T. Campbell, Sheri Fabian, Bill Glackman, Kevin Haggerty, Mark Israel, Darrell Kean, Louise Kidder, Katarina Kolar, John Lowman, Anthony McIntyre, Russel Ogden, John Russell, Juan Tauri, Will van den Hoonaard, and Dalia Vukmirovich. We especially thank Dalia Vukmirovich and April Chai for their assistance in tying up some of the many loose ends that needed tying as we entered the home stretch and were finalizing the book for submission to the production team at SAGE.

At SAGE, numerous individuals have played a role in making the book what it is, and we have been blessed with a group of incredibly effective and capable people. We have always held SAGE and the books they produce in the methods area in high esteem—in our view they are second to none in that realm—and have been nothing but impressed with the professionalism we encountered in working with them. Leah Fargotstein, our acquisitions editor, coordinated extensive reviewer feedback across ten different disciplines, took us to the point of consensus regarding what our final submission for publication would include, and has kept the entire process on track. Claire Laminen, editorial assistant, was wonderful to work with both in dealing with bureaucratic and management issues, as well as ensuring we had access to appropriate resources to complete our writing. The efforts of copy editor Agnes Preethi also were much appreciated; it was a pleasure working with someone who became involved with the material and made some great suggestions that improved the book. We also thank production editor manager Olivia Weber-Stenis and the design, permissions, and marketing folks who ensured this book made it into your hands.

Mostly, however, we thank the faculty who will consider this book for their courses in universities and colleges across the country and internationally, and our students, whose questions and feedback help us speak to them. In the end it is only because of all of you that we had the opportunity to deal with the challenge and the great fun of figuring out what to include in this book and how best to explain it. Our hope, of course, is that you enjoy this book as much as the two of us have enjoyed collaborating on creating it.

The authors and SAGE would also like to thank the following people for their thoughtful input during the development of this book:

Rhonda Breitkreuz, University of Alberta

Regina Conway-Phillips, Loyola University Chicago, Niehoff School of Nursing

Mustafa Demir, State University of New York at Plattsburgh

Karen H. Larwin, Youngstown State University

Mark Malisa, University of West Florida

Cathryn Molloy, James Madison University

Michael Rich, Emory University

Jon Wergin, Antioch University

Kenneth C. C. Yang, The University of Texas at El Paso

Finally, we are also accessible via the internet. You can email Ted at palys@sfu.ca or visit his webpage at www.sfu.ca/~palys/, and/or email Chris at atch@shaw.ca and see his website at www.academic-freedom.ca. Both websites contain links that might be of interest to professors and students.

Ted Palys and Chris Atchison

Vancouver, BC

1 August 2020

ABOUT THE AUTHORS

Chris Atchison is an accomplished health and social science researcher who has spent over two decades designing, conducting, and administering a wide range of regional and national, interdisciplinary research initiatives. He has published and taught extensively in the area of mixed-methods research within the social and health sciences and is a leader in the development of computer-assisted research design and analysis techniques. Throughout his career Chris has focused much of his attention on developing innovative methods for the study of a wide variety of social justice issues in an effort to help provide a space for the voices of stigmatized, marginalized, and disenfranchised groups to be heard. He has contributed to projects in areas ranging from youth labor regulation, social welfare, health-care provision, mental illness, Aboriginal identity and achievement, and sex worker safety and security.

Ted Palys is a social science researcher, methodologist, and Professor at Simon Fraser University in Vancouver, Canada. His methodological interests go beyond the pragmatics of design and analysis to include implications of research policy changes on the sociology of knowledge. One such focus was on the impacts of the development of national codes of ethics and review and how institutions deal with legal threats to research confidentiality (see *Protecting Research Confidentiality: What Happens When Law and Ethics Collide*, 2014, with coauthor John Lowman). He was one of five academics from across the country appointed by the Presidents of Canada's federal granting agencies to advise them how to improve Canada's federal ethics policy's consideration of research in the social sciences and humanities. More recently, his concerns with surveillance capitalism as the economic model for the internet have led him into the realm of internet governance and the threat that model holds for our ability to protect research participants while doing research in controversial areas that often have the greatest need for empirically derived information on which to develop and evaluate law and policy alternatives.

PERSPECTIVES ON RESEARCH

Sociology, psychology, criminology, business administration, education, political science, nursing, social work, communications, health studies, human ecology, and the rest of the social and health sciences each have a designated academic "turf." But this book deals with something these otherwise diverse disciplines have in common—a belief in the desirability of trying to obtain the best possible answers to research questions that involve exploring, describing, understanding, explaining, and sometimes bringing about change through the systematic study and analysis of attitudes, beliefs, behaviors, and artifacts, i.e., research.

You may be one of those students who is interested in research, enrolled eagerly in your research methods courses, and is simply interested in learning something about how it's done. If you fall into this category, then no problem; this book is written by two "keeners" who love doing, teaching, and talking about research and are eager to share what we know.

But we've also taught enough research methods courses to know that there are students at the other end of the spectrum as well, i.e., those who have been dragged kicking and screaming into a required course (as research methods courses often are) and wondering what they might have done in a previous life to have been sentenced to this semester of pain. What we have found among this latter group is that they are often people who are not interested in research as a career, are more interested in what they see as a more applied or professional vocation, and, because of that, write off "research" as an esoteric or arcane pursuit that is only of interest to academics and has nothing of relevance to offer them.

We suggest quite the opposite is true, i.e., that "research" is one of the most fundamental things you can learn about, and that it is relevant to absolutely any walk of life you might wish to enter. Surely there is no more basic human process than (1) being curious about something we want to understand or having a question we want to answer; (2) identifying and gathering the information we have decided is "relevant" to our question or concern; (3) making sense of the information; and (4) forming some tentative conclusions on the basis of it. Who doesn't do that? Your physician does that when you go in to complain about the pain in your side and they start asking questions and poking around to try and diagnose the source of the problem. The courts do that when they interview witnesses and examine forensic evidence to try to determine guilt or innocence. Your mechanic does that when they try to figure out why your car is making that pinging sound whenever you accelerate. Journalists do it when they gather information to write stories and engage in analysis about events in the news. You did that when you tried to figure out what university or college to attend and what program of study to pursue. It's also one of the reasons that Google has become one of the largest companies on the planet.

Asking questions and trying to figure out what is going on and why things happen the way they do is a fundamental part of being human; there seems to be no end to the questions we pose and the information we wish to access. We may not always call these activities "research" or the processes we follow "research methods"—in fact, most of the time we don't—but people and events engage our curiosity, and we try to understand. In doing so, we gather information, decide who and which parts of it we believe, form conclusions, and act on them. The main difference is thus not in what we do—because we all do "research" every day in our own particular way—but in the extent to which we reflect on how we know what we know and on the rules or principles we use to determine whether what we believe is a "fact" or something else, e.g., a rumor, speculation, hearsay, guess, or simply wrong.

NO ROYAL ROAD TO TRUTH

There are many misconceptions people have about research as a way of understanding the world. One of the biggest is the idea that there is only one "right" method of research. Those who subscribe to this view include all those researchers who only learn one method in the first place. We have a hard time understanding that approach; it makes as much sense to us as a carpenter who refuses to use any tool but a hammer. When all you have is a hammer, you are immediately limited only to jobs that require hammering; it makes far more sense to us to decide first what you would like to build and then use tools appropriate to the task.

Similarly, contemporary researchers require a full range of observational and analytic strategies in order to arrive at the best answers to their questions about the world, not because they will necessarily use them all on any given job but because it is the job that should dictate what tools are used to complete it. Although we understand that some students become interested in research because they love to do statistical analysis with large databases or can't wait to immerse themselves in an ethnography of some interesting cultural group, limiting your research to only one method will severely limit what you do and what you find because of the artificial limits it imposes on what you *can* find.

The beginning point for us is always the research question you want to ask; research design then involves deciding what information and method will best help you answer that question. Accordingly, our job in this book is to acquaint you with some of the range of methods and approaches that are available to allow you to make those decisions. We begin by outlining two very broad perspectives involving **quantitative approaches** and **qualitative approaches**. Although much has been written in years past about which of these approaches is "best" or why one or the other tradition is most deserving of the title "science," this book goes beyond those debates.

While the two perspectives can be distinguished on many different dimensions, there also are many similarities to which both these grand traditions subscribe. In the next two sections, we examine quantitative traditions and qualitative traditions separately to understand the internal logic of each approach and to highlight the unique strengths that each perspective brings to research. We then conclude the chapter by looking at the common ground that both approaches share and discuss how employing the two in combination can act symbiotically to produce research that is more than the sum of its parts.

QUANTITATIVE TRADITIONS

Although quantitative approaches have a long philosophical lineage, their contemporary forms are often traced to the mid to late 19th century. Individuals such as Auguste Comte (in sociology and social psychology) and Wilhelm Wundt (in psychology) noted the tremendous theoretical and technological advances that had occurred in the natural sciences and believed that natural science methods could be of service to the social sciences as well. The metaphors they used to describe the challenge to social scientists were permeated with natural science imagery. For Comte, for example, "societies and groups [are] organisms—analogous to biological or physical organisms—that exist and behave in accordance with objective and external laws" (Faulconer & Williams, 1985, p. 1181).

A Positivist Epistemology

Comte, Wundt, and others embraced an **epistemological** tradition known as **positivism**, which championed the view that the only way to truly understand the world and develop dependable knowledge was to avoid philosophical reflection and rely solely on observation of concrete phenomena. Within the social and health sciences, this would mean focusing on observable behavior and avoiding references to anything we cannot see, such as thoughts and perceptions.

A Realist Perspective

An attribute strongly associated with positivism is its **realist perspective**. Most vigorously applied in the context of positivism, realism's more extreme version of direct or naïve realism subscribes to the view that there is a (i.e., one) reality out there that exists independent of the researcher that can be understood and awaits our discovery (e.g., Chakravartty, 2011; Filstead, 1979). Naïve realists thus aim to uncover *the* facts and to understand *the* laws or principles that account for those facts. The challenge is to think of the "right" theoretical concepts and develop techniques that are sufficiently precise to measure and test them. For Donald T. Campbell, a noted methodologist you will be hearing about more than once in this book, realism was the foundation for his notion of evolutionary epistemology, which posited that, as long as we commit ourselves to constantly subjecting our theories to empirical test, successive generations of scholars will bring us ever closer to knowing those ultimate laws that govern human behavior (see Campbell, 1974; Palys, 1990).

Just Another Organism

As you might expect from the emphasis on humans as biological organisms, references to Charles Darwin's evolutionary theory were frequent among turn-of-the-20th-century positivists. Psychologist John B. Watson (1913), for example, was clearly impressed by Darwin's work and its impact on the biological sciences. A prime reason for this advance, said Watson, was that Darwin resisted the temptation to treat humans as a special entity and instead saw them as just another biological organism, subject to the same scientific principles as any other.

We can see this as an example of a principle in the sciences known as Occam's razor, which expresses the idea that any theorizing we do should be as simple as possible: if two theories both explain some phenomenon but one does so more simply (involving fewer concepts and/or less complex mechanisms) than another, then the theory that does so more simply is preferred. According to that view, if human behavior can be explained using the same principles that govern the behavior of other organisms and without resorting to abstract notions like "consciousness" or "attitudes" or "alienation," then so much the better.

Inputs and Outcomes

Positivism's mechanistic purity also was sought with respect to the variables that were to be included in any analysis. The world was seen to be made up of causes (or predictors) and effects (or outcomes) like billiard balls being knocked around a table. We see the causes (e.g., the white cue ball hits a red ball), observe the effects (e.g., the red ball moves and falls into a pocket), and can develop principles to describe that action (e.g., the angle of incidence equals the angle of reflection, as any physicist or pool player knows) without worrying about what is going on "inside" either ball.

Similarly, early positivists felt that organisms could be treated as "black boxes": any invisible processes that might go on inside (such as thinking in humans) were deemed irrelevant; all that *really* counts is what goes in (the predictors or causes) and what comes out (the effects or outcomes). Only those causes external to individuals were deemed "legitimate" to scrutinize, largely because such forces and processes are most amenable to observation and measurement. We can't see people's thoughts or motives, but we *can* see what people *do*. If we can understand the relation between causes and effects, who cares what happens in between?

Don't Get Too Close

Natural science perspectives on "objectivity" also were adapted to the quantitative cause. Positivists suggest that the route to objectivity requires investigators to *depersonalize* the research situation, like the proverbial Martian who naively investigates these strange beings called humans (see Lofland, Snow, Anderson, & Lofland, 2006). "Good" data are thought to be dispassionate data, far removed from their source. The closer one comes to dealing with people on a one-to-one basis, the more dangerous the situation becomes, since one might be tempted to resort to metaphysical concepts such as thoughts, perceptions, attitudes, and values.

Indeed, many quantitatively oriented research textbooks suggested that the worst fate that can befall anyone who engages in field research is for them to "go native" or overidentify with those being studied. This is said to occur when researchers become so attuned and sensitive to the culture or group they're investigating that they take on the perspective of the group's members, leaving their ostensibly more appropriate detached, analytical perspective behind. Hagan (1989) makes the common argument that the appropriate attitude for researchers is studied neutrality; we should neither love nor hate the groups we study and should always maintain some social distance.

Social Facts

The idea of detachment also is consistent with the quantitative preference for aggregated data, where you compile responses from many persons so that general trends or patterns across people are made visible. The desirability of aggregated data also can be seen in the quantitative attachment to social facts. According to Durkheim (1968 [1938]), the important social facts of life, and hence the appropriate causal variables to study, were social practices and institutions such as education, religion, the law, and the economic system. We clearly did not cause them; they existed before we did. They influence us all, although the nature of their effects may vary. And even had we not been born, they still would exist and still would influence whoever happened to be here. For example, if you were born in the United States, you were born into a capitalist economic system; the United States still would be capitalist even if you had not been born here. That system is a social fact of your life; it has affected you in ways that differ from the effects of being born in, say, a communist state such as the People's Republic of China or Russia.

Thus, for Durkheim, social facts are the most appropriate causal factors for social scientists to investigate because they exert their influence coercively and do so even when we try to resist:

> *A social fact is to be recognized by the power of external coercion which it exercises or is capable of exercising over individuals, and the presence of this power may be recognized in its turn either by the existence of some specific sanction or by the resistance offered against every individual effort that tends to violate it. (1968 [1938], p. 250)*

He continued,

> *The most important characteristic of a thing is the impossibility of its modification by a simple effort of the will … Social facts have this characteristic. Far from being a product of the will, they determine it from without; they are like molds in which our actions are inevitably shaped. (Durkheim, 1968 [1938], p. 253)*

To measure the effects of social facts, Durkheim recommended relying on official rate data (e.g., birth rates, divorce rates, suicide rates, crime rates). Such data deal with matters relevant to and affected by "social facts," are outside the influence of researchers or of the individuals the data described, and describe "reality."

A Deductive Approach

For classic positivists, the ability to predict is the acid test of understanding: if you truly understand a phenomenon (e.g., hurricanes, depression, birth rates, sexual safety), you should be able to predict its presence and absence or rise and fall. Not surprisingly, therefore, quantitative researchers prefer the hypothetico-deductive method (often referred to more simply as deduction or the **deductive method**), which involves making predictions and assessing their success in an ongoing process of theory refinement.

Chapter 2 discusses this approach in greater detail; here we need only note that it involves beginning with a **theory**; deducing a hypothesis (prediction) from the theory; gathering data to test the prediction (and hence also the theory that gave rise to it); and then either looking for another situation in which to test the theory (if the prediction is borne out) or revising or discarding the theory (if the prediction proves inaccurate). In the ideal situation, the effects of certain variables can be assessed with all other influences held constant, making the classic experiment a method of choice (see Chapter 5).

Researcher-Centered

You should see from all the above that, for strict quantitative approaches, the researcher is the star of the show. The emphasis on taking a deductive approach brings with it the idea that it is theory that tells you what the important variables are to consider. It is the researcher who will determine which theory to test, pick the situation to test it in, design the study, and do the research to see whether the theory is supported empirically or not. Research participants—often referred to as "human subjects" in quantitative publications—have a minimal role beyond responding to whatever stimuli are presented to them. Subjects' thoughts about what they do are of little interest because their motives and perspectives are suspect; they are too close to the situation to view it with the detached objectivity the researcher seeks. Any interaction beyond the standardized set of procedures that comprise the research is considered problematic because it introduces error and thereby contaminates the results. Many quantitative methods—the classic experiment being the foremost example—sometimes even require that subjects be kept completely in the dark as to what hypotheses are being tested or even to deceive them about what the "real" purpose of the study is, ostensibly to ensure that subjects' behavior is "natural" and not a reflection of their desire to respond in a socially desirable fashion because someone is watching what they do.

QUALITATIVE TRADITIONS

Qualitative approaches follow their own logic that departs in several key respects from the choices made within quantitative traditions. Schutz (1970), who was writing in German in the 1930s and whose works were not translated into English until the 1960s and 1970s, is illustrative. He disagreed with positivists' choice to investigate a mechanistic world from the aloof stance of the knowledgeable social scientist, but his disagreement wasn't based on a belief that such a science would necessarily give "wrong" information. Rather, he felt that in the long run, such an approach was inherently incomplete and thus inevitably would fall short of a comprehensive understanding of human action.

His position is reminiscent of a story known as "the drunkard's search" (e.g., Farris, 1969). The story involves a researcher who is walking down the street one night when he comes across a rather intoxicated individual who is down on his hands and knees, looking for his house keys on the ground under a street lamp. The researcher joins in to help, but after another 15 minutes, neither has been able to find the keys. "Are you sure this is where you lost them?" asks the researcher.

"Actually … I lost them over there … closer to the house," says the fellow who lost his keys, pointing to a dark spot close to the house, about 50 feet away.

The researcher's jaw drops when he recognizes the futility of what they have been doing. Exasperated, he asks, "Then why are we looking over here?"

The response: "Because this is where the light is."

Analogously, Schutz argued that the first trick to gaining an understanding about humans and human behavior is to look in the right place and not to choose methods simply because a certain approach is easier, is associated with some prestigious field of inquiry, or is expedient to adopt in the short term. The choice should be made on the basis of what is, over the long haul, the right thing to do.

A Human-Centered Approach

The methodological "right thing to do" for Schutz was to acknowledge that social scientists, in trying to understand *human* behavior, face challenges fundamentally different from those faced by the natural scientist:

> The world of nature, as explored by the natural scientist, does not "mean" anything to the molecules, atoms and electrons therein. The observational field of the social scientist, however, … has a specific meaning and relevance structure for the human beings living, acting, and thinking therein. By a series of commonsense constructs they have preselected and pre-interpreted this world which they experience as the reality of their daily lives. It is these thought objects of theirs which determine their behavior by motivating it. (Schutz, 1970, pp. 272–273)

And while the complexity this cognitive life creates might be challenging, it also creates great opportunity because, unlike gall wasps or the chemicals in a test tube, we can talk to humans, they can consider our questions, and we can learn from what they say. Schutz and others working within the qualitative tradition believe that when we study humans we must view them as thinking, motivated actors, while also acknowledging the challenges that arise because, as humans, social and health scientists are part of the very entity they seek to understand. A philosophy that expresses this view is known as **phenomenologism**.

Phenomenologism

Phenomenologists maintain that any effort to understand human behavior must take into account that humans are cognitive beings who actively perceive and make sense of the world around them, have the capacity to abstract from their experience, ascribe meaning to their behavior and the world around them, and are affected by those meanings. W. I. Thomas (1928) stated that "perceptions are real because they are real in their consequences"; that is, in many situations the influence of "reality" (if indeed such a thing exists independently of our experience of it) pales in comparison to the influence of our perceptions of the situation—indeed, those perceptions define our "reality."

As an example, many Americans these days seem deeply concerned about violent crime. Consistent with these concerns, many citizens and their elected representatives call for more punitive sentencing, more caution in the granting of parole, and "special measures" that would give courts greater leeway to incarcerate particularly nasty people and habitual offenders for a long, long time. Yet the "reality" of the situation in the United States is that, at least as measured by the rates reported by the FBI, violent crime in the United States has been dropping steadily for more than 20 years.[1] Which is more important in accounting for Americans' behavior regarding violent crime: the "reality" of the situation or people's perceptions of it?

Phenomenologists argue that any science of human behavior is destined to be trivial and/or incomplete unless it takes people's perceptions into account. Any approach that defines itself as phenomenological makes understanding human perceptions its major research focus: if perceptions are real in their consequences, and if they are a major determinant of what we do, then clearly they are what we must set out to understand.

Numbers Create Distance

The shift to phenomenologism affected many other aspects of theory and method. For example, a central aim of positivism was to establish functional relations among

---

[1] Tables showing data back to 1996 can be seen at https://ucr.fbi.gov/crime-in-the-u.s/2015/crime-in-the-u.s.-2015/offenses-known-to-law-enforcement/offenses-known-to-law-enforcement.

explanatory concepts, expressed, ideally, in mathematical (quantitative) form. In contrast, many phenomenologists believe that imposing a quantitative measurement just removes researchers further from directly understanding human experience. The more we listen to people explaining, in their own words, the nature of their experiences, the better our understanding.

Understanding Equals *Verstehen*

In contrast to quantitative researchers who emphasize the ability to predict as the acid test of understanding, researchers who adopt a phenomenological approach embrace Max Weber's concept of *verstehen*, which involves the more intimate and empathic understanding of human action in terms of its interpretive meaning to the participant. While researchers who embrace strict positivism seek general principles of behavior, Weber argued that, in themselves, such principles can't account for action in context:

> An "objective" analysis of cultural events, which proceeds according to the thesis that the ideal of science is the reduction of empirical reality to "laws," is meaningless ... The knowledge of social laws is not knowledge of social reality but is rather one of the various aids used by our minds for attaining this end ... Knowledge of cultural events is inconceivable except on a basis of the significance which the concrete constellations of reality have for us in individual concrete situations. (Weber, 1968a [1949], p. 91)

Weber didn't completely dismiss quantitative research or the theories associated with it; he just felt that we had to go beyond blanket assertions made by strict positivists to account for action in context.

Validity Comes From Closeness

Researchers who adopt qualitative approaches believe that understanding people requires getting close to "research participants" or "informants" or "collaborators." You must spend time with them, get to know them, be able to empathize with their concerns, and perhaps even be one of them, if you hope to *truly* understand. Key here is the notion of **rapport**—the development of a bond of mutual trust between researcher and participant that is considered to be the foundation upon which access is given and valid data are built.

What degree of closeness is "appropriate," however, is a matter of ongoing debate within the community of people engaged in qualitative research. For most researchers, establishing rapport is possible as long as you are respectful, trustworthy, and spend a lot of time with the person or group that will be the focus of the research. Others question just how close you can get to people who are not like you, believing that you can never understand a group of which you are not a part—e.g., that male researchers can never truly understand what it means to be a woman or that Caucasian researchers can never know what it means to "grow up Black." By implication, therefore, for these researchers, only women should research women and only African American researchers should do research on issues of importance to Blacks.

We have some empathy for these views, particularly as they apply to subordinated or minority populations who are often misunderstood and miscast by those from the dominant group. We all should be aware of the limitations of our experience. That said, we would not impose predefined limits on what topics are "appropriate" for any given person to study. Both causing and grappling with ethical issues surrounding the nature of the relationship between researcher and researched are strong traditions among those who do field research. We discuss some of these in Chapter 4; choices as to the different roles that researchers may occupy in any given research project appear throughout the book.

An Inductive Approach

Associated with the view that closeness is desirable is the idea that researchers should *listen* to their participants/collaborators, aim to understand categories and theoretically important dimensions from the perspective of their experience, and incorporate those understandings into the analysis. Accordingly, more phenomenologically oriented researchers emphasize **inductive approaches** (where observation in the field *precedes* the generation of theoretical concepts; see Chapter 2).

Instead of beginning with theory and assuming that there's one theory that will eventually account for everything, a strict qualitative approach typically involves beginning with individual case studies trying to understand each situation on its own terms and leaving open, for the moment, the question of whether generalizable theoretical concepts can ever be drawn together in anything resembling a grand theory. For people engaged in qualitative research, theory isn't something you start with; it's something you build.

A Preference for Field Research

The qualitative preference for an inductive approach is accompanied by a priority being attached to doing research in "the field," i.e., where behavior can be examined in context. There are two main reasons for this. First is simply that, according to qualitative perspectives, behavior only has meaning in context, and hence "in context" is the only place where behavior can legitimately be observed.

A second related reason for preferring field research is that if the reason we do research is to understand the behavior of people in the world, then field research is the most valid option because it is only in field-based research that we duplicate the contextual conditions that shape behavior and give it its meaning. As noted methodologist Howard Becker (1996) explained,

> When we watch someone as they work in their usual work setting or go to a political meeting in their neighborhood or have dinner with their family—when we watch people do things in the places they usually do them with the people they usually do them with—we cannot insulate them from the consequences of their actions. On the contrary, they have to take the rap for what they do, just as they ordinarily do in everyday life. An example: when I was observing college undergraduates, I sometimes went to classes with them. On one occasion, an instructor announced a surprise quiz for which the student I was accompanying that day, a goofoff, was totally unprepared. Sitting nearby, I could easily see him leaning over and copying answers from someone he hoped knew more than he did. He was embarrassed by my seeing him, but the embarrassment didn't stop him copying, because the consequences of failing the test (this was at a time when flunking out of school could lead to being drafted, and maybe being killed in combat) were a lot worse than my potentially lowered opinion of him. He apologized and made excuses later, but he did it. What would he have said about cheating on a questionnaire or in an interview, out of the actual situation that had forced him to that expedient?

Constructionism

Recall that classic positivists embraced a philosophical perspective known as **realism**. Phenomenologists, in emphasizing the role of human perception in understanding human behavior, adopt a contrasting perspective or position known as **constructionism**. As described by Schwandt (1994),

> [C]onstructivists are deeply committed to the view that what we take to be objective knowledge and truth is [actually] the result of perspective. Knowledge and truth are created, not discovered by mind. They emphasize the pluralistic and plastic character of reality—pluralistic in the sense that reality is expressible in a variety of symbol and language systems; plastic in the sense that reality is stretched and shaped to fit purposeful acts of intentional human agents. They endorse the claim

that, "contrary to common-sense, there is no unique 'real world' that preexists and is independent of human mental activity and human symbolic language." (p. 125; the last sentence quotes Bruner, 1986, p. 95)

To illustrate, suppose we follow Becker's illustration and decide to study the phenomenon of "cheating," known in some universities as "academic dishonesty." A realist approach to studying cheating would affirm that there are behaviors we consensually recognize as "cheating" and that some people are more or less likely to cheat than others. Given this perspective, our attention might turn to trying to measure either "frequency of cheating" or how likely a given person or group of persons is to cheat; investigating why some people are more likely to cheat than others; or why some situations result in more or less cheating than others.

In contrast, a constructionist looking at cheating wouldn't deny the usefulness of any of these approaches. But they also would encourage us to take a step back and look at "cheating" as a socially constructed concept. Why do we consider "cheating" something worth asking about? Why do we consider some behaviors where one person seeks the help of another "cheating" (e.g., looking over another person's shoulder to see what answers they put down in an examination) but not others (e.g., hiring a tutor or studying together)? We also might want to interview people who have been identified as cheaters about how they perceived their actions: Did *they* consider it "cheating" or did they call it something else? How did they come to engage in that behavior?

The realist, then, takes the existence of certain behavior categories as a given, being prepared to assume that there are such things as "cheating," "aggression," and "crime," along with other supposed givens such as "birth," "death," and "taxes." Constructionists, on the other hand, are at least as interested in why these categories interest us, whom or where we decide to sample in order to investigate the phenomenon firsthand, where the boundaries of the phenomenon are, what meanings the terms have for us, and how those boundaries and meanings change over time. To be a constructionist is not to deny that certain phenomena exist, but to insist that their existence cannot be completely understood unless you understand why, how, and to whom they are applied.

One implication of this perspective is that many of the research results or "truths" we take at face value and perceive as enduring may be little more than transient relationships that reflect the prevailing social order. While realists may be content to try to assess *the* effects of race, poverty, daycare, being gay, winning the lottery, or taking illicit drugs, constructionists argue that we can understand such matters only if we also understand something about how they're construed and the context in which they occur.

Emphasizing Process

A distinct difference in emphasis also follows from either seeing the important elements of the world as essentially stable and awaiting discovery (the realist view) or seeing the world as something that is actively constructed, deconstructed, and reconstructed on an ongoing basis (the constructionist view). According to those who hold the latter view, our constructions of the world—and hence the world itself—are open to change.

As we've seen, positivist researchers working quantitatively tend to emphasize the measurement of *outcomes* in their research. This is consistent with the positivist division of the world into causes and effects and with the view that there are real, monolithic forces that rule our lives. But constructionists consider the world a more ephemeral, transient place whose dynamics are more directly contingent on the meanings and understandings we use to negotiate our world. Accordingly, constructionist-oriented qualitative approaches are also characterized by greater attention to *processes*, particularly the processes by which constructions arise and, by implication, the processes by which constructions can be changed.

Participant-Centered

All of these objectives are well-served by more collaborative approaches in which, ideally, the researcher will begin the research with an open mind and without preconceived theory, will spend much time with participants in the field, and will look to participants to guide them in the identification of important questions that will focus the research and possibly assist in interpretation. How far this goes will depend on the individual researcher. Some see the researcher as no more than an instrument whose job is to represent the views of participants in their own words. Others believe that researchers have a role to play because while any given participant has a unique history and experience that the researcher does not, the researcher's social position makes it likely that, at the end of the research, they will be the only one in the setting who has systematically learned from *all* of the participants in a setting and thus should have the broadest and most comprehensive view.

BRIDGING APPROACHES

Thus far, we've seen that numerous differences traditionally have characterized quantitative and qualitative approaches to research. Table 1.1 outlines these differences—at least as they've been associated with each approach historically.

TABLE 1.1 ● Comparing Quantitative and Qualitative Approaches		
	Quantitative Approach	**Qualitative Approach**
Philosophical considerations	Positivist epistemology	Phenomenological epistemology
	Natural science model: humans are just another organism	Human-centered approach: people's ability to think and abstract requires special consideration
	Realist perspective	Constructionist perspective
Epistemological priorities	Preference for a deductive approach: start with theory and create situations in which to test hypotheses	Preference for an inductive approach: start with observation and allow theory to emerge
	Human behavior can be extracted from its context to be studied	You must look at behavior in situ; behavior only has meaning in context
Role of researcher	Researcher and theory decide what is important to study and how results will be interpreted	Often more collaborative approach where research participants can help identify research focus and aid interpretation
	Objectivity is achieved through social distance and a detached, analytical stance	Valid data come from closeness and extended contact with research participants
Implications for methods	Emphasis on observable variables that are external to the individual; social facts	No variables ruled out; internal, perceptual variables expressly considered
	Quantitative measures are preferred for their precision and amenability to mathematical analysis	Direct, qualitative verbal reports are preferred; quantifying responses is a step removed from people's words and perceptions
	Preference for larger samples looking for patterns across many cases; paying more attention to "the forest"	Preference for case study analysis; paying more attention to "the trees" and trying to figure out what forest they are a part of
	Emphasis on causes and effects: what goes in and how it comes out; predictors, outcomes	Emphasis on processes: perceptions and their meanings and how these emerge and change
How do you define success?	The criteria for understanding is the ability to predict what will happen in any given situation	The criterion for understanding is *verstehen*: understanding behavior in context in terms meaningful to the actor

Each element in the table has been discussed in the preceding pages, so you should now be able to define and explain them and understand why and how each is characteristic of one or the other of the extremes of the two perspectives discussed in this chapter. In addition to looking at the dimensions along each row of the table, have a look down each column as well, and try to get the sense of each set of approaches as an internally consistent package where each element makes sense in relation to all the other components.

The two columns of Table 1.1 show how the two traditions *can* be very different, and the fact we have given each one its own space for pedagogical reasons may seem to magnify the differences between them. But there are no rigid borders dividing them. No rule says a researcher doing a more quantitative study cannot take an inductive approach, or that someone undertaking a more qualitative project cannot be motivated by a desire to answer theoretically specific research questions and collect aggregate data across numerous respondents. Indeed, methodological mixtures involving aspects of both approaches are becoming more and more commonplace.

And although Table 1.1 highlights some of the differences between qualitative and quantitative approaches, difference does not have to imply disagreement, inconsistency, or incompatibility. In fact it is quite the opposite: notwithstanding superficial differences between the two approaches, they actually share a similar underlying logic and, when used together, can complement one another very well. Probably most important among these is that both traditions are committed to an empirical approach to the generation of knowledge, i.e., affirming that our understanding of the world should come not from philosophizing or speculation, but from data that comes from interacting with and observing the world we seek to understand. Both approaches also value theory *and* data, even though they differ in their preferences of which comes first. The two traditions also share a desire to explore, describe, and understand the world, both for its own sake and because of a shared belief that the moral and political debates we engage in about what policies and laws should be enacted to improve the social condition should be based on evidence and not on misinformation, stereotype, or blind dogma.

In the next portion of this chapter, we revisit Table 1.1 in order to ask what a third column of entries might look like if we were to think of the two traditions not as separate entities requiring a choice of one or the other, but rather as alternatives that can be pursued individually or in combination. We do so under five broad themes—(1) philosophical stance; (2) epistemological priorities; (3) the role of the researcher in relation to participants; (4) implications for particular methods; and (5) criteria for determining success.

Philosophical Stance

We introduced you earlier to the epistemological traditions of positivism and phenomenologism and the related dichotomy of realism and constructionism. Researchers who are open to mixing methodological approaches reject the idea that researchers must proclaim allegiance to one tradition or the other. They feel that social and health-related phenomena are often better studied using both qualitative *and* quantitative methods and have sought to ground their approach in an epistemological position that is capable of seeing a middle ground between direct realism and constructivism.

Philosophically, the limits of positivism and phenomenologism are subsumed in mixed methods approaches as pragmatism. This philosophical tradition, with roots in the late 19th century through the works of Charles Sanders Pierce, John Dewy, and William James, played a major role in the emergence of symbolic interactionism (e.g., Cooley, 1902; Mead, 1934). Pragmatism is not committed to any single system of philosophy or view of reality. The central position advanced within pragmatism is the rejection of traditional dualisms of realism *versus* constructivism, free-will *versus* determinism, subjectivism *versus* objectivism, and induction *versus* deduction in favor of taking whatever position works best in a particular situation (Johnson & Onwuegbuzie, 2004).

Pragmatism envisions a method of inquiry based on a dialectic relationship between the processes of discovery and action as opposed to the search for a single truth or correct answer. Pragmatists favor eclecticism and pluralism as opposed to dogmatism when it comes to theoretical, methodological, and analytical approaches to understanding the social world. Pragmatists are results- or outcome-oriented and less concerned with prior knowledges, laws, or rules governing what constitutes valid knowledge (Maxcy, 2003). They are concerned with finding the best or most complete answers to research questions through the best method or combination of methods and have a strong commitment to praxis (i.e., theory informing practice). To that extent, pragmatic traditions can be seen to favor the more human-centered approach that is more characteristic of qualitative traditions, not as a choice over a natural science model, but simply because it is more inclusive. At the same time, Occam's razor, a principle prioritized more highly within quantitative traditions, reminds us to be economical and efficient in our theorizing.

As for the realist-constructionist dichotomy, a philosophical position that appreciates the kernel of truth residing in both positions is fallibilist realism or critical realism (e.g., see Cook & Campbell, 1979; Manicas & Secord, 1983). This perspective acknowledges that we cannot deal with reality directly, but only through our constructions of it. Yet the task of science is to construct theories that aim to represent the world. In doing so, certainly it is true, as the constructionists argue, that there are different ways we can describe the world that are all equally "correct"—for example, surely it is equally "correct" to say "humans are social organisms" or "humans are biological organisms" or "humans are economic organisms"—and which metaphor(s) we pursue will have implications for what kinds of research questions we pose, the theories we develop, and the actions that arise from the understandings we generate (e.g., what kinds of policies or laws or other interventions we implement). But not *all* explanations are equally correct. We also have to acknowledge there are statements we can make about humans that are clearly and demonstrably "wrong"—for example, surely it would be "wrong" to say that "humans are asexual" or "adult humans do not care for their young." But if it's possible for us to be wrong, then there must be something that we can be wrong about, i.e., there must be a reality that exists independent of our analysis of it (see Bhaskar, 1986).

Stated another way, although our constructions *are* social and historical products (i.e., knowledge at any given time is "produced" by a community of scientists and flavored by its historical context), it is *not* the case that "anything goes." We should indeed be able to develop rational criteria by which the adequacy, or at least the utility, of our formulations can be judged. And it is a reasonable endeavor to collect evidence through empirical inquiry; we need only remind ourselves that while "facts" may exist, their meaning and relative importance are negotiable—there are both realist and constructionist elements to knowledge.

Epistemological Priorities

Two different issues stand out in Table 1.1 with respect to epistemological priorities, by which we refer to broader issues about how one approaches the research process as opposed to the more detailed choices of specific methods that we consider below. The first of these involves the deductive-inductive dichotomy. Although we discuss those processes in more detail in Chapter 2, we'll note here that deductive approaches operate in the belief that research should begin with good theory, which researchers then go about testing by finding (in the world) or creating (e.g., in a lab) situations where the theory is supposed to apply, and then seeing whether predictions that arise from the theory find support. If so, the theory collects one gold star and the researcher goes on to the next test. Inductive approaches, in contrast, operate in the belief that good theory arises from observing behavior in context, so you begin by going into contexts that you are interested in for one reason or another (see Chapter 2), observing the phenomenon of interest, and developing theoretical speculations on the basis of your direct observation in the field.

When we see that both approaches involve a perpetual interaction between theory and data and between observation and abstraction, identification of "where the process began" seems trivial. Nor do you have to proclaim allegiance to one or the other; mixed methods approaches encourage researchers to open the door to a more comprehensive understanding while benefitting from the often offsetting advantages and disadvantages that various methods entail. You should not be surprised, therefore, to hear that many mixed methods investigations are often simultaneously inductive *and* deductive, which allows the types of questions that researchers work on within this perspective to be more layered, nuanced, and comprehensive than those that inspire single-method studies. We will be giving you many examples of exactly that sort of boundary crossing throughout the book as we discuss particular methods.

Table 1.1 also notes the quantitative preference for extracting phenomena of interest from their context in order to study them under more controlled conditions, as well as the qualitative assertion that behavior must be observed in context in order to be understood. Far from seeing these in opposition, we see each setting as appropriate for the questions they seek to ask, part of a broader research repertoire, and hence note here simply that the two in combination contribute complementary information allowing for a more comprehensive understanding.

Decontextualizing social processes by looking across many cases in order to arrive at "overall" or "general" patterns or *ceteris paribus* ("all else being equal") truths through such methods as surveys and experiments is a mainstay of quantitative techniques. They are extremely useful for probing general theoretical issues where assertions about the strength of relationships or differences are being tested and when they involve gathering descriptive information about how different goods—and injustices— are distributed throughout society. In turn, the more qualitative emphasis on examining how phenomena of interest play out in the day-to-day world is not only itself a source of important data to spur understanding and subsequent theorizing but also offers sites in which theories can be tested and qualifications to general theories developed.

Role of Researchers

The two traditions have quite different emphases as outlined in Table 1.1 when it comes to the role of researchers in relation to those they study. Within quantitative traditions, the researcher is clearly the star of the show. Researchers decide what is important to study, design the research, interpret the results, and write the reports. They are guided in these efforts by their colleagues and the literature and see "objectivity" as something that you accomplish by staying aloof from the people you are studying. The logic of this seems quite compelling; when the objective of your research is to find overall patterns across large numbers of cases, then the researcher brings the expertise to design that research, they and/or the literature (and theory) define what the important questions are to investigate, and unlike the participants, the researcher is the only one who gets to see the bird's eye view that aggregation across many cases allows. Qualitative traditions emphasize quite the opposite. When your interest is in doing case studies in the field to build theory inductively, then the research design and analytical skills the researcher brings address only half the challenge; determining what the important questions are to ask and understanding the implications of what you are observing is built by a more collaborative approach characterized by mutual trust that exposes the researcher to insights they, particularly as an "other," may not previously have considered.

Although the two types of relationship may seem to conflict, we suggest they are actually an accurate reflection of the multiple roles that researchers need to have in their repertoire, and that part of the complexity of research involves being able to go back and forth between those two roles. We see great value in both of them. Researchers bring research design expertise that provides an opportunity to produce valid and useful data that help achieve research objectives. However, ignoring participants is a foolhardy move, particularly when engaged in research that seeks to inform about some niche of life—many research injustices have arisen and much ill-will generated when researchers imposed their understanding on people who are not like them—and/or promote social change involving the group under study. You will see examples of these issues arising on numerous occasions during the book, as each method brings its own challenge to how to manage the researcher–participant relationship.

Implications for Methods

We saw how researchers working within quantitative traditions tend to emphasize the search for very general descriptions of human behavior in the hope of unearthing general laws while those working within qualitative traditions are more interested in understanding specific cases and how general principles play out in specific contexts. This often leads them to pose different research questions and to look in different places for answers and explanations. But are they not opposite sides of the same coin? General laws are of limited use if they cannot shed light on specific contexts; and context-specific understandings are typically of limited interest unless they can be located within broader principles of human behavior. Each offers only a partial understanding of the world; any comprehensive understanding of a phenomenon will require us to be able to explain *all* the data that are relevant and not simply cherry-pick that subset of information that serves a smaller purpose.

The general idea that propels this section is that more data, and more diverse data in terms of the ways it is collected and the sources it is collected from, is a desirable goal. While social and health researchers have been mixing multiple methods of data collection within a single study for well over a century (Maxwell & Loomis, 2003), Donald T. Campbell, with various collaborators, is widely regarded as one of the first to formally encourage their use in order to avoid becoming too method-bound since every method has both strengths and limitations, and relying on only one method means you have the benefit of its strengths, but are imprisoned by its limitations. *Unobtrusive Measures: Nonreactive Research in the Social Sciences* (Webb, Campbell, Schwartz, & Sechrest, 1966) expressly pointed out the benefits to be gained by encouraging and implementing methodological pluralism. In another classic article, Campbell (1969c) encouraged researchers of different disciplines to collaborate and enjoy the benefits that would accrue from the diversity of approaches they would bring, and his notion of the "experimenting society" and quasi-experimentation that we discuss in Chapters 6 and 7 was based in large part on the analytical power that could be mustered by strategically combining different types and sources of data (e.g., Campbell, 1969b; Cook & Campbell, 1979).

Denzin (1970, 1978) built upon these ideas when he coined the term triangulation, which is a research strategy that permits us to validate our observations by drawing upon multiple sources or perspectives within the same investigation. He suggested there were four distinct ways this triangulation could occur:

1. Theoretical triangulation involves employing multiple theories throughout the design, collection, and analysis process. Proceeding in this manner would involve a researcher or group of researchers developing research questions from different theoretical vantage points and thereby studying a phenomenon through multiple lenses.

2. Investigator triangulation refers to the practice of several different researchers contributing in the study to collect, analyze, and interpret data and observations. This practice is thought to improve both the credibility of the observations and the resulting interpretation of the research. One place you see investigator triangulation is in the progressively more common

practice of multi-, trans-, and interdisciplinary research collaboration that brings together teams of researchers from different disciplines in order to research a problem of common interest (e.g., see Campbell, 1969c; Leavy, 2011).

3. **Methodological triangulation** involves employing multiple methods to study a particular phenomenon in order to overcome the deficiencies and biases that may result from employing a single-method approach. Certainly this book, which extols the virtue of combining qualitative and quantitative approaches, exemplifies this approach.

4. **Data analysis triangulation** refers to the practice of employing several different methods of analyzing and interpreting data in order to improve the validity of the conclusions by ensuring the robustness of your results.

Early writings by Campbell and his colleagues in the more quantitative realm and Denzin in the qualitative realm set the stage for the emergence of what some (e.g., Johnson & Onwuegbuzie, 2004; Johnson, Onwuegbuzie, & Turner, 2007) have labeled a "third paradigm" of research—mixed methods. Johnson et al. (2007) define this as "the type of research in which a researcher or team of researchers combines elements of qualitative and quantitative research approaches (e.g., use of qualitative and quantitative viewpoints, data collection, analysis, inference techniques) for the broad purposes of breadth and depth of understanding and corroboration" (p. 123). Researchers adopting this perspective encourage an eclectic approach to the research process that draws upon the complementary strengths of qualitative and quantitative techniques. Proponents believe that the best answers to any research problem or set of problems come when we consider multiple questions, viewpoints, perspectives, positions, and standpoints instead of one.

How Do You Spell S-u-c-c-e-s-s?

Although Table 1.1 focuses on how the two traditions differ in their definitions of success—with quantitative traditions emphasizing a statistical criterion and the ability to predict while the qualitative traditions have emphasized *verstehen*—there is an even more fundamental criterion that is common to both traditions. Both approaches share a similar underlying logic about how arguments about the validity of a particular conclusion will be evaluated, which is that any explanation will be accepted to the extent that it is the best one available, where "best" is defined as the one that does a more complete job of explanation than any **rival plausible explanation**. The way rival plausible explanations are handled will differ within the different traditions—those working quantitatively are more likely to use either experimental or statistical techniques to rule out alternative explanations while those working qualitatively are more likely to go back and gather more data from the same or another context that will address the rival plausible explanation—but both traditions assert a "superior" explanation will be the one that explains the most, does so most simply, and leaves the fewest or least serious rival plausible explanations (see Palys, 1989) in its wake. Stated another way, both traditions subscribe to the view that no matter what methodological approach you employ, your job as a researcher is always to be your own best critic and to anticipate as much as possible what rival plausible explanations might be brought forth to critique your interpretation. If you don't, then someone else probably will.

A Third Way?

With our review of qualitative and quantitative traditions complete, we are ready to replace Table 1.1 with Table 1.2, which summarizes in tabular form all that we have explained above. As you can see, far from seeing the two as incompatible alternatives one must choose between, we appreciate the contributions of both traditions and see both as necessary parts of the contemporary researcher's repertoire. It is very much also giving you an indication of the kind of approach you will see in this book—a review of both qualitative and quantitative techniques that emphasizes each method's strengths and limitations, as well as many examples of mixed methods studies that seek to combine the two, whether in the context of any one study, or more broadly in a program of study. While you will in all likelihood make your own choices about which type of research you prefer to do, understanding that "other" research that you may not do will at the very least make you a more responsible reader of the literature and make you a better colleague because of your ability to contribute to and appreciate the contributions those other researchers make.

SUMMING UP AND LOOKING AHEAD

This chapter introduced you to qualitative and quantitative traditions in research, as well as the mixed methods approaches that are becoming more and more prevalent among social and health researchers working individually and in teams. If you haven't taken a course in research methods before, you might feel slightly overwhelmed by now. But fear not; these themes will crop up on several occasions in the rest of the book, giving you lots of chances to review and understand them.

TABLE 1.2 ● Beyond Quantitative and Qualitative Approaches

	Quantitative Approach	Qualitative Approach	Bridging Approaches
Philosophical considerations	Positivist epistemology	Phenomenological epistemology	Pragmatic approach that emphasizes using whatever mix of approaches allows you to best address your research questions.
	Natural science model: humans are just another organism	Human-centered approach: people's ability to think and abstract requires special consideration	The emphasis here is on a human-centered approach that offers more comprehensive explanations, while Occam's razor reminds us to ensure we are not getting more complex than we need to.
	Realist perspective	Constructionist perspective	Critical realism embraces constructionism while also noting we can be "wrong," which suggests there is a reality independent of our constructions.
Epistemological priorities	Preference for a deductive approach: start with theory and create situations in which to test hypotheses	Preference for an inductive approach: start with observation and allow theory to emerge	Both approaches encourage a dialectical relationship between theory and data; the only difference between the two is in where you start. Any given project can have both deductive and inductive elements.
	Human behavior can be extracted from its context to be studied	You must look at behavior in situ; behavior only has meaning in context	No reason you can't do both. The former answers purely theoretical questions while the latter helps you look when the variables of interest compete in real-world contexts. Both are important parts of a broader strategy that values methodological diversity.
Role of researcher	Researcher and theory decide what is important to study and how results will be interpreted	More collaborative approaches where research participants can help identify research focus and aid interpretation	The nature of the researcher-participant relationship will vary depending on the types of methods chosen and the overall objectives of the research.
	Objectivity is achieved through social distance and a detached, analytical stance	Valid data come from closeness and extended contact with research participants	Both positions are important—getting close helps you understand meaning, while striving for independence of observation and analysis allows you to step back and bring a perspective people embedded in the situation may not see, i.e., gives a role for both researcher as analyst and participant as knowledgeable collaborator.

(Continued)

Table 1.2 (*Continued*)

	Quantitative Approach	Qualitative Approach	Bridging Approaches
Implications for methods	Emphasis on observable variables that are external to the individual; social facts	No variables ruled out; internal, perceptual variables expressly considered	Combined approaches maintain a broad conception of evidence with the emphasis on whatever will help answer the research question(s). All data need to be accounted for.
	Quantitative measures are preferred for their precision and amenability to mathematical analysis	Direct, qualitative verbal reports are preferred; quantifying responses is a step removed from people's words and perceptions	Encourages us to stay connected to what people say, while quantitative analysis offers analytical power in describing broader patterns. The two together often complement one another with each source helping interpret the other.
	Preference for larger samples looking for patterns across many cases; paying more attention to "the forest"	Preference for case study analysis; paying more attention to "the trees" and trying to figure out what forest they are a part of	Different but complementary; each implies the other. General patterns are not interesting unless they can help you understand particular cases; particular cases are less interesting when they cannot help you understand broader issues and implications.
	Emphasis on causes and effects: what goes in and how it comes out; predictors, outcomes	Emphasis on processes: perceptions and their meanings and how these emerge and change	Depends in part on interest, but they can also help inform each other. For example, in evaluation research, step 1 is to find out whether an intervention makes a difference; but step 2 is to look more closely to see how/why it happens.
How do you define success?	The criteria for understanding is the ability to predict what will happen in any given situation	The criterion for understanding is verstehen: understanding behavior in context in terms meaningful to the actor	The criteria for success will depend on the methods being used; both are important in their respective contexts. In both cases, however, researchers seek for explanations that are demonstrably superior to any rival plausible explanations that might be offered.

The chapter described how quantitative traditions have embraced a perspective known as positivism. This perspective borrows a direct realist epistemology or way of knowing from the natural sciences and posits that human beings can and should be scrutinized in the manner of any living organism because they are subject to and shaped by the same laws of nature. Along with this comes a preference for observable variables, which, in its most orthodox versions, eschewed unobservables like thoughts and perceptions. Much research focuses on the impacts of social facts—megavariables whose monolithic impact is felt by all of us—whose effects can be measured through rate data and where aggregate tendencies reveal social impacts unaffected by the idiosyncrasies of any single case. Emphasis is placed on being aloof and dispassionate in the interests of maintaining objectivity and independence of analysis. The hypothetico-deductive method is the foundation of this tradition: researchers specify a theory, deduce a hypothesis, and then gather data to test the hypothesis and, hence, also the theory. The trick is to be inventive in our theorizing and to look for general principles or laws that guide and shape human action. "Good" theory is thought to be simple, to be capable of being expressed in precise mathematical form, and to accurately reflect the relationship between causes and outcomes.

Qualitative traditions, in contrast, argued that people's perceptions not only should not be avoided, but rather should be the focus of analysis: "Perceptions are real because they are real in their consequences" (Thomas, 1928). We must understand those perceptions if we want to understand human behavior: what people think about the world influences how they act in it. Acknowledging that people construct reality implies that there are actually many "realities" and possible realities that exist, and that we negotiate on an ongoing basis. "Understanding" or *verstehen* involves being able to explain unique behavior in context, after investigating the ways in which reality is constructed and negotiated. You must get close to the people you study in order to understand them. "Good" theory is not imposed; rather, it emerges inductively from direct observation and contact with people in context.

Rather than seeing the two traditions as in conflict with one another because of their historically different foci and choices, we see them as two grand traditions, each of which sheds a partial light on the world we are interested in studying, and whose differences counterbalance and often complement each other in a broader empirical strategy. This approach is very much in keeping with the push for greater diversity of methods Donald Campbell and his colleagues affirmed in *Unobtrusive Measures* and that Norman Denzin encouraged in his discussions of triangulation. Mixed methods approaches encourage us to rise above the forced dichotomies that underlay and propelled qualitative–quantitative rivalries for many years and allow us to achieve more comprehensive understandings that use the advantages each tradition brings to counterbalance the limitations of the others it is paired with. Future chapters will see us fleshing out the various ways such techniques can be combined and analyzed.

It is noteworthy how significant shifts in the academy also have helped propel these developments. One involves changes in academy personnel. As science slowly democratizes, with progressively greater representation from women, members of the LGBTQIA community, Indigenous peoples, Third World academics, and others, new voices are heard, and methodological models that embrace diverse voices and experiences are encouraged. Such research also has benefited from developments in digital technologies that facilitate data gathering and analysis involving a wide array of sources and allow members of research teams to communicate more easily in order to exchange views, monitor their collective progress, and write up and share the results of their research. While the lone researcher of yesteryear is still with us, research *teams* crossing disciplinary, institutional, and international boundaries are becoming more and more commonplace. Contemporary researchers do not need to duplicate all the different expertise around the table, but they do need to know how to talk to each other and contribute to each other's work. Our objective in this book is to show you how that can be done.

Key Concepts

Case study analysis 16

Constructionism 13

Critical realism 18

Data analysis triangulation 23

Deduction 7

Deductive approaches 7

Dichotomy 18

Direct or naïve realism 5

Epistemology 4

Evolutionary epistemology 5

Fallibilist realism 18

Go native/overidentify 6

Hypothetico-deductive method 7

Induction 18

Inductive approaches 12

Investigator triangulation 22

Methodological triangulation 23

Mixed methods 18

Occam's razor 5

Phenomenologism 10

Positivism 4

Pragmatism 18

Qualitative approaches 4

Quantitative approaches 4

Rapport 11

Rate data 7

Realism 13

Rival plausible explanations 23

Social facts 6

Theoretical triangulation 22

Theory 8

Triangulation 22

Verstehen 11

STUDY QUESTIONS

1. Consider the dimensions of difference between the quantitative and qualitative approaches shown in Table 1.1; explain in your own words what each dimension entails.

2. Now go to Table 1.2 and explain in your own words how the final column resolves any apparent tensions between qualitative and quantitative traditions.

3. Outline the differences between realism and constructionism as ways of perceiving the world. Give an example of how a person's perspective on this issue might be evident in research. How does critical realism (also known as fallibilist realism) offer a resolution to the conflict between those two perspectives?

4. Outline some differences you see between positivism and phenomenologism.

5. Why have qualitative researchers preferred field-based case study research? Explain how this approach fits into qualitative perspectives.

6. What are "social facts," and what role do they play in positivist inquiry?

7. What is evolutionary epistemology, and why does it make sense within a realist epistemology but not a constructionist one?

8. Compare and contrast the approaches that might be taken by a realist and a constructionist if each set out to study the effects associated with being a child of divorce.

9. Table 1.1 outlines some of the differences between quantitative and qualitative approaches. But what are some of their similarities?

10. What four modes of triangulation were articulated by Denzin (1970)? Explain each one.

11. In what sense do mixed methods approaches reflect the philosophical tradition known as pragmatism?

12. What changes in the research enterprise have contributed to interest in and the ability to do multimethod, multidisciplinary, and multiperspectival research?

GETTING STARTED: DEVELOPING RESEARCH IDEAS

CHAPTER OUTLINE

The fact that you're reading this book suggests that you have some interest in the social and/or health sciences. You may even have articulated more specific interests for yourself, for example, studying juvenile delinquency, organizational dynamics, the socialization process, immigrant life, or sexual health. Still, that's only the beginning. Doing research involves translating general interests into specific researchable questions and then designing concrete research procedures that reflect those questions and allow you to collect the information necessary to answer them. Indeed, one of the first truisms you learn about research is that it is not an activity you can do in the abstract—"doing research" ultimately involves gathering very specific information from specific samples of individuals, groups, or social artifacts in particular places at a particular time. In this chapter, we will take you through some of the first steps in that process, in which we outline the different approaches to theorizing and look at some ways research ideas arise.

CAN YOU SOLVE THIS?

Let us begin by telling you about a provocative little YouTube video we found entitled, "Can you solve this?,"[1] in which an interviewer poses a problem to people passing by. The problem is posed thus:

> *I'm going to give you a three-number sequence, and I have a rule in mind that those three numbers obey that I want you to figure out. The way you can get information about my rule is to offer three numbers of your own that you think follow my rule. I will tell you whether they follow my rule or not, and then will invite you to tell me what my rule is.*

It sounds simple enough and the interviewer begins by offering three numbers that follow his rule: "2, 4, and 8."

The first person offers back 16, 32, and 64, and the interviewer says, "Yes, that follows my rule." When asked to report the rule, the fellow says, "Double each number." The fellow is stunned when the interviewer says, "That is *not* my rule."

The next several people offer different numbers. One says "3, 6, 12," while the next says "10, 20, 40." The first person tries again and says "5, 10, 20." In each case, the interviewer says, "Yes, that follows my rule." But when each person suggests again

---

[1]The video is at https://www.youtube.com/watch?v=vKA4w2O61Xo.

that the rule is "Double each number," the interviewer again says, "No, that is not my rule." Other people make more guesses: "100, 200, 400" says the next person; "500, 1,000, 2,000" says the next. The interviewer acknowledges that each sequence follows his rule. But what is the rule? "That you double each number?" "No," says the interviewer, yet again.

Do you have a theory about what the rule is? What numbers would you try next? Before we tell you what the rule is that the interviewer had in mind, we want to describe three forms of logical reasoning that parallel different approaches to research and have implications for the ways researchers go about generating and testing theories.

THREE APPROACHES TO THEORIZING

In logic, a distinction traditionally has been made between three different processes of logical reasoning: deduction, induction, and **abduction**. Let's consider each of these in turn.

Deductive Logic

Deduction involves reasoning from the general to the particular or from premises to conclusion. Often these are stated as if/then propositions. *If* the premises are correct, *then* the conclusion follows. The classic example from philosophy, illustrated in Figure 2.1, is (1) all men are mortal; (2) Socrates is a man; (3) therefore Socrates is mortal. There is an implicit "if" there with respect to the premises, i.e., *if* all men are mortal, and *if* Socrates is indeed a man, *then* the conclusion that Socrates must be mortal follows. Of course, it may well be that one or more premises are not true, in which case we still end up with a conclusion that follows logically, but is invalid. For example, we might say (1) all immigrants are criminals; (2) my friend Louise is an immigrant; (3) therefore Louise is a criminal. The problem here, of course, is that while the logic is correct, the premise that all immigrants are criminals is not true; so that while your friend Louise may well have come to the United States as an immigrant, it does not necessarily follow that she is also a criminal.

The hypothetico-deductive method reflects this logic. The method involves (1) developing theories about a phenomenon; (2) expressing hypotheses (predictions, if/then statements) based on these theories; (3) creating or observing conditions where we can assess whether things happen as the theory predicts they should; and then (4) looking for new situations in which to test or expand the theory if it succeeds or revising the theory or even abandoning it entirely if its predictions are not supported

FIGURE 2.1 ● Deductive Logic

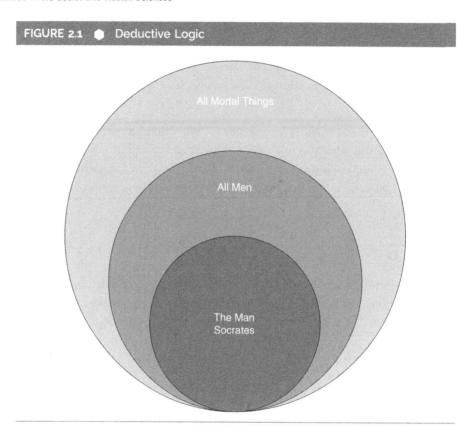

All Mortal Things

All Men

The Man
Socrates

(e.g., Shank, 2008b). As you know from Chapter 1, this deductive model of science has been preferred by many people who engage in quantitative research who often go so far as to call it "the" scientific method. Its strength is that it encourages us to take our speculations and subject them to some real-world test. The logic is quite elegant: If a theory is true, then in a certain situation covered by the theory, some particular result should occur. If it does, we give points to the theory (metaphorically) and look for a new test in a new situation covered by the theory; if it does not, we abandon the theory or at least reevaluate the range of situations to which it applies.

One limitation of the hypothetico-deductive approach to theory building is that we can never "prove" a theory because we can never test every single situation in which a theory might potentially apply; all we can do is keep on finding new ways and new situations in which to test the theory. The more such tests the theory meets, the more confidence we have in it. Conversely, when a theory's predictions are *not* observed, we start to lose confidence in the theory. A mixture of positive and negative findings may at some level be more confusing, but also may provide us with clues about where and in what circumstances a theory applies, and when it does not.

Another difficulty with deductive logic and the hypothetico-deductive method arises when we do not give other explanations an opportunity to be tested. Kuhn (1970/2012) made the point when he talked about how observations are often theory-laden and thereby do not allow us to see that another state of affairs—another theory that could also explain the result—is actually true. We can illustrate the problem by going back to the YouTube video referred to at the beginning of this chapter.

Note what the people who were interviewed did when they were asked to participate. Each of them first heard the sequence the interviewer gave—2, 4, 8—and presumably came up with the theory, which does seem both obvious and quite reasonable, that the second and third numbers simply double the number preceding it. They then take a situation where the theory should apply and offer three numbers that follow the theory—10, 20, 40 and 16, 32, 64 and 100, 200, 400—and in each case hear "Yes, that follows my rule." However, note that in doing so, the guessers are not taking into account that there are other theories that could also be operating that might also account for the observed sequence.

Inductive Logic

A second form of reasoning illustrated in Figure 2.2, *induction*, begins with specifics and uses these to generate general principles. You *start* by observing, in other words, and then move from observation to theory rather than the other way around. A strength of inductive logic is that it arises from observation, such that any consistent patterns we identify are rooted in the real world. But there are problems associated with inductive reasoning. One is that, unlike deductive logic where, if the premises are true, the logical conclusion must follow, with inductive reasoning the best you can do is make probabilistic statements based on what you have seen. This in turn brings up the problem that what has been true up to now is not necessarily true from here on. While our inclination when we see a number sequence that goes 1, 2, 4, 8, 16 is to say that the next number will be 32, who is to say that the sequence does not then reverse itself to 16, 8, 4, 2, 1 in a continuing wave formation or start anew with triples this time, i.e., 1, 3, 9, 27. There may well be "safe" generalizations. For example, because we see the sun rise every morning and set every evening we are confident in saying that day and night will continue (and no doubt the planet would be in big trouble if that were not the case). And although these examples are trivial, the dynamics of the world we are trying to understand can also change overnight …

FIGURE 2.2 ● Inductive Logic

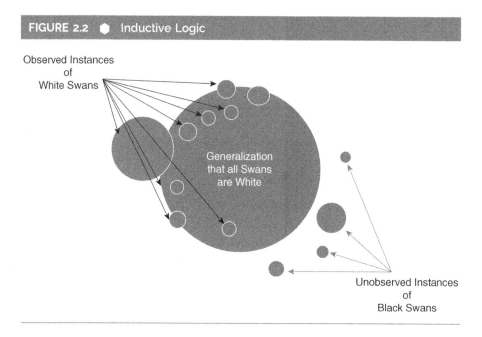

as it did when terrorists destroyed New York's World Trade Centre on the date that has become known simply as 9/11 or when Edward Snowden revealed the extent of the NSA and CIA's spying on Americans.

Another limitation to inductive approaches is simply that there are many ways we can be "wrong" about our inferences. For example, we might go to the park and observe the swans and see they are all white. Our inductive logic might lead us to say (1) every swan we have observed is white; (2) therefore, we conclude all swans are white. But we can be wrong, as we realize as soon as we observe our first non-white swan. Indeed, falsification is just around the corner whenever we do a simple generalization in that way. As this example suggests, the problem arises by focusing too narrowly on one option, which unfortunately means that we can feel completely correct and yet be completely wrong either by being lazy and not looking for new examples or by maintaining ideological blinders that cause us to only look for and see information that is consistent with our beliefs or theory—this type of error in inductive reasoning is also known as *confirmation bias*.

One of the fascinating aspects of the "Can you solve this?" video is how unwilling people are to accept they are wrong. After hearing the interviewer give the example of

2, 4, 8 and guessing 16, 32, 64 and being told that "Doubling each number" is *not* the rule the interviewer has in mind, their first inclination is nonetheless to do more of the same, and they offer further examples that follow exactly the same pattern … 5, 10, 20, then 20, 40, 80, and then 100, 200, 400. Interestingly enough, tunnel vision or confirmation bias is associated with very poor decision-making in other realms. It is a major factor in wrongful convictions, for example (e.g., MacFarlane & Cordner, 2008), as well as in misdiagnoses (and malpractice law suits) in the medical realm (e.g., Redelmeier, 2005). It is also a major reason why researchers who do qualitative research, who favor more inductive approaches, always preach both fascination with and the wisdom of looking for negative cases … instances that violate your theory … seeing those as even more informative than confirming instances.

Abductive Reasoning

A third form of reasoning illustrated in Figure 2.3, *abduction*, accommodates and goes beyond both deductive and inductive logic. It is somewhat different from the other two in several respects. First, it is less oriented toward prediction and hypothesis testing and more interested in inference and explanation—explaining the why and how of what *did* happen rather than speculating on what *will* happen. Shank (2008a) cites 19th century American philosopher Charles Pierce as an early proponent of abduction, which he explained using the following form:

Some event, X, is surprising to us.

But if some explanation, Y, were in place, then X would be ordinary.

Therefore, it is plausible that X is actually a case of Y.

The key takeaways here are the idea that abduction seeks to offer "explanations," and further that the measure of the adequacy of an explanation is its "plausibility." Abduction is also known as "Inference to the best explanation" (Douven, 2017), which captures well the idea that abduction urges us to consider which of various different explanations best accounts for whatever has been observed. In doing so, it parallels the processes we use in many different research and other life situations.

Douven (2017) gives a number of simple examples of abductive reasoning at work. In one, we learn that Tim and Harry recently had a terrible argument that ended with them terminating their friendship. But then a mutual friend tells you that she just saw the two of them jogging together. What would account for this? Note how the example is dealing with a specific case and that you are asked for a plausible

FIGURE 2.3 ● Abductive Logic

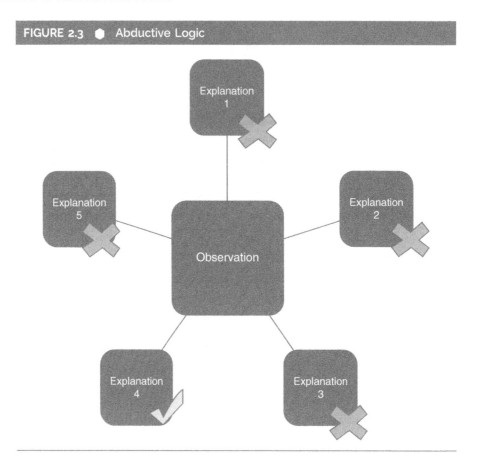

explanation. The trick with abduction is to have as many rival plausible explanations as possible and then to decide through a process of elimination which of the explanations best accounts for the evidence. In the example given, the possibilities are pretty thin because very little information is given. We might posit that Tom and Harry resolved their argument and rekindled their friendship. Another possibility is that, even though their friendship has ended, they may have other dealings—e.g., a business they share—that needs attention and does not give them the luxury of ignoring one another. Another possibility is that the mutual friend may have mistaken the identity of one or both of the joggers they saw. Note how in each case the pull is to gather more information that would allow you to decide on the plausibility of each alternative.

In the case of the "Can you solve this?" video, an abductive approach would see any given person first thinking about what all the possibilities are when the interviewer gives the example of 2, 4, 8 exemplifying his rule. One possibility has been mentioned, i.e., that the progression starts with a number that is doubled and then redoubled. But there are many other rules that could be in effect. Some examples of rules that could potentially be operative with 2/4/8 include (1) list three even numbers; (2) list three single digit numbers; or (3) list three different numbers of increasing value. Once we start gathering some of the different possibilities, our attention can then turn to figuring out ways to determine which of the possibilities is most plausible.

It is in the closing portion of the video where we finally see someone being interviewed change tack. As the video proceeds and the people being interviewed become more exasperated at being told their theory is incorrect even though the numbers they are offering are consistent with the interviewer's rule, one of them then says, "Well, now I'll tell you three numbers that don't fit the rule, and see what you say: 2, 3 and 7!" Much to his astonishment, the interviewer says, "That fits my rule." Interestingly, the fellow's first response is, "So the rule is that anything I say is okay?" But the interviewer says, "No, that is not my rule." Nonetheless, the fact that 2, 4, 7 does fit the rule is now immediately informative. It immediately eliminates the "doubling" explanation and also eliminates the "even numbers" possibility we suggested, but leaves the other two, i.e., that the rule might be either "three single digit numbers" or "three numbers of increasing value." How might we decide between those? All we need do is suggest the numbers 8, 9, and 10 because that sequence violates the "single digit" rule but not the "increasing magnitude" rule. If 8, 9, 10 were suggested, and the interviewer were to respond with, "That fits my rule," that would eliminate "All single digit numbers" as the possible rule, while leaving "Each number is larger than the one before it" as the most plausible rule that we have come up with. Are there still other plausible options? Possibly. And that is one of the challenges to abductive reasoning—there might always be some other more plausible alternatives that we have not yet thought of and ruled out.

Although Shank (2008a) has argued that abduction is particularly well-suited to qualitative research, we would go a step further and suggest that abduction is a reasonable model for all research. The notion of "rival plausible explanations" appears throughout this book as a concept that underlies all the methods we will discuss (see Palys, 1989 for an early statement of this rationale). In any piece of research, the researcher must be sensitive to "what else" might be going on other than whatever putative explanation is being offered. The challenge for the researcher is always to manage and control those rival plausible explanations as part of showing why the explanation offered is the most plausible.

WHERE DO RESEARCH IDEAS COME FROM?

Our description above of the three approaches to logical reasoning (summarized briefly in Table 2.1) sets the stage for telling you some of the different places that ideas come from for research. From deductive logic and the hypothetico-deductive method, you should start to appreciate the role of theory and theory development in suggesting research designed to test and thereby potentially extend or constrain a theory's reach. From inductive logic we start to see the role that raw observation in particular settings can play in theory generation and in providing fodder for further inquiry. The explanation of abductive reasoning should sensitize you to the central role that rival plausible explanations—identifying them, managing and controlling them, and testing for them—play in encouraging our creative juices and providing new routes of investigation. Noted methodologian Donald T. Campbell once talked about a "tribal" model of knowledge in which the role of each generation of researchers—who he referred to as "disputatious questioning truth-seekers"—was to come up with new rival plausible explanations and new ways of looking at the world that would go beyond the vision of their predecessors (e.g., Campbell, 1979b, 1986). Consider yourself encouraged.

Connecting With the Literature

If there is a "tribal" or collective element to the research community—which we believe there is—then "the literature" is where we store our tales of discovery. While

TABLE 2.1 ● Summary of Approaches to Theorizing		
Deduction	**Induction**	**Abduction**
Also known as the hypothetico-deductive model, research begins with theory, from which hypotheses are deduced and then tested by gathering data. Sometimes known as a "top-down" approach.	Research begins with observation, from which empirical generalizations can be induced, and then, through analytic induction, attempts to develop a full-blown theory that adequately reflect the observed reality are made. Sometimes known as a "bottom-up" approach.	Moving away from prediction and hypothesis testing; research considers which of various different explanations best explains an observed phenomenon.

literature most often refers to things like books, book chapters, and journal articles, it can also include background sources such as encyclopedias; magazines; newspapers; government reports and information; reports from industries, NGOs, and associations; law reports, legal cases, and court transcripts; videos, audios, and images; datasets; and maps or spatial data. In short, any collection of published materials on a topic can be considered part of "the literature." Since such a wide array of materials can be considered literature, one of the first challenges we are faced with is getting access to these materials.

Real and Virtual Libraries

There are several places you can go to locate literature on a topic you are interested in. One is the library—the heart of every university. If you are uncertain about what to do once you get to the library, ask your librarian about tours or look on your school's library website under the "help" section where you are likely to find a wealth of guides, references, and answers to "frequently asked questions" that will help you familiarize yourself with the physical and virtual resources your library has to offer. Books, journals, media, databases, and other materials are *not* filed randomly, and a working knowledge of what's available, where things are, and how to find them is invaluable. Knowing the general area in the library that contains material related to your topic of interest still provides splendid opportunities for browsing.

Increasingly, however, library buildings and the physical books and journals they hold are being supplemented and sometimes replaced with virtual materials that you can acquire from your institution's online library catalogue. The catalogue of your institution's library holdings provides you with a comprehensive list of all of the books, articles, reports, guides, FAQs, and digitized collections relating to your topic of interest that your institution owns. While searching your library catalogue is a great place to begin your quest for literature on your topic, it often reveals just the tip of the iceberg when it comes to the depth and breadth of extant literature on a topic because catalogue searches do not search all available databases, they do not map to specific disciplines, and they only return findings for materials that are owned by or accessible to your institution.

A second, and arguably more lucrative, place to start looking for literature is in *subject-specific databases*. Subject-specific databases generally catalogue materials published in a single academic discipline or a group of related disciplines. One major advantage of subject-specific database searches is that you can fine-tune or "*scope*" your search to find materials that have been produced by people working in specific disciplines such as health science, epidemiology, anthropology, or criminology. Another advantage is that they provide you with valuable metadata or descriptive information about the resource such as title, author, keywords, abstract, number of pages, number and content of citations, and citation ranking. This metadata is vital for helping you sift through thousands or even tens of thousands of sources to locate the select few pieces of literature that are most relevant for your literature review objectives.

While databases offer a very powerful and efficient way to locate literature on your topic, using them is often time-consuming, more technically difficult, and dependent upon your institution having a paid subscription to access the database you want to use. Beyond this, it is important to keep in mind that the database you use can greatly impact the efficiency and success of your search for literature. Some databases are restricted to certain types of literature, published by specific publishers, within a particular set of fields or subfields. The larger and more comprehensive databases give you direct access to a wider array of literature (e.g., all materials from multiple disciplines as opposed to just books, articles, and reports published in the social or health sciences). Table 2.2 lists some of the most popular and inclusive databases that are used within the health and social sciences.

A third place to begin your search for literature is Google Scholar. Google Scholar is a publicly accessible web search engine that indexes the full text and metadata of literature across an array of publishing formats and disciplines. What sets Google Scholar apart from databases is that it provides a single catalogue of the tremendously large array of literature that is archived on the internet. In fact, the literature catalogued in Google Scholar is exponentially more than all of the subscription-based databases (such as the ones listed in Table 2.2) combined. Since the search engine that powers Google Scholar is built upon a sophisticated algorithm, it tends to be efficient, easy to use, and provides you with access to the most popular literature. Moreover, because it catalogues materials archived across various public and private domains of the internet, it is excellent for locating literature outside of standard academic publications or "gray literature" such as preliminary reports; institutional, internal, technical, and statistical reports; research memoranda; market research reports; reports of commissions and study groups; conference proceedings; and technical and commercial documentation.

While Google Scholar is an impressive search tool, it is important to keep in mind that it is not mapped to specific disciplines and it doesn't allow for use of more sophisticated search techniques, so it is not uncommon to return hundreds or thousands of items in your search results that you then have to sort through in order to locate the handful of materials that will be most useful for your literature review. Moreover, the sophisticated algorithm that the search engine is built upon is

TABLE 2.2 ● Popular Subject-Specific Databases	
Database	**Database Description**
Criminal Justice Abstracts	Major criminology database: covers crime trends, prevention and deterrence, juvenile justice, legal issues, psychology, and more.
EconLit	The American Economic Association's electronic database, the world's foremost source of references to economic literature.
ERIC (Education Resources Information Center)	Online digital library of education research and information.
JSTOR (Journal Storage)	Multidisciplinary digital library of books and other primary sources and current issues of journals.
LexisNexis	World's largest electronic database for legal and public records related information.
MEDLINE/PubMed	A bibliographic database of life sciences and biomedical information. It includes bibliographic information for articles from academic journals covering medicine, nursing, pharmacy, dentistry, veterinary medicine, and health care.
Project Muse	Digital humanities and social science content for the scholarly community. MUSE provides full-text versions of scholarly journals and books.
PsycINFO	Comprehensive database of abstracts of literature in the field of psychology produced by the American Psychological Association. Contains citations and summaries from the 19th century to the present of journal articles, book chapters, books, and dissertations.
PubPsych	Open access information retrieval system for psychological resources.
Scopus	Abstract and citation database of peer-reviewed research literature (book series, journals, and trade journals) from life sciences, social sciences, physical sciences, and health sciences.
Semantic Scholar	A multidisciplinary artificial intelligence backed search engine designed to retrieve the most important scholarly papers and to identify the connections between them.
Sociological Abstracts	Major sociology database with an emphasis on sociocultural topics.
Web of Science	Multidisciplinary database, including coverage of criminology, psychology, law, labor, gender, political science, policy, sociology, and more.

proprietary, so the searches are "optimized" in such a way that the results are geared toward most popular or newest (or some other unknown factor) as opposed to the best or most relevant for your needs. Finally, and perhaps most importantly, unlike the materials located by academic databases, those located by Google Scholar are

TABLE 2.3 ● Main Advantages and Disadvantages of Different Sources of Literature

	Advantages	Disadvantages
Catalogue and library search	<ul><li>Gives you a comprehensive list of books, articles, reports, etc., that are available through your institution</li><li>Searches books and articles at same time</li><li>Particularly good for book searches</li><li>Good for getting you access to actual holdings</li></ul>	<ul><li>Does not search all databases</li><li>Does not map to specific discipline</li></ul>
Subject-specific databases	<ul><li>Mapped to a specific discipline</li><li>Search limiters unique to discipline, allow fine-tuning of search results</li><li>Records search history and search sets</li><li>Can use subject headings that are key to a literature review</li></ul>	<ul><li>Time-consuming</li><li>More difficult due to technical search aspects</li><li>Access to these databases is often by paid subscription only</li></ul>
Google Scholar	<ul><li>Provides catalogue of a lot of literature</li><li>Helps you identify the most popular literature</li><li>Efficient due to use of algorithms</li><li>Great for searching for known items and when using unique terminology (words)</li><li>Excellent for locating literature outside of standard academic such as repositories, legal rulings, and grey literature</li></ul>	<ul><li>Database not mapped to specific discipline</li><li>Does not allow for use of more sophisticated search techniques</li><li>Searches are optimized so they will be biased</li><li>Emphasizes new or popular first</li><li>Proprietary algorithm makes it hard to know how searches are being done and what is and is not being located</li><li>Does not actually provide access to the actual materials, only links to materials that are often stuck behind pay walls</li></ul>

frequently locked behind pay walls making it more difficult and expensive to actually access them. Table 2.3 summarizes some of the advantages and disadvantages of different sources.

Take a Broad View of Your Topic

Your initial review of the relevant literature will sometimes be cursory and sometimes quite exhaustive, but you do owe it to yourself and to your colleagues to have a look at what's been done in your area of interest. By familiarizing yourself with the literature, you can find out what theory, research, and/or policy has been constructed; you can see how others have approached finding answers to particular research questions, the problems and successes experienced by others in the area, and what gaps in theory and research remain.

Of course, "the literature" is a big place, and one big question you have to address is the one of "which literature?" you should look at. One of the biggest mistakes novice researchers make is that, when they examine "the literature" on a topic, they construe the topic too narrowly and too concretely. Suppose, for example, that you're interested in understanding the decisions made by customs officials at border crossings. How do they decide whether to wave someone through without further scrutiny or pass the person on to their colleagues for more detailed questioning and examination? What makes customs officers suspicious about some people but not others? What makes them decide to look through a person's suitcases, take a person into an interrogation room, or search or even dismantle someone's car?

If you begin your literature search by looking for studies that deal with that specific situation—customs agent decision-making with respect to the identification of individuals who warrant further scrutiny—you'll find very little. Many people would mistakenly leave off searching there, saying, "Gee, I guess there's nothing on this topic, so I'll just have to start off on my own."

But stopping there is quite inconsistent with the spirit of doing research. Any piece of research involves constantly working back and forth between theory and data, that is, between the abstract and the concrete. Seen in this manner, a researcher would rarely be interested in the decision-making of customs officers per se, unless they are doing a project in collaboration with those providing border services. But in most cases, if that's as far as our interest goes, we might as well look at when people choose to mow their lawns or why some people prefer chocolate and others vanilla when they buy ice cream. The question to be asked is, "What makes the decision-making of customs officers more 'interesting' (from a research perspective) than someone's choice of ice cream?"

Let's first consider what it is that customs officers' work involves. They are government employees whose job involves security and social control. They are the first Americans that a border crosser meets, and their job involves keeping apparently "nasty" people or other perceived "undesirables" (e.g., people who are escaping prosecution; people who are trying to bypass "normal" immigration channels; "terrorists") out of the country; keeping nasty things (e.g., unsafe products) out of the country; and ensuring that people who bring goods into the country pay the relevant duties and fees. In the process of executing their jobs, customs officers have an incredible amount of power: you must answer any question they ask, they can seize your car or other belongings, and they can subject you to processes that most of us consider invasive and undesirable (e.g., interrogation, body scans, strip searches). But if they interrogated, scanned, and searched every would-be border crosser, there would soon be lineups miles long and many exasperated people would be calling for their heads. Instead, customs officers are given discretion and are expected to use that discretion wisely. Perhaps only one in ten persons is asked more than a few simple questions (e.g., Where do you live? How long have you been away? Do you have any goods to declare?), and only a small sample is subjected to more detailed searches of their persons or belongings (e.g., people who fit the profile of a "drug mule" or "terrorist"). But where in the literature can we look beyond "customs officers"?

One "trick of the trade" that Howard Becker (1998) calls the "Bernie Beck trick" is a very useful device here. The trick gained its name because Becker had the office next door to Beck's when both were at Northwestern University in Chicago, which led to Becker hearing Beck pose a certain challenge to his students many times over the years when they would come in and tell Beck there was "no literature" on a topic or had completed their research and did not know where to go next. The challenge was: "Tell me briefly what your research is all about, but without using any of the identifying characteristics of the actual case." If he were to issue the challenge to someone studying customs officers, it would have been gone something like this: "Tell me what your research is about, but without using the words 'border,' 'customs officers,' or 'screening.'" In response, the researcher might say, "Well, basically I'm looking at a situation where one individual has to form an impression and make a discretionary decision very quickly about another individual in very ambiguous circumstances with very little if any feedback as to whether the decisions they make are 'correct'."

Given this more general description, you should see that there are now several "relevant" literatures that the researcher might look at, including (1) the various literatures on how people make decisions in an atmosphere of uncertainty (since, after the person leaves without being checked, we can never know for sure whether they did indeed smuggle something into the country or import a dangerous weapon); (2) the "impression formation" literature, which deals with factors people take into account when "sizing up" another person they meet for the first time; these might include studies that look at both "lay people" and "professionals" (e.g., social workers, clinical psychologists); and (3) the "discretion" literature, which looks at the use of discretion by agents of social control (e.g., police officers, judges, parole boards, psychiatrists). And, of course, this is not to say that you should forget about checking for any existing literature on "customs officers" as well, since the results of such studies might help us understand more about who these people are, how they are trained, how their job is defined, how they perceive their job and their role, and so on, which would be useful in placing them in the larger realm of individuals who make decisions in the theoretical realms you've identified.

You might think of other areas that could be relevant to the study of customs officers and their decisions (e.g., whether and how stereotyping and racist or classist attitudes enter into the decision-making process or a study of interview techniques). But the above discussion should suffice to show that "the relevant literature" for such a study includes far more than just whatever research deals with that specific decision by that specific group. Belonging to the community of scholars who engage in research means always looking for ways to benefit from the work of others, whether for positive reasons (e.g., to incorporate methods they've used or to include factors shown to be important) or negative ones (e.g., to avoid repeating mistakes and pursuing dead ends). And as this text argues, your search for "relevant" literature should cast a necessarily wide net.

Additional Techniques for Searching the Literature

It should be clear by now that the quality of your literature review will depend on the quality and relevance of the literature that goes into it. Knowing where to go to find literature and developing better ways to construe your topic once you start looking for literature is only half the battle. Becoming skilled at finding literature also requires that you employ specific search strategies and techniques to help you scope your search so that you are able to locate the most relevant and important literature. There are several important search strategies and techniques that you can employ.

The most basic search strategy and one that most people start with when they begin to delve into the literature is the *simple subject search*. Articles and books frequently have 3–8 broad subject headings assigned to their bibliographic record as metadata. These subject headings are the most basic and universal way of classifying a particular piece of literature. Searching literature by subject will return materials that are specifically ABOUT your topic instead of just mentioning it.

While subject searches are a good way to start to narrow down the literature to locate relevant materials, they frequently return quite a broad array of materials, many of which are not directly relevant to your interests or needs when it comes to writing your literature review. In order to start to restrict the scope a bit more, it is a good idea to identify a narrow set of *keywords* or terms (and their synonyms and antonyms) that are most associated (or not associated) with the topic, problem, or question that your literature review is structured around. Combining subject and keyword searches will most certainly yield fewer results while generating more relevant materials for your literature review. Depending on how successful your keyword restricted search is on helping you retrieve literature, you may find that you have to narrow down or expand your list of terms.

As you search you will likely find better keywords as you go. Looking at the metadata associated with keywords that you identify as being potentially most useful is a great way to cycle your search by revising your keywords. Beyond combining subject and refined keywords in your searches, you can further restrict the scope of your searches by directing the search engine to restrict searches to specific disciplines, languages, date ranges, study types, and geographic regions. From here you can order your search results by date in descending (i.e., newest to oldest) or ascending (i.e., oldest to newest) order, allowing you to locate the most contemporary literature or helping you to quickly locate the seminal source that everyone else quotes or references.

As you become more comfortable using more elaborate combinations of subjects and keywords and restricting the scope of your searches, you will probably want to start to take advantage of some more advanced techniques such as the use of **Boolean operators**. Boolean operators allow you to combine keywords with modifiers in order to generate more complex searches. There are numerous Boolean operators, but the three main ones are AND, OR, and NOT. To illustrate the way they work, imagine you are at a restaurant with family and friends and have just finished dinner, and the waiter comes to check on whether anyone is interested in coffee (apologies to the tea drinkers) and/or dessert. The waiter finds that people fall into one of the four groups as illustrated in the Venn diagrams shown in Figure 2.4.

Figure 2.4(a) shows the situation where people want coffee AND dessert, i.e., the area in the overlap where both elements are present. Figure 2.4(b) shows the most inclusive situation where people are happy with whatever arrives, coffee OR dessert. Figure 2.4(c) and (d) show where people want one, but NOT the other.

Now instead of coffee and tea, imagine you are doing a library search because you are assigned a paper on research methods. A search for research AND methods would retrieve all literature containing the keyword research AND methods. Similarly, the OR operator placed between keywords will broaden your search to literature that contains any of the two or more keywords (e.g., research OR methods will return all literature related to research OR methods). Placing the NOT operator between keywords will narrow your search to materials indexed at one keyword and not another (e.g., methodology NOT methods will only return literature related to methodology). You can join multiple operators together to narrow your search even further (e.g., research AND [methods OR methodology] will return all literature indexed as research methods and research methodology).

There are two other handy variations you can employ as well. The first is when you are looking for an exact phrase. If you were to put the keywords SOCIAL AND

FIGURE 2.4 ● Boolean Operators AND, OR, and NOT

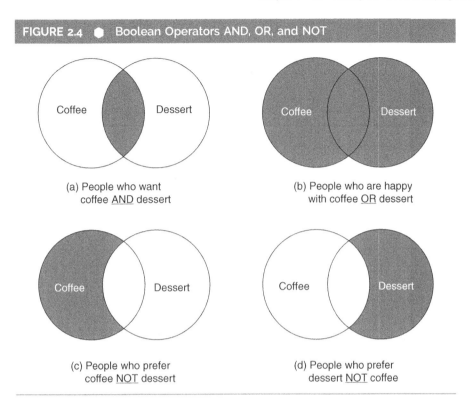

(a) People who want
coffee AND dessert

(b) People who are happy
with coffee OR dessert

(c) People who prefer
coffee NOT dessert

(d) People who prefer
dessert NOT coffee

HEALTH RESEARCH METHODS in a search engine, the default assumption is that the words are separated by OR, such that you would probably get back thousands of links for all sources that include the word SOCIAL, thousands more that contain HEALTH, thousands more for RESEARCH, and so on. But if you were to put quotation marks around the phrase, so that it appears as "social and health research methods," then only those links that include that whole exact phrase will be returned.

A second variant is useful when various forms of a word are possible, and you want to ensure that all the various possibilities are included in the search. The operator that is used there is the asterisk (*), which is essentially a wildcard saying that you are open to receiving whatever variations on the root word exist. So, for example, if you were to make method* your search word, the search engine will include method, methods, methodology, methodologist, methodologian, and any other word out there that begins with METHOD. Placing the wildcard in the middle of a keyword instructs the search engine to retrieve results with multiple spellings of your keyword. For example, behavio*r will return literature indexed with the keywords behavior and behaviour, which would ensure that you retrieve links that include both the American (behavior) and British/Canadian (behaviour) versions of that word.

And of course these can be combined with other Boolean operators. For example, research AND method* will return items indexed at research method, research methods, research methodology, and so forth.

Creating and Managing a Personal Digital Archive

We recommend that you always download and save a digital copy of relevant materials you find in the course of your searches of the literature. There are several reasons for this. First is that it is far lighter and more convenient to have a library of files at your disposal on your laptop or flash drive than to haul around heavy things like books or stacks of photocopied articles. Second is that the biggest challenge you face these days with all of the information at your disposal is actually going through and managing it, and it is far easier to do so with electronic materials than physical ones. Third is that developing your own electronic archive of readings in the substantive areas you are interested in will be an invaluable tool as you move through your career.

The two of us now manage our materials as much as we can electronically by downloading documents, or scanning and creating our own pdf or docx documents, cataloguing them with a citation software such as Zotero or Mendeley, and then incorporating them as part of a "project" in an analysis program known as NVivo. We will be talking more about NVivo in Chapter 13, which deals with the analysis of nonnumeric data, where the program is already well-recognized as among the best nonnumeric data analysis software programs available, but the program's usefulness as an information management tool is only now being more fully recognized (e.g., Palys & Atchison, 2012).

Briefly, incorporating documents into NVivo involves creating an overall "project" into which all "data"—documents in this case—are imported. Two very powerful processes are enabled by doing so. The first is that all of the documents within the project are searchable, which is rather like having your own personal search engine that only goes through the materials that you have included within the project shell. The second is that you can do anything electronically that researchers formerly would do with highlighters—tagging particular sections with the concepts they include, noting interesting quotes, making memos or notes (annotations) of your thoughts about particular passages of your material, and so on, so that any tagged passage or thought you had about that passage can be retrieved at will. The program also introduces new options that would not be possible manually, such as autocoding, word cloud coding, running a network analysis of bibliographies to help identify seminal authors in a field, and so on. These will be described in greater detail in Chapter 13 on "analyzing nonnumeric data." Suffice it to note for now that these possibilities arise because the "data" the program is capable of managing can be any sort of text, audio, or image file, which makes it as useful for managing your literature as it is for managing qualitative data.

Theory as a Source of Research Ideas

Theory is also an important source of research questions simply because that is what good theory is supposed to do. A theory is essentially a set of *conceptually grounded propositions* and a delineation of their *interrelationships* that, taken together, purport to explain a phenomenon or set of phenomena. One function of theory is to help make sense of the world or of a particular class of phenomena. In doing so, theories also guide research, which makes them both powerful and constraining.

Perhaps an example will help here. Suppose we're interested in explaining why some people do not use condoms when they have sex with casual sex partners. An infinite number of factors could potentially "explain" failure to use a condom during casual sex—everything from not having one available, to individual religious beliefs, to lack of knowledge about the "risks" that can be associated with not using condoms.

A theorist takes a particular subset of these factors and tries to offer a convincing explanation of why and how they combine to generate condom use or avoidance. These speculations, made public, give theorists and others a research direction to pursue by offering propositions that can be tested. For example, advocates of health belief theory (HBT) such as Rosenstock (1974) theorize that health-related behaviors are the result of a rational decision-making process whereby people evaluate (1) the severity of risk associated with a particular behavior; (2) the degree to which they believe they are susceptible to such risk; and (3) the benefits and barriers (practical and psychological) they expect to gain from acting in a particular way to avoid or reduce such risks. A researcher guided by this theory would thus want to seek information not only about the type and frequency of sexual activities people engage in but also about (1) the severity of risk they believe they are or would be exposed to if they did not use a condom; (2) the extent to which they believe their own behavior choice—to use or not use a condom—creates or mitigates risk during casual sexual encounters; and (3) the benefits or other consequences they feel arise from their choices.

But while it makes logical sense to ask about the elements a theory you are advancing or testing says are important, note that there is also a downside to this focusing of attention. Because HBT focuses on individual cognitive processes as determinants of sexual safety behavior, researchers employing this theory focus all their energies on measuring people's opinions and beliefs about their likelihood of risk and completely ignore other cultural, social, and situational factors that also might play a significant role in a person's risk-taking behavior. For example, some other health researchers began to look toward social ecology theory (Bronfenbrenner, 1979) to help fill in what they saw as theoretical gaps in explaining health behavior in general and condom use in particular. Social ecologists maintain that health behavior such as condom use is influenced by a combination of personal factors (e.g., individual knowledge, attitudes, skills, and beliefs), your relationships (e.g., ties to family and friends), organizational factors (e.g., educational, occupational, religious, recreational organizational structures), community factors (e.g., belonging to and participation in organizational activities), and policy frameworks. As this suggests, an important dimension on which theories vary is in their prospective *comprehensiveness*.

In sum, "good" theories are useful devices because they help coordinate research by *providing a research focus* and by *implying hypotheses* that can be tested empirically. Their weakness is that they may blind you to other factors or other perspectives that are beyond the scope of the theory. This suggests an important consideration when researching or testing a given theory is whether the test is solely of elements internal to the theory or whether the situation allows for other, potentially competing or rival plausible explanations to be considered as well.

Applying Theory to Situations

Many research ideas emerge from theory. If a theory states that some set of events *should* go together, you can test the theory by thinking of a specific situation in which the theory should be able to predict or account for what occurs. For example, cognitive dissonance theory (see Festinger, 1957) suggests that people will feel differently about things after they have committed themselves to a course of action than before. In a now-famous field experiment, Knox and Inkster (1968) decided to test that theoretical proposition at their local racetrack. They approached two groups of bettors—some who were in the lineup waiting to place their bets, and others who had just finished placing their bets—and asked them how confident they were their horse would win. Sure enough, those who were asked *after* they had placed their bet how confident they felt about their wager expressed significantly greater certainty about whether their horse would win than those who had not yet made it to the betting window, even though the difference between the two situations was less than a minute.

Extending or Limiting a Theory's Coverage

Another procedure for generating research ideas is to try to *extend the coverage* of an existing theory. One person might have posited a theory that explains a certain social dynamic within business organizations. You'd be making a significant contribution by showing that the same theoretical principles also apply to illicit markets run by drug dealers or organized crime. Conversely, you'd also be making a contribution if you were to *point out limitations* to the applicability of existing theories. Theories of aggression, for example, have typically been developed to account for aggression toward minority groups and/or sources of frustration. But do these theories also account for violent behavior toward intimates, child abuse by parents, or wife assault by husbands?

Offering Alternative Explanations

Yet another source of research ideas involves trying to formulate *alternative explanations* for a given phenomenon, as is very much in keeping with the abductive reasoning we outlined above. For example, early criminological theories (e.g., Lombroso, 1911) saw those who went through the justice system as "born criminals" and tried to ascertain the ways in which "criminal" differed from the rest of us. But later theorists (e.g., Rubington & Weinberg, 1968) demonstrated that many, if not most, of us have indulged in "criminal" behavior at various points in our lives. This finding shifted the research focus of interest from identifying who the "born criminals" in society were, which was based on the assumption that some people do criminal things while others do not, to the ways that society reacts to criminal activity and the process by which some persons or actions are labeled "criminal" while others are not.

Wagner (1984) refers to this process of theory development as *variation* and offers numerous other examples of theorists building on one another's work by offering competing explanatory mechanisms for similar phenomena. Also, note how one role of theory in science is to generate research possibilities; if a theory doesn't suggest research possibilities, it's not a very good theory. Perhaps even more importantly, in order to be considered "scientific," a theory must be capable of being tested and disproved. If there are no data that can possibly lead us to say, "Oh, I guess we were wrong," then we are not talking about theory or science, but about faith, ideology, and dogma.

A list of ways that theory can be a source of research ideas is summarized in Table 2.4.

TABLE 2.4 ● Different Ways Theory Can Be a Source of Research Ideas

Theory as Source of Ideas

Theory as explanation of a phenomenon
Theory A explains part of a phenomenon BUT it is limited in its scope. Is there a theory that explains more or more completely explains the phenomenon?

Test of theory
A good theory will generate hypotheses. If we test them, can we find support? How well does this theory explain this phenomenon?

Extend coverage of theory
A theory explains one phenomenon, but can it explain other phenomena as well?

Alternative theoretical explanation
Which theory offers the best explanation of this phenomenon?

Inductive Sources of Research Ideas

We've seen that theories are an integral starting point when employing a deductive approach to science and that they can be very useful for those who take a more abductive approach. But what about for those employing more inductive approaches? Inductivists place no less emphasis on theory than deductivists, but they disagree over whether theory should *guide* or *emerge from* the research process. Recall that, for deductivists, you *begin* with theory, and then "good" theory suggests or implies what to research. In contrast, inductivists argue that such theory—particularly when it is not grounded in thorough observation—is unlikely to be profound and may represent little more than a premature imposition of theoretical blinders that says more about the theoretician than about the phenomenon under consideration. They suggest that ideas and theories should emerge from interacting with and observing the phenomenon itself.

Recall that, from within qualitative perspectives, the inductive (grounded) approach to data gathering and theorizing is encouraged, and "intimate knowledge" of the phenomenon under consideration is not considered a liability. Accordingly, while some individuals schooled only in more quantitative approaches might be worried if you are "too close" to a phenomenon of interest because of the propensity to "overidentify" and the concern that you might be unable to remain "appropriately" detached and analytical, researchers working within a qualitative framework are more likely to recognize that those who have undergone particular life experiences may bring special insights to their research because of having experienced a phenomenon from the "inside" (e.g., Faulkner & Becker, 2008).

Starting From Where You Are

Consistent with this view, Lofland, Snow, Anderson, and Lofland (2006) suggest that one way to begin research is to "start from where you are"; that is, to begin with your own life situation and the concerns and issues that arise therefrom. Dozens of examples can be cited of researchers who did exactly that:

> *For example, Gary Alan Fine's* Gifted Tongues *(2001), a study of high school debate and adolescent culture, was connected to his son Todd's distinguished career as a high school debater. In a similar vein, John Irwin's interest in* The Felon *(1970), in* Prisons in Turmoil *(1980), and in* The Jail *(1985) was intimately related to his own felony conviction at the age of 21 and the five years he spent in a California state prison. And Mary Romero's study of domestic workers (*Maid in the U.S.A. *1992) may be said to have had its origins in the fact that as a teenager she had worked as a domestic, as had her mother, sister, relatives, and neighbors. (p. 10)*

Starting from where you are has several advantages. You bring (1) an interest in the research topic, because of its meaningfulness to you, that will help sustain you through the persistence of effort required to actually complete a piece of research; (2) insights into those aspects of the phenomenon with which you are familiar that, ideally, will allow you to ask "good questions" in a manner that is meaningful to people in that milieu; and probably (3) knowledge of at least some others who are in the same position as you, which may help provide access to needed research sites and to an initial sample of people you can approach regarding their experiences.

At the same time, there are also potential potholes in this road that need to be avoided. The first is that, as an insider, you come with baggage—beliefs about "how things work," or "what the problems are," that you will have to get past to ensure that people who do not think like you are included and feel free to express their views. Associated with this is the idea that you have to be open-minded about what you will find and ensure this is not just pseudo-research whose answer is a foregone conclusion because you only look at things and talk to those who will confirm your point of view. Less malevolent, but equally problematic, is that you and your participants' familiarity with the situation may make you less likely to ask questions about things that "everyone knows" to be true, which may or may not be the case: what you believe "everyone knows" may not in fact be shared by "everyone," and it is often the case that what "everyone knows" to be true isn't.

Starting from where you are also can be problematic because of role conflicts that can emerge from making part of your life a research site. Suppose you're employed as a nurse, for example, and want to do a study regarding doctor–nurse relationships. Information derived from interviews with doctors and nurses in the ward where you work might be problematic when and if your role as a researcher creates role conflicts in relation to your duties as a nurse. For example, as a researcher, you are normally expected to keep the source of everything you hear confidential; as a nurse, there may be reporting requirements associated with your role in which you are supposed to report certain categories of behavior to your union, hospital officials, or supervisor. Even if you *are* able to compartmentalize your role for the duration of the study——something you are ethically obliged to do to ensure your primary interests are those of the research participants—once the study is completed, you go back to your former role. But you now have information you might not otherwise have obtained about certain people, information you can't simply "forget."

A third potential problem arises when you are so embedded in a situation that you are unable to rise above it. The trick in starting from where you are is to use the insights to be gained from your own experience, but then to activate your "sociological imagination" (as Mills [1959] termed it) and be able to see yourself as one instance of many, thereby helping to contextualize your own experience. This is sometimes easier said than done. There is a saying, "If you want to know what water is, don't ask the fish" (see Hagan, 1989, p. 157). It's sometimes very difficult to see what's "interesting" about our lives, in the social or health science sense, when we are too wrapped up in experiencing them.

Observation as a Source of Ideas

As you might expect, research ideas within the inductive framework emerge through observation coupled with the natural curiosity of the social or health scientist who inevitably asks "Why?" or "How?" You might begin with a particular phenomenon that interests you (e.g., unemployment, criminality, depression, the availability of organic food, people buying memberships in fitness centers, the surge of interest in "designer" dogs) and then try to suggest and test out factors that might influence it. Where does it come from? Who does it? Is there more of it in the summer than the winter? Are the patterns the same or different in the United States and Australia?

It was observation of this sort coupled with asking "Why?" that led Emile Durkheim to formulate his classic work (1951) on suicide. He began by observing that countries differ in their predominant religious affiliation and that they also tend to differ in their suicide rates. This observed covariation ultimately led him to formulate his ideas that suicide is affected by both social regulation (norms) and social integration and group solidarity.

Intensive Case Studies and Experience Surveys

Systematic observation in the context of *intensive case studies* is another useful source of research ideas, still within the inductive framework. Many of Jean Piaget's theories on child development emerged from observing his own children, for example, while many of Sigmund Freud's came from his discussions with clients. Similarly, if you're new to an area of research, an *oral history* or broader *experience survey* may suggest research ideas. If you want to study prejudice and discrimination toward minority groups, for example, you could talk to a Japanese person who lived in the internment camps in California during World War II, a Jew who lived in Germany at the same time, to Muslim women in North America who choose to wear the hijab, or a Maori in New Zealand. Be careful, though, not to let this process steer you away from a review of the relevant literature. Also don't assume that the first person you talk to is necessarily representative of their group. When doing this sort of exploratory research, talk to and observe as diverse an array of people and situations as possible.

Table 2.5 summarizes the different ways that inductive approaches can be a source of research ideas.

TABLE 2.5 ● Different Ways Inductive Approaches Can Be a Source of Research Ideas
Inductive Approaches as Sources of Ideas
Starting from where you are Beginning with your own life situation. The trick here is to see your situation as part of a bigger phenomenon by seeing yourself and your situation as one of many.
Observation/experience In our daily lives and when engaged in more systematic observation, we come across phenomena that arouse our curiosity and lead us to ask "why?" or "how?" it came about.
Case study/experience survey Research ideas also can arise when we look at particular cases or people who have undergone life experiences that interest us.

Ideas From the Research Process Itself

A third general place research ideas arise is during the actual process of doing and reading about research.

Replication

Replication of prior research can serve a useful function. Although most professional journals aren't interested in publishing a straight replication for its own sake (e.g., Kelly, 2006; McNeeley & Warner, 2015), situations may arise where the replication provides interesting information. For example, many older studies that looked at sex differences might be interesting to replicate now that the sex roles in our society have supposedly undergone a major transition over the last few decades. Similarly, studies based in Canada or Europe might be replicated in the United States if you had reason to speculate that some aspect of the US social context might yield different results.

When Technologies Open New Doors

A special occasion arises when new technologies open doors that previously were closed and thereby provide new opportunities for replicating earlier research with newly accessible samples or moving into areas that were previously inaccessible. There is a wealth of research that was conducted during the mid to late 20th century that needs to be replicated. This research involves looking at the impact of new technologies on social and health related phenomena and developing a better understanding about how digital technologies have affected the kinds of data available to address our research questions.

Another door that has opened with the advent of digital technologies and the internet is with research methods themselves. There were decades of study that went into advising us on how to design a mail-out questionnaire so that it will be most inviting, for example, or how to make an engaging survey on paper. Digital technologies have fundamentally changed the look, feel, and mode of administration of the traditional paper-and-pencil survey, yet very little research has been done devoted to see which of the old rules still apply.

The internet and the wide array of digital technologies that surround it also have brought together communities of persons, particularly through blogs, podcasts, instant messaging, and social network and media spaces, who otherwise would be very difficult to locate in any significant numbers. Chris does research involving the sex trade, for example; in this field much research has been done on sex trade workers, but very little had been done regarding their clients because of difficulties in locating and contacting them. With the opportunities afforded by the internet, Chris ended up conducting one of the first large-scale studies of sex worker clients when more than 500 clients responded to his solicitations to participate in an anonymous internet-based survey of persons who had paid for sex (see Atchison, 1998; Atchison, Lowman, & Fraser, 1998). As new technology develops and becomes more integrated into our daily lives, there is no end to the new research possibilities that will arise for members of the social and health science communities to pursue.

Challenging Prior Research

You also can generate new research by *challenging prior research*. For example, earlier research into the day-to-day lives of sex workers found that a very high percentage of women who sell sexual services had experienced violence on the job. Tamara O'Doherty (see 2011a, 2011b) did not doubt that result, but wondered whether that finding was true throughout the sex industry. She soon had the opportunity to interview a small sample of women who worked in off-street venues such as massage parlors and escort agencies and found that violence in off-street venues was actually quite rare. This suggested that violence is not something that is integral to the industry, but, rather, varies depending on other ecological and situational factors, which she proceeded to investigate in subsequent research.

Clarifying Underlying Processes

The idea of "clarifying underlying processes" arises because many treatments, therapies, and programs actually comprise multiple interventions. Given an overall finding that a certain treatment, intervention, or program is effective, a useful next step would be to determine *which* aspects of the intervention, treatment, or program actually produced the observed effect. One researcher might find, for example, that a particular group therapy program led to some positive social outcome for the participants. But what *specifically* about the program led to that success? Was it the individualized attention? The opportunity to practice new skills? A change in self-concept? The presence of social support? An overall finding that a new therapy is effective can be followed by research that attempts to analyze the processes involved in an ongoing process of program development. For example, Chris is currently involved in a large-scale evaluation of a population-based screening and monitoring tool used to assess and identify special learning needs of students known as response to intervention (RTI). A central objective of the evaluation is to obtain an in-depth understanding of RTI processes in diverse contexts as they unfold over time and to examine diffusion of the RTI model within school systems. By better understanding the processes underlying RTI, the research team hopes to be able to inform the development of RTI policies and practices that can effectively address adoption and implementation inequalities.

Resolving Conflicting Results

Occasionally the literature contains conflicting results, and you may want to do research that attempts to *resolve the conflict*. For example, the business literature that deals with the effects of job enrichment shows mixed results from study to study; sometimes job enrichment leads to more positive job satisfaction, while other times job enrichment either has no effect or sometimes even has a negative effect on job satisfaction. Malka and Chatman (2003), and Saari and Judge (2004) are among those who have tried to account for these conflicting results by focusing on the needs and interests of the employees whose jobs were being enriched. They found it useful to distinguish between employees for whom the job or career itself is intrinsically rewarding versus those for whom their job is simply a job and valued only to the extent it gives them the time and/or money to be able to indulge in other domains of life they value more highly.

Employees who looked to the job itself as a source of satisfaction became more satisfied with their jobs the more enriched the job became—greater responsibility, more autonomy, and so forth—while increasing extrinsic rewards such as income on its own tended to have little or no effect on their job satisfaction. The prototype here would be the workaholic, i.e., someone who loves what they do and is happy to do more because of the satisfaction it affords. In contrast, employees for whom jobs were instrumental to satisfaction in other domains responded positively to extrinsic rewards such as more income or longer holidays, while showing reduced job satisfaction in response to job enrichment. If a job is important only because it provides a source of income that allows a person to do the things that are really important to them—spending time with family and friends, traveling, or acquiring material possessions of one sort or another—then greater responsibility only gets in the way, while greater income is the key to their heart.

Analogy

Research also may be generated on the basis of *analogy* to other domains. William McGuire (1973), for example, took the immunization model from biology and tried to apply it to the realm of attitude change. In biology, organisms are immunized against various diseases by giving them vaccines that actually contain weak strains of the disease. When McGuire tested out this same logic in the attitude area, he found similarly that people who were first "immunized" by hearing samples of arguments that might be used against their own position were much less likely to change their attitudes than were those who had not been "immunized" when both were exposed to arguments in opposition to their own opinion.

Surprises: Anomaly and Serendipity

The terms **anomaly** and **serendipity** refer to research that begins or is redirected because an unexpected and surprising state of affairs arises. Anomalies are situations that should *not* exist according to the theory that's guiding the research. An anomaly is "a fact that doesn't fit" and hence requires explanation for the deviation.

In his classic *The Structure of Scientific Revolutions*, Kuhn (1970/2012) argues that anomaly is a significant contributor to scientific innovation, although a state of affairs must first be *recognized* as an anomaly before the real process of discovery begins. He provides several examples of anomaly in the natural sciences but also notes a number of instances where the same state of affairs clearly existed prior to someone's "discovery" of the anomaly. Yet the anomalous situation had been ignored, rationalized away, or otherwise not appreciated by the earlier researchers.

Similar to anomaly is serendipity. While anomaly refers to unearthing disconfirming evidence in the process of an ongoing inquiry, serendipity refers to unexpected findings that are virtually stumbled upon while looking for something else, such as the prospector who digs for gold and strikes oil. Once again, Kuhn (1970/2012) notes that recognition of the event precedes "discovery" and that the history of science is replete with examples of individuals who ignored outcomes or considered them a mistake instead of taking the inferential leap required for discovery.

In sum, it helps to be in the right place when puzzling anomalies and surprising outcomes occur, but you also need to be open enough to recognize their significance. A comprehensive understanding of the relevant literature makes both more likely.

The Supplied Problem

Many studies come about because someone *gives* you a problem. Such is particularly the case in applied settings, where myriad questions require systematic, empirical answers: Is our program effective? How can we better meet our objectives? What will happen if we change our intake criteria? How can we decide who has the best chance to benefit from our program?

For example, the two of us were approached a few years ago by a corporation that publishes magazines in the health and fitness area and was interested in gaining a better understanding of the production, marketing, and consumption of health food products—anything "organic" or "green" and including assorted vitamins and supplements. They envisioned doing a series of studies with health food producers, retail store owners, and consumers and asked us to design, implement, and analyze the Web-based survey that retailers from across the country who distributed their magazines would be asked to complete, as well as to advise them on the interview research their employees would be doing with retailers and manufacturers. We agreed to do so in large part because of our interest in how digital technologies can be incorporated into research processes more so than in their marketing objectives per se. It was actually an interesting example of two different groups—the corporation and us—coming in with different focal interests, but with sufficient common ground that the process and product benefitted both groups.

Cultural Folklore, the Common Wisdom, and "Common Sense"

Much of what we feel we "know" is based on traditional, speculative, or polemical belief that has never been verified empirically. A valuable role of research is to help refute or confirm our beliefs, assuming we believe that truth is a priority and that important decisions should be based on evidence rather than on speculation or stereotyping.

Immigration policies, for example, have often been the subject of heated debate, and this has particularly been the case recently with the Trump administration in the United States as well as in Canada and many other countries in Europe. Politicians who favor limited immigration often point to one or two isolated examples of immigrants who get in trouble and wonder aloud whether their country can really "afford" as many immigrants as it takes, given all the social costs and problems allegedly associated with them. But *are* immigrants a burden on a country? In Canada, the decision was made to address the question empirically. A study undertaken by Statistics Canada entitled *Canada's Changing Immigrant Population* (Badets & Chui, 1994) examined census data, addressed that very issue, and concluded that, at least at that time, such fears were unfounded. As the press reportage of the time explained:

> *Amid widespread fears that Canada's immigration system lets in criminals and layabouts, Statistics Canada has published a study showing immigrants are more hard-working, better educated, and more stable than people born here. (Mitchell, 1994, p. A1)*

TABLE 2.6 ● Different Ways the Research Process Can Be a Source of Research Ideas		
Research as a Source of Ideas		
Replication Can a previous finding be reproduced?	*Clarifying underlying processes* What part of this process is most responsible for the changes we have observed?	*Anomaly and serendipity* Why are these strange or unexpected things happening?
New technologies Have things changed since this new technology or social development came along?	*Resolving conflicting results* Why do two different studies show opposing results? Can they be reconciled?	*Supplied problems* What is the answer to this person or group's question or problem?
Challenging prior research Do the findings from previous research still apply in this context?	*Analogy* Can research done in one field or domain produce similar results or be extended to another domain or field?	*The common wisdom* Is what we think we know about this phenomenon really true?

Clearly, therefore, research has a significant role to play in going beyond stereotype. Gathering data and thereby providing systematic evidence about what "everyone knows" to be true—and often isn't—is an important role for research that attempts to facilitate the development of social policy and/or simply sets out to better inform us about ourselves.

A summary of the different ways that the research process itself can be a source of research ideas is illustrated in Table 2.6.

SUMMING UP AND LOOKING AHEAD

In this chapter we have outlined some of the issues that you must address even before beginning the research process. One of the first involves getting an idea of what to research. Three different approaches to reasoning—inductive, deductive, and abductive—were introduced not only to explain in more detail a concept introduced in Chapter 1 as one on which researchers' preferences often differ but also to show the various ways that different perspectives contribute to achieving general scientific goals and the role that each can play in generating research possibilities.

We then discussed the usefulness of connecting with the literature—both in the library and through internet-based sources—and encouraged researchers to avoid conceptualizing their research too narrowly. The "Bernie Beck trick" offered a way to think about your research to take you beyond its concrete specifics to a more conceptual understanding of the phenomena you are investigating. Subsequent sections of the chapter outlined various ways that more inductive approaches can generate research ideas, as well as how the research process itself can generate many research ideas.

It's pretty tough to do any research if you don't even have a topic. The emphasis on this chapter was on how to get those creative juices flowing in identifying viable topics for research. In the next chapter we discuss the first steps that are required to now turn those ideas into a specific feasible project.

Key Concepts

Abduction 33

Anomaly 61

Bernie Beck trick 46

Boolean operators 48

Google Scholar 42

Keyword search 47

Real and virtual libraries 41

Replication 58

Serendipity 61

Sociological imagination 56

Starting from where you are 55

Wildcards 49

STUDY QUESTIONS

1. Differentiate between *inductive, deductive*, and *abductive* approaches to reasoning in your own words.

2. What role do *theories* play in empirical research, and in what sense are they both *uplifting* and *constraining?*

3. What do practitioners of the inductive and deductive approaches agree on and disagree on with respect to the role of theory?

4. From the deductive perspective, one begins with a theory, generates hypotheses that are implied by the theory, and then gathers data to test the hypothesis (and hence the theory). If the data do *not* support the hypothesis, we say that the theory has been refuted or disproved. If the data are consistent with the theory, we can say that the theory has been "supported," but we do *not* say that it has been "proved." Why?

5. Some researchers suggest that "starting from where you are" is a good place to begin doing research. What are some of the advantages and disadvantages of "starting from where you are"?

6. Social scientists argue that a good place to begin your research is by *reviewing the literature* in the relevant area. What benefits are gained by doing so?

7. What are some of the strengths and limitations of using Google Scholar for your search of the literature?

8. A researcher is interested in getting information about different types of interviews, and particularly regarding focus group and oral history interviews. How can the researcher make sure that their search will include the exact phrases "focus group" and "oral history" rather than those individual words? What effect would using the words AND, OR, or NOT between those two phrases have on the results that are produced?

9. What is "the Bernie Beck trick" and how is it useful?

10. Locate three empirical articles from refereed journals that relate to the research topic or question you have developed and briefly discuss how each of these articles relates to your research topic and provide a short justification for why you selected these particular articles.

11. Go to your favorite news website (e.g., BBC News at http://www.bbc.co.uk/news/) and identify three social or health-related stories that interest you, and how each of the three stories you have identified could be made into a researchable topic.

12. Identify five social and/or health science databases (other than Google Scholar) that you could use to locate refereed journal articles and other academic literature.

GETTING SPECIFIC: WHAT'S THE PLAN?

CHAPTER OUTLINE

CONSTRUCTING A RESEARCH PROPOSAL

Getting an idea about something you might like to research is one thing, but as you will hear us say several times in this book, research does not happen in the abstract. Ultimately, those ideas have to be given life in the real world, which means making decisions about who/what/when/where/how. O'Leary (2014) reminds us that there are very few projects that get off the ground these days without getting someone's approval. You may need the approval of the Instructor in the course you are taking right now before you can begin a term research project. Alternatively, you may need your supervisor and committee's approval for an Honor's or Master's thesis you hope to undertake. Sometimes you even need to do multiple proposals for the same project—one for the admissions board, another for your thesis committee, the next one for a funding agency, the one after that for your institution's research ethics board, another to the people you are asking for access to their business, agency, club, ward, or organization. A proposal is essentially your answer to the question, "So, what's the plan?"

As is true of every well-written paper, a research proposal will have an introduction, a body, and a conclusion. The goal is to explain how the proposed study and its guiding questions are important, relevant, and interesting and to show that the techniques you have selected are ethically and methodologically sound enough to allow you to complete the proposed study given your resources and limitations. The important thing to keep in mind is that you are not writing the proposal for yourself, although you may well benefit from doing one because of how it forces you to think through the specifics of your project. Odds are you are writing it for someone else—your course instructor, or thesis supervisor, or the Institutional Review Board (IRB), or the granting agency or organization you hope to access—which immediately means you are actually giving a sales pitch. The number of pages you have to outline your proposed research, the amount of detail that is expected, and the final list of topics you are expected to address (e.g., whether a budget is required or not) will vary depending on who is funding the research, if anyone, and the purpose of your proposal.

Butler-Kisber (2018) uses the metaphor of a map for the role that a proposal plays. A proposal is your description of how you get from "here" to "there," which means that you will have to begin with some sense of where "here" is. It matters, in other words, whether you are beginning your drive from Chicago or Boston. You also will need to identify where "there" is. If Chicago is your starting point, then the roads you take and the map you need to get to Los Angeles is different than the one you will need to drive to Nashville. Your job in a proposal is to convince whoever you are writing it for that you know where you are going and can be entrusted with the keys to the car.

Although the particular elements that are included or emphasized will vary depending on the specifics of your proposed project, several interrelated components are common to nearly all proposals. These include a critical discussion of academic or background *literature* that offers a convincing *justification* for conducting the research, clearly stated **research questions** or **hypotheses,** a discussion of the specific *research design* and *data analysis strategies* that will be used to derive an answer to your research question(s) or decide the adequacy of your hypotheses, and a discussion of any *research ethics* issues that pertain to your research. We consider each of those elements below. While detailed consideration of all of those elements and more will take us the rest of this book to articulate, outlining the various elements of a proposal here will allow us both to outline what you need to do to get your term research project or thesis project underway and to highlight how and where these elements are addressed in subsequent chapters.

DEFINING "HERE": THE LITERATURE REVIEW

While it is always important to pursue new, exciting, and novel topics, ideas, and questions, remember that research is ultimately a communal enterprise. A well-written literature review situates a project and provides clear evidence that allows the audience to better assess why the topic and research questions are important and how your proposed research fits into the larger academic context. Your literature review should provide a clear and concise synthesis of the major trends in theory, research, policy, and practice and identify questions or areas of concern that are considered to be the most important or relevant for the community currently working in the area. Recall from Chapter 2 that the point of a literature review is not simply to regurgitate what others have said about your topic but to think critically about what has been said and to identify and highlight the consistencies and disagreements in theory, research, policy, and/or practice that are evident and relevant to your project. Once you have accomplished this, you will be in a much better position to identify the flaws or gaps in knowledge that need to be remedied. It is by highlighting these flaws or gaps that you begin to lay the foundations for your own study.

The approach you take to structuring your review is a matter of personal style, preference, and a consideration of your audience. Different audiences are likely to be partial to a particular style of writing over another and may be more or less sympathetic to a particular perspective on social or health research. That said, it would not be unusual for a literature review to address some or all of the following basic questions:

- Are there particular problems or controversies surrounding the topic?

- What is the history behind these problems or controversies? How have they arisen?

- What theories have been developed around the topic and what do they say?

- What methods have been used to study the topic?

- What research has been done on the topic? What gaps exist that should be addressed?

- What policies or practices have been developed in relation to the topic?

- Are there consistencies in existing theory, methodology, research, policy, and practice relating to the topic, or is there disagreement?

- Are there flaws in the existing theory, methodology, research, policy, and practice that you feel you can remedy through your proposed research? What are these flaws and how will your research resolve them?

Stylistically, the literature review is similar to a discussion paper like the ones you would write for a theory class; the objective is to critically synthesize and assess academic books or articles that have been written in your area of interest. Your literature review should be a free-flowing discussion of the major themes and controversies that are highlighted among books or articles that you feel are well-suited for helping you provide a solid critical overview. It is important to note that literature reviews are different from annotated bibliographies in that the latter are simply itemized summaries of articles and books while the former are critical discussions of major themes that are present within a series of articles and books.

Quite often students ask us how many pieces of literature or how many articles they need to include in the literature review of their research proposal. Although we understand the basis of the question, in many ways it is the wrong question to ask, because there is no magic number. You need enough books or articles to demonstrate that you have a good understanding of the topic area, within whatever constraints you are operating. In some cases this may be 8 or 10 books or articles; in other situations it might be 30, 40, or 50, with the number expanding or contracting depending on the forum you are writing for. The one you do for ethics review or community funding organizations will have hardly any literature at all. These review committees are typically happy with a one- or two-paragraph intro that simply identifies the topic area and otherwise cuts to the chase and goes directly into methods and the ethics issues that are relevant to your research. Your course instructor may want you to be similarly succinct and minimalist if you are writing a proposal for a term research project. In contrast, your thesis supervisory committee or a potential funder may want a more elaborate literature review that shows you have a broad command of the literature and can explain how your potential contribution will contribute to it.

Justifying Your Research

Suggesting that you have to justify your proposed study and explain its potential contribution is another way of saying that you need to explain to your reader why they should care. Just because you feel something is important, relevant, or interesting does not mean that your audience will share your beliefs or passion without some explanation of the potential contribution it can make to our understanding. If you cannot convey to readers why they should care about the particular topic, then you are unlikely to get the support, guidance, advice, or funding necessary to realize your goals.

There are several ways that you can go about justifying your study. It is often impossible to know who is going to be reading your research proposal and even more difficult to know exactly how to engage them. Fortunately, you do not need to place all of your eggs in one basket when it comes to elaborating the justifications for your particular research design, topic, and questions. You can justify your study on a number of different grounds in an effort to engage as diverse an audience and range of sensibilities possible. The easiest way to do this is to ensure your literature review draws specific connections between your proposed research and the development of theory, method, policy, and/or practice.

Contributing to Theory Development

One of the most common ways of justifying a study is to situate the research topic and questions within the theoretical literature in the area and to point to the contribution that the proposed research will make to the development of theory. For instance, in his dissertation proposal that involved a study on prostitution and the role of the male sex buyer, Chris pointed out that by further describing, exploring, and understanding the population of men who buy sex, the research community would be better equipped to develop theories of masculinity and gender that were informed by empirical evidence rather than conjecture or stereotype:

> *Risk-based research authorizes researchers as expert speakers about sex buying at the same time as it de-legitimates male sex buyers as speakers and active subjects capable of framing the problems in different ways. Aside from one phenomenological investigation conducted by Holzman and Pines in the early 1980's, sociologically informed research into the nature of the socio-cultural context of sex buying has not received much attention within the theoretical or empirical literature on the client. The primary focus of [the proposed] research will be the development of a qualitatively and quantitatively informed understanding of risk decision making processes involved in the male purchase of sex. More specifically, … I hope to be able to obtain an interpretive understanding of the attitudes, behaviours and decision making practices of male sex buyers that is grounded in both an empirical investigation of self-reported attitudes and behaviours and an in-depth account of the lived experiences and varied and multiple socially and culturally informed meanings that male sex buyers attribute to the risk decisions that are pertinent to their purchase of sex.*

A Different Methodological Approach

Another potential way to justify the pursuit of a particular topic or a research design is to point to the methodological contributions that the design will make. For example, if all the studies on student satisfaction with their research methods classes are based on the analysis of aggregate statistics collected from year-end surveys, it is likely this method will produce a limited understanding of students' experiences with those classes. Such surveys are necessarily superficial in what they ask, and rarely ask for details about the students that might be useful in understanding, for example, what sorts of professors, teaching styles, and classes appeal to what sorts of students. Instead of doing yet another aggregate survey, you could propose sampling a smaller number of students and conducting interviews that would offer a more in-depth understanding of how beliefs about education and preference for different teaching styles influence the way students rate their professors and courses.

Implications for Policy or Program Development

You also can justify your proposed study in terms of the policy applications that could emerge as a result of the data acquired from the study. For example, Bob Menzies has done historical research looking at what archival records can reveal about the way that visible minorities were treated in mental health facilities that were developing in the late 1800s and early 1900s, i.e., a rather esoteric pursuit. However, as Menzies would argue in a grant proposal, understanding history is important because many of the problems of the past still exist and beg attention:

This project will make a significant contribution to the historical understanding of medical and social ordering by offering a unique approach to understanding the institutional treatment of racial and ethnic minorities. To the extent that problems of racialization and ethnocentrism remain entrenched in contemporary society, the work has both historical and contemporary relevance. It will help to expose both the manifest and implicit means by which the dimensions of race and culture get played out in the operations of our therapeutic and regulatory institutions. In addressing the practices of the past, we can learn much about the conflicts and prejudices that continue to plague our social order.

A second example comes from graduate student Tammy Dorward, who wanted to look at the important role that "community" plays in the development of Aboriginal programs. She did so by doing a case study of how "the community" was defined during the development of what has proven to be a highly successful Native justice program (VATJS—Vancouver Aboriginal Transformative Justice Services). Her thesis proposal was explicit and succinct in identifying her policy interests:

My goal will be to critically analyze the concept of "community" as it was developed and implemented in the development of the VATJS and to explore the implications of that concept, and my analysis of it, for future programme development.

Addressing Gaps in the Literature

One of the most common ways to justify research is simply to point out gaps in the literature that you then propose to fill. For example, when MA student Daniel Reinhard submitted his thesis proposal on mobility patterns of homeless people for ethics review, his contextualization of the problem pointed out that despite all the attention that homelessness was receiving, there was still much about that we did not know about the variety of ways that people who are homeless manage time and space:

Previous research has yet to conclusively document the kinds of settings the homeless spend their time in. Most research that has looked at how the homeless travel has focused on the sheltered homeless as those in shelters are easier to reach and have a semi-fixed address from which to base calculations regarding their range of mobility. Furthermore, much of the research that has been done in this area has studied homeless mobility as an individual's journey from their last home to the current homeless shelter in which they reside.

...

Understanding the rationale and scope of mobility for survival strategies of the homeless is necessary to further grasp why some homeless persons willingly remain unsheltered (a factor influencing and possibly influenced by mobility; see Wasserman & Clair, 2009) and for understanding preferences in kinds of survival strategies between individuals. Additionally, the local Homeless Count this year found more homeless than any previous year despite the Mayor promising to eliminate street homelessness (Quinn, 2016); given this, more research on homelessness is warranted.

Similarly, when Abby Kolb prepared a dissertation proposal for her supervisory committee for a project on women gang members, her literature review noted how little attention had been paid to the role of women in gangs and how stereotypical the research that did include them appeared to be.

Gang scholars who use traditional approaches to create causal models for understanding gang membership have largely ignored women's involvement and experiences in gangs (Bachelor, 2009). While there have been some exceptions (see Cohen, 1955; Thrasher, 1927), these examples have generally minimized the role of women in gangs by explaining away their motivations for joining the gang and remaining affiliated. Those theorists who have discussed women's affiliation with gangs and their role in the gang have tended to masculinise, feminize or sexualize (see Miller, 2002; Moore & Hagedorn, 2001; Young, 2009) their existence. Gang-affiliated women tend to be dichotomized as either liberated feminists seeing equality through delinquent acts and violent means or weak victims of sexual exploitation (Bachelor, 2009).

Abby went on to elaborate the various components she envisioned for her research, each component of which was justified by its connection to the literature. This involved noting gaps in the existing literature that she proposed to address, identifying methodological challenges to overcome, and identifying some of the theories that she intended to incorporate into her interviews and analysis.

Multiple Sources of Justification

As you can see, there are a variety of ways to go about justifying researching a particular topic or researching specific questions within the body of your research proposal. While the approach you take is largely a matter of personal style, preference, and a consideration of your audience, it is wise to attempt to address the following general questions:

- Why is the topic worth studying?

- Why are the research questions that have been developed worth answering?

- What practical significance does the proposed study have?

- What will be accomplished by the completion of the proposed research project?

- In what ways does the proposed study contribute to the general understanding of the topic or to the construction of social theories?

- What contribution is the research expected to make to the advancement of knowledge or to the development of new methods?

- What contribution is the research expected to make to wider social policy or practice?

Setting Up Your Project

However much space you get, remember that the purpose of your literature review and justification is to set up your project, so what you want to do is to insert "hooks" to issues or variables that will appear in your research. The way Abby Kolb began her proposal was a perfect example of that; noting the dearth of attention paid to female gang members described a key aspect of the literature that simultaneously opened the door for her to look at gender in her own research. By setting it up in that way, when she gets to the point of identifying what questions she will address in her research and the gender issue pops up, the reaction of the reader is, "Of course, that makes sense," rather than, "Gender? Where did *that* come from?"

Does your research begin to explore an important social or health issue? Then contextualize the issue and give us some information that convinces the reader that this is something we need to know about, perhaps because it is serious and on the rise or because it's important but little is known about it. Are you trying to resolve a debate in the literature? If so, then explain the two (or more) conflicting positions and what distinguishes them in a way that starts to set up how you will make some determination of the plausibility of each. Or are you trying to fill a gap in the literature? Then explain where the gap is and why it would be useful to fill it. As this suggests, the introductory literature review is always a selective look at the literature that summarizes what others have done in a way that also helps to set up the question(s) and/or hypotheses that will guide your research at the outset.

DEFINING "THERE": RESEARCH QUESTIONS AND HYPOTHESES

While a literature review gives readers a picture of the state of the art in your area of interest, a well-crafted review will take readers by the hand and lead them to a research question or set of hypotheses that your proposed research will now set out to address. In many ways the articulation of research questions and/or hypotheses is the most important element of your research because doing so helps define what or who is "relevant" to include. The metaphor of going on a trip is again useful here. While it may help us to know that we are currently in Chicago, in the absence of a destination, there is not much we can do to prepare for our trip. It will make a big difference depending on whether we are going to Los Angeles or Berlin. It is only once you decide on a destination that focused preparation can begin. Only then does it become reasonable to decide what mode of transportation to use, whether you need a passport, what clothes to bring along, and what route to take to get there.

As with research ideas, research questions and hypotheses can emerge from a number of different sources. Sometimes they arise more inductively from our own observations and interests. On other occasions someone will give us a research question they would like us to answer or that we determine more collaboratively with an individual, group, or agency. Other times it is theory that provides us with a research question or hypothesis. We will consider each of these options in turn.

Research Questions

The biggest trick with respect to developing a research question is to ensure that what we come up with is indeed "researchable" and that we are open to whatever answers we might find. Some examples of researchable questions include the following:

- Why do people buy lottery tickets?

- How does free access to medical care affect the physical health of a population?

- Have legislative changes regarding prostitution affected the street trade?

- What impact has the UN Declaration on the Rights of Indigenous Peoples had on government policies regarding the rights of Native peoples?

- How does extended exposure to a minority group affect attitudes toward that group?

- Through what verbal and nonverbal means is occupational status preserved and displayed in business organizations?

Notice how each of these questions is quite focused and implies some real-world situation that we can look at to ascertain an answer. The first one is probably the vaguest ("why" questions tend to be the toughest), but even here, we might start off by tracking down some people who buy lottery tickets and asking them why they do so, or propose a theory that predicts which individuals or groups will be more or less likely to buy them. We might proceed by comparing those who buy lottery tickets with those who never do, or those who buy frequently with those who buy less often, or those who buy lottery tickets with those who engage in other forms of gambling (e.g., racetrack betting, bingo, playing the stock market). The information obtained may not provide the ultimate answer to our question, but there *is* real-world information that can help inform the answers we do derive. This process of "posing a researchable question" may seem straightforward, but it's actually related to one of the most common mistakes people make when they undertake a piece of research.

The difficulty arises when a would-be researcher chooses a question that is not actually *researchable*, that is, no empirical answer can be derived. Consider the following questions:

- Is capitalism or socialism the better economic system?

- Is democracy the best political system?

- What teaching style is best?

- How should we respond to domestic terrorism?

- Are quota systems fair?

- What should we do about pornography?

These are not *empirical* questions; they are questions of value, philosophy, law, or politics. Answers to questions like these cannot be determined without specific criteria by which to identify the "right" answer. Research *can* be done in such areas, but these questions are not researchable in their present form. Look at them again. In each case, the questions are asking you to make value judgments, using words like "better," "best," "fair," "appropriate," and "should." Although value judgments may well be of interest to us, and the research that we do may lead us to develop opinions about what we believe an "appropriate" course of action might be, researching such questions would require us to specify the criteria that will be used in making those judgments. Specifying criteria *does not* make answering such questions any less of a political, moral, or philosophical process, since the very choice of criteria embodies these dimensions, but it *does* require us to make that aspect of the process more explicit and, hence, more amenable to scrutiny by ourselves and others.

Researchable questions are specific, limited in scope, related to some empirical "reality" (i.e., there must be some sort of evidence that can be consulted), and should have specific evaluation criteria, so that you can tell whether you are getting closer to an answer. These criteria emerge from social negotiation and debate and will undoubtedly reveal something of the researcher's personal leanings. One recurring problem is researchers' failure to recognize the values implicitly embedded in their choice of variables to investigate. The researcher who evaluates organizational interventions on the basis of changes in productivity alone, for example, is effectively accepting productivity as the only important indicator of a "successful" intervention. Other researchers might evaluate the same interventions by looking at changes in group cohesiveness, worker safety, or job satisfaction. Each approach makes an implicit value statement about what is "important" to observe. Your obligation is to make "what you say" the result of a conscious decision whose rationale can be articulated.

If you are conducting your research in a collaborative environment where you are working with other researchers or community/organizational partners, your research question(s) may arise from consultation with "relevant" stakeholders—people that you recognize as having a legitimate stake in the outcome of your research. Doing so will help ensure your results "speak" to their interests, perspectives, and concerns. Conversely, when you are working independently, you have to ensure that you remain aware of the multiple influences you as a researcher have on the research process while also acknowledging how the research process influences you, i.e., being reflexive about what you bring to the table that might influence the results of the research.

Problems can arise when a researcher seizes upon a research question prematurely. That is not likely to happen with more deductive research, since the theory you want to test and the literature concerning what has been done so far have implications for the kinds of research questions you will ask. But remember that more inductive research is more typically emergent in that regard, i.e., it's not until you are in the situation and talking to stakeholders and others who inhabit the setting that you get a sense of what the important questions to ask are.

The Emergent Question

In contrast to the more deductively minded who emphasize beginning with theory and the hypotheses they imply, more inductively oriented researchers believe the place to start is often in the field at a particular site where you can watch, talk to people, and look for a focus to your research—something "interesting"—that will act as a sort of conceptual hub around which the research will then proceed. This is especially true when embarking on a new area of research where you are still trying to get your bearings, trying to figure out just what are the important and meaningful questions to ask. Book-length reports such as William Foote Whyte's (1943) classic *Street Corner Society* or Michael Duneier's (1999) *Sidewalk* often describe this process in their early chapters, but it is rare to see it discussed in more article-length or chapter-length treatments. An exception is Howard Becker's (1993) *"How I Learned What a 'Crock' Was."*

Becker's article recounts the beginnings of a study that eventually was published as a book (by Becker, Geer, Hughes, & Strauss, 1961) in which Becker and his colleagues set out to understand the socialization process that occurs during the years students are in medical school. The University of Kansas Medical Centre was chosen not because it was in any way "special," but because it was for the most part "typical"—or certainly not "atypical"—and unremarkable. The research began with Becker not sure what he would do other than to "hang around" with some of the medical students and observe them in their routines of taking courses, interacting with supervisors, doing rounds, giving examinations, and so on. The turning point came about a week later from a comment that Chet, one of the students, made:

> *One morning, as we made rounds, we saw a very talkative patient, who had multiple complaints to tell the doctor about, all sorts of aches, pains and unusual events. I could see that no one was taking her very seriously and, on the way out, one of the students said, "Boy, she's really a crock!" I understood this, in part, as shorthand for "crock of shit." It was obviously invidious. But what was he talking about? What was wrong with her having all those complaints? Wasn't that interesting? (pp. 30–31)*

You can tell a lot about people from the in-groups and out-groups they identify, who they love and hate. An intense declaration like "She's a crock!" is another way of saying "She is wasting my valuable time" or "How am I ever going to become a doctor with patients like her taking up my time?" But what sort of interests was this patient violating? In response, Becker asked Chet a very simple and straightforward question, which was, "What's a crock?" Chet's first reaction was to return with a look that said, "Are you kidding? Any fool knows what a crock is!" But Becker persisted: "Seriously, when you called her a crock, what did you mean?" Not used to being asked to define so basic a term, Chet fumbled around for a bit and then came up with the idea that "crocks" were people with a psychosomatic illness.

This seemed reasonable, but the next task was to employ the definition. Soon they came across a patient who had a gastric ulcer, at which point the attending physician used that patient as an opportunity to give the students a brief lecture on psychosomatic illness, with ulcers as the example. As this was what Chet had said made someone a "crock," Becker said only, "Crock, huh?" But no, Chet indicated that patient was not a "crock." But why not? He did have a psychosomatic illness. Another student overheard and intervened: "He's not a crock. He really has an ulcer." The other students in the group were involved now, too, with discussion ensuing among all of them about what exactly a "crock" was, different definitions being offered, and Becker trying them out as they went from patient to patient until they came to one definition—that a "crock" is a patient that has multiple complaints but no apparent physical pathology—that held up in test after test on succeeding patients thereafter.

But arriving at a consensual definition of a "crock" was not the end of it. As Becker points out in the article, being able to identify a crock was one thing, but he still had to find out "why students thought crocks were bad. What interest of theirs was compromised by a patient with many complaints and no pathology?" (p. 32) Although we will leave it to you to read the "crocks" article if you are interested in more of the specifics, in general, "crocks" proved to be the doorway that opened discussion into medical students' desires to make use of limited time to maximize the amount of "practical experience" they could amass. Given that crocks were time-consuming and you could learn everything you needed to know about how to deal with a "crock"—of whom there were many—from your first one, any successive ones were not a good use of your time. After that your time was better spent with other patients, who would give you an opportunity to get as much varied experience as possible with the "sights, sounds, and smells of disease in a living person" (p. 33). It also explained much of their other behavior, such as why they often switched patients with each other ("I'll trade my heart attack patient for your diabetic.").

Of course Becker and his colleagues were focusing on the would-be doctors in their research, but we also can see how such a concept could open the door to understanding the experience of some patients. How many of us know or have heard about someone who has a long list of complaints and goes from doctor to doctor, no doubt being dismissed as a "crock" by many who then shuffle them out the door, only to finally be diagnosed at some point along the way by some physician somewhere who finally diagnoses the problem correctly? Looking at it in that way, "crock" becomes a medical shorthand for "I don't have the faintest idea what's wrong with you," with "crock" becoming the way for physicians to rationalize that the problem is not with them and their diagnostic skills, but with a hypochondriac patient who bothers them for nothing.

The "crocks" article is a beautifully concise example of that transition moment that comes from extended contact with a person or group and being patient in waiting for that "aha" moment where a pivotal event or comment or dilemma arises that then becomes the focus of study because of the way that it crystallizes the dynamics of the person or group or situation you are trying to understand. There is a saying among qualitative researchers that the ideal focus is where you are able to see "the universe on the head of a pin," i.e., where the social dynamic surrounding some process you focus on becomes the lens through which you can see everything important about your phenomenon of interest. In this instance, focusing on what a "crock" was allowed Becker to better understand the doctor–patient relationship through the eyes of the medical students as a limited opportunity to bring life to the illnesses and conditions they were reading about in their textbooks and the implications that objective had on their behavior. It also should encourage you to take the time to interact with the people or site you are interested in understanding—we are always astonished at how many researchers work exclusively with databases and have never actually met a real person or been to a real place with whom/where the phenomenon of interest happens—and to be patient in allowing that "aha" moment to arrive.

You should see that embedded in this way of doing research is very much of a constructionist perspective on how to approach the analysis of any given situation. Our tendency when a teacher points at a student and says, "He's lazy," is to look at the student and ask, "Oh, just how lazy is he?" and we might even develop a "Laziness" scale to measure exactly how lazy the student is. But as Becker's experience with the medical students shows, the existence of the category and the way it is used tells you as much about the teacher doing the categorizing as it does about the person being categorized. His experience also shows how important it is to *listen* to what people share with you, to pay particular attention to the way they categorize others and draw boundaries that include some people and exclude others. Examples are everywhere. When sex workers call someone a "good trick" (or a bad one), or when students say their instructor is a "great professor" (or a terrible one), they are telling you as much about what they think sex work or "getting an education" is all about as they are about the persons they are pointing at. Are there terms you can think of that students or other members of your profession use that are similarly evaluative or that create "insiders" and "outsiders" in the same way?

Hypotheses

Notwithstanding the centrality of research questions to the process of actually doing research, different research traditions emphasize different ways to get to that point. For more deductively oriented research that follows the hypothetico-deductive method, there is a big reliance (almost by definition) on theory, which helps by generating hypotheses, which guide the research process by providing a focus. Hypotheses also can arise simply from your observation of the world when you think you understand it enough to speculate about how some phenomenon of interest arises.

Expressing a hypothesis involves making a specific statement about a phenomenon of interest that is open to empirical test. Your hypothesis may be seen as your specu- lative answer to a research question you are posing. In the context of deductive (theory-guided) inquiry, the hypothesis states what your guiding theory says *should* happen in a particular situation if, in fact, the theory is true and, as such, represents a test of the theory in one particular situation to which it should apply.

Each hypothesis will mention at least two variables and will state how those variables might be related. Here are a few examples:

1. A communicator's perceived objectivity will influence the extent to which an audience is persuaded by their arguments.

2. Work groups that are run on a democratic basis will have higher worker morale and group cohesiveness than those run autocratically.

3. Educational techniques that emphasize student–teacher interaction will result in higher rates of learning than unidirectional lecture techniques.

4. Providing the elderly with information about safe sex practices will reduce the transmission of sexually transmitted diseases in that population.

In sum, a hypothesis is a testable prediction about what should happen if a theory of interest has merit, or simply if your speculations about a phenomenon are reasonable.

Any research project will involve recognizing, structuring, or creating a situation in which you can gather information to discover whether the evidence supports or refutes your assertion about the relationship(s) among two or more variables. At times, this can be a challenge, particularly when you are at the whim of available data, but the basic idea is to put your money where your mouth is and place your bets *before* the dice are thrown. Researchers from the deductive tradition have been the most adamant about the virtues of hypothesis-oriented inquiry. Why? Three main reasons are cited.

Hypotheses as Instruments of Theory

Scientific epistemology affirms that dependable knowledge requires an ongoing interaction between theory and data. Although authors like Kerlinger (1973) sometimes assert emphatically that theory is *the* aim of science, theory is actually judged by its ability to account for data. Hypotheses are thus crucial to scientific inquiry, since they provide a link between theory and data. A theory specifies relationships among constructs in the abstract; the hypothesis applies the theory to a concrete situation, bringing the theory into contact with the real world so that its viability can be assessed. While it is sometimes the case that pragmatic considerations preclude a theory being fully tested, until that occurs, the theory is no more than speculation. For example, many of the implications of Einstein's relativity theory were put on hold for decades until the technology required to test them could be created.

Hypotheses Imply a Test

Since a hypothesis represents a concrete specification of a testable state of affairs, the deductive tradition affirms that you can proceed to gather relevant evidence to establish the truth or falsity of the proposition. This tradition asserts that the true nature of reality can be made to reveal itself unambiguously through empirical inquiry; that is, we can create or observe a situation in which the truth or falsity of a hypothesis (and hence of the theory that gave rise to it) can be assessed (e.g., Stinchcombe, 1968).

Others have more reserved views of how much can be accomplished. Popper (1959) argues that although disconfirming evidence allows us to *falsify* our hypotheses (and hence our theories), *confirmatory* evidence (i.e., results consistent with our prediction) can "provide support for" but *not* "prove" them. There are two reasons for this. First, a supportive datum is only a single victory in a theoretically infinite series of challenges that can be made to the theory; "proof" would require showing that a theory is correct in *all* situations in which it might be used to predict. In contrast, a pattern of disconfirmation is more quickly set. In other words, it takes a long time to get to the Hall of Fame, but not long at all to be banished to the minor leagues.

Second, as Cook and Campbell (1979) have explained, although a given result may be consistent with a theory, the theory that gave rise to the prediction may not be the *only* theory that can account for that result. We showed exactly that in our discussion in Chapter 2 of the "Can you solve this?" video. While the number sequence 2, 4, 8 was indeed consistent with the rule (or theory) that you start with a number and then double it each time, there were other rules/theories that also were consistent with the sequence. Paying attention to the rival plausible explanations that might exist for any given observations we make—as abductive reasoning encourages us to do—encourages us to be as exhaustive and creative as possible in identifying those plausible alternatives and actually testing them out rather than only seeking evidence that can confirm, but not falsify, our theory.

Hypotheses Make Us Place Our Bets

A third important quality of hypotheses is that they are public. "Stating your hypothesis" implies an attitude of self-disciplined honesty: putting your money where your mouth is. If you think you understand the dynamics underlying some social or health phenomenon, tell us *ahead of time* what will happen in any situation you choose. Articulate your theory. Explain what your theoretical constructs mean to you and how you will observe or measure them. We ask gamblers to indicate their bets *before* the dice are thrown; we chastise pseudo-scientific astrologers, whose predictions are so vague that they are always "right" no matter what happens; and we roll our eyes at conspiracy theorists who can see conspiracies in any set of facts. Surely the foundations of knowledge are valued more highly than mere money; surely the sciences are capable of more than the vague and self-serving accounts of mystics.

There are numerous fringe benefits to be gained by this attitude. It promotes the communal nature of science by allowing others to comment on our efforts. The possibility of critique and review is afforded only by the public presentation of our research logic. And if we view science as dynamic—as an ongoing process—then we should value components that enhance that process by fostering communication and debate.

Operationalizing: The Bridge Between Concepts and Data

Recall that one thing that both qualitative and quantitative approaches have in common is the commitment to both theory—abstract concepts that we think help us make sense of the world—and data—real-world evidence that we gather that we feel sheds light on those concepts. Sometimes we start with the concept and look for opportunities to employ it in a more deductive approach—something like "social capital," for example, that you hear a lot about in sociology these days (e.g., Bourdieu, 1977; de Vaus, 2002). Other times we begin more inductively by observing concepts that the people who participate in our research employ, such as when Becker heard the medical students refer to some patients as "crocks." By then working with the students to define what they meant by a "crock," Becker and his colleagues came to understand the importance of "clinical experience" in the education that the medical students were receiving in the process of being socialized into the doctoring profession. The notion of "developing indicators for" or "operationalizing" variables addresses the question of how we travel back and forth between those abstract and concrete levels. Normally, this process will see you considering two types of definitions: nominal definitions and operational definitions.

Nominal (or Constitutive) Definitions

The **nominal definition** (sometimes called the constitutive definition) involves articulating what you mean by the concept under scrutiny. It's a bit like supplying a dictionary definition, although the nominal definition is often linked to your theoretical stance. For example, a radical feminist inspired nominal definition of violence might be "any act that is designed to restrict or repress an individual's physical, psychological, intellectual, or emotional well-being." Conversely, researchers working from within a harm-reduction perspective might define violence as "any act that results in direct physical or psychological harm."

Nominal definitions are not always so straightforward and, because they are socially constructed, they cannot be "right" or "wrong"; they can only be more or less useful. This poses a bit of a problem insofar as, if definitions cannot be right or wrong, does that mean that anyone can define anything any way they want? Yes and no. There are times someone comes along and changes the world by arguing that we need to pull the gauze from our eyes and see the world a different way. But for the most part, having a definitional free-for-all makes definitions irrelevant, makes communication between researchers difficult, and often ends up in pointless debate where groups of researchers argue about something when, at the bottom of the debate, the fact is that they are simply talking about different things. For example, the extent to which "poverty" exists in the United States clearly depends in large part on how you define "poverty." What is important is that researchers articulate their definitions, are aware of the values inherent in their choices, and pay heed to any empirical evidence that sometimes can be used to make the claim that one definition is more useful than another. It is also a reason for connecting with the literature relatively early in your research—and especially if you are following a more hypothetico-deductive approach—to see what indicators others have used for the concepts that will provide the foundation for your research.

Operational Definitions

While the nominal definition is in many ways your articulation of what you are trying to capture in your research, the operational definition is your articulation of *how* you will do so. It involves giving specific empirical meaning to a concept by delineating the specific indicators or operations that are to be taken as representative of a concept. The trick here is to be specific about how you will derive, create, identify, measure, or record the indicator and to choose one or more indicators that best approximate your nominal definition.

The notion of finding indicators might still sound somewhat foreign to you, but it's analogous to processes we engage in every day when we make inferences and draw conclusions about the people we meet. If you meet someone for the first time, the number of questions that person asks about you, the amount of eye contact they make, and their tone of voice may be seen as indicators of how interested that person is in you. If the other person laughs at your jokes and the space between you begins to shrink, those may be taken as indicators that you like each other. In each case, you are observing concrete actions (e.g., two people holding hands) and, on the basis of your observation, inferring the existence of some underlying construct or variable (i.e., the two people like each other).

Of course, there are times when these indicators may be erroneous. A person may hold another's hand to restrain them rather than to demonstrate affection. Someone who asks a lot of questions about you may not be particularly interested in you, but may want to divert attention away from themselves. Similarly, people sometimes laugh at your jokes only out of politeness or to relieve tension, and the space between you may be shrinking only because the other person cannot hear what you are saying. But despite such exceptions, these indicators are probably, in general, fairly accurate ones and, hence, overall, fairly useful, particularly when used in combination.

At the same time, we also can envision bad or poor indicators of a concept. If we took "a person running" to be an indicator of "a crime having just been committed," we would likely be wrong more often than we were right and would probably get on the wrong side of many joggers, soccer players, and people in a hurry. Similarly, many people are so socially insensitive that when someone they are attracted to does anything short of telling them to "get lost," they perceive the other person as "coming on" to them or otherwise encouraging further interaction.

Much the same occurs in the social and health sciences, although the process varies depending on whether the researcher follows an inductive or a deductive approach. Deductive researchers begin with a variable of interest (e.g., liking) and then try to generate a list of indicators that can be used systematically to classify people on that dimension. Researchers taking a more inductive approach may see a behavior they wish to focus on and then will start to record specific instances of it in all its variation before providing some encompassing concept that unites them and/or will look to see what persons in the research setting identify as indicators of important concepts that arise.

In either case, the indicators might be behavioral (e.g., whether two people hold hands or how much eye contact they make with each other); archival (e.g., the content of letters the two people exchange); physiological (e.g., changes in galvanic skin response that occur for one person when a second enters the room); or self-report (e.g., answers to the question "Do you like that person?"). None of these indicators is itself "liking"—we never observe pure reality, only our constructions of it—but each can arguably be linked to our understanding of that construct. Demonstrating this linkage involves assessing the **epistemic relationship** between the theoretical variable and the particular indicator or measure we have chosen to represent it.

Although researchers who take an inductive or deductive approach may differ in the *way* they go about operationalizing variables, the central point here is that all researchers operationalize. The main requirement is that researchers articulate their constructs and operationalizations in a way that affords communication between researchers and is amenable to public scrutiny. This says little more than that "being empirical" requires a commitment to both theory (abstract explanatory concepts) and data (real-world evidence) and a consideration of how well the two coincide.

Evaluating Operational Definitions

There is no reason to believe that researchers are blessed with inherently greater insight about people or human behavior than anyone else. If social and health scientists have any special insights, it is because they subject their insights to the rigors of empirical method before they espouse their beliefs. Empirical method requires researchers to present some sort of argument to show why their choice of indicators or operations makes sense. This is generally done in one of two ways: by citing tradition or by demonstrating that the operation does the job you want it to do.

By Citing Tradition. Science is a communal enterprise. Thus, establishing connections between you and other researchers—by noting the ways in which your conceptualizations and operationalizations are similar to and/or different from those of other researchers—is an important responsibility. One benefit to connecting with the literature is that other researchers have often done the job of validating their measures for constructs that you want to include. Using measures others have used also enhances your ability to compare or extend results associated with that or those particular measure(s) or procedures. This is particularly helpful when your results depart from what others have found because it gets rid of the problem of not knowing whether the different results were due to the simple fact that you operationalized the concept differently.

For example, for many years, laboratory researchers looking at aggression often used something called the Buss Shock Apparatus. Participants were told that they could use this apparatus to deliver one of five levels of electric shock to another participant (who was generally an employee of the experimenter's and who never actually received any shocks). The average level of shock delivered was taken as an index of aggression. Similarly, in the field of interpersonal dynamics, a participant's tendency to engage in cooperative or competitive behavior was typically assessed with the "prisoner's dilemma." There are also many attitude scales, personality measures, and aptitude tests that have been validated and made available for general use.

There are also many standardized ways to define many other variables of interest to researchers. Survey researchers, for example, tend to have fairly standard ways of asking about age, income, education, and other **demographic variables** that are routinely included in surveys to allow the researchers to describe their samples. You can see examples of these and many other types of surveys and survey questions by going online to the Roper Center site at Cornell University in the United States,[1] the Survey Question Bank coordinated by the UK Data Service at the University of Essex in England,[2] and/or the General Social Survey site operated by Statistics Canada.[3]

Notwithstanding the benefits to using standard measures, the downside to doing so is when it starts to encourage **mono-operationism** (also known as mono-operation bias) and mono-method bias (e.g., Campbell, 1969a; Cook & Campbell, 1979; see also our discussion later in this chapter), that is, respectively, an overreliance on one particular measure of a construct and/or of always using a particular method to measure it (e.g., by self-report questionnaire).

---

[1] https://ropercenter.cornell.edu/.
[2] https://ukdataservice.ac.uk/.
[3] https://www.statcan.gc.ca/eng/survey/household/4501.

By Empirical Demonstration. In the event that the measure(s) you are using have not been validated in any way, then it will be your job to provide the evidence that the epistemic relationship between the theoretical construct and its operational indicator is solid, i.e., the measure is reliable and valid.

Reliability. "Reliability" is generally synonymous with consistency, whether of the same phenomenon over time or of judgments about the same phenomenon across different observers. Many constructs that interest social scientists are considered to be relatively stable. For example, attitudes, aptitudes, personality traits, personal values, cognitive styles, and organizational processes may change to some degree over time but are generally fairly consistent, particularly over shorter periods and in the absence of significant relevant life events.

For example, imagine that we administer a test of mechanical aptitude to a person one week, and it reveals them to be a prospective Thomas Alva Edison. We administer the same test to the same person a week later, and on this second occasion it reveals that they would probably have difficulty figuring out how to operate a light switch. If this occurred, we hope you would be more than a little surprised. Given that the attribute you are dealing with is a reasonably stable one, any legitimate measurement of that attribute should classify the person consistently over repeated measurements. In fact, researchers often test a measure of some attribute by administering it to the same group of people on two successive occasions. This procedure, known as **test-retest reliability**, reveals whether classifications on the attribute are indeed consistently (i.e., reliably) produced. You will see more of this when we discuss reliability in the context of measuring attitudes in Chapter 9.

A second reliability strategy is known as **inter-rater reliability**. If you have adequately specified what a particular construct means to you, other researchers should be able to read your explanation (or be trained in your procedures) and then proceed to make the same judgments you would. If they cannot, then you have not explained it clearly enough. You will see more of this when we discuss content analysis in Chapter 12.

Validity. Although the demonstration of reliability is considered a prerequisite to validity, the two terms are not synonymous. Rather, they should be seen as two successive hurdles. If a measure fails the reliability hurdle, there is no use going any further, since in most cases it cannot be valid. If the measure is shown to be reliable, its validity remains an open question. Consider a variable like shoe size. Shoe size is a relatively stable attribute, at least among adults, and we could develop a technique of measuring shoe size (as shoe manufacturers have) that would let us score individuals consistently (i.e., reliably) both over time (test-retest) and across observers (i.e., inter-rater). But shoe size is probably invalid as an indicator of intelligence or creativity.

Operationalizations are considered to be valid for some purpose. To demonstrate validity, you show that your particular operationalization accomplishes the purpose for which you intend to use it. Your challenge is to pick a relevant criterion in which the construct is embodied and then show that the operationalization is indeed related to that criterion (convergent validity), but not related to other constructs you do not want to measure (divergent validity).

For example, if you develop an operationalization for a construct like "love" (as did Rubin, 1973), people who proclaim themselves to be "in love" should score or be classified differently on your measure from persons who do not declare themselves to be "in love" (as Rubin in fact showed). You would also want to show that it's loving itself you are assessing most directly, as opposed to related but different constructs (e.g., liking, infatuation, respect) or clearly unrelated constructs (e.g., the tendency to respond to questions in a socially desirable manner).

If both the operationalization (e.g., Rubin's measure of "loving") and the independent criterion (e.g., self-reports of whether the persons were in love) are obtained at about the same time, then we speak of concurrent validity. In predictive validity, administering the operational measure and observing the criterion occur at different times, as when standardized tests such as the Scholastic Assessment Test (SAT), Law School Admissions Test (LSAT), or Graduate Record Exam (GRE) are used to predict academic success.

Assessments of validity will be dealt with in greater detail later in this book (see Chapters 6–9). Here, we need to note only that empirical requirements recall the legendary Missourian who says "Show me." Recall also that operationalizations are never considered valid in a general sense, but rather are demonstrably valid (or invalid) for some purpose and within demonstrated constraints. Thus, if a procedure is shown to be a valid predictor of success in graduate school, that is all it's good for. A measure that has been shown to differentiate between criterion groups may not be valid for categorizing individuals. And if the validation process involves criterion groups that are clearly different (e.g., a group of neo-Nazis is shown, as expected, to have more authoritarian attitudes than a group of civil libertarians), the measure's validity must still be considered tentative with respect to finer distinctions.

Caveats Regarding Operationism

As we saw earlier, the process of research in the social and health sciences involves a continuing interaction between theory and data. Theoretical constructs are important entities in this scheme, and the operational definitions we choose represent our pragmatic attempts to gather information about the world that bears on our theoretical conceptions. Listed below are a few final admonitions.

Mono-Operation Bias

Rarely can a single operationalization of a construct fully capture the richness of a theoretical construct. We do a disservice both to our theoretical constructs and to the research process if we repeatedly deal with only a single operationalization of a particular variable of interest to us. This problem is referred to as **mono-operation bias**.

Similarly, since all methods of gathering information have their respective advantages and limitations, we run the risk of producing method-dependent results if we always use, say, self-reports or archival sources. This problem is referred to as mono-method bias.

Researchers should use multiple operationalizations and multiple methods whenever possible. If you get the same results even when the theoretical construct is operationally defined in three different ways, you can draw conclusions more confidently than if you have defined it in only one way. And if the results *differ* depending on which operationalization is used, the inconsistency is provocative. Multiple operationalizations may also help resolve previous inconsistencies in the literature, by showing the relationships that exist among the respective operationalizations. You will see these issues again in several chapters in this book, but most notably in Chapter 13 when we discuss the search for more diverse measures of human attitudes and behaviors.

Definitional Operationism

A particularly despicable example of mono-operation bias has been termed definitional operationism (e.g., see Campbell, 1969a; Cook & Campbell, 1979). This process involves essentially imposing a definition by fiat and ignoring the theoretical issues inherent in that choice. Rather than discussing the theoretical construct "intelligence," for example, and attempting to deal with the considerable difficulties of generating measures of that construct, definitional operationists seize on a particular operational definition—such as a particular IQ test—and consider it to be definitive of the construct. The result is a tautological and hence trivial statement: "The scores from the IQ test are my operational definition of intelligence. What is intelligence? It is what the IQ test measures."

Besides being obviously circular, this data-oriented approach must also be considered antiscientific: it implies a contentment with manipulating numbers without considering the theoretical constructs that underlie them and, hence, deflects rather than encourages embellishment and revision. Operationalizations are a means to an end, *not* an end in themselves.

BRINGING IT HOME

Methods: The Road From Here to There

Methods provide the framework and tools that take you to your research destination—tentative answers to your research questions and/or tests of your hypotheses. Your goal in the methods and data collection section of your research proposal is to provide a convincing argument for why you feel that the particular measure you have developed and the data collection technique or techniques that you have selected are the best suited for your proposed research. Again, there is no template for how you should go about doing this, but there are several key questions that you need to consider in order to present a solid argument for the decisions you have made, including the following:

- What are the key concepts or variables in your study, or how will you go about identifying them?

- How will you conceptually and operationally define the central concepts or variables in your study?

- In what respect do your definitions and measurement techniques duplicate, build on, or differ from those used in previous studies of this topic?

- What specific data collection technique(s) will you use to collect the data necessary to answer your research questions and address your research objectives, or how will you determine what those will be?

- Why have you selected the data collection technique(s) that you have?

- How do you know that the observation/measurement device you plan on using for your study will give you the best information or data for answering your research questions?

- Once you have completed your observations, what procedures will you implement to store the research data?

- What procedures will you implement to ensure that the data remain secure and confidential?

Proposals will vary in the extent to which measurement instruments can be specified. In more exploratory and inductive research you may be able to do little more than list a few themes that might be addressed for starters, with everything else to be determined on a collaborative basis depending on where your conversations with research participants lead you. In other areas you may be able to specify more concretely what you will ask.

Analysis, Expected Outcomes, and Benefits of the Study

Once you have presented a clear and well-defended argument for what or who you will study and how you will make your observations or collect the data necessary to answer your research questions, you need to shift your attention to thinking beyond the project to envision the type of analysis you will do and what some of the expected outcomes of this analysis are likely to be. Many students find this section of the proposal very difficult to write because they find it hard to envision what the data they will be collecting will look like, and they often have not yet been exposed to the range of qualitative, quantitative, or mixed-data analysis techniques available to help researchers make sense of their research observations and data. In order to begin to think about this, you will want to read through Chapters 13 and 14 to get a feel for how data are handled at the analysis stage.

By this stage in the proposal writing process you have already designed and discussed the data collection techniques that you plan on using to answer your research questions, so you should have a very clear idea of what the possible format of the information you will be collecting will look like. For instance, if you plan on using a self-administered questionnaire or quasi-experimental design in order to gather observations, you already know that the information you get back will be in a fairly structured format with many of the responses or observations already defined and ordered. Conversely, if you plan on conducting lengthy personal interviews, case studies, oral histories, or micro-ethnographies, you will most likely have to deal with large amounts of open-ended textual information and field notes.

Regardless of whether you have quantitative or qualitative data or both, making sense of it will involve a process of data reduction where you take the volumes of information that you have collected and organize and synthesize them into core components or themes that help you to best go about answering your research question(s). The point is to make the information accessible and understandable so that you can bring to light certain patterns that speak to your research questions. For the purposes of the research proposal, you are generally required to provide your audience with some indication as to how you think you will go about doing this.

In order to accomplish this, there are several key questions that you should address in your research proposal:

- How will you organize the data to make them ready for analysis (e.g., transcription, data entry, coding, cleaning [correction/synthesis/editing])?

- How will findings be analyzed and reported (e.g., by hand or using a data analysis program)?

- What specific analysis procedures are you planning on using or what kind of analysis do you plan to conduct? Are specific hypotheses being tested? How do the analyses connect back to your research question(s)?

- What is the purpose of the analysis?

- What are the projected findings, conclusions, and implications of the proposed research?

- How will the findings be disseminated?

- What effect might your analysis have on or for the population that you are studying?

Acknowledging Potential Limitations

Far too often, both novice and experienced researchers construct research proposals that promise the moon and the stars without taking into account that there are likely to be methodological and practical constraints that will prevent the delivery of such lofty promises. A well-thought-out and convincing research proposal will clearly detail the potential limitations of the project.

In the limitations section of your proposal, you acknowledge the potential weaknesses of your design that have been brought about by the compromises you have had to make in order to construct a realistic project. Limitations can include potential problems obtaining access to people or settings, possible respondent refusal, equipment failure or technological support issues, limitations on personal skills and expertise, restricted budgets and time frames, and cultural and linguistic barriers.

For example, perhaps you realize that to fully understand the effects of long-term exposure to images of gaunt and unhealthy women in fashion magazines on women's health practices, a longitudinal study where you follow a group of women from adolescence to adulthood would be optimal. As a student who may be heavily burdened by a full course load and student loan debt, you may not have the time or financial resources to conduct such a study, so instead you have opted to design your research around a more manageable qualitative cross-sectional design, i.e., a one-shot study where you make comparisons between women based on the extensiveness of exposure or between those who subscribe to such magazines versus those who do not. It is in the limitations section of your proposal where you should acknowledge this fact but make the argument that in spite of this, the data that you will get from your study will be an acceptable first step in understanding some of the ways that these images are affecting women's health. By doing this you address potential criticisms before they are made and you lay the groundwork for future research.

SOME FINAL ADVICE

When you are asking people for something, you will always do better when you are on your best behavior. In the context of proposal writing, it means following the guidelines you are given in terms of things like word limits, recommended headings, content requirements, and submission deadlines. You also should be meticulous about your writing—your proposal should be grammatically flawless and easy to read, and there should be zero typos in it. In many ways a proposal is like a trial run or audition. If you cannot put your ideas in logical order, write in an engaging and understandable way, explain why you would make this choice as opposed to that one in your design in your proposal, or explain to your reader in your proposal why your project is important and should be approved and/or funded, then reviewers infer that it's unlikely you will be able to do so when they let you in the program or give you the okay to go ahead or give you the funding. We suggest you try and get a hold of any successful proposals that you can, as they will give you a bit more concrete idea of what you are aspiring to and may offer something of a template you can adapt to your own project.

While those are all the things for you to aspire to, Gray (2014) also gives us a list of things to *avoid* in proposals. These include the following:

1. *Topics that are too big* and give every indication you are trying to address life, truth, and the universe in one proposal. One trick of being an effective researcher is being realistic about what you can accomplish and not biting off more than you can chew. Successful careers are made by having a broad interest or goal that you aspire to take a significant shot at, coupled with the understanding that it takes many smaller and more manageable steps to get you there.

2. *Topics that are too small.* Somehow it always seems the Goldilocks solution is the one that works the best—neither too big nor too small—but indeed it's true, don't be trivial. Sometimes the importance of a topic will simply jump out at you because it is clearly an important social issue, but sometimes you will need to explain why something that seems trivial in fact is not. The question to ask yourself is the "so what?" criterion, i.e., why should your reader care whether your research is ever done?

3. *Questionable feasibility.* Reviewers want to know you will be able to do the project and do it well. Do you have access to an appropriate research site? Are there people on hand who have expertise in that area and can guide you and act as resources as you go through the research? Check into these things before you write the proposal. Although institutional ethics policies typically require you to get ethics approval before you begin your research, it is permissible to get in touch with prospective research sites in order to ensure that access is possible under conditions that both you and your prospective participants feel comfortable agreeing to.

4. *Dependency on another project.* You want to be able to exercise control over your project and cannot do that if your project getting done requires some other project to be done and have a particular outcome first. If that project has problems, you are toast, and remember that Murphy's Law is active in the research realm as much as any other domains of life. One of the reasons that we prefer to have our students do actual research projects in methods classes we teach is that we want students to understand what research is really like, which is rarely like the idyllic way it sounds when people are creating the "perfect" study in a proposal. S**t happens.

5. *Unethical.* Do not propose or get involved in a project where you feel uncomfortable ethically. Your job is to ensure that no one is harmed when you do your research, and that includes people who may not be the nicest people in the world. You may love the idea of talking to a serial killer or finding out how a sexual predator can possibly justify what they do and still sleep soundly at night, but it takes a particular kind of person to be able to listen to those explanations in a relatively nonjudgmental way without feeling the urge to dial 9-1-1. Be realistic about who you are and what you can handle.

SUMMING UP AND LOOKING AHEAD

While the previous chapter talked about where ideas for your research might come from and discussed different places you can find relevant literature, the current chapter outlined the basic elements needed for a research proposal. Chapter 2 thus offered the first crucial elements—a preliminary research idea and a review of the literature—but at that point we hit something of a wall, because what you outline next depends on what kind(s) of design you will create and what kind(s) of data you will gather. Your alternatives here are sufficiently voluminous that it will take us the rest of the book to explain them. Chapter 4 will outline ethical issues you need to consider and the ethics review process you will encounter, while Chapter 5 discusses the various approaches to sampling you will need to consider as you decide from whom and/or what you plan on gathering your data. Chapters 6–8 then discuss three different classes of research design—experiments, quasi-experiments, and case study designs—you can use to frame your research, while Chapters 9–12 offer specific methods you can use singly or in combination to gather your data. Chapters 13 and 14 then discuss how to analyze that data. Your research proposal will include your explanation of why you made the choices you did.

Although our aim is to do research in the broad sense, getting it done ultimately means addressing a specific, researchable question in a particular setting at a given time. The "researchable question" in more quantitative work is the beginning of the research design process, but in more qualitative studies is more likely to be more of a preliminary question that will evolve as you make contact with those who will be the focus of your research. Notwithstanding the fact that some research is done simply to find out what a good research question would be, serious research cannot begin until the researcher has a focused issue on which to concentrate their energies. Put bluntly, it's difficult to search for an answer if you do not know what the question is.

Once particular variables have been isolated for analysis, a next step in some cases, but not all, will be to specify a hypothesis for test. Although there are often good reasons for asserting a hypothesis, particularly when engaging in the deductive process of theory testing, there are at least as many situations where the researcher and the phenomenon under investigation would be ill served by engaging in such hypothetico-deductive inquiry. This is particularly so with respect to more inductive research approaches, where priority is placed on ensuring that the research question(s) being posed and any hypotheses being expressed have meaning within the context being investigated.

Having a research question is a key turning point in the research process because it is the point where the rubber hits the road—where our abstract concerns and objectives start to become more concrete as we now start looking at where specifically we will look, what specific data we will gather, and so on. Whether you engage in specific hypothesis testing or not, another issue that must be addressed concerns the links between your theoretical interests or position and the actual measures or indicators that you take as representative of the concepts that are implied by your research question(s). The literature can be useful in identifying these operationalizations, or they emerge at the site from observation, collaborative strategizing, or the development of valid and reliable instruments. The issue here is one of considering and assessing the epistemic relationship that exists between your theoretical (conceptual) interests and those concrete indicators that you use in your research.

The notion of operationalization reflects science's dual commitment to theory and data. Deductivists and inductivists may argue about whether you should begin with the theoretical constructs and operationalize them or with exploratory observations from which grounded theoretical constructs can emerge. Researchers engaged in finding answers to qualitative and quantitative questions may argue over whether variables of interest are most adequately described verbally or according to some numerical scale. But all researchers believe in an interplay between theory and data. And part of the turf that invariably comes with this dual commitment is the issue of how to move back and forth between these two levels of interest. The operational definition is little more than the procedural articulation of a variable of theoretical interest. All researchers operationalize, since all are committed to an ongoing dialectic involving both theory and data, and hence must at some point be explicit about the particular data in which our theoretical concepts live.

Taken together, the issues described in this chapter offer a conceptual framework for approaching any given piece of research—you find a topic, determine your objectives, devise a particular question or set of questions, connect with the literature, and start thinking about how you will operationalize your terms (where the literature will again offer you some help). For some researchers, theory will provide the questions and much of the design can be done from your desk; for other researchers, and particularly those in the field, the whole process may be a more collaborative one that emerges from interaction at the research site. How it happens will differ, but it will happen.

It is important when you are writing a research proposal to recognize that you will need to remain flexible and willing to change as your design unfolds. The point is not simply to put together a proposal that looks like it might work, but rather to sketch out a well-thought-out design that demonstrates that you have given each step of the process careful thought and attention and that as a result you have produced a sound design that anticipates potential problems and incorporates methodological techniques that dramatically improve the chances that the research will be successful. It is impossible to anticipate all the potential road closures and detours that you may confront during the journey through conception, design, implementation, and analysis. Like any cross-country road trip, the process of research is full of twists and turns, bouts of car sickness, and truly amazing and serendipitous discoveries. The point is to prepare yourself for these possibilities by familiarizing yourself with the landscape and the roadways so that you arrive at your destination safely and securely with a whole bunch of interesting stories to tell.

We are almost ready to start talking about gathering data. But before we do so, Chapters 4 and 5 will guide you over a crucial bridge between thinking about research and actually going out and doing it—Chapter 4 discusses the ethical principles that guide social scientists' efforts, while Chapter 5 reviews sampling considerations when deciding on whom or what to focus.

Key Concepts

Concurrent validity 90
Convergent validity 90
Definitional operationism 91
Demographic
 variables 88
Divergent validity 90
Epistemic relationship 87
Hypotheses 69

Hypothetico-deductive
 method 82
Inter-rater reliability 89
Mono-method bias 91
Mono-operationism 88
Nominal definition 85
Operational definition 86
Operationalizing 85

Predictive validity 90
Reflexive 78
Reliability 89
Research questions 69
Stakeholders 78
Test-retest reliability 89
Validity 89
Variables 82

STUDY QUESTIONS

1. "Should the use of magic mushrooms (psilocybin) be decriminalized?" is a good question, but is it a *researchable* question? If so, explain why; if not, indicate why not and how you might change it into one.

2. Should you feel obliged to specify a formal hypothesis when doing research? What, in your own words, are the strongest arguments for both sides? Are positions on the inductive–deductive issue related to positions on the hypothesis issue?

3. Select a particular research topic that interests you and develop three researchable questions to explore, describe, understand, or explain something about that topic that interests you. Once you have done this, make a list of the approaches that you could use to study each of your research questions.

4. Select a research topic or question that interests you and in 250 words or less provide a convincing justification for why this topic or question is important and why research needs to be conducted in relation to it.

5. Locate three empirical articles from refereed journals that relate to the research topic or question you have developed in Question 3 or 4 above and briefly discuss how each of these articles relates to your research topic and provide a short justification for why you selected these particular articles.

6. Go to your favorite news website (e.g., BBC News at http://www.bbc.co.uk/news/), and identify three social or health-related stories that interest you, and how each of the three stories you have identified could be made into a researchable topic.

7. Because of budget tightening in the healthcare system, a local hospital decides that it will begin a program of research to identify strategies to improve the quality of service they offer in the Emergency area. Before they begin identifying the different strategies they will try out, they know that they will need to operationalize the term that will become the fundamental measure of whether they are successful or not—quality of service. Suggest what you think would be an appropriate nominal definition of "quality of service" as well as three different ways that it could be operationalized in the hospital setting. What are some of the strengths and limitations of each of the potential indicators that you identify?

8. How do *nominal* and *operational* definitions relate to *hypotheses?*

9. On what bases might one justify the choice of any given operationalization?

10. At the library, locate two recent empirical articles, one each from two of your areas of interest. What concepts are being scrutinized in each study? How are they operationalized? Evaluate the *epistemic relationships* created. What values are implicit in the authors' choice of variables and operationalizations? On what basis (or bases) do the authors justify their choice of operationalization?

11. What is *definitional operationism*, and why is it problematic?

12. Do both inductive and deductive researchers engage in operationalization when they do research? In what ways do they differ in how they do research?

13. What is the purpose of a research design?

14. What are some things to avoid when outlining in a proposal the studies you want to conduct?

ETHICS IN SOCIAL AND HEALTH RESEARCH

After some beginning lessons about "science" and "empiricism," followed by a discussion of the preliminary stages of conceptualizing research, we're almost ready to tackle the procedural aspects of doing research. Our emphasis thus far has been on the *strategy* of investigation. But as Schatzman and Strauss (1973) remind us, the conscientious researcher "needs both strategy and morality. The first without the second is cruel; the second without the first is ineffectual" (p. 146).

There are at least two major reasons we should strive to maintain the highest ethical standards in our dealings with research participants. One is simply that the reputation of the research enterprise, and the integrity people attribute to researchers, arises in large part because of the relationships we establish with those who participate in our research. When one of us does something less than honorable, we all feel the effect. The second reason is a pragmatic one: the information research participants provide is the fuel that makes the research machine run, and without the active involvement of humans willing to share aspects of their lives with us, we would be a pale shadow of what we are now.

The fragility and special nature of our relationship with participants is underlined when we consider how little we actually offer those who participate in our research compared to other professions who also have duties to those in their care. People share information about themselves with a lawyer in order to obtain legal advice, with a medical professional in order to be cured, and with a spiritual adviser—a priest, Elder, minister, rabbi, or imam—in order to seek absolution and feel closer to their God. In contrast, people who participate in social and health science research often get very little in return other than perhaps an opportunity to vent on some issue of interest to them or some vague promise that we will "give them voice" and thereby hopefully contribute to better social or health policy, practice, or procedure. It is actually considered unethical for us to make incentives to participate so large that people are tempted to participate only *because* of the incentive, which leads to us to offer no more than token amounts or gifts or a simple thank you. As a reflection of this, although people usually initiate interactions with lawyers, physicians, and spiritual advisers, prospective participants rarely approach us—unsolicited—about participating. Instead, we are the ones to approach them in an effort to enlist them in our work, knocking at the doorway of their lives, hoping they will let us in. With anything less than complete trust that we will protect their welfare, it is far easier for someone to say "no" when we ask them to participate.

Notwithstanding the moral and pragmatic desirability of proceeding ethically, we also have to acknowledge that researchers of all stripes—those who work for corporate interests, or for the state, or in academe—have at times failed to live up to that standard.

FORMALIZING CODES OF ETHICS

Biomedical Horror Stories

The contemporary formalization of principles of research ethics is most often traced to what was undoubtedly one of the most grotesque examples of experimentation with humans that history can offer: the Nazis and the medical research they performed on the Jews and others they had incarcerated in concentration camps during World War II. As the postwar Nuremberg trials revealed, the Nazis' experiments included such procedures as severing and exchanging limbs between live people made all the more torturous by a lack of anæsthetic. Or, with clipboards and observational protocols in hand, the researchers would place their captives in ice baths and watch to see how long it took them to die from hypothermia.

The Nuremberg trials resulted in development of the "**Nuremberg Code,**" which was the first contemporary statement of research ethics to articulate ethical standards for conducting biomedical research involving human participants. That code subsequently "became the foundation of the *Declaration of Helsinki*, adopted by the World Health Organization in 1964 and revised in 1975. It was also the basis for the 'Ethical Guidelines for Clinical Investigation' adopted by the American Medical Association in 1966" (Berg, 2007, p. 55).

Although the scale of the Nazi experiments was unprecedented—the Holocaust Museum reports that at least 7,000 people were victims of Nazi experiments conducted across eight different concentration camps[1]—their heartlessness was not. For example, beginning in 1932, the United States Public Health Service (USPHS) undertook the Tuskegee syphilis study, which ended up being a 40-year longitudinal study of the consequences of untreated syphilis. The USPHS did not infect anyone with syphilis in the Tuskegee study; rather, it identified a group of men who had contracted the disease and, without their consent, decided it would be useful to observe systematically their deterioration over time. When the study began, there was no known treatment for the disease. However, even after a cure was identified, the researchers made sure that the men in their sample—all of whom were African American—received no treatment, since doing so would have "spoiled" the study (Devlin, 2018; Reverby, 2012).

Even if we were to assume that the Tuskegee syphilis study initially may have had legitimate aspirations for furthering scientific understanding of syphilis in the 1930s when no cure yet existed (although we still cannot ignore the lack of consent), there is nothing that could justify continuation of the study—and simply watching the men degenerate and die—after a cure had been developed. The scientific gains were minimal while the potential human cost was huge. To continue the study was no less than a denial of the dignity of the participants as human beings, as the US President Bill Clinton declared when he made a formal apology to the eight participants still alive in 1997 and the surviving families of the others (Lahman, 2018).

---

[1]https://www.ushmm.org/collections/bibliography/medical-experiments.

Nor does the list of biomedical horrors perpetrated in the name of science end there. It was only recently discovered that the US Public Health Service did another study on syphilis in Guatemala over a 3-year period (1946–1948). Unlike Tuskegee, in Guatemala, researchers actually infected more than 2,000 research subjects—sex workers, mental patients, prisoners, and soldiers—without seeking their consent (Reverby, 2012). Other examples include the two Brooklyn physicians who injected live cancer cells into their unsuspecting geriatric subjects; the CIA-sponsored LSD/brainwashing experiments conducted on psychiatric patients in Montreal during the 1960s; the US and Canadian pharmaceutical researchers who used prison inmates as test subjects in risky drug trials; and the government and church authorities who used Native American children attending residential schools as subjects in a variety of experiments without their or their parents' consent.

The stories seem to go on and on (e.g., Berg, 2007; Bronskill & Blanchfield, 1998; Collins, 1988; Lahman, 2018; "Native Kids Used for Experiments", 2000). All too often, overzealous researchers have mixed the "noble" motives of science with self-interest, an overblown sense of self-importance, and a dehumanization of their "subjects"—who all too commonly were members of socially vulnerable groups such as Jews, Blacks, Indigenous people, psychiatric patients, the poor, the drug addicted, the homeless, street-based sex workers, the elderly, and citizens of the Third World—and have forgotten about such fundamental ethical issues as consent and human rights. Clearly, in these cases, the research never should have been done in the first place; no gain in knowledge can justify the denial of human dignity that is involved when human beings are treated as no more than means to an end.

Complexities in the Social Sciences

In the social sciences, questions about the possible formalization of ethics guidelines began in the late 1950s. Unlike the biomedical domain, the discussion did not arise initially from horror stories of social science research, but from new sensibilities about the sorts of issues that social scientists were facing. One issue dominating the debate involved complexities arising from the growing professionalization of social science fields of study. In his 1959 presidential address to the American Sociological Association (ASA), Talcott Parsons noted the growing interest among sociologists in applied issues and, believing these would create new conflicts of interest, suggested that "perhaps a working code of relationships particularly needs to be worked out" (Parsons, 1959, p. 558). In the 1960s Project Camelot—in which the CIA was surreptitiously funding research devoted to discovering how to generate insurgency that might topple Third World governments and thereby showing they were willing to masquerade as anthropologists if it suited their purpose in foreign lands (Horowitz, 1967)—left sociologists and anthropologists concerned about maintaining academic freedom and ensuring independence from government.

Sociology did not jump at the opportunity to develop a formalized code of ethics, however, which was seen as a double-edged sword. Most of the 1960s were spent debating whether developing a disciplinary code of ethics was desirable. Some members of the ASA argued that "ethics regulation" was best left in the hands of individual researchers who would remain accountable for their actions (e.g., Becker, 1964; Freidson, 1964; Roth, 1969). Their worry was that the creation of an external standard would undermine academic freedom by taking the locus of ethical decision-making from researchers and handing it to bureaucrats who might or might not understand the research process. As Galliher (1973) cautioned,

> *Even after giving due weight to all the likely costs and risks to the profession, the unavoidable question sociologists must answer is whether a sociology that only poses approved questions in an approved fashion is either empirically or morally sound. (p. 99)*

Others argued the opposite, i.e., that, far from *impeding* academic freedom, a formalized code of ethics would help *preserve* it by serving as a buffer against third-party intervention into the research process (e.g., Schuler, 1967). When and if a government were to point to this or that isolated example of an ethics violation and propose seizing control of the research-regulating apparatus that most codes of ethics represent, researchers could point to their disciplinary code and say, "Thanks, but no thanks; we are already regulating ourselves."

A Shifting Locus of Responsibility

If part of the intention of the development of formalized codes of ethics was that it would protect academic freedom by keeping external efforts at regulation at bay, then the strategy in the long run has proven a colossal failure. In the 1970s, the idea that anyone but the researcher should be driving the ethics bus was laughable. How could anyone possibly predict all the things that could happen during a research project? Who but the researcher would have the knowledge and experience to make responsible ethical decisions as issues arose? How could academic freedom survive any other way?

Several decades later, much on the ethics landscape has changed. One of the more visible shifts saw control and judgment of ethics decision-making move from a more decentralized approach—outlining "guidelines" that should be "considered" by the researcher who was the final decision-maker—to a more centralized set of "standards" or "codes of conduct" where the respective associations or boards were the final arbiters of ethical practice instead of researchers. The period also was marked by significant federal intervention, largely because of some of the scandals discussed above involving biomedical researchers.

Government Intervenes

The idea of centralizing ethics regulation and placing government in a watchdog/overseer role seems to have originated in the wake of the Tuskegee scandal at the US Department of Health and Human Services with the establishment of the Office for Protection from Research Risk, which more recently became the Office for Human Research Protections. And although the primary concerns arose in relation to biomedical research, the social sciences and humanities were taken along for the ride (see Schrag, 2017) with little effort made to accommodate the diversity of methodologies, perspectives, and research contexts that characterize the humanities, health, and social sciences. It was "one-size-fits-all," with the "one size" reflecting a biomedical, experimentalist, quantitative model, with little attention or concern over how these principles would translate into other epistemologies and approaches. Although the general principles that appear in codes of ethics are very similar across diverse disciplines, simply taking a common practice that makes sense in one research context and imposing it on another can create a very unethical situation, and yet that is exactly what happened in the United States (e.g., see Adler & Adler, 2002; Christians, 2000; Hamburger, 2005), Canada (e.g., Haggerty, 2004; Social Sciences and Humanities Working Committee on Research Ethics, 2008; van den Hoonaard, 2001), Australia (e.g., Israel, 2004a, 2004b, 2015), and Great Britain (e.g., Pearce, 2002), all of which now have centralized governmental regulatory systems in place.

The Common Rule

The regulatory system for ethics in the United States is embodied in what is known as "The **Common Rule**" in the *Code of Federal Regulations*, or more specifically, 45 CFR 46.102(d) and (f). The regulations, which were initially formulated in 1991 and significantly revised in 2018, apply to all "research" that involves "human subjects" in institutions that seek federal research funding. "Research" is defined as "a systematic investigation, including research development, testing and evaluation, designed to develop or contribute to generalizable knowledge," while a "human subject" refers to "a living individual about whom an investigator (whether professional or student) conducting research (1) obtains information or biospecimens through intervention or interaction with the individual, and uses, studies, or analyzes the information or biospecimens; or (2) obtains, uses, studies, analyzes, or generates identifiable private information or identifiable biospecimens"[2] (see also Devlin, 2018).

As these definitions suggest, not all research is subject to review. Instead, the definition offered in the federal rule is a pragmatic one that defines the jurisdiction of the Common Rule and the range of activities to which it does and doesn't apply. Moreover, much research done in the social sciences and humanities is now being recognized as sufficiently innocuous as to be permissible with no or minimal ethics review. Research done in educational settings to evaluate student performance or new teaching techniques, for example, is not subject to review, nor is data that is non-identifiable as to its source or is so innocuous that there would be no negative consequences to disclosure of the information gathered (e.g., most marketing surveys, or observation in public settings where no one is identified) or involve "benign behavioral interventions."[3] Nor does all research that requires review need to be reviewed by the full Institutional Review Board (IRB); the Common Rule allows for "expedited" review for research that involves no more than "minimal risk" to prospective research subjects. Although the regulations do not identify who at an institution can determine whether a project is exempt, they do make clear that this determination cannot be left up to the researcher. In most cases, the IRB or its delegated authority would make that determination.

An ongoing challenge for IRBs is to have a membership with sufficient disciplinary and methodological diversity of expertise to be able to provide thoughtful and sensitive ethics review. Lahman (2018), for example, laments that reviews are often inadequate when IRB membership does not include persons with expertise in the methodologies you want to use. Although this would seem a rather fundamental requirement, IRBs are in general fairly small (the minimum size permitted is five), and the range of methods practiced in a diverse institution can be extensive. A related concern, and often the source of this inadequacy, is insufficient support for IRBs by institutions, which leads to overworked and underappreciated IRB members faced with mountains of paperwork.

---

[2]https://www.ecfr.gov/cgi-bin/retrieveECFR?gp=&SID=83cd09e1c0f5c6937cd9d7513160fc3f&pitd=2018
0719&n=pt45.1.46&r=PART&ty=HTML#se45.1.46_1102.

[3]For a full list of exemptions, see https://www.ecfr.gov/cgi-bin/retrieveECFR?gp=&SID=83cd09e1c0f5
c6937cd9d7513160fc3f&pitd=20180719&n=pt45.1.46&r=PART&ty=HTML#se45.1.46_1104.

Limited qualifications of IRB members also can go in the opposite direction and result in an *overextension* of IRB jurisdiction known as "ethics creep" (Haggerty, 2004). Concerns here abound with respect to an overbureaucratization and over-monitoring of research and how this can undermine academic freedom, a practice discussed with biting humor by Shea (2000) in an article entitled "*Don't talk to the humans.*" Lahman (2018) summarizes the critique thus:

> *The current state of U.S. IRB review has been called ethical imperialism, mission creep, nanny-state, ethics police, and more. Research ethics boards are seen increasingly as simultaneously broadening and deepening their ethical domain by reaching into areas of human interactions with scholars who work to acquire knowledge not historically seen as generalizable such as music, theater, oral history, journalism, and literature disciplines, while also deepening the level of review. (p. 59)*

Finally, concerns also have been expressed that "ethics review" on some occasions appears to be no more than "liability management" dressed up as ethics. Adler and Adler (2002), who have done various studies that focus on illegal behavior, lament seeing a growing bureaucratization of the ethics review process coupled with a reticence about going the distance to protect research participants. Ironically, they believe this makes many kinds of socially valuable research more difficult to do in an ethical way. Their article entitled "*Do university lawyers and the police define research values?*" sees them wondering aloud just who it is that is being protected:

> *What are we really being driven by here—an ethical imperative to protect the rights of people or an unethical imperative designed to keep universities, publishers, and sponsoring agencies from being sued? (p. 42)*

One place this liability-driven approach is apparent is in relation to consent forms. Menikoff, Kaneshiro, and Pritchard (2017) of the Office for Human Research Protections note that, "consent forms have been growing longer and can be difficult to understand. They too often appear to be designed more for protecting the legal interests of institutions conducting research than for helping someone make a decision about participation." The authors note approvingly that the 2018 revisions encourage researchers to have a short synopsis that highlights major points at the beginning in an effort to increase understanding.

Implications for the Sociology of Knowledge

We continue to be concerned about the regulatory process for ethics that now exists in the United States, Canada, Australia, Britain, and many other countries because of the impact these highly bureaucratic regimes appear to have had on the sociology of knowledge for reasons that have nothing to do with ethics per se (e.g., Fitzgerald, 2004; Katz, 2007; Shea, 2000). While many US authors have emphasized the censorship aspects of ethics regulation (e.g., Hamburger, 2005), few have considered the repercussions that contemporary ethics regulation has had for whose voices are being heard and whose are missing in the great social discussion to which researchers are supposed to contribute. Social groups that are most likely to be affected are the socially marginalized and vulnerable who have shown for decades their willingness to speak to social and health scientists who want to learn about their niche of life and point of view as long as their conversations are confidential, but who would be most concerned about prosecution, suppression, and stigmatization if they were to be identified. This includes not just those who have broken or who are breaking the law that criminologists often talk to but also those who walk in the shadow between illegal and legal, or who are the whistleblowers that help shed light on injustice or the illegal behavior of those for whom they work, or who are harassed by legal authorities who themselves are treading the boundary between legal and illegal, or who suffer from health conditions that would affect their reputation, employability, or insurance benefits.

British author Robert Dingwall (2008) draws attention to the role of independent observer that the university has occupied and the perspectives that would be lost if researchers were to become simple agents of the state:

> In the contemporary world, citizens depend upon a great deal of expert knowledge in order to make good judgments about each other and about the social institutions that they encounter. The quality of that knowledge depends crucially on free competition between information providers. If what has traditionally been the most disinterested source of information, the universities, becomes systematically handicapped in that competition, then all citizens lose out. When we give up doing participant observation with vulnerable or socially marginal groups because of the regulatory obstacles, then a society becomes less well-informed about the condition of those who it excludes and more susceptible to their explosions of discontent. How helpful is it when the only ethnographers of Islamic youth in the UK are undercover police or security service agents? (p. 10)

The result is a shallower research enterprise relying more and more on existing public data sets that have been prepared by institutional authorities to serve their own ends and a progressively greater denial of voice to those most affected by what those institutions do. It is still too early to tell, as of this writing, whether the changes in the Common Rule introduced in 2018 will result in a more proportionate approach. Ideally, more sensitive and ethically challenging studies will get the attention they deserve while properly expediting more innocuous studies in which risks are minimal to nonexistent and the bigger danger is of undermining academic freedom.

ETHICS PRINCIPLES

One concern about the centralization of ethics policies and the review process is the extent to which it has turned the discussion about ethics away from one that focuses on education, debate, and discussion about ethical principles throughout the research process to one that focuses on ethics review and how to be "approved" or to "get through" ethics. Although review does focus on key moments in the researcher–participant interaction—soliciting participants, initial contact, acquiring consent, collecting and managing data, and avoiding conflicts of interest—it would be naïve to think that your problems are behind you after having been approved. Surprises arise, particularly in field-based research where researchers are confronted with the messiness of the social world. We agree with Cresswell (2016) that sensitivity to ethics issues needs to extend from the very first decision of whether to do the research, to final decisions about how to best translate and mobilize the research findings in various professional, public, and policy settings.

Is the Research Worth Doing?

The choice at the beginning of any research project involving human research participants is whether to do the research at all. This "basic ethical dilemma" involves balancing two important and sometimes conflicting obligations: to science and to participants. Our **scientific obligation** is to *do* research in the *best* way we know how. Being a social or health scientist involves a commitment to the value of knowledge and understanding. Our social mandate is to understand all aspects of society not only as an end in itself but also to contribute to the development of rational policy. Since much of our research involves human participants, we also have a **humanistic obligation** to treat people with dignity and to safeguard their interests. People typically volunteer to participate only because we enter their lives and ask them to do so, for little or no direct personal gain, which only increases our obligation to ensure that no harm comes to them. That responsibility rises exponentially when the participants do not even know they are participating in a piece of research, as often occurs, for example, when we do observational research in public settings, in archives, or perhaps even after a person's death.

We have noted already some of the biomedical research that clearly involved greater cost to participants than was justified by the research. Research in the social sciences is not without risks—and some research can pose considerable risk, particularly in relation to maintaining confidentiality—but in the social sciences and humanities at least we do not kill people. The more typical situation arises with those studies that challenge us to consider where exactly we should draw the line between ethical and unethical.

Stanley Milgram's obedience research (e.g., Milgram, 1963, 1974) is often discussed in this regard. His research dealt with an important social behavior: blind obedience to a presumably legitimate authority figure. However, to obtain his data Milgram deceived his participants by telling them his experiment was about the effects of punishment on learning, when "really" (from Milgram's perspective) it was about how obedient ordinary people would be when ordered to deliver what they believed were real and painful electric shocks of increasing severity to another human being (who was actually an employee of the experimenter and "in" on the deception) every time they made a mistake in a learning task.

Many were surprised and disturbed that 65 percent of Milgram's participants were completely obedient to the end, even when every indication was that they had certainly hurt, and may even have killed, the other participant. Perhaps even more disturbing were their rationalizations for doing so, along the lines of "I was only following orders" and "It was not *my* responsibility to decide," which were chillingly reminiscent of the rationalizations of the Nazis charged and tried at Nuremberg following World War II and of US Private Lynndie England after her involvement in the abuse and torture of prisoners at Abu Ghraib prison in Baghdad, Iraq. The guilt and stress that participants felt during their participation was considerable. You get a feeling for what it must have been like for the participants when you read Milgram's (1963) original account of how "real" the situation was for the participants. His general characterization of the atmosphere created is as follows:

> *In a large number of cases the degree of tension reached extremes that are rarely seen in socio-psychological laboratory studies. Subjects were observed to sweat, tremble, stutter, bite their lips, groan, and dig their fingernails into their flesh. These were characteristic rather than exceptional responses to the experiment … Full-blown,*

uncontrollable seizures were observed for 3 subjects. On one occasion we observed a
seizure so violently convulsive that it was necessary to call a halt to the experiment.
(p. 375)

Milgram presents evidence from the debriefings that always followed participation that his research subjects accepted the deceit and felt they had learned from the experience. But *was* the infliction of deception and stress he routinely induced warranted? Milgram argued that it was and received various awards for his research from such prestigious authorities as the American Association for the Advancement of Science; in contrast, critics such as Diana Baumrind (1964) believed what he had done was despicable and that his research would sully our reputation for many years to come. The fact Milgram's work is now commonly cited in research methods texts as an example of "unethical" research more than 50 years later suggests perhaps Baumrind was correct in her assessment.

Informed Consent

One core ethical principle is that of **informed consent**, that is, the notion that it is important for researchers to get consent from people before involving them in research, and that their consent, when and if they give it, should be based on honest and complete information regarding what their participation will involve and any risks this might entail. Although it is a consideration to be addressed in all research, this principle is particularly high on the list for those who do biomedical research. In the biomedical realm, this most often involves a written agreement in the form of a contract that the research subject is expected to sign in order to participate. This practice is consistent with the accounting culture that exists in the medical community and the highly regulated process of clinical trials necessary to develop and distribute new drugs and treatments. Such research often takes place in hospitals and other medical facilities and operates in a very legalistic context (e.g., for establishing the effectiveness and risk of newly developed drugs), and the range of risks can be considerable. People have the right to choose whether to participate in drug trials or experimental procedures that may benefit them, particularly in "last resort" situations. Our ethical obligation is to ensure each person understands the potential risks and benefits and can make an informed choice about whether to participate nonetheless.

In contrast, in the social sciences and humanities, and especially with more qualitative forms of research, the process of informing the prospective participant and obtaining consent is more likely to be done orally, a provision that is also allowed by the Common Rule. There are three main reasons for doing so. First, the ideal researcher–participant relationship is one built on mutual trust and rapport; signed consent forms impose a legalism that undermines that ideal. Second, it raises the question of just who is being protected through such a form. If "research ethics" is all about the protection of the rights and interests of research participants, why is the participant the one asked to sign their name on the dotted line? And third, consider how important confidentiality becomes in research. In order to do research in relation to some of society's most controversial and important social issues, people need to trust they can share information with us that, if it were to be disclosed and known to be about them, could lead to them losing their employment, reputation, insurability, citizenship, and/or freedom. Part of protecting personal information is to avoid creating needless paper trails—like consent forms with peoples' names and signatures on them—because these can undermine your ability to protect their information.

Rather than asking participants to sign a form, many researchers will give a written information sheet that outlines what participation in the study would involve and any promises and safeguards the researcher and their university propose. The idea is to inform prospective participants, in language they understand, about any considerations a reasonable person would want to know before deciding whether to participate. It is often a good idea for the researcher and prospective participant to read through the sheet together, with the participant encouraged to ask any questions about the study and any prospective risks and benefits and how they will be addressed. We think of it in terms of how we would want a family member or close friend treated and what we would want to make sure they know before deciding whether to participate. You want to be both clear and realistic about what is being offered, making neither grandiose claims about the prospective utility of the research nor any promises you are not prepared to keep.

But informed consent is not always required in research. For example, when observational research is done in public places, the participants might never even know that they were part of a study. Of course, this begs the question of where "public" ends and "private" begins. Consider, for example, the covert participant observation research Lofland and Lejeune (1960) conducted at Alcoholics Anonymous, where researchers actually joined a group and surreptitiously kept notes of the group's activities and dynamics. Is an AA meeting "public" because anyone can walk in and participate? Or is it "private" because the people who go there for help have an expectation of privacy once they have taken the courageous step of sitting down and seeking help for a serious problem? Similar issues face us today online. Is an internet chat site such as Ask.fm or discussion board such as Reddit "public" because anyone can use them? Or are they "private" because of some tacit social expectation that only those who are serious about the topic will join? And if we do go in as researchers, is it reasonable to "lurk" in the online space without drawing attention to our arrival and intentions? Or are we obliged to announce our presence? Is it any more ethically acceptable if the researchers ensure that no one is ever named or otherwise identified?

Perhaps the most famous and controversial study of this type was Laud Humphreys's (1970) *Tearoom Trade*, in which Humphreys played the role of a "watch queen" in order to observe intimate homosexual encounters in public washrooms. This choice in itself gave some observers cause for pause because of the intimacy of the behavior he was observing, notwithstanding that it was happening in a "public" place. Even more controversial was his next step, when Humphreys surreptitiously took down license plate numbers, used a contact in the Department of Motor Vehicles to find out where the men lived, and then (in disguise) interviewed them in their homes to discover more about who they were in their lives away from the tearooms. Was the lack of consent justified by the knowledge that was produced and/or the confidentiality that was maintained? Would it make any difference to you to discover that homosexuality was illegal in most of North America at the time and that Humphreys's research went a long way to dispelling many of the homophobic stereotypes that were prevalent? As was the case with Milgram's experiment, there were researchers who lined up on both sides of the controversy surrounding Humphreys's field research.

Even when you set out to ensure a fully informed consent, pragmatic problems can arise. The information to be conveyed might be too technical or esoteric for prospective participants to appreciate fully, or some attribute of them might virtually preclude the assurance of communication (e.g., in the study of young children or some psychiatric patients). Your challenge is to identify and communicate those aspects of the study that might "reasonably" affect someone's willingness to participate in terms they can understand. This will vary from population to population. Guardians or other advocates of the prospective participant(s) can and should be brought in as appropriate, although their approval should be sought in addition to, rather than instead of, the consent of the actual participant wherever possible.

In some circumstances, securing informed consent can be virtually impossible or highly impractical. When coding archival records or photographs of crowds, for example, it may not be possible to identify or contact all the people involved. Lack of identification may not be a problem since it also implies anonymity, although you also would want to ensure that subsequent accounts avoid inadvertently providing identifying information through other clues (e.g., personal characteristics, place of work, geo-id, or tags). When people can be identified but not contacted, precautions normally should be taken to ensure confidentiality (e.g., by blurring or pixelating faces if pictures are used).

Of course, mere difficulty or impracticality of getting consent does not in and of itself excuse the researcher from the need to obtain it, particularly when our presence in the setting is not a passive one. Simply observing a setting without consent is one thing—in that case the main issues likely will surround whether the situation is "public" or "private" and the expectations of those who inhabit the site—but going into a situation and actively manipulating it is another. Facebook discovered that when a Facebook employee and two Cornell University researchers published a study involving 689,003 Facebook users that involved manipulating the positivity or negativity of users' newsfeeds. The results, published in the *Proceedings of the National Academy of Sciences* (Kramer, Guillory, & Hancock, 2014), were framed as an illustration of how emotional contagion can spread through social media despite the absence of in-person interaction and nonverbal cues.

The backlash when the study was published was considerable as some of the headlines of the time reveal. In a *Forbes* magazine article headlined, "Facebook Manipulated 689,003 Users' Emotions for Science," Kathryn Hill (2014) asked, "So is it okay for Facebook to play mind games with us for science?" Her answer was in the negative as she noted with disdain that the Facebook study was never subject to ethics review, with the company justifying its intervention by saying that the study did not violate the terms of service that users agreed to when they started their Facebook accounts. In another article in *The Atlantic* entitled, "Everything we know about Facebook's secret mood manipulation experiment: It was probably legal. But was it ethical?," Meyer (2014) notes that although two of the three authors of the study were from Cornell University rather than Facebook, the Cornell ethics review board decided against reviewing the study because the manipulation had already been done. This meant the Cornell researchers were only dealing with "secondary data" whose acquisition was assumed to have been done legally by Facebook and which in that case would be consistent with the Common Rule. Nonetheless, he also makes clear it is unlikely the Cornell IRB would have approved the original study had it gone through ethics review, which leads to more questions about the ethics of using secondary data generated by unethical means.

Facebook has faced considerable criticism in recent years on more than one occasion for its careless handling of people's personal information and the way it has permitted other commercial and political interests to exploit that information for their own aggrandizement and to improve Facebook's bottom line (e.g., Cadwalladr &

Graham-Harrison, 2018; Confessore & Kang, 2018; Sanders & Patterson, 2018). While there were lessons to be learned through the "emotional contagion" scandal, we wonder whether Facebook's takeaway from the experience is (1) don't do manipulative research on Facebook users without their consent; or (2) continue doing manipulative research, but don't publish the results in journals where people can discover what is being done to them. We hope it is the former, but it appears much more likely to be the latter (e.g., see McNamee, 2019).

The PNAS editor's "expression of concern" draws our attention to the fact that while academics are held to a high ethical standard through both disciplinary and federal codes of ethics, the corporate world is not. With more and more attention being paid these days to "big data"—compiled for the most part by large web-based corporations—and with many academics enticed by the range of research questions such databases allow us to pursue (see Chapter 12), we do wonder whether further regulation is warranted for such partnerships. Cornell University's decision to treat the database as "secondary data" and thereby turn a blind eye to the conditions under which the data were gathered in the first place would seem to represent a loophole that allows unethical research to come in through the back door. Doing so allows university-based researchers to be subject only to legal limits to their behavior—a far lower standard than our codes of ethics would allow—and thereby promote an erosion of integrity we should be loath to accept.

Protecting Confidentiality

While informed consent is often touted as the primary ethical principle in the biomedical community, **confidentiality** is more often our priority concern in the social sciences and humanities. People have a right to keep information about themselves private or to share it only with those whom they trust to safeguard it. When we approach people and ask them to divulge information about themselves, and especially when that information could cause them embarrassment or harm if it were to be released, it is incumbent on researchers to take every precaution to ensure that identifiable information—information that can be linked to a specific source—is protected. In order to provide that protection, however, it is important to consider where and how threats to confidentiality might arise and, hence, what we are protecting ourselves and our participants against.

"Loose Lips Sink Ships"

By far the most pervasive threats to confidentiality are those that come from our interactions with people in the milieu we are researching. These are what you might call relatively "low-grade" threats because they disappear most times with a simple "no," but they occur frequently and must be prevented. They arise most commonly when multiple people are being interviewed in one setting—a given organization, community, or family, for example. Some of the participants inevitably will be curious about what another research participant said. It may be quite well-meaning: a concerned parent might fish for hints about what their uncommunicative child divulged to the researcher about illicit drug use or something as apparently innocuous as what they said about their career plans. Or it may be more maliciously motivated: a respondent might give the impression that they are an "insider" on some issue and look for confirmation from you that another person divulged a particular opinion, allegiance, or point of view as a way of justifying a vendetta or other campaign of action against the person.

Researchers need to be very careful not to say anything to any one person that another person told them, or in many situations even whether some specific other person participated (or did not). This may sound very simple, but guarding against it requires considerable vigilance. The problem arises because we want to appear competent, intelligent, and "in the know" so that people will respect us as interviewers and feel confident giving us information. But if we start sharing what others have told us, even if the information seems innocuous, we begin to tread on very dangerous ground. Our typical status as "outsiders" to the setting means we are less likely to know enough about the internal dynamics of the setting to make good choices about what is safe to share and what is not. Things that to us seem innocent may have significant consequences within the setting we are researching. The best way to inspire confidence in research participants is to show them how vigilant you are in safeguarding the information that others give you; it tells them that you will show the same vigilance with their information and that they really can trust you. Conversely, if you are sloppy with others' confidences, why would they believe you will be careful with theirs?

Procedural Protections

When engineers learn to design a bridge, they are taught to neither underbuild nor overbuild. This requires them to have a good understanding of the place the bridge will go—how solid is the ground underneath? what range of weather conditions will it have to endure? how high do the winds ever get? how much traffic does it need to hold at peak time?—and then to design something that is safe within those parameters. If they underbuild, they run the risk of the bridge falling down and killing those who are on it. If they overbuild, they end up spending tens of millions of your taxpayer dollars for nothing.

Researchers face an analogous challenge when it comes to confidentiality protections. The trick is to be thoughtful and careful and to know enough about what you are getting yourself and your research participants into so that you understand the probable or likely risks without getting hysterical and seeing possible or potential threats in every shadowy corner or, conversely, ignoring real risks that you need to mitigate. When the data are gathered anonymously or anonymized very soon after collection, there is little danger to participants for a violation of confidentiality and hence the researcher should simply guarantee to their participants that their identities will remain unknown. However, if the source of the information is identifiable and a disclosure would bring harm to the participant—if, for example, disclosure of the information could lead the participant to lose their job, be jailed, or lose insurability—then that is when you need to build a stronger bridge. In this section, we look first at some of the procedural protections you can use to protect your participants' data and then move into some of the ways that more law-based strategies can be implemented.

The easiest way to protect the confidentiality of respondents is simply never to obtain or record participants' names in the first place. This immediately safeguards against any effort to determine their identity by providing them with **anonymity** from the moment you begin gathering data. There are many kinds of research—particularly more structured kinds of research such as structured interview and questionnaire-based studies in which numerous respondents are all being asked roughly the same questions—where this is the easiest rule to follow. If you have never gathered identifying information in the first place, and if the information you gather is not sufficient to identify specific individuals indirectly, then there is no threat to worry about, and you can simply guarantee confidentiality to your participants when you inform them prior to asking them for their consent to participate.

In situations where you must obtain people's names, either because you need them ahead of time in order to know whom to approach or because the circumstances of the situation lead you to obtain that information, you should anonymize your records at the first opportunity ("**redact**" is the formal term) and then destroy your original digital recordings or records (or give them to your participants if that is what you promised to do) according to whatever plan was approved by your IRB. Sometimes you may need to keep some form of identifier that allows you to distinguish between respondents; in that situation use **pseudonyms**, that is, invented names that are used consistently through your notes so that you can keep together all the quotations from the person you'll call "Kim" and be able to differentiate "Kim" from "Pat." Should your notes ever inadvertently fall into the wrong hands, no one but you will know who "Kim" and "Pat" "really" are, and with the passage of time, your memory of who was assigned what pseudonym will no doubt fade as well. Some people allow participants to choose their own pseudonyms, but we advise against it; the fewer people who can connect a given transcript with a given person, the better, including the participant (e.g., see Palys & MacAlister, 2016). In the event you are generating more quantified and structured data that are maintained in digital files, your options are simply to delete any identifying information from the file as soon as is practical or to keep identifying information in a separate file, preferably in a different order than exists in the "content" file, but linkable through some designator included in each file that only you know about.

Regardless of what form of data you have—but the more sensitive the data, the more you are advised to do this—researchers save their data on hardware-encrypted drives or in files using **encryption** software such as the freely available VeraCrypt. Both of these options provide as good an assurance as you can get that no one else will be able to make use of the data to identify particular respondents. One thing we like about software encryption solutions such as VeraCrypt is that they allow you to encrypt anything from a single file to an entire drive on any laptop or desktop computer. More commonly, however, you create "containers" of any size that are essentially virtual drives into which you can place files. We recommend putting all your data on hardware-encrypted drives or in software-encrypted containers and even having multiple encrypted drives or containers to make the task of anyone trying to break your encryption even more difficult by obfuscating where the sought file(s) might be. Always using encrypted drives or containers ensures your data are safe even if your portable drive or computer is lost or stolen; the person who finds or who stole your drive or computer may delete your data, but will never be able to read it.

Other strategies for anonymizing, encrypting, and hiding computerized data are given by Boruch and Cecil (1979). Although the specific technologies they describe are in many cases obsolete, the conceptual guidelines they provide for devising anonymizing strategies are as relevant today as they were at the time that book was written. More contemporary strategies that better consider the strengths and weaknesses of current technologies can be seen in Aldridge, Medina, and Ralphs (2010). A website that offers very helpful suggestions we encourage you to check out is that of the Electronic Frontier Foundation who offer up-to-date information regarding ways of protecting information from electronic surveillance.

And finally, although high-tech, computer-based approaches can create a challenge to third parties who might be interested in your data, another line of defense is offered by going precisely in the opposite direction, that is, the "old school" low-tech solution of using a notebook of sorts (especially for qualitative field note data), which can be hidden more easily than your computer's hard drive. The thing to do here is to seek and pursue approaches that are appropriate for the kinds of data you are compiling. The greater the harm that can come to participants if the data were to be revealed, the greater the level of protection you should seek.

Dealing With Legal Threats

Far less common are more formal efforts by third parties to acquire information from confidential research sources through legal means such as subpoenas. The literature contains a few dozen examples of legal threats to confidentiality that have arisen in the United States in the last 40 years out of what is no doubt hundreds of thousands of research projects that have been carried out in that time (see Cecil & Wetherington, 1996 and Lowman & Palys, 2001a for a sample of cases).

Asserting Privilege. When a legal challenge to research confidentiality is made, it is generally for one of two reasons. In a criminal trial, the prosecutor in the case may have reason to believe the researcher has information that would be useful in establishing the guilt of an accused. In a civil action, the lawyer for either side might have reason to believe a researcher has information that will either help their own client or undermine the case of the person or corporation on the other side.

The presumption in court is that all of us are obliged to give evidence when we are subpoenaed and have information that is relevant to a court proceeding. Many academics appear in court willingly as expert witnesses when we are asked to bring the expertise we have developed through our research to advise the court on its implications for some case. For example, Chris, who has done extensive research in relation to the sex industry, was recently an expert witness in a case where the defendants were arguing that the laws as currently constructed caused sex workers to work in conditions that violated their constitutional right to safety and security of the person. As this suggests, being asked to help the court is not necessarily a problem in and of itself. But we reach a line in the sand that must not be crossed when we are asked to disclose information that can be tied to particular individuals, particularly when disclosure of that information could result in our participants losing a job, ending a marriage, being incarcerated, feeling humiliated, diminishing their reputation, and/or making them uninsurable. In that situation our job is to resist, and we do so by invoking a researcher–participant "privilege."

To say that some relationship has "privilege" means that persons in that relationship are exempt from the normal requirement that all of us have to testify when asked to do so in a court of law when and if information discussed in the context of that relationship becomes of interest to the court. The lawyer–client relationship is protected by a privilege, for example, so that you can go and talk freely to your lawyer and seek legal advice without fearing that they will be subpoenaed and appear on the witness stand the next day giving evidence against you. Because privileges can interfere with the court's search for truth—evidence that might otherwise be useful to a court adjudication is not available—privileges are very rarely granted. However, some socially valued relationships simply could not exist without assurance that what is said in the context of that relationship will remain confidential. Some of these are recognized in statute; any others have to be asserted in court.

Statute-Based Protections. One way to protect information is to write the protection into law. In the United States, the first research participants to enjoy **statute-based protection** were those who participate in research conducted by the Census Bureau. As the Bureau explains on its web pages,

> *It is against the law for any Census Bureau employee to disclose or publish any census or survey information that identifies an individual or business. This is true even for inter-agency communication: the FBI and other government entities do not have the legal right to access this information. In fact, when these protections have been challenged, Title 13's confidentiality guarantee has been upheld.*

In the 1970s, similar protections began to be extended to other researchers who were doing research in the public interest that involved looking at behavior that was against the law. Cases began to appear in the late 1960s and 1970s in which legal authorities (police, grand juries, and prosecutors) tried to acquire confidential research information from researchers in order to prosecute a research participant or someone known to the research participant for violations of law. Former President Richard Nixon and former Director of the FBI J. Edgar Hoover were known to go after those they perceived as enemies of the state, particularly within the anti–Vietnam War movement. The FBI threatened the Kinsey Institute on sex research with subpoenas in the late 1960s if they did not share information about sexual practices that might be used to embarrass war resisters or leverage cooperation from prospective informants (e.g., see O'Neil, 1996; Palys & Lowman, 2014), but Kinsey refused and the FBI withdrew.

By 1970, however, when significant numbers of Vietnam veterans were returning with heroin addiction, Congress heard testimony asserting the need for research into the phenomenon along with concerns about the ability to do that research because it involved illegal activity and thereby aroused police interest. Congress responded by passing the *Comprehensive Drug Abuse Prevention and Control Act of 1970*, part of which gave the Secretary of Health, Education, and Welfare the power to authorize

> *… persons engaged in research on the use and effect of drugs to protect the privacy of individuals who are the subject of such research by withholding from all persons not connected with the conduct of such research the names or other identifying characteristics of such individuals. Persons so authorized to protect the privacy of such individuals may not be compelled in any Federal, State, or local civil, criminal, administrative, legislative, or other proceedings to identify such individuals.[4]*

The resulting mechanism—**Certificates of Confidentiality** (CoCs)—is administered by the National Institutes of Health (NIH). Over the years, CoC protection has been expanded beyond the realm of "addictions" to include a broad range of "health" research (Wolf, Patel, Williams, Austin, & Dame, 2013). As of 2017, all research that is funded by NIH automatically receives a CoC, while all others who engage in "health" research even if it is not funded by NIH are eligible for one by application if the data gathered are "sensitive" and their source identifiable or potentially identifiable.

Statute-based protections also have been developed for some criminological research. "**Privacy certificates (PCs)**" are administered by the Department of Justice via the National Institute of Justice. They work somewhat differently than CoCs insofar as they are only available for research that is funded by NIJ or one of its sister agencies and are required of all who receive funding from NIJ. Unlike CoCs, which focus on protecting the identities of participants, PCs protect "identifiable information." And while CoCs allow the researcher to make exceptions to the coverage as long as these are conveyed to the participant, PCs do not allow for any limitation to the protection other than "future crime."[5]

---

[4]Comprehensive Drug Abuse Prevention and Control Act of 1970, Pub. L., No. 91–513, 84 Stat. 1236, 1241 (1970).
[5]See https://www.nij.gov/funding/humansubjects/Pages/confidentiality.aspx.

A recent review of the two protections suggests both have done a formidable job of protecting research participants from legal threats, with CoCs doing the best job of establishing broad availability of protection, while PCs seem most successful at actually delivering that protection and avoiding legal challenge (see Palys, Turk, & Lowman, 2018).

Thanks to the existence of these protections, many sources of legal threat have all but disappeared. And yet they still do appear. Criminological research that is not funded by NIJ is not eligible for PC protection. Moreover, because CoCs must for the most part be applied for, many sensitive "health" projects do not seek the protection, leaving them exposed to the risk of legal threat. And of course there is also a very broad range of research that involves sensitive information but is neither "health" nor "criminologically" focused that is not eligible for either of the statute-based protections. Where statute-based protection is not available, researchers can end up in court, where they are forced to argue through the **common law**—law as it is interpreted in court—that their participants should be protected through maintaining the confidentiality of their data.

Common Law Protections. The two types of privilege that are generated through the common law are known as "class" and "case-by-case" privileges. They differ in how well-established they are and where the onus of proof lies when a challenge arises. An example of a **class privilege** is the lawyer–client privilege that has been recognized by courts in the United States and other countries for a very long time. There is no specific law that says attorney–client privilege exists; instead, it is a privilege that has come to be recognized by the courts as fundamental to the constitutional right to a fair trial. How could you have a full and frank discussion with your lawyer to generate a legal defense if you were worried about your lawyer showing up the next day as a witness for the prosecution? To say it is a "class" privilege means that the court is prepared to assume it exists without the need for every lawyer and client to prove they deserve it every time the confidentiality of their communications is challenged. If anyone were to argue that any given communication between a lawyer and their client should be revealed, the onus of proof would be on the challenger to demonstrate what compelling reasons exist in this case for the privilege to be set aside.

When no statute-based or class privilege exists, the standard academic response is still nonetheless to resist disclosure. The law still allows for the possibility of a privilege to be recognized on a case-by-case basis. However, in such instances, the onus is on the person claiming the privilege—the researcher in this case, on behalf of the participant—to demonstrate why the privilege should be recognized. The most common legal defense in the United States involves making the claim that the work of academics is highly similar to the work of journalists—both gather information from people and other sources that is intended to provide insights into society and its workings that is disseminated through public forums, much of which would not be possible unless the sources of our information are convinced that no harm will come to them for sharing that information—and thus should be constitutionally protected via the First Amendment.

The United States v. Microsoft. An exemplary case for our consideration is one that was decided by the US Court of Appeals in 1998 involving Microsoft Corporation, the maker of the Windows operating system and a variety of other software and hardware. The company was accused of antitrust violations—engaging in predatory behavior designed to nullify unfairly their competition. A case in point was their Internet Explorer browser. As the internet was coming into popular existence in the mid 1990s, one of the first browsers to capture public interest and to be available for free was a browser known as Netscape Navigator. By 1997, Netscape Navigator was used by 80% of the market, with Internet Explorer less than 20 percent. Within just a few years, however, those numbers were reversed. Regulators alleged this dramatic shift was the result of the predatory practices of which Microsoft now stood accused. In defense, Microsoft claimed the turnaround was because of the brilliance of its managers coupled with poor decision-making by their counterparts at Netscape.

It also just so happened that, around that time, two researchers—Michael Cusumano of MIT and David Yoffie of Harvard—were doing research at Netscape that included interviews with current and former Netscape employees. Microsoft's lawyers discovered that a book based on those interviews—eventually titled *Competing on Internet Time: Lessons from Netscape and the Battle with Microsoft* (Cusumano & Yoffie, 1998)—was in the works and subpoenaed the professors' research notes, all the recordings and transcripts of interviews, and all correspondence with participants, believing these would buttress their case. However, Cusumano and Yoffie had promised their participants complete confidentiality. As the justices of the First Circuit of the US Court of Appeals would later explain,

> *As part of their research for* Lessons, *the respondents interviewed over 40 current and former Netscape employees. Their interview protocol dealt with confidentiality on two levels. First, the respondents signed a nondisclosure agreement with Netscape, in which they agreed not to disclose proprietary information conveyed to them in the course of their investigation except upon court order, and then only after giving Netscape notice and an opportunity to oppose disclosure. Second, the respondents requested and received permission from interview subjects to*

record their discussions, and, in return, promised that each interviewee would be shown any quotes attributed to him upon completion of the manuscript, so that he would have a chance to correct any errors or to object to quotations selected by the authors for publication. (In Re: Michael A. Cusumano and David B. Yoffie, 1998)

Clearly billions of dollars were at stake. In addition to showing the agreement that enabled them to acquire the information they did, Cusumano and Yoffie's lawyers argued that,

... they are sufficiently like journalists for the protection afforded to journalists' materials to be applied here; that the information which they procured is confidential because of their interview protocol; and that forcing them to disclose the contents of the notes, tapes, and transcripts would endanger the values of academic freedom safeguarded by the First Amendment and jeopardize the future information-gathering activities of academic researchers. (In Re: Michael A. Cusumano and David B. Yoffie, 1998)

In the end, the Court of Appeals agreed. In many ways, cases such as this come down to a balancing of interests—in this case the right of Microsoft to evidence that would be of use to the company in addressing the charges against it *versus* the needs of the research community to be able to gather information about important social issues without research participants having to worry that what they say today will be used against them in court tomorrow. On the one hand, the court agreed that Microsoft likely would benefit from having the information. Microsoft had not merely gone on a "fishing expedition" in the hope they might find something relevant; the book, and presumably the interviews underlying them, dealt squarely with Netscape's behavior during the browser wars with Microsoft and thus was likely to include content relevant to Microsoft's defence. The book itself included some quotes that even suggested that might be the case. On the other hand,

The opposite pan of the scale is brim-full. Scholars studying management practices depend upon the voluntary revelations of industry insiders to develop the factual infrastructure upon which theoretical conclusions and practical predictions may rest. These insiders often lack enthusiasm for divulging their management styles and business strategies to academics, who may in turn reveal that information to the public. Yet, pathbreaking work in management science requires gathering data from those companies and individuals operating in the most highly competitive fields of industry, and it is in these cutting-edge areas that the respondents concentrate their efforts. Their time-tested interview protocol, including the execution of a nondisclosure agreement with the corporate entity being studied and the furnishing of personal assurances of confidentiality to the persons being interviewed, gives chary corporate executives a sense of security that greatly facilitates the achievement of agreements to cooperate. (In Re: Michael A. Cusumano and David B. Yoffie, 1998)

Anticipating the Wigmore Criteria. Just because a researcher asserts privilege does not mean that it will be recognized, and at times it has not been. Palys and Lowman (2002, 2014) note several losses, two of which resulted in the researchers spending time in jail for contempt of court. This led the authors to suggest that, although the likelihood of being pulled into court on a subpoena is small—there are thousands upon thousands of projects that do not generate legal attention for every one that does—researchers would do well to ensure that they are prepared for the sorts of evidence that the courts will ask them to produce. A useful template for how to prepare is given by the Wigmore criteria, which reflects the sort of decision-making process the courts go through when deciding whether to recognize a researcher–participant privilege in any given case (see Palys & Lowman, 2002; Traynor, 1996).

The Wigmore criteria or **Wigmore test** comprises a set of four criteria developed by John Henry Wigmore (1905), a former Dean of Law at Northwestern University. Wigmore offered the test after reviewing all the legal decision-making regarding confidentiality and privilege that had appeared up to that point in legal decisions in the United States, the UK, and Canada. The Supreme Court of Canada has formally stated it will use the Wigmore criteria to adjudicate whether a privilege should be recognized given the circumstances in the case at hand (Palys & Lowman, 2000), while the US Supreme Court has recognized the Wigmore criteria as providing an appropriate decision-making template for the courts to apply (Palys & Lowman, 2002; Traynor, 1996). Perhaps most importantly, when Palys and Lowman examined the few losses that have occurred in US courts, they could easily identify in each instance at least one of the Wigmore criteria on which the claim for privilege failed.

The criteria specify that

1. The communications must originate in a *confidence* that they will not be disclosed;

2. This element of *confidentiality must be essential* to the full and satisfactory maintenance of the relation between the parties;

3. The *relation* must be one which in the opinion of the community ought to be sedulously *fostered*; and

4. The *injury* that would inure to the relation by the disclosure of the communications must be *greater than the benefit* thereby gained for the correct disposal of litigation (Wigmore, 1905, p. 3185; italics in original).

A successful claim of privilege requires evidence that speaks to all four requirements (e.g., Crabb, 1996; Daisley, 1994; Jackson & MacCrimmon, 1999; O'Neil, 1996; Palys & MacAlister, 2016; Traynor, 1996; Wiggins & McKenna, 1996). Researchers who are dealing with sensitive information where the possibility of subpoena is legitimate should consult competent legal help; we emphasize "competent" because we have found there are actually very few lawyers who are up-to-date with the law of privilege *and* who understand the academic enterprise and its ethical requirements.

A Tale of Two Researchers. If you are eligible for a CoC because you are doing "health" research where confidentiality is crucial to the acquisition of reliable and valid data or are doing criminological research that is funded by NIJ and thereby eligible for a PC, then you should definitely take the time to secure that protection. But if you are not in one of those situations and are gathering data that are sensitive and would be harmful to participants if they were to be disclosed, then you owe it to your research participants to try and anticipate as much as possible the Wigmore criteria to make your research as impervious to threat as possible. The wisdom of doing so is illustrated by a story we can tell you about two researchers—both graduate students who happened to be subpoenaed in the early 1990s and both of whom were directed by a legal authority to divulge confidential research information—who met with very different outcomes.

The first researcher is Russel Ogden, who was pursuing a Master's degree in criminology at Simon Fraser University in Vancouver, Canada. Ogden became interested in assisted suicide and euthanasia, which was illegal throughout North America at that time. It was also a time when the HIV/AIDS epidemic was at its most horrific—there were no effective treatments, which meant that all you could look forward to once diagnosed was being treated as a social pariah and left to face a lonely gradual deterioration over a period of a few years followed by certain death. Ogden set out to learn about assisted suicide and euthanasia as it was playing out in the community of HIV/AIDS sufferers in Vancouver. Part of his research involved interviewing people who had observed and/or played an active role in an assisted death.

The second researcher is Rik Scarce, who in the early 1990s was in the PhD program in Sociology at the Pullman campus of Washington State University. Scarce's interest was in the community of animal rights activists, and a group he had extensive contact with was ALF—the Animal Liberation Front. Scarce had been a journalist prior to working on his PhD, had already written a book on the radical environmental movement entitled *Eco-Warriors* (Scarce, 1990), and intended to do a more scholarly treatment of the topic for his dissertation.

One of the first differences between the two researchers seems to be the quality of supervision they received. Ogden's supervisor was Simon Verdun-Jones, a Yale-educated lawyer. Although by the early 1990s there had never been a case in Canada where a researcher was subpoenaed and asked to divulge confidential research information, Verdun-Jones nonetheless encouraged Ogden to design his research in a manner that anticipated the Wigmore criteria while meeting all of SFU's policy requirements with respect to ethics review. In contrast, Scarce did not even know that he was supposed to submit his research for ethics review, and consequently did not. There is thus one clear contrast from the first moment their research began—Ogden was doing a project that was authorized by the institution, consistent with policy, had an existing paper trail that included documentation of how important maintaining confidentiality would be to ensure that participants would feel comfortable sharing information about illegal behavior, and anticipated the sort of evidence a court would be looking for if a legal challenge to Ogden's promise of confidentiality were to arise. In contrast, Scarce's project had not been reviewed and thus did not have an official institutional stamp of approval, although it should be noted that, as far as we can tell, Scarce's research was done in a manner completely consistent with the American Sociological Association's code of ethics.

But then comes the moment that seems to come from nowhere that changes your life. In Ogden's case, it was when the Vancouver Coroner read an article about assisted suicide in a Vancouver paper that included mention of Ogden's research. The article led him to wonder whether Ogden might know something about a death he was currently investigating. The Coroner issued Ogden a subpoena with the intention of asking him whether he knew anything about the assisted death written about in the paper and, if so, the identity of the two persons—a friend and a physician of the deceased—who were there at the time of her death (Palys & Lowman, 2014). For Scarce, the moment came some time after he returned home from a vacation to find that the animal care facility at Washington State had been vandalized to the tune of about $100,000, and that the prime suspect in the case was the member of ALF who had house-sat and cat-sat for Scarce while he and his family were away. In his case the subpoena came from a grand jury—a setting often referred to as a "prosecutor's dream" because there is no judge present, you are not allowed a lawyer, and the prosecutor can thus ask pretty much anything they want—that was looking into who might be charged with the crime (Scarce, 1990, 2005).

It is interesting that those also were the moments both researchers were formally abandoned by their respective universities. Rather than jumping in with legal assistance to defend the respective attacks on their research participants and academic freedom, both universities did little to nothing to help. After first denying him any assistance at all, SFU offered Ogden a token amount on "compassionate" grounds when Ogden's advisor made a final plea for assistance, but otherwise left Ogden to find his own representation (Lowman & Palys, 2000). At WSU, meanwhile, Scarce's university used the fact that he had not gone through ethics review to deny him legal representation, and as the victim of the vandalism, seemed more interested in helping legal authorities put pressure on Scarce to identify the perpetrator, if indeed he even knew who it might have been, than on defending academic freedom and Scarce's research participants (Scarce, 2005).

It is also important to note that neither researcher was abandoned completely. Ogden's department stood behind him and wrote letters that almost all members of the department signed urging the university to recognize the importance of the case and fund Ogden's legal defense. Two members of the department also led the charge afterward to have the university recognize, however retroactively, the error of its ways (see Palys & Lowman, 2014). Scarce's department sent similar urgings to WSU's administrators, while fellow graduate students and faculty members at the university began what today would be called a "crowdfunding" initiative to fund his legal defense (see Scarce, 2005). By hook or by crook each researcher thus was able to muster legal representation; both also were determined never to disclose information that would be harmful to their research participants. From that point on, however, things proceeded quite differently. We use the four Wigmore criteria to highlight differences in the legal status of the respective claims for privilege the two researchers made.

Criterion 1: Establishing a Shared Expectation of Confidentiality. The first criterion tells us that a prerequisite for claiming privilege is that the two or more people involved in the relation must have a shared understanding that their communication was, in fact, confidential. As Wigmore (1905) wrote, "The moment confidence ceases, privilege ceases" (p. 3233). In practical terms, this means researchers should ensure there is a clear "expectation of confidentiality" that is shared by researcher and participant and that the research record includes evidence that speaks to that understanding.

In the few US cases where things have gone badly for researchers (e.g., see Cecil & Wetherington, 1996; Lowman & Palys, 2001a; Palys & Lowman, 2002, 2014), it is noteworthy that none had evidence regarding this first element. In Scarce's case, Scarce's failure to go through ethics review meant he also had no record of the pledge he had made to participants, nor was there any formal indication or approval that showed he was engaged in an activity that was university-approved and being executed in accordance with the canons of his discipline. Nor had he kept records of his and the participants' understanding regarding confidentiality in field notes.

In cases where a researcher–participant privilege *was* recognized, the opposite held true. For example, when the Vancouver coroner subpoenaed Russel Ogden and asked him to identify research participants who may have witnessed the death, Ogden presented evidence showing that he had completed a proposal and undergone a research ethics review. He also was able to produce copies of the pledge of confidentiality he had made to prospective participants. These established that Ogden was indeed engaged in "research," that appropriate officials at the university believed his plan reflected the highest ethical standards of his discipline, and that he and his participants shared the understanding that their interactions were completely confidential.

A matter of no small legal importance with respect to Ogden's pledge was that it was unequivocal. Anything less runs the risk of being treated as a "waiver of privilege" by the courts. For example, in Atlantic Sugar v. United States (1980), corporate respondents to an International Trade Commission questionnaire were told that the information they provided would not be disclosed "except as required by law." A US Customs Court later used this exception to justify its order of disclosure of research information from researchers, saying they were the law and "required" the information.

Criterion 2: Establishing That Confidentiality Is Essential. Because claims of research-participant privilege are decided on a case-by-case basis in the absence of statute-based protections, general claims about the importance of confidentiality to research are not enough. Researchers also should be ready to demonstrate that confidentiality is crucial *to the specific research project* in which confidentiality is being challenged (Daisley, 1994; Jackson & MacCrimmon, 1999; Palys & Lowman, 2000, 2002). Traynor (1996) suggests that the necessity of confidentiality should be addressed in research proposals, thereby showing that confidentiality was part of a considered plan and neither capricious nor rote. For example, Ogden's research proposal explained why he believed it would be impossible to gather reliable and valid data and to meet the ethical standards of his discipline unless he offered complete confidentiality to participants.

Claims that confidentiality was "essential" can be weakened by behavior that is inconsistent with—or can be depicted as inconsistent with—such claims. For example, in the *Scarce* case, the court seemed skeptical about his claim of privilege when it became known that Scarce and the research participant who was the prime suspect in the case were friends outside the research context. Was the researcher truly claiming privilege because of the research relationship? Or was he using it out of convenience and his allegiance to a friend? The claim of privilege was undermined further when it became evident the researcher's wife was at a key breakfast meeting where information about the vandalism may have been shared, when the wife had not been shown in evidence to be part of the research team (*In re Grand Jury Proceedings: James Richard Scarce*, 1993; O'Neil, 1996; Scarce, 1994, 1999). While Scarce was adamant no such conversation occurred, court decisions sometimes turn not on the basis of what *did* happen, but on what *could* have happened during a particular interlude. If confidentiality is important, then your actions should be consistent with that claim, and "confidential" conversations do not happen when people who are not part of the research team are present.

In contrast, Russel Ogden only strengthened his claim for privilege by asking participants directly—and recording their answers—how important the provision of confidentiality was to their participation. All participants who had witnessed or participated in an assisted suicide or euthanasia stated that confidentiality was vital to their participation. They would divulge information to Ogden *only* if he promised to keep the fact of their involvement in an assisted death and participation in the study confidential. The coroner found this evidence persuasive, recognizing that the information he sought never would have existed in the first place had it not been for Ogden's guarantee, which he now was obliged ethically to honor (Inquest of Unknown Female, 1994).

Criterion 3: Establishing That the Community Values the Relationship. The third criterion asks whether the relationship under scrutiny is so socially valued that "the community" believes it should be protected. That is a fairly easy criterion for research to meet. Governments, corporations, and institutions set aside billions of dollars every year for research because we believe that advancing knowledge and gathering information that allows us to create better informed policy and law is a valuable thing to do. Various other "communities" can be considered as well, depending on the specifics of the case, such as the community of which participants in the research at hand are members; those who engage in policy formulation and implementation and who value independent research that contributes to that task; and the broader citizenry, who benefit from the knowledge created through research. Much of this information would come from expert testimony when and if the researcher is subpoenaed. However, there is also evidence that can be gathered and material that should be retained as one goes through the process of preparing for and executing the research.

For example, any research that has satisfied peer review, secured funding, and/or undergone ethics review must clearly be valued by the research community. Court decisions, too, often make reference to and reflect the high value that society places on academic research (e.g., *Dow Chemical v. Allen*, 1982; *In Re: Michael A. Cusumano and David B. Yoffe*, 1998; *Richards of Rockford v. Pacific Gas and Electric Co.*, 1976). In Ogden's trial, an internationally renowned criminologist testified about the importance of confidentiality to research such as Ogden's. A nurse who had worked with Vancouver's HIV/AIDS community for years also testified about how important confidentiality was within that community, especially given the hysteria about HIV/AIDS at that time. In Scarce's case, in addition to many colleagues and associations from his own university and beyond who offered support, the American Sociological Association submitted an *amicus curiae* ("friend of the court") brief that outlined the importance of confidentiality to the research enterprise, its importance in allowing social scientists to contribute to social understanding, and affirmed that Scarce was behaving in a manner consistent with the highest ethical standards of the discipline.

Criterion 4: A Balancing of Interests. Any well-designed social or health science research on a sensitive topic that anticipates the evidentiary requirements of the Wigmore test should satisfy the first three criteria easily. The fourth criterion sees the court balance the social values upheld in the researcher–participant relationship against the costs that would be incurred by withholding relevant evidence in the case at hand. In Ogden's case, this came down to Ogden's need to maintain his ethical pledge to participants and the impact a disclosure would have on the research enterprise if Ogden complied *versus* the coroner's need for the evidence to make an accurate determination of the Unknown Female's identity and cause of death in the inquest at hand.

But note the asymmetry here: until a "class" privilege is recognized, researchers have to make their decisions ahead of time and can only hope they are correct in their speculation of the range of circumstances that might arise, while the courts make their decisions after the fact on the basis of the concrete facts that are presented to them. The US Supreme Court recognized this paradox in a case involving a claim of therapist–client privilege (*Jaffee v. Redmond*, 1996):

We part company with the Court of Appeals on a separate point. We reject the balancing component of the privilege implemented by that court and a small number of States. Making the promise of confidentiality contingent upon a trial judge's later evaluation of the relative importance of the patient's interest in privacy and the evidentiary need for disclosure would eviscerate the effectiveness of the privilege. … [I]f the purpose of the privilege is to be served, the participants in the confidential conversation "must be able to predict with some degree of certainty whether particular discussions will be protected. An uncertain privilege, or one which purports to be certain but results in widely varying applications by the courts, is little better than no privilege at all."

Researchers face exactly this dilemma. We can see what decisions the courts have made and feel some degree of confidence that research can meet the Wigmore criteria and that the judiciary has been very respectful of the rights of research participants. But with the balancing exercise that is involved in the Wigmore test and that courts apply even when not formally engaging Wigmore (e.g., recall the balancing exercise described in the Microsoft case), all we really know in advance is that the law will be made after the fact on the basis of a situation we can only guess at. Who can predict at the outset of their research when a situation will arise in relation to a research project that might be of interest to a legal authority and what the specific legal issues will be involved in that case? And yet, researchers must make their decisions ahead of time.

Other Confidentiality Considerations

The Intersection of Ethics and Law. The ideal course of action for any researcher is to do their best to be ethical *and* legal, as Cusumano and Yoffie and Russel Ogden and many other researchers who have been subpoenaed have demonstrated is possible. However, if a statute-based protection is not available, and the winds of chance blow a subpoena in your direction, the fact that the law is effectively made up well after your research is over creates the possibility that the "ethical" thing to do—to fulfill your duty to protect your research participants and their right to confidentiality—may conflict with the "legal" thing to do—to give identifying information to a court when a legal order for disclosure is given and all legal means of resistance have been exhausted. Because of this, researchers who want to gather sensitive information from participants must decide ahead of time what they will do if, in that last instant, law and ethics point in different directions.

Criminology as a discipline would not be possible unless researchers were prepared to take a nonjudgmental approach to many of the people they study, and the same is true of many other disciplines. How can epidemiologists understand the spread of disease if persons who have them are unwilling to talk to researchers because they will be reported if they admit exposure? How can political scientists understand the development of political attitudes and social policies if members of fringe groups see the researcher as a prospective agent of the state? If we believe that studying these difficult and controversial areas is a prerequisite to the positive, rational, and humane development of law and policy, ensuring research participant confidentiality is safeguarded so that they do not pay a price for their altruism and our benefit is a fundamental ethical requirement; to do any less seems exploitative. This stance is reflected in the draft *Code of Ethics* of the Academy of Criminal Justice Sciences, which states,

> *Confidential information provided by research participants should be treated as such by members of the Academy, even when this information enjoys no legal protection or privilege and legal force is applied. The obligation to respect confidentiality also applies to members of research organizations (interviewers, coders, clerical staff, etc.) who have access to the information. It is the responsibility of administrators and chief investigators to instruct staff members on this point and to make every effort to insure that access to confidential information is restricted.*[6]

Other disciplines say much the same thing. For example:

> *[P]riority must be given to the protection of research participants, as well as the preservation and protection of research records. Researchers have an ethical responsibility to take precautions that raw data and collected materials will not be used for unauthorized ends. … Researchers have a responsibility to use appropriate methods to ensure the confidentiality and security of field notes, recordings, samples or other primary data and the identities of participants. (American Anthropological Association Principles of Ethical Responsibility, 2012)*

> *As citizens, researchers have an obligation to cooperate with grand juries, other law enforcement agencies, and institutional officials. Conversely, researchers also have a professional duty not to divulge the identity of confidential sources of information or data developed in the course of research, whether to governmental or non-governmental officials or bodies, even though in the present state of American law*

---

[6]Online at https://www.acjs.org/page/Code_Of_Ethics.

they run the risk of suffering an applicable penalty. (American Political Science Association Guide to Professional Ethics in Political Science [2nd ed.], 2012)

Sociologists take all reasonable precautions to protect the confidentiality rights of research participants. … Confidential information provided by research participants should be treated as such by sociologists even if there is no legal protection or privilege to do so. … To ensure that access to confidential information is restricted and respected, it is the responsibility of researchers, collaborators, and administrators to instruct and supervise staff and research workers to ensure they take the steps necessary to protect confidentiality. (American Sociological Association [ASA] Code of Ethics, 2018)

However, all these codes also enjoin researchers to understand the law as it relates to their work, to consider possible limitations to confidentiality that may arise from either legal and/or ethical considerations, to make an ethical choice about how these will or will not affect their work, and to be honest and forthcoming to research participants about these choices.

In our view, the question we need to ask ourselves for any piece of research we do is whether we believe the rights of our participants and the knowledge we are gaining outweigh any other foreseeable concerns or interests that might arise in the research. If the answer to that question is yes, then one proper ethical course is to give an unqualified pledge of confidentiality, and, having made that decision and the promise that goes with it, we are ethically obliged to keep it. If the answer is no, you would give up the information if ordered to do so, then in our view the proper course of action is to not do the research because you would have to limit confidentiality, and that would be placing research participants at risk for your benefit—i.e., downloading the problem to them—when you have a duty to protect them from harm and not throw them to the wolves when the going gets tough.

In the cases of Ogden and Scarce, both researchers understood their obligations and both were prepared to go to jail if they had to in order to protect their participants and maintain the integrity of their pledges to participants, who would not have taken part without those pledges. In Ogden's case, the Coroner accepted that Ogden met the Wigmore criteria and recognized a researcher–participant privilege in that case. In contrast, the Scarce case did not end well, with the researcher escorted to jail for contempt of court. Incarceration for contempt is supposed to be "coercive" rather than "punitive," so in theory you stay in jail until the judge becomes convinced that further incarceration will not persuade you to disclose the information sought by the court. The first researcher to be incarcerated for failure to disclose when ordered by a court was Samuel Popkin, a Harvard political scientist who went to jail for 8 days in 1972 when he refused to identify his sources for the *Pentagon Papers*, a secret study of America's involvement in the Vietnam War (see Popkin, 2001). Scarce was the second, and he would spend 159 days in jail (see Scarce, 2005 for his discussion both of the case and his incarceration). While his case serves as an exemplar of how not to prepare for research on a controversial social issue, both Scarce and Ogden stand as beacons of integrity in their willingness to put themselves in harm's way to ensure that those who participated in their research were not harmed, something we all benefit from.

Is It Ever Reasonable to Limit Confidentiality?

A Realistic Appraisal of the Situation. We find there are three major reasons some researchers have cited for limiting their pledge of confidentiality. The first is purely pragmatic and reflects a realistic assessment of the risks that exist in some situation. For example, when we do one-on-one interviews, the information gathered in that interview is very much within our control and our responsibility to protect. However, when we do group interviews—sometimes known as focus group interviews (see Chapter 10)—we can encourage the various people in the group to respect each other's privacy outside the interview setting, but we have less control over what members of the group will do. Accordingly, we need to remind participants that while we will do everything on our part to maintain confidentiality, there are also elements beyond our control they should consider when deciding what to share with us.

A related concern we have these days with respect to digital technologies is the extent to which digital has become synonymous with "hackable." Ever since Edward Snowden's revelations about the extent of NSA and CIA surveillance of Americans' communications and the extent of cooperation they were receiving from companies such as Google, Facebook, Verizon, and so on (e.g., Greenwald, 2014; see also Palys, 2016; Zuboff, 2015), researchers pretty much have to operate on the assumption that any digitized communications that are not created with end-to-end encryption are very likely to be recorded somewhere and retrievable. In such situations, explaining to prospective participants that confidentiality may be limited would be a wise move.

At the same time, merely informing the participant about a risk does not take the researcher off the hook from protecting the participant from that risk. If we had no choice but to use the hackable technology, then we would do so and would warn our participant about that possibility, but we also would feel obliged either to refrain from asking questions that could cause the person harm if disclosed or look for a non-connected technology as an alternative. For example, when recording an in-person interview on a sensitive topic, a stand-alone digital recorder with no network connectivity would be preferable to using a recording app on your smartphone; the former would create a file you would then want to encrypt before putting in any network-connected device, while the latter would be hackable from the moment of its creation and may or may not be retrievable even if you were to delete it from your phone (because either your phone provider or internet service provider may have it on its servers).

(Un)Anticipated Third-Party Harm. A second scenario of interest occurs where a researcher learns of some horrific fate that will befall an innocent third party and the researcher considers violating confidentiality for the higher ethic of preventing harm to an innocent individual. The key thing to consider here is whether or not such revelations of prospective harm are anticipated (e.g., Palys & Lowman, 2014). If they are *not* anticipated, then it makes little sense to refer to them in informed consent statements. For example, it would be a tad absurd and somewhat offensive to start off interviews with parents by saying something like, "These interviews about your children's teachers are completely confidential unless you tell me that you are going to kill one of them." We assume the best of our interviewees unless there is reason to believe otherwise, and a pledge of confidentiality about their views of teachers is exactly that, a pledge about their provision of that information. Any plot to kill one of the teachers would be beyond the realm of what we would normally anticipate in such a project, and the researcher would have to figure out some ethical way to try and prevent that harm without violating the rights of the participant they are still obliged to protect.

The decision-making becomes a bit more challenging in situations where we might well *anticipate* getting information involving harm to third parties. For example, in the literature on prisons, there has been an ongoing debate regarding the effects of solitary confinement on prisoners. One set of researchers argued that there is really no problematic effect to solitary confinement per se, while another group of researchers argued that the effects of solitary confinement can be very debilitating and in particular may lead prisoners to become more violent to themselves (i.e., suicidal, self-mutilating) and/or others (i.e., assaultive).

If we wanted to do research in which we assessed what happens to prisoners who are placed in solitary confinement, it seems unlikely that prisoners would tell us about these tendencies if they knew we would inform authorities about anything unseemly they disclose. Imagine you are a prisoner placed in solitary confinement, whereupon a researcher comes up to you and says, "I would like to interview you about the effects of solitary confinement. I am particularly interested in hearing whether you have any intention to harm yourself or others. However, I should warn you that if you tell me anything along those lines, I'll be obliged to tell prison authorities."

If you were a prisoner who was planning on doing harm to yourself or someone else, would you tell the researcher about those desires, knowing that the researcher would then go and tell prison authorities? We suspect not. And yet that is exactly the position in which Ivan Zinger and his colleagues (Zinger, 1999; Zinger, Wichmann, & Andrews, 2001) placed their participants in research conducted in three maximum security prisons concerning the effects of solitary confinement. In the end, Zinger found that prisoners in solitary were no more likely than inmates in the general prison population to report a desire to harm themselves or others and, because of that, sided with researchers who had argued that there are no terrible effects to solitary confinement. Given that Zinger was at that time an employee of Corrections Canada (where the research was done) and that his results place a stamp of approval on Corrections Canada policies—"Problems with the use of solitary confinement? What problems?"—we can only see the limitation of confidentiality in this case as an exercise in self-interest (see Lowman & Palys, 2001b; Palys & Lowman, 2001).

To the extent that other researchers follow Zinger's lead and routinely limit confidentiality, we can envision a huge credibility gap arising in situations where self-interest leads a variety of authorities to want to find nothing, that is, to do research "with eyes wide shut." Imagine wanting to study police interrogations in order to determine whether and how frequently they violate the rights of accused and limiting confidentiality by telling officers that any violations will be reported to superiors. Or imagine studying the ways that forestry and mining companies circumvent environmental regulations and telling employees that anything they tell you might be subject to subpoena. We can imagine the headlines now: "Police Always Follow Procedure, Says Study"; "Study Finds Resource Companies Always Respect Environmental Regulations." How comforting.

We don't mean to minimize the difficulties and ethical soul-searching that can characterize such situations, but remember again that there are two things we need to consider whenever we undertake a piece of research. One is what it takes to ensure that the data we end up with are valid and reliable, i.e., the scientific obligation. If we end up with data whose validity is questionable, then we have wasted everyone's time and perhaps placed people at risk for nothing. Indeed, that is our biggest concern with Zinger's research regarding the effects of solitary confinement; however important the question he addressed and however thoughtful other elements of his research design may have been, his decision to limit confidentiality made the value of the information he gathered questionable. So why gather it in the first place?

The second part of the equation involves the humane considerations that we have for our research participants and those around us. And on that score we have to consider whether hearing about some things and gaining some kinds of knowledge are worth it. Zinger began his research by noting that 19 prisoners died in custody in Canadian prisons from suicide or homicide in the year preceding his research. To what extent did solitary confinement contribute to that number? Could more humane policies or procedures or the simple banishment of forced solitary confinement reduce that number? Do we want to know or don't we? By limiting confidentiality, Zinger will never know. Is the long-term benefit of potentially saving 19 lives per year worth going into this research with an unqualified guarantee of confidentiality? In our view, that is exactly the question that has to be answered. Because the validity of the data depends on the guarantee of confidentiality, the choice is between deciding that the benefits are worth it and doing the research with full confidentiality or deciding that it is not and withdrawing from the research. This does not prevent researchers from taking actions designed to try to avoid the harm that otherwise would result, but they must do so in a way that respects the rights of the informant as well.

Mandatory Reporting. A third reason researchers might limit confidentiality is when a mandatory reporting law known at the outset of the research is relevant to them. For example, many states have a **mandatory reporting** requirement when anyone hears about a child in need of care because of ongoing abuse. Another widely known criterion for mandatory reporting arose at the University of California at Berkeley in *Tarasoff v. Regents of University of California* (1976). In that case, Prosenjit Poddar, a student, told a psychologist at the University who was treating him that he planned to kill Tatiana Tarasoff after she rejected his marriage proposal. Mr. Poddar repeated the threat several times, which led the psychologist to tell Poddar he would have to take steps to restrain him if the threats continued. At that point, the client stopped attending therapy. The psychologist informed campus security who interviewed Poddar, thought he seemed rational, and left after he promised he would stay away from Ms. Tarasoff. Instead, Poddar soon thereafter bought a gun and killed Tarasoff. Her parents sued the university for negligence for failing to inform them or their daughter about the threat. The case ultimately made its way to the Supreme Court of California, where the court majority decided that,

> [O]nce a therapist does in fact determine, or under applicable professional standards reasonably should have determined, that a patient poses a serious danger of violence

to others, he bears a duty to exercise reasonable care to protect the foreseeable victim of that danger. (Tarasoff, 1976, at 31)

Although a decision of the California Supreme Court is not binding on other states, many other states nonetheless have since adopted Tarasoff-inspired mandatory reporting laws. There is wide variation in the requirements from state to state, however, and the decision itself remains very controversial (see Bollas & Sundelson, 1995; Herbert & Young, 2002).

Researcher Conflicts of Interest

Being "ethical" as a researcher means that you have a primary obligation to consider things from research participants' perspectives and to ensure participants' rights are safeguarded. In many cases the interests of researcher and participant coincide. Researchers become researchers for many different reasons, but two we frequently hear include the desire to understand something deeply and well for its own sake (whether as a general motive or to understand some specific domain) and to generate knowledge that will help produce some social good. Research participants are also typically altruistic; none of them gets any direct or large reward for participating. So in that sense, both researchers and participants often share the belief that something is important, and both hope their actions will produce knowledge that will benefit the greater good.

However, it would be naive of us to assume that the interests of researchers and research participants always coincide. Occasions may arise when it is in the researcher's self-interest to gloss over the details in order to ensure a ready supply of research participants from whom they can gather information. And these days many university researchers engage in entrepreneurial interests in addition to their university "day job": consulting; creating standardized tests that are used in schools, hospitals, prisons, and other institutions; and other product development such as pharmaceuticals, software, and educational materials. Concern arises over the conflicts of interest these activities may bring to the underlying research, for example, where development of a particular product can result in considerable wealth being generated from patents, royalties, fees, and commissions, or where a favorable evaluation may result in an increase in share value. In these situations the university researcher is no longer an "independent" researcher who is simply following knowledge for its own sake with no stake in the outcome.

This conflict of interest is particularly problematic when the researcher is in a position of power relative to the research participant—or when the gatekeeper who has allowed the researcher access to the participants is in a position of power over the participants—and is especially worrisome in the case of captive audiences who depend on the researcher for other rewards. For example, it used to be that many psychology departments would require students—especially the hundreds or even thousands who take Introductory Psychology at some universities—to participate in research in return for partial course credit, in part because it gives students the experience of what it is like to be a research participant but also to keep up the supply of bodies required for faculty member and graduate student research. The practice still continues in many places, but there is now more effort made to ensure that students have reasonable options if they would rather decline the opportunity.

Of course, many of those studies entail little or no risk whatsoever; the major one is probably the possibility of dying of boredom. However, other "captive" situations are far more problematic, as the following incident reveals:

> We used prison inmates in a number of research projects and always asked for their consent. However, in retrospect, it seems to me that since I also sat on boards that made recommendations for parole and had other important influences on their prison lives, it might be questioned whether they really felt free to refuse in view of their high need in these areas. (APA, 1973, p. 47)

Ethics problems arise when the power differential between researcher and participant is considerable. They are exacerbated when the prospective risk to participants or the possible cost to them if they refuse to participate is high, for example, where the researcher is also the teacher who hands out grades, the healthcare provider who is also responsible for treatment, or the prison authority who is also responsible for maintaining discipline or making recommendations for positive rewards like day passes or parole. From an ethical perspective, it is incumbent on the researcher to seek out independent advice on how best to deal with any appearance of conflict of interest—conflict that would be evident to any neutral third party looking at the situation. The most common ways of doing so are taking steps to alleviate the conflict—for example, by divesting yourself from one side or the other of the conflict, such as by divesting yourself of shares in the company, or getting an independent decision-maker involved who has no vested interest in the outcome and is not in any way dependent on or related to the researcher.

Conflicts of Role

A woman was sitting on a riverbank one day, soaking up the sun, when suddenly she saw a man in the river in danger of drowning, calling for help.[7] She bravely jumped into the water, swam over to the man, dragged him out, and saved him by giving him artificial resuscitation. But no sooner had she sat down to catch her breath when another body appeared in the water, and she jumped in again and saved that person as well. Both were thanking her profusely when suddenly a third body appeared and in she jumped again. But no sooner than she had finished saving that person, yet another appeared in the water! However, this time, instead of jumping into the water, she began to walk upstream.

"Hey!" called someone who had been watching all of this unfold. "Aren't you going to save that guy as well?"

"Hell, no!" she replied. "I'm going to go upstream to find out how all these people are ending up in the river in the first place!"

It is difficult to be in two places at once, as is the case with the woman in our story. She can be the first responder who jumps in and saves people, or she can don a researcher's cap and head upstream to find out what is causing the situation, but she cannot be in both places at the same time. An analogous situation arises when the individual doing the research occupies two different roles with respect to the participant where the duties associated with the two roles come into conflict.

We have already described how the primary ethical duty of the researcher is to protect their research participants. With respect to confidentiality, this typically means putting your judgmental hat aside and listening to whatever it is that the participant wants to share with you, and sometimes what people tell you is not pretty. This is especially true in regards to many of the social and health problem areas that are most important to understand—poverty, addiction, disease, abuse, oppression, exploitation, harassment, bullying, prejudice and discrimination, corruption. For anyone who has a duty of confidentiality, the bar that might justify a disclosure is set very high.

However, there are now many professionals—including, for example, social workers, physicians, teachers, nurses and counselors—whose professional codes of ethics call on them to report certain kinds of behavior to authorities, with lower triggers for disclosure than were outlined in the *Tarasoff* case, for example. These often are

---

[7]We first came across this story in Stan Cohen's (1985) Visions of Social Control. He attributes it to social activist Saul Alinsky. We offer our own version of it here.

"helping" professionals whose inclination and obligation, going back to our allegory of bodies in the river, is to jump in the river and save whoever is floating downstream. There are many situations where their professional codes of ethics do not clash with codes of research ethics, but many others where they will, and confidentiality is one of those areas.

If left unmanaged, the main problem with these role conflicts is that they can put the researcher in a policing role—as was the case with Ivan Zinger in his study of the effects of solitary confinement—instead of simply trying to understand the situation, which is what research is supposedly all about. Researchers should avoid being put in a position of becoming informants for authorities or leaders of organizations.

Balancing and Combining Ethical Principles

Although not exhaustive, the list above describes some of the major principles you need to consider before undertaking your research. The role of the researcher is to treat research participants with care. A general rule we always try to apply is to ask what standard we would expect a researcher to follow if the participant was a family member or close friend.

And of course there are many issues we haven't discussed in this relatively intro-ductory treatise: situations that arise in particular research contexts that pose unique dilemmas and have been the subject of considerable debate. Where does "encour-agement to participate" end and "coercion" begin? What ethical safeguards should researchers practice when they are dealing with cultures and groups other than their own? Is concern about privacy outmoded when tens of millions of people put the intimate details of their lives on Facebook and line up to participate in reality TV shows that leave nothing of their personal lives to the imagination?

Our main intention in this chapter has been to try and convey something about some of the main ethical principles that researchers bring to their work. But if "being ethical" involved no more than following a bunch of principles or rules in relatively predictable scenarios, then everything would be easy. We're all intelligent people; we all want to be ethical; we all have a sense of right and wrong. However, problems arise for at least three main reasons, all of which suggest that it's not as easy as it looks.

First is that the very nature of research involves some degree of unpredictability. If we knew exactly what was going to happen, there would be no need to do the research. The implication is that, instead of relatively *certain* costs and benefits, we are often weighing our best *guesses* of costs and benefits in particular situations that arise as the research unfolds.

A second source of difficulty is that ethical principles do not exist in isolation. All of them operate in any given situation and sometimes they conflict. "Being ethical" thus involves not simply following a set of rules but trying to find a way to resolve competing demands, balancing and trading off different "goods," and making decisions based on the perspective and best interests of our research participants.

An implication of the above is the third difficulty, i.e., that there are rarely any clear-cut "right" and "wrong" ethical answers. Add to this the fact that researchers and participants are individual human beings who differ from one another, have different belief systems, and value ethical principles differently—because of the value systems they bring to the research—and part of the "problem" is to recognize that there are potentially different ways to deal with situations, more than one of which can be ethically defensible.

Indeed, far too much time is spent by would-be ethicists arguing about what the "right answers" are, as if these were things that could be determined absolutely once and for all, when (arguably) the more important issue is whether the *process* of ethics consideration engaged in by the researcher has adequately taken into account the perspective of participants and the specifics of the case as they are known. At bottom is the question of whether the research can survive mechanisms of accountability that revere two core principles: whether we adequately consider and protect the rights of the research participant, whose dignity we value and without whose participation the research enterprise would not exist, and whether it is respectful of the academic freedom of the researcher, which is a cornerstone of the research enterprise and without which the social value of research would be undermined.

Beyond some reading that discusses ethics issues and some of the more contentious debates that have raged in the social and health sciences on these issues, your ethics education will come in large part from a frontline involvement with research where you meet real people and, we hope, take the time to know your research participants as people. And notwithstanding the general principles that books like this espouse, ethics considerations always come down to case-by-case considerations that involve a unique mix of the people who are your participants, the specific issue you are researching, your own perspective and interests, the norms and standards of your discipline, the social and legal context in which you are operating, and on and on. There are few simple answers, and you owe it to yourselves and your participants to give these matters deep consideration.

SUMMING UP AND LOOKING AHEAD

In this chapter we have attempted to convey some of the many complexities that must be faced whenever we do research with human participants. If there is a central point to this chapter, it is to think about the relations you allow to exist between researcher and researched.

We began by examining the Common Rule that governs the regulation of ethics by the IRBs in the United States, noting that similar federal policies exist in Canada, Britain, and Australia, to name a few. We noted how there has been a trend toward more extensive and more centralized ethics regulation over time, at least in part because of some particularly horrific examples of overzealous researchers trampling research participant rights. Although we generally support the idea of ethics review because of the opportunity this allows for an independent look at the proposed research by a third party, concerns arise to the extent these third parties are themselves involved in conflicts of interest that lead them to advance views and interests that can be at odds with the rights and interests of research participants and the ethical obligations and academic freedom interests of researchers.

Research participants are a crucial resource to science disciplines that attempt to understand human action, and, particularly when we are in a more privileged position than our research participants, and especially when we are in a position of power over participants, we must live up to our obligation to maintain their dignity and treat them with care. In this regard, we introduced several major ethics principles that transcend disciplinary boundaries, including the balancing of scientific and human considerations that influence whether we engage the research in the first place, the principles of informed consent and the maintenance of confidentiality, and issues of researcher, IRB, and institutional conflicts of interest and researcher conflicts of role.

Key Concepts

Academic freedom 107
Anonymity 120
Certificates of Confidentiality 124
Class privilege 125
Common law 125
Common Rule 108
Confidentiality 118
Conflict of interest 143
Conflicts of role 144

Encryption 121
Ethics creep 110
Gatekeeper 143
Humanistic obligation 112
Information sheet 115
Informed consent 114
Mandatory reporting 141
Nuremberg Code 105
Privacy certificate 124

Privilege 123
Pseudonyms 120
Redact 120
Scientific obligation 112
Secondary data 117
Statute-based protections 123
Wigmore criteria 128

STUDY QUESTIONS

1. According to the chapter, what is the "basic ethical dilemma"? Why is it a dilemma?

2. What does each of the following concepts mean, and how can you ensure that they are implemented in your research: informed consent, confidentiality, anonymity.

3. Look up a recent issue of a journal in your area of study, pick an article that interests you, and evaluate it in terms of the ethical principles outlined in this chapter.

4. Is an AA meeting "public" because anyone can walk in and participate? Or is it "private" because the people who go there for help have an expectation of privacy once they have taken the bold step of sitting down and seeking help for a serious problem? Does it make it any more acceptable if the researchers ensure that no one is ever named or otherwise identified? If so, can researchers go anywhere and watch anything as long as no participant is ever identified?

5. Seek out the ethical guidelines of the discipline or career for which you are studying. Are the principles discussed in this chapter included among the guidelines of your discipline? What new issues arise that are not dealt with here?

6. What is the difference between anonymity and confidentiality? What procedures can you follow to ensure confidentiality? What legal mechanisms exist for the protection of the confidentiality of research participants?

7. What are the three sources of privilege? How do they differ?

8. What are the Wigmore criteria, and why is it beneficial to know them? Give some concrete suggestions on how you can integrate your knowledge of the Wigmore criteria into your research.

9. Describe some of the ways ethics regulation has changed over the last 40 years.

10. Go to your university's or college's website and read the ethics policy. What does your institution do to ensure there is no institutional conflict of interest?

11. How many IRBs are there at your university or college? Who are the members of the IRB that you would be applying to? Do they represent the full range of research done at your institution? Are there committee representatives who have expertise in both qualitative and quantitative research traditions?

12. The Common Rule encourages research ethics boards to have at least one "community member" on the board. Who is/are the community member(s) at your institution? In what way might the presence of this/those person(s) be beneficial for researchers and research participants? In what ways might it be detrimental?

13. Discuss the question of the rights of researchers in relation to the rights of participants, and generate your own criteria for how conflicting interests might be resolved (1) when the researcher is in a position of power over participants and (2) when the researcher is dependent on an agency and/or participants for continued funding and access.

14. This chapter has argued that, while researchers should make every effort to be both "ethical" and "legal," situations might arise where those two are placed in conflict, that is, you must choose between acting ethically but in violation of a particular law (e.g., you can live up to your ethical obligation to protect the rights of your research participants only by defying a court order to disclose confidential research information) or to act legally but in violation of an ethical obligation (e.g., follow a court order to disclose confidential research information even though this brings harm to your participant). Put yourself in these situations. Which do you believe is more important? What does your discipline's code of ethics say about that issue?

15. In the 1950s and 1960s when formalized codes of ethics were first being developed in the social sciences, some researchers opined that formalizing a code of ethics was the best thing a discipline could do because it would protect academic freedom and keep third parties who would undermine discipline-based control at bay. Others argued the opposite, i.e., that it was a slippery slope that would ultimately undermine academic freedom and end up with nothing better than socially approved questions being asked in socially approved ways to the benefit of no one. We now have the benefit of hindsight. Sixty years later, who do you think was right?

16. You are undertaking a study in a psychiatric clinic for which you have signed an agreement guaranteeing confidentiality to the caregivers you are observing. You soon begin to notice cases where patients are apparently being denied their rights to refuse treatment, and you see two instances of what you perceive as physical abuse. Revealing this information to another authority would be a violation of the confidentiality you guaranteed. What would you do in this situation?

5

SAMPLING AND RECRUITMENT

Research does not happen in the abstract. Although we can talk about research in general terms and can identify abstract principles that are useful for guiding decisions as the research is being designed, done, and interpreted, in the end any given piece of research involves gathering specific data from specific sources in specific places at specific times. Each one of those choices is a **sample** of all of the choices that we could make in doing our research. To do research, we inevitably sample from among all the possible questions we could ask, all the behaviors (or other attributes) we could observe, and all the people or situations we could approach. Our choice of methods is a sample of all the methods we could use, our analysis of the data is a sample of all the analyses we could perform, and the pattern of findings we choose to focus on in our final write-up is a sample of all the possible patterns we might have identified and all of the different ways we might have gone about presenting this information.

These facts of research life arise simply because we cannot do everything at once. Although our general interest might be in "healthcare service delivery," in the end out of all the places we could go to study healthcare being delivered—in a clinic; at a physician's office; in a home care program; at an out-patient facility—we may choose to study service delivery in a hospital. And because we cannot go to every hospital, we decide to go to the one that is located near where we study or work. Once we get there, because we cannot watch every single delivery of every single service within the hospital, perhaps we decide to focus on services delivered within the emergency room. And because we cannot use every single method available to us, perhaps we decide to interview people as they are awaiting service and as they leave, or observe them as they go through the process, or simply look at completed files after the patient becomes a "former" patient and walks out the door. If we have the resources, we might be able to focus on two or three areas of the hospital and incorporate more than one method, but these will still be subsets of all the places that deliver health services and of all the methods we could employ.

In a literal sense, when we get to the end of our research, we could write an article about "what happened in the emergency room of Grey Sloan Memorial Hospital when we were there the week of November 13 and talked to 50 of the 333 people who went through their Emergency Room that day." But who cares? Although it may be perfectly reasonable for Grey Sloan Memorial to do in-house research that focuses only on that hospital as part of its interest in improving service delivery, most of the time when we do research in one research site we hope that what we learn there will help us understand a broader class of sites—not just Grey Sloan Memorial, but perhaps hospitals more generally, or service providers even more generally. Will the knowledge of what came of our research in that part of the hospital with those specific people on that specific day be useful to the administrators of Grey Sloan Memorial now that the day is over? Should a hospital administrator sitting in Minneapolis or Miami be interested in the results? Might the study be of interest to individuals in other kinds of settings where other types of products and services are delivered—prisons, social agencies, the tire installation center at Costco, the beer vendor at a St. Louis Cardinals baseball game? These are all questions that ask about the generalizability of our results beyond the original context of our research. The answers to them will depend on how we construct our research, and what theoretical concepts we or others who read our research invoke to explain what we have found. These all involve sampling issues and need to be understood as such.

OUR APPROACH TO SAMPLING

Before we start explaining different procedures available to you and when you might use them, there are three points we need to make to contextualize our approach to sampling, given our belief that sampling is probably one of the most misunderstood areas of the research process.

There Is No One "Best" Sampling Method

The sampling chapters in many methods books try and sell you on the idea that some sampling methods are inherently better than others. Brancati's (2018) assertion that "Random sampling is the gold standard for data collection" expresses a commonly held belief. We disagree. Anyone arguing there is one "best" method probably only has one type of research and sampling objective in mind.

Simple random sampling is most certainly the method of choice if we have a huge bag full of marbles and want to make an educated guess regarding the proportion of marbles that are red, green, and blue by looking only at a sample of them instead of counting every single one. But people are not marbles, and populations of interest to social and health scientists are not as easily defined as populations of marbles in a container. And although there are some sampling situations in the social and health sciences where a randomly chosen sample is indeed the best way to go—as we will describe below—most times such a sample is not only impossible to acquire but also a waste of time and resources to pursue even if we could acquire one, for the simple reason that employing it often would be counterproductive to answering our research questions and achieving our objectives (i.e., what we need or want to be able to do with our research findings).

In our view there is no one "best" sampling procedure across the broad range of research that is done in the social and health sciences. The "best" sampling procedure and the "best" sample in any given situation will depend on your research question(s) and objectives, your (and the literature's) understanding of the phenomenon under scrutiny, and on practical constraints. Ultimately, the most important principle is how you connect with the person(s) or other sources of information that best allow you to address whatever research question you pose (Gorden, 1980). As O'Leary (2014) phrased it more recently, "No matter what the scenario, it is absolutely crucial to figure out who [or what] might hold the answer to your research question and how you will open up opportunities to gather information from those in the know" (p. 181; bracketed words added). Depending on how you formulate that question, the right place to look and the "best" way to sample will vary. The "best" sampling method is the one that best allows you to achieve your objectives and answer your research question(s).

All Sampling Is Purposive

A second point, which follows from the first, is that all sampling is purposive, i.e., there are certain objectives the researcher is trying to accomplish in any given study, and the nature of these objectives will have implications for the sampling procedure that is most appropriate in that context. Although this may sound obvious, we mention it because it will help explain why our discussion not only eschews the idea of one best sampling procedure but also will depart from the "usual" division of sampling procedures into "probabilistic" and "nonprobabilistic" procedures.

We have abandoned that dichotomy for two main reasons. First is that such distinctions are often accompanied by discussions that extol the virtues of random sampling for the purpose of choosing samples that are theoretically **representative** of the larger population from which they were drawn. While there certainly are research questions for which a formally representative sample is highly appropriate, the types of research questions that require such a sample are but a minor part of the research that is done in the social and health sciences. Indeed, we suspect these are far outnumbered by situations where random/representative sampling would be redundant or downright self-defeating. Accordingly, we would rather focus on the purpose that probabilistic sampling procedures serve—to acquire a theoretically representative sample—and discuss them in that limited context.

Second is that we reject the label "nonprobabilistic" for the second set of procedures. Labeling these procedures on the basis of what they *are not* gives the impression we wish they could be and implies a second class status because of it. We would rather refer to them in a more positive way by focusing on what they *are* and what they seek to achieve. One implication of this shift is that we will distinguish the range of procedures typically grouped as "nonprobabilistic" into two subgroups. One of these subgroups will be called *quasi-probabilistic procedures* because their major role is to offer a reasonable approximation of a truly random sample in situations where a probabilistic procedure would be ideal, but is unavailable. The second group is distinguished because representativeness is not their priority; we will refer to this group of procedures as *purposive*, *targeted*, or *strategic* sampling procedures, because that is what they seek to do—focus on the specific site or group of people or things that will allow you to generate answers to the particular research question(s) you are addressing.

Let's Get Real

Finally, most discussions of sampling do not take into account situational factors that influence the kind of research that can actually be done. The pragmatics of everyday life, however mundane that might sound, is one such factor. Regardless how beautiful the sampling strategy looks in your proposal, one thing you quickly learn about research, and especially field-based research, is that you can never completely assess the feasibility of your sampling plan until you get to your research site and see what you will have access to and what will work in that setting at that time.

Sometimes you don't even get to the place you planned first. If the funding or grant fell through, or you engage in self-funded research with limited resources, you may not be able to afford a visit to your preferred site. Even if you can get there, you may not have the connections to get you past the front door. Most organizations will have some kind of gatekeeper with whom you will have to negotiate access. Even with access, gatekeepers will sometimes seek to constrain what you can and can't look at and/or who you can and can't talk to, leaving you the challenge of how to make the best of a less-than-perfect situation. And even if you do have unlimited access, although you may think your proposed research is the most important study that can be done, people at the research site who are the envisioned participants in the research may not share your enthusiasm, such that the 30 people you hoped would volunteer to be interviewed are nowhere to be found.

As this discussion suggests, we do believe it is important for you to understand sampling well enough to develop Plan A—the ideal plan that would be most wonderful if the sampling gods were amenable. But you also need to understand the logic of sampling well enough to make justifiable decisions to implement a Plan B when and if Plan A falls apart, which it often will, because of factors beyond your control (i.e., don't take it personally). Our goal in this chapter is to outline the range of sampling procedures you have at your disposal, as well as to outline some of the respective advantages and trade-offs that can be associated with those alternatives depending on where and how they are deployed.

THE SAMPLING PROCESS

If we start at the point where you enter the research situation with an interest in some phenomenon and some research question that you want to pursue answers to, then the sampling decisions you face come in what we envision as a two-step process. The first step is an orienting one in which you decide on a research site and source of data that is consistent with your objectives. Once you get there—and please forgive us if we conveniently ignore until later chapters all the complexity and negotiation that may involve—comes a second step where you make more specific decisions at that site about who and/or what will be your primary sources of data.

It may well be that the pervasive misunderstanding we see regarding sampling comes from the fact most chapters on sampling jump directly to step two and talk about sampling in the abstract. When sampling in the abstract, statements about "gold standards" may make some sense. But research is not done in the abstract, and it is those contextual elements that nudge us in one way or the other with respect to the sampling decisions that make the most sense. The sorts of "contextual" elements we have in mind are the aspects we made note of above, i.e., in particular, your objectives and whatever specific decision parameters exist at your chosen site.

Step One: Framing the Sample
When It Just Doesn't Matter

Part of the difficulty involved in talking about sampling comes from the varied considerations that come into play before you even begin doing your research. For example, one issue is how you envision the phenomenon you are interested in. Psychologists, for example, have long been on a search for "laws of human behavior" that apply to everyone, i.e., cultural universals. If that is the case, i.e., you believe that the principles you are looking for will be true of everyone, then it doesn't matter who you sample because everyone is ostensibly interchangeable. Any humans will do.

The logic of it is similar to a health technician who gets your physician's request for certain blood tests to be conducted. If that happens to you, we hope your technician did not read one of those chapters that talks about the random sample as the "gold standard" and starts poking holes in random locations all over your body to acquire samples of your blood for analysis. Fortunately for those of us who are not all that keen about needles, the technician need only take one blood sample from anywhere on our body, because all our blood is the same, no matter where the sample is taken from. This is one of the several reasons why psychologists do so much of their research with introductory psychology students: if the behavioral principles or laws you are looking for are universals, then it makes a lot of sense to stick with a sample that is close by, not very costly, and allows you to acquire huge numbers of participants very quickly.

Some psychologists even go a step further and search for principles that are universal even across species. Many experiments that tried to understand how humans learn were not done with humans at all. The belief was that basic principles of learning are universal, so that the way you learn that questioning your partner's integrity is a quick way to end a relationship follows the same fundamental principles by which a rat learns to turn left in a maze in order to get a food reward. And if that is so, then pigeons and rats are as good as any other organism to include in an experiment. In many ways, they are even better than introductory psychology students: you can buy them in any number from a supplier and they always show up for their appointments. As outlandish as sampling rats, pigeons, and fish might sound, the huge profits generated by casinos from Las Vegas to Atlantic City are monuments to the fact that people's behavior in response to different reinforcement schedules when pulling the lever on a slot machine is indeed exactly the same as that of a pigeon pecking a target to receive grain or a rat pressing a lever to get a food pellet.

Of course, if your interests are in trying to understand how students evaluate their professors, or the factors people consider when deciding whether to report a sexual assault, or how welcoming military officers will be of transgender recruits, then these are all clearly cases where people's views are *not* all the same and where they will hold those views for what is likely a variety of different reasons. In that case, then it *will* matter where we look and who we speak with or what we look at, and we need to consider both our objectives in doing the research and the different sampling methods at our disposal.

When Sampling Does Matter

Is it too much of a truism to say that all research has to happen somewhere and at some time? We won't get into a discussion of secondary data sources just yet (but see Chapters 9 and 12). That, too, can be thought of as a research site, but our interest right now is in how to gather new data rather than to rely on something some other person or organization has compiled. One of the first questions you have to address is what site will give you access to a sample that will allow you to address your research objective(s). Stated another way, if you want to catch some fish, step one is to find out where the sort of fish you want to catch can be found, and go there.

But as we have suggested above, where "there" is will depend on your research question(s) and objective(s), and the fact of the matter is that any given area of interest can be pursued in all sorts of equally legitimate ways. Different disciplines have different issues that interest them and different methods they favor. And even within disciplines, there can be significant differences between institutions in how they think of the discipline and what methods and procedures they think it is most important that you be exposed to.

To illustrate, let's take just one possible topic of study and brainstorm a bit about the different ways we might investigate it. There is much attention being paid these days to the practice of journalism, accusations about "fake news" and assertions of "alternative facts," allegations against social media companies regarding media manipulation they have both perpetrated and allowed, and the harassment, imprisonment, and murder of journalists that has become all too frequent in different countries. Suppose you are a student in Communications who is interested in the general question of how the news is produced out of the infinite number of events that happen in the world on any given day and how different news organizations ensure the accuracy of their stories. The sample you pursue and the sampling procedures that you follow will depend on what you want to know.

If you are wondering about the general population's confidence in the journalistic profession and the credibility they attach to different news organizations, then you might consider doing broad social surveys. Because it would be impractical to contact every person in the country to ask them that question, you would probably look to acquire a large sample of people who you hope collectively will mirror the views of the broader society, something that is best achieved by a straight random or quasi-random sampling procedure. A subquestion of interest to you might be whether there are differences among population subgroups in how they view those issues—those with differing political perspectives, people from different ethnic/cultural groups, people from different economic or educational backgrounds, in which case you will also need to make sure you have a way of distinguishing those groups in your analysis. If some of the groups you are interested in comparing are quite small relative to the size of other groups, then you may want to adapt your random sampling procedure to sample certain groups more extensively to make sure that you have reasonable numbers on which to base your analyses.

Alternatively, you may be interested in finding out how the people who define "the news" for us each day—newspaper editors and TV producers and the reporters they work with—have been affected by these developments. That might also get you thinking about doing a large-scale survey or interview or mixed methods study with individuals in those positions in a wide variety of media outlets. However, we suspect many researchers would prefer a more fine-grained analysis involving one or more detailed case studies of editors/producers/reporters of a more limited array of media that have generated the most attention in these media debates—perhaps the CNN and FOX networks and/or the *New York Times* and *Washington Post* newspapers. Your focus might be on anything from their views on recent challenges facing journalists to a mix of interviews and observation that will give you a better understanding of how "the news" is created on any given day.

Yet another researcher might be interested in putting contemporary newscasts in a more historical context and begin looking to see whether they can find archived broadcasts or previous editions of a newspaper or magazine they are interested in. The sampling decisions you make with these archives will parallel those we discussed above regarding people. Are you interested in a broad spectrum of media, one particular medium, or some number in between? Are you interested in the making of the news in general, or of how the process of defining the news has changed, or the transitions that a story goes through from piquing someone's interest to making front-page headlines to becoming tomorrow's fish wrap? All of these situations call for different kinds of sampling and recruitment strategies; your challenge is to find and implement whichever one(s) help you achieve your objective(s).

Step Two: Getting Down to Business

Remember that one of the central tenets of our approach to sampling is that every piece of research is a case study in the sense that all research is bound in space and time, which applies equally to all sorts of methods and approaches. To take the biggest first, to us the census may involve several hundred million participants, and in most cases actually is considered a "**population**" rather than a "sample," but is nonetheless nothing more than a case study of a complete country—a snapshot—of a moving target at one point in time. To go to the other extreme, we would call a small-scale oral history of the evolving relationship between you and your partner a case study as well. All those myriad studies in between—a program evaluation at the local hospital; content analysis of an extremist group's discussion board after the most recent school shooting; a survey of workers at a manufacturing plant during an economic downturn; interviews about gaming culture with women who play video games; or a field experiment to determine how frequently wallets left in obvious places are actually returned to their owners—are research site/cases in our view as well. Although our loose use of the term might cause more than one methodologist to roll their eyes, the thing that all of these examples of research have in common is that we typically do them as researchers in order to try and unearth truths that go beyond the specific case at hand. We always end up taking a sample of the world, in other words, and do so sometimes because we simply want to understand that corner of the world, but more often because we hope that studying one small part of the world will help us understand something more than that.

We come back to the idea that different kinds of samples and sampling procedures will be more or less appropriate depending on our research questions and objectives. If our questions/objectives are such that we will need/want to be in the position to make statistical generalizations that extend to the larger population, the "best" sampling strategy (or set of strategies) are ones that will allow us to do that, which for the most part sees us working in the domain of probability sampling. Conversely, if we are interested in more substantive types of generalizations—as is the case when we want to use the data to generate new theory or to arrive at a more complete and nuanced understanding of a phenomenon or set of phenomena, the "best" sampling strategies will lie more commonly among the strategic/purposive techniques. And regardless of which direction we emphasize in any given project, we must remain mindful that what we produce will always be limited to the time and space when/in which we produce it. With that as our backdrop, let us now discuss some of the many options available to you.

WHEN STATISTICAL GENERALIZATION IS THE OBJECTIVE: PROBABILISTIC TECHNIQUES

Consider the situation where you are a polling researcher who wants to figure out what degree of support different candidates have for an upcoming election. Or perhaps you have just been hired by the registrar at your university or college who wants to know how interested current students would be in seeing the institution develop an internship program that would allow them to get some job experience in their chosen disciplines and professions prior to graduating. Alternatively, let's say you are a historian who has been granted access to an archive of all the files that were kept in a 100-year-old asylum that was just demolished. Or maybe you work for a dating service, want to understand what people of different ages look for in a prospective mate, and have access to 150,000 online dating profiles in which people express their preferences and priorities.

All of these situations present a problem that is like the marbles-in-a-bag problem we alluded to earlier. You do not have the resources or the time to talk to every single person or read every file in each one of those settings; instead, you decide that you want to speak only with a subset of the larger population or look at a subset of files—a sample—in the hope that looking at that smaller group will allow you to be confident making statements about the broader group on the basis of what you observed in the smaller sample. This type of problem is best addressed by probabilistic sampling methods, all of which are based on notions of random selection.

Probabilistic Sampling: The Vocabulary

This family of sampling techniques is known as probabilistic because they are based on probability theory. Understanding them requires that we spend some time reviewing the language that is relevant to this approach.

The Meaning of "Random"

Before we go any further, it's worth dwelling on that word "**random**" a bit, because it is an important sampling concept that has a more precise meaning in research than it has in our everyday lives. In casual conversation we may talk about how random something is when we find it unusual or when someone says something to us that comes out of nowhere ("That was so random!"), or when we make a choice haphazardly or arbitrarily without giving any serious thought ("I was preoccupied and made a random choice off the menu."). But random in the social and health sciences has a very specific referent with respect to sampling: a sample is random if and only if every member of the population from which it is chosen has an equal likelihood of being selected.

Think of it as you would a lottery. When people buy lottery tickets, each ticket has as much chance as any other of matching the winning numbers. Similarly, if we were to number every member of a human population and then use a random number generator to pick which people will be in our sample, then that choice is random because every person in the population would have had an equal opportunity of being selected.

We as researchers cannot make random choices—using that term in its methodological sense—on our own. It turns out that people are incredibly poor at recognizing random events or doing things randomly (e.g., Kahneman, Slovic, & Tversky, 1982; Mlodinow, 2008). If we went to a shopping mall determined to randomly choose people in the mall on our own, the sample would not meet a research standard of randomness. If left up to you (or anyone), any sample you choose will be influenced by you and your "biases," if we can employ that word in a very nonjudgmental way simply to refer to deviations from the random. As we wander through the mall trying to make our random selections, our social selves will notice some persons more than others, make more eye contact with some persons more than with others, feel more comfortable in the presence of some persons than with others, and so on. Similarly, people cannot generate random number sequences when asked to just start speaking out numbers as randomly as possible; they favor some numbers more than others and repeat numbers less frequently than random models would predict (Mlodinow, 2008).

We know from the above that any random selection that is done will have to be outside of us—by using a random number table or random number generator or dice or whatever. Fully random sampling has another requirement as well, which is that we need to begin with a list of every possible element in our population of interest. What this suggests is that we need to begin with a very well-defined population; fortunately there are situations where such lists exist. In that regard, we chose the examples with which we started this section quite carefully. Pollsters who are interested in tracking voter sentiment during election campaigns and predicting results have access to voter's lists that define the population from which they can sample. Researchers commissioned by the registrar to gage student interest in practicum programs would have access to the registrar's list of currently enrolled students. Our fictitious historian who was looking at the asylum archives had or could easily create a numbered list of every file in their possession and could then sample from that population of files. The hypothetical dating service employee would have access to the company's client database listing all of the people who have used the service.

Given that you are in such a situation, and your objective is to draw a sample that will allow you to generalize back to every member of the broader population, then random sampling is the way to go. We see this type of situation most commonly in survey research and especially the type of research done by national polling organizations. At election time, each of the political parties and every media organization seems fixated on the idea of tracking sentiment toward the various parties in the interest of knowing who is doing well, who is losing ground and why, what effect last week's leaders debate had on their respective parties' fortunes, who will win the election, and so on. The "well-defined population" in this instance is the American electorate, which in the end is defined as "all US citizens 18 years of age and older who are registered and thereby eligible to vote," which for the 2016 Presidential election comprised about 157 million people (United States Census Bureau, 2017). On the basis of samples of only a few thousand people, many national polling organizations do an astonishingly good job of generalizing back from that comparatively small sample to the population as a whole. And yet, the 2016 election was like no other, and the polling results showed it. Although most polling organizations seem to have done a decent job of predicting the national popular vote (which Hilary Clinton won by approximately 48–46 percent), almost nobody predicted that Donald Trump would win the Presidency on the basis of the Electoral College vote (major polling organizations were predicting with anywhere from 71 percent to 99 percent confidence that Clinton would win).

We will talk more about the 2016 Presidential election and what methodological lessons can be learned from it in Chapter 9 when we talk in more detail about survey methods. For the moment we merely note that when a researcher is faced with a research problem of this sort—going from an identified whole population (American voters) and choosing a sample that will allow them to generalize back to the population as a whole—then ensuring a representative sample is the primary objective, and the best way of doing so is to utilize a **probabilistic sampling** technique.

Representativeness

Probabilistic techniques are the best ones to use if you want to obtain a representative sample of some target population. A sample is **representative** of some larger group when the distribution of relevant attributes in the sample mirrors the distribution of those attributes in the population. Thus, if our target population is 52 percent female, 47 percent male, and 1 percent transgender, then a "representative" sample of 100 people drawn from the target population would contain approximately 52 females. The same would be true of all other variables—if 80 percent of the population is right-handed, 23 percent prefer the Republican party, and 13 percent own Toyotas, then a representative sample of 100 people should include about 80 right-handed persons, 23 who say they prefer the Republican party, and 13 Toyota owners. Probabilistic techniques minimize **sampling error**, i.e., the difference between the sample and the population.

Units of Analysis or Sampling Elements

Any study involves a choice of **units of analysis** or sampling elements, that is, the units or elements about which information will be gathered. If we wish to find out how people in North Dakota feel about the state government's approach to education issues, for example, the individual person is our unit of analysis. If we wish to determine the attention given to environmental issues in *The San Francisco Chronicle* by doing some form of newspaper content analysis, individual issues of or individual articles in that newspaper become our unit of analysis. Units of analysis or sampling elements aren't inherent or inevitable divisions among entities; they're defined by the researcher, depending on their research interests. Your unit of analysis might be the individual person, family units, larger groupings (e.g., university departments, census tracts, electoral ridings), or even whole countries; it is little more than a statement of what "things" you want to study.

The Universe

A **universe** is a theoretical aggregation of all possible sampling elements. If our sampling element is the individual British citizen, our theoretical universe is "all citizens of Great Britain." If our unit of analysis is the newspaper, our universe is "all newspapers." The notion of "universe" is not especially practical, since your universe is generally so amorphous and huge that it's impossible to define in detail. Its major role, instead, is to keep us attuned to two ideas: (1) that there's often a much broader realm to which our theorizing or conceptualizing refers and, we hope, applies; and (2) that we must consider the limitations of our empirical pursuits. To continue with the example of the election survey, the universe would have been "all voters."

The Population

A more practical and perhaps less presumptuous term is **population**. Like "universe," "population" refers to an aggregation of sampling elements, but "population" delineates the exact boundaries that define our sample elements. While "all Oregonians" might be our universe of interest, we might define our population as "all people over 18 years of age who are US citizens and resident in the state of Oregon on January 1, 2020." For the example of the voting survey, the population might be "all US citizens who are eligible to vote in the 2020 Presidential election." The term "population" is thus more precise than "universe" in delimiting who or what *specifically* makes up our *target group* for this study at this time. Defining our population of interest is thus Step 1 when engaging one of the probabilistic sampling procedures, since it requires us to specify, in no uncertain terms, who or what is "eligible" for participation in our research, as well as defining the population to which we want to be able to generalize our results.

Sampling Frame

The **sampling frame** is a complete list of all the sampling elements of the population we wish to study. If our population of interest is "all students enrolled on a full-time basis at the University of California at Davis as of February 1, 2020," our sampling frame is the list of all students who fit the description. If our population of interest is "all divorce cases adjudicated in Texas courts during 2019 in which child custody was contested," our sampling frame is a list of all such cases.

Although the sampling frame's list of all elements would *ideally* reflect our population exactly, it typically does *not*. Many lists are imperfect to begin with, and others quickly become obsolete. For example, in the voting survey example, given that our population was "all US citizens who are eligible to vote in the 2020 Presidential election," the voters list—all persons whose names appear on the list of registered voters—might seem an obvious choice for a sampling frame. But some people who are actually eligible to vote will not be registered to do so, and some others who are technically ineligible nonetheless may appear on the list. Thus, even something as current as a voter list starts out as a good but imperfect list of eligible voters. Nonetheless, in this case, the voters' lists would be a good starting point for us if our intention is to chart voter preference during an election campaign, since it is only those on the list of voters who are actually eligible to vote. On the other hand, if we wanted to focus on eligible voters because one aspect of our study involved assessing which eligible voters do *not* end up appearing on voter registration lists and why, then the list of voters would be a poor sampling frame to answer that question.

Given that all the preceding prerequisites have been met—we have a well-defined population, are interested in drawing a sample that will allow us to generalize our results back to that broader population, and have a complete and accurate sampling frame from which to sample—then we can proceed with one of the several equally effective probabilistic techniques.

PROBABILISTIC SAMPLING TECHNIQUES

Simple Random Sampling

Simple random sampling is the best way to identify a representative sample. It minimizes **sampling error** (deviation of the characteristics of the sample from the characteristics of the population) and, because the probabilities are known, allows us to calculate the degree of sampling error that might exist. Recall from our earlier discussion that two criteria are essential for selection to be considered random: (1) nothing but chance must govern the selection process; and (2) every sampling element must have an equal probability of being selected. If these criteria are met—for example, by numbering every entry in the sampling frame and using a random number generator or table to select a sample—the resulting sample will be representative of the population included in the sampling frame, within some margin of error.

Sampling Error

"Sampling error" refers to the extent to which the sample's characteristics deviate from those of the population. There are two types of sampling error: **systematic error** and **random error**.

Systematic error occurs when aspects of your sampling procedure act in a consistent way to make some sampling elements more likely to be chosen for participation than others. For example, if you are interested in the opinions of *all* the students at your university or college (i.e., the entire population of students enrolled that semester), but place ballot boxes for a referendum only in the buildings where arts classes are held, you've made voting easier for arts students than for science students. This systematic bias all but ensures that arts students' opinions will be *overrepresented* while science students' opinions will be *underrepresented* in the final result. Similarly, when we survey city dwellers by using the city's list of homeowners as our sampling frame, we systematically bias the resulting sample to reflect the views of wealthier and possibly older people (i.e., those more likely to own homes) and systematically ignore younger and less wealthy people, as well as all renters, the transient, and the homeless.

Random error has no systematic bias involved but merely reflects the vagaries of chance variation. If we flip a coin 100 times, we may *expect* (theoretically) to see the coin fall heads-up 50 times and tails-up 50 times, but we wouldn't find it particularly unusual if the coin were to fall heads-up 53 times and tails-up 47 times. Such things happen, purely as a result of chance variation. You may hear such expressions of sampling error when poll results are reported. For example, pollsters who conduct election surveys might state that, "These results can be expected to reflect the 'true' situation plus or minus 3 percent 19 times out of 20."

Assuming you use a random sampling method, the amount of sampling error you incur depends on the size of your sample: the bigger the sample, the smaller the sampling error. Suppose the members of the city council in UniverCity are trying to decide where to put the new Art Gallery they are planning to build. Two different locations have been debated—one downtown and another in the suburbs—and the council is at a stalemate, with five council members voting for each alternative. Instead of casting the deciding vote, the mayor suggests they look to the residents of the city for guidance. The council hires us to take the pulse of the city and to report back on what the people want.

The first problem we have to deal with is the sampling frame problem, which also highlights the distinction we made earlier between the "universe" and the "population." Sometimes it is easy to demarcate a population and attendant sampling frame. If our universe is "voters" and our population is "all voters in the 2020 Presidential election" and we have access to lists of all eligible voters (our sampling frame), then there is a very good correspondence between our universe and our population. But to go back to our municipal example, our universe there would be "residents of UniverCity." This may sound simple enough. But it is highly unlikely that every single inhabitant of any given city will have been enumerated other than in the census, so the question remains as to how we can define our population and attendant sampling frame from which to sample.

In these situations, researchers look for solutions that are "good enough" to accomplish their objective. One possibility is that the UniverCity council might give us access to taxation records, which would allow us to use that list to contact a random sample of taxpayers. But "taxpayers" are not the same as "residents," so in this situation we have a bit of a mismatch between our universe of interest and the population we had to settle for in order to have a sampling frame from which we could sample. All non–tax-paying residents of the city will be left out, such as renters and the homeless, which probably means that our sample will also tend to under-represent minorities, recent immigrants, the poor, and younger respondents who are less likely to have the wealth needed to buy property and appear on taxpayer rolls. At the same time, not all property owners are residents, which means we will be including people in our sample who should not be. If it turns out these people are more likely to be wealthy individuals who hold investment properties in different places, then we would be overrepresenting wealthier people in our sample. In this municipal situation it is unlikely that any sampling frame we could find would be perfect. The reason this is important is because, even though random sampling is the best way to gather a theoretically representative sample that allows us to generalize the results we obtain from the sample back to the population, the population we are generalizing to is only as good as our sampling frame.

Let's press on and assume that we do acquire an acceptable sampling frame and we're confident that we have a good handle on the population whose views we hope to capture. From this list, we randomly sample 10 people and find that 7 of them, or 70 percent, would prefer to see the Art Gallery built downtown. If the 10-person sample was indeed randomly chosen, we can expect (in theory) that these people are representative of our population of interest, within some margin of error. Chapter 9 looks at some of the mathematics associated with computing the sampling error. For now, we need to only know that, with a sample size of 10, our estimate that 70 percent of the population would like to see the Art Gallery built downtown must be qualified by stating that the "real" figure could be as low as 34 percent or as high as 94 percent (e.g., see Gray & Guppy, 1994, p. 145) given so small a sample. Why such a wide range? With a sample of only 10 people, it wouldn't be unusual, simply due to the unpredictability of chance, to get a "weird" result that would be unlikely to repeat itself twice in a row.

If we take such a result to the city council members, they won't be impressed. Being "95 percent confident" that the "real" figure is somewhere between 34 percent and 94 percent (a range of 60 percentage points) is not much better than saying that overall, people might agree or disagree with the decision. You might as well have flipped a coin. The council will send us back to the field to draw another sample.

The degree of sampling error you incur relates most strongly to the *absolute* sample size you draw rather than to the *proportional* sample size (e.g., Warwick & Lininger, 1975). Table 5.1 shows the relationship between sample size and the margin of error when sampling is completely random. In each case we assume (just to have a number to work with) that 70 percent of the sample indicates a certain preference (e.g., that the Art Gallery should be built downtown). If we were to increase the sample size from our original 10 to 50 and in that situation find that 70 percent support the downtown building site, this bigger random sample allows us to be a little more

TABLE 5.1 ● Margin of Error by Sample Size

If 70% of a sample agrees, then with	The population value might be		
A sample size of	As low as (%)	As high as (%)	Size of confidence interval (high-low)
10	34	94	60% (±30%)
50	55	83	28% (±14%)
100	59	78	19% (±9.5%)
250	64	76	12% (±6%)
1,000	67	73	6% (±3%)

From Gray and Guppy (1994, p. 145). Reprinted with permission.

confident in our data, and we see in Table 5.1 that this larger sample allows us to say that the "true" figure in the population is now 95 percent likely to be between 55 percent and 83 percent (a range of 28 percent). At least now we could say with reasonable confidence that a majority of the population is in favor of locating the proposed Art Gallery downtown. The city council may be happy with that, or they may want something more precise, in which case we could increase our sample size yet again. A sample of 100 would reduce the range to 19 percent (roughly 70 ± 10 percent). Increasing the sample size to 1,000 reduces our confidence interval to a mere 6 percent: if 70 percent of that 1,000-person sample supports a downtown location, we could be 95 percent confident that the "real" figure is somewhere between 67 percent and 73 percent (i.e., 70 ± 3 percent).

If we push for greater and greater accuracy, and hence require a larger and larger sample, we eventually face the need to acquire a huge sample, which would require equally huge resources to contact and interview. Indeed, we soon reach a point of diminishing returns, where whopping increases in sample size produce only very small gains in accuracy. Gray and Guppy (1994) explain that "the rules of probability theory tell us that we reduce our margin of error by one half if we quadruple our sample size" (p. 144). It follows that, to go beyond the figures shown in Table 5.1, we would have to increase our sample size from 1,000 to 4,000 in order to reduce our 95 percent confidence interval to 3 percent (i.e., ±1.5 percent), or to 16,000 to reach ±0.75 percent, or to 64,000 to reach ±0.375 percent, and so on.

At some point, such increases simply aren't worth the improved confidence they bring us. Each researcher must determine where that point is, considering such factors as the available resources, how precise the estimate needs to be given the importance and consequences of the answers we seek to our research questions, and how the available funds might otherwise be spent. The researcher must also keep in mind how accurate other elements of the process will be. It would be silly to spend many thousands of dollars to increase sampling accuracy from plus or minus 1.5 percent to 0.75 percent, for example, when small changes in the wording of a question can easily cause results to vary as much as 5–10 percent or more. Forgetting those other elements of the process produces nothing but a specious scientism and a spurious sense of precision that simply does not exist (see Chapter 9 regarding the substantial impact that even small changes in wording can have).

Systematic Sample With Random Start

A type of random sample with a slight twist to it is the **systematic sample with random start**. Like simple random sampling, this technique also requires a sampling frame in which each element is numbered and appears only once. But instead of randomly sampling from the entire list each time, you begin at a *randomly determined starting point* and then sample every n^{th} element on the list.

To illustrate, assume you have a voters list with 10,000 names on it and wish to draw a random sample of 500 people from that list. Your **sampling ratio**, in other words, is 1:20 (or 1 in 20). To do a systematic sample with random start, you would first randomly choose a number from 1 to 20. Suppose you open up a spreadsheet program such as Microsoft Excel® or Open Office Calc®, place your cursor in the first cell of the table (A1), type RANDBETWEEN(1,20), hit enter, and the program (or function) generates the number 13. That's your random start: the first person you sample is number 13 on your voters list. The systematic part is dictated by your sampling ratio of 1:20; that is, you now systematically pick every 20th person on the list. Thus, given that you began with person number 13, the next one you sample will be number 33, then 53, then 73, then 93, and so on through the sampling frame, until you come to your 500th sample person, who would be number 9,993 on the original list of 10,000 people.

Stratified Random Sampling

A third type of probabilistic sample is the **stratified random sample**. In this procedure, the researcher first divides the population into groupings (or *strata*) of interest and then samples randomly within each stratum. This technique is used when there is some meaningful *grouping variable* on which the investigator wishes to make comparisons and where the probabilities of group membership are known ahead of time.

Suppose a researcher wants to survey a representative sample of students who have declared a major in the Faculty of Arts at Washington State University (WSU). Suppose further that we know that 10 percent of WSU's Arts students are sociology majors, another 30 percent are psychology majors, 5 percent are English majors, and the remaining 30 percent are in other Arts disciplines. Just to keep the numbers easy, suppose there are 1,000 students with declared majors in the Faculty of Arts. They are represented by the "population" drawing in the upper portion of Figure 5.1.

FIGURE 5.1 ● Proportional and Disproportional Stratified Random Sampling

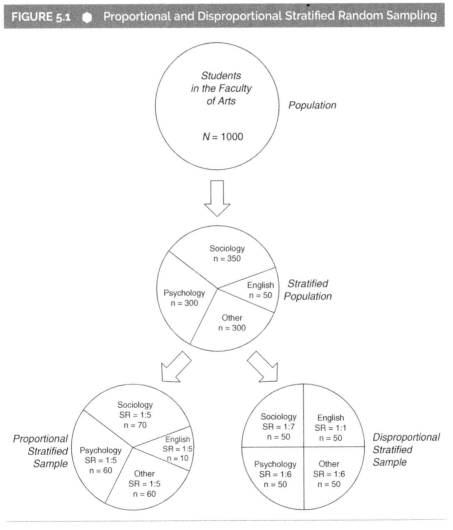

Note: SR = sampling ratio.

A researcher who is interested only in "polling students from the Faculty of Arts" could get a list of the 1,000 students from the registrar's office (i.e., a sampling frame) and then draw a simple random sample or a systematic sample with random start. If properly done, the sample should contain, within the limits of sampling error, roughly 35 percent sociology majors, 30 percent psychology majors, and 5 percent English majors, while roughly 30 percent of the sampled students should have majors that don't fall into any of these categories and are therefore labeled "other."

But suppose our researcher wants to *compare* the responses of the four groups (sociology, psychology, English, and other). Since 5 percent of the students in our example are English majors, we would *expect* to find 10 English majors in a randomly drawn sample of 200 of these students. But the vagaries of chance might leave us with more or fewer than 10 English majors in the sample. If the researcher wanted to ensure that the sample is exactly representative of the population with respect to the grouping variable of interest, stratified random sampling is more appropriate than simple random sampling.

The first step in this technique involves stratifying the population according to the grouping variable of interest, as shown in the section of Figure 5.1 labeled "stratified population." The researcher then performs simple random sampling *within* each stratum. Actually, the researcher has another choice to make: whether to use proportional or disproportional stratified random sampling.

Proportional Stratified Random Sampling

In **proportional stratified random sampling**, the same sampling ratio is used within each stratum. In our example, this approach produces the following result: the proportion of students with different majors in the sample is exactly the same as the proportion of students with different majors in the population; and the students within each stratum of the sample are theoretically representative of the students within the corresponding population stratum (e.g., the sociology majors in the sample are representative of sociology majors in the population), within the limits of sampling error. At the end of this study, the researcher's conclusions will apply both to "students in WSU's Faculty of Arts" (since the sample as a whole is proportionately representative of the population, within the limits of sampling error) and "WSU students majoring in sociology, psychology, English, or any other arts discipline" (since each stratum of the sample is representative of the corresponding stratum of the population, within the limits of sampling error).

But in an example like this one, while the researcher has obtained stratified samples that are theoretically representative of each stratum within the population, their ability to make conclusions about each stratum, and especially to compare strata, is impaired. It all comes down to that qualifying phrase "within the limits of sampling error." The main problem arises from including the English majors, of whom only 10 are sampled. As our earlier discussion of sampling error revealed, any result based on a sample of only 10 is bound to be very tentative, since our 95 percent confidence range would require us to specify that the result could be inaccurate by plus or minus 30 percentage points, which is not a very precise conclusion. There are two ways to get around this problem: (1) we can increase the overall sample size, so that even the smallest group is still large enough for analysis; or (2) we can use *disproportional* stratified random sampling.

Disproportional Stratified Random Sampling

When the researcher is primarily interested in *comparing* results between the strata rather than in making overall statements about "students in the Faculty of Arts," or when one or more of the subgroups are so small that a consistent sampling ratio would leave sample sizes in some groups too small for adequate analysis, a **disproportional stratified random sample** might be drawn.

Here, the researcher still begins by stratifying the population into subgroups of interest and then taking a random sample within each stratum. But a different sampling ratio is used within each stratum, so that equal numbers of students end up in each of the strata samples. If the researcher wants a sample of 200 students from the population of 1,000 students (i.e., an overall 1:5 sampling ratio), *proportional* stratified random sampling will yield 70 sociology majors, 60 psychology majors, 10 English majors, and 60 students with majors in "other" arts disciplines. But with *disproportional* stratified random sampling, the sample of 200 might include 50 majors of each type (to create an optimal comparison using equal numbers of students from each group), chosen by using different sampling ratios within each stratum. In such a case, overall statements about "WSU students majoring in arts subjects" would be tenuous without further adjustment (since the sample as a whole is no longer representative of the university's arts students), but the researcher could make statements *comparing* the subgroups, since each subgroup (or stratum) of the sample is representative of that subgroup in the population. In sum, we end up with the alternatives depicted in the bottom portion of Figure 5.1.

QUASI-PROBABILISTIC TECHNIQUES

Multistage Cluster Sampling

Each technique discussed so far requires a sampling frame. But, as we have seen, a sampling frame isn't always available. Does the lack of a sampling frame prevent researchers from drawing a probabilistic sample that, in theory at least (within some margin of error), comprises a representative sample? No. One probabilistic technique *doesn't* require a sampling frame. Known as **multistage cluster sampling**, instead of randomly selecting a sample from a sampling frame, this technique involves random sampling of clusters within clusters until you reach the desired unit of analysis.

Suppose the San Francisco Bay Area, California city council is evaluating a proposal to change the color of transit system signage throughout the Bay Area and want to get a sense of how receptive Bay Area residents would be to the proposed change. However, they decide that they really don't want to spend the large amount of money that it would take to put together a sampling frame to do a pure random sample of all the residents. Instead, they just want the views of a group of citizens who reflect the full diversity of the Bay Area population and without any obvious systematic bias in who is surveyed. In this instance, a quasi-random sample is "good enough" to be able to answer the research question. With no sampling frame, how can we find a sample of people who could at least be considered an "unbiased" sample and might even meet the "representativeness" criterion?

Multistage cluster sampling begins by acknowledging that people (our unit of analysis) generally live in residences, that residences exist on blocks, that blocks are part of neighborhoods, that neighborhoods make up municipalities, and that most major American cities actually comprise a collection of municipalities. Thus, if we first prepare a list of the 101 municipalities that make up the Bay Area (i.e., including San Jose, Oakland, Santa Rosa, Hayward, Berkley, etc.) and then take a random sample of these municipalities, that sample of municipalities is formally representative of the population of municipalities that make up the Bay Area. We can then get maps of each of our sample municipalities, divide them into neighborhoods, and take a random sample of neighborhoods within each of the municipalities we sampled in step 1. Because the neighborhoods are representative of the population of neighborhoods in the municipality from which they were drawn and because the municipalities were randomly chosen to be representative of all communities in the Bay Area, the neighborhoods we've sampled must be representative of all the neighborhoods in the Bay Area. Neighborhoods comprise individual blocks, so we can randomly sample blocks within each of our sample neighborhoods and then randomly sample residences within blocks; finally, we can randomly sample the people within the sampled residences.

By conducting random sampling within each cluster, we end up with a sample of people that is theoretically representative of the population of people in our sample residences, which in turn is representative of the population of residences on our sample blocks, which in turn is representative of the population of blocks in our sample neighborhoods, which in turn is representative of the population of neighborhoods in our sample communities, which in turn is representative of the population of communities that make up the Bay Area. Our sample of people is thus theoretically representative of people who live in the Bay Area—and we found them *without* a sampling frame.

While this approach obviously can get somewhat laborious, it *does* allow us to acquire a formally representative sample—an even better description would be to call it an "unbiased sample"—when no sampling frame is available. Multistage cluster sampling can be very useful, but it should be used only when a sampling frame is unavailable, since it's ultimately not as good as the true probabilistic techniques. To appreciate why that's the case we must go back to the concept of sampling error. Remember that there will always be *some* sampling error whenever we draw a random sample, although the bigger the sample, the lower that error is likely to be. For a simple random sample, we sample only once and can easily compute the probable degree of sampling error. But for a multistage cluster sample, we're actually taking samples of samples of samples, and since all sampling involves some degree of error, we thus *accumulate* error with each successive level of sampling. Mathematically, there is no easy way to be able to determine just what amount of sampling error we have.

Quota Sampling

A final quasi-probabilistic procedure is **quota sampling**, a technique that made Gallup (as in Gallup Poll) a household word after George Gallup correctly predicted the result of the 1936 US presidential election. Quota sampling is still used by some pollsters, especially marketing researchers who want a heterogeneous sample that has some of the characteristics of a formally representative sample but is not drawn randomly.

To do a quota sample, the researcher must first know something about at least the demographic characteristics of the population to be studied. Such information is usually provided by census data. Suppose that we want to ask people about child-rearing

TABLE 5.2 ● Hypothetical Population Breakdown by Sex and Education			
	Completed High School or Less (%)	Some Postsecondary (%)	Completed Postsecondary (%)
Male	30	15	5
Female	35	10	5
Total	65	25	10

practices and that we know from earlier research that attitudes about these practices vary with the respondents' sex and educational background. We begin by acquiring census data that show how those characteristics are distributed in the population. Suppose we do so and find the breakdown shown in Table 5.2.

For the sample to be formally representative, 30 percent of our respondents should be males who have completed high school or less, 10 percent should be females who have obtained some postsecondary education, and so on. As with stratified random sampling, quota sampling starts with a target population that has *known* characteristics. But with stratified random sampling, we'd now proceed to randomly select people from within each category. In contrast, the quota sampler would merely go out and find (for a sample of 100, for example) 30 males with a high school education or less, 35 females with some postsecondary education, and so on. Since *any* 30 males with a high school education or less will do, the researcher might look for them in shopping malls, at pool halls, at union meetings, at laundromats, or just about anywhere.

The quota sampling technique assumes that all people within a given stratum are equal and that, for example, all males with a high school education or less will have pretty much the same attitudes regarding the phenomenon of interest. While such an assumption may not be indefensible, it's still fairly tenuous. Quota sampling's major strength is that it ensures a heterogeneous sample with respect to relevant background variables. Ironically enough, the limitations of quota sampling were revealed by the very same person who made them famous—George Gallup. Although Gallup made his name with this technique in the 1936 US presidential election and successfully used it again in 1940 and 1944, he suffered huge embarrassment in 1948, when he predicted that Thomas Dewey would be the next US president. The American public voted instead for Harry Truman (see Figure 5.2). Gallup subsequently abandoned quota sampling techniques in favor of probabilistic procedures.

FIGURE 5.2 ●   Dewey Defeats Truman

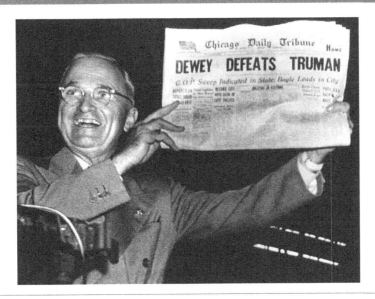

CAN SAMPLING PROBLEMS BE OVERCOME BY SAMPLE SIZE?

As noted earlier, probabilistic samples receive that name because the sampling techniques used to obtain them conform to the rules of probability theory, particularly its basic requirement that the probability that any given person or element will be selected must be known, or at least knowable. When the population is known and sampling is random, these techniques ensure a theoretically representative sample, within the limits of sampling error.

Sampling error in this context varies according to two factors: the nature of the procedure followed (it must be random) and the sample size. Assuming that the first criterion (random sampling) is met, then the larger the sample size, the smaller the sampling error, and the more confident we can be that we've obtained a truly representative unbiased sample.

But if we violate that first criterion by failing to use a random sampling procedure, the principles and mathematics of probability theory cannot be applied because we have no idea of the likelihood that a given element will be sampled. As a result, we can't compute or estimate how much sampling error exists. Thus, as sample size increases, we have no way of knowing whether we can be more and more confident that our estimates of the population's characteristics are getting more and more accurate or whether we're merely acquiring a bigger and bigger biased sample.

Huge samples in themselves—no matter how big they might be—do not ensure representativeness; it's *how* you sample that's most important. An excellent illustration of this point arose in relation to a little experiment that was created in relation to the 1992 State of the Union address given by then-US President George H.W. Bush (senior). After Bush's speech, the CBS program *America on the Line* coupled its postspeech discussion with a "viewer call-in poll." Viewers who owned touch-tone phones[1] were encouraged to call and offer their reactions to the speech through a computerized system that would compile all the responses. A total of 314,786 people phoned to express their opinions. Now, 314,786 people is a lot of people, far more than the 2,000–3,000-person samples used in most national surveys. It's hard not to be impressed when a poll's source states that the poll captures the opinions of more than 300,000 people. But can this particular huge sample genuinely be considered statistically representative of the broader population of Americans?

One way to address that issue considers it on a purely rational basis, asking whether there's any reason to believe that the sample *is not* statistically representative. If there is, we should be able to at least speculate on its deficiencies. The CBS phone-in sample clearly was not chosen randomly; people "volunteered" themselves for participation in a very particular social context. In order to have participated in the poll, a person would have to be home that evening, own a television, have the television on, have enough interest in current affairs to watch the CBS news instead of whatever was on the other channels, be interested enough in politics to listen to a presidential speech, care enough about having their opinion heard to actually phone the CBS number, understand English well enough to understand the survey questions, and be free to spend the required time on the phone answering questions. It's doubtful that people who met all these criteria are representative of the general American public. Thus, despite the mammoth sample size, it seems unlikely that a sample of opinion drawn in the manner of the CBS phone-in poll would be representative of the broader population.

---

[1] Although less than 30 years ago, at that time only a very small portion of the population owned cell phones (which were about the size of a brick) and while many landline phones had push buttons, many homes still had "rotary dial" telephones and thus could not participate in the CBS call-in poll.

We also can address the representativeness issue empirically. The ideal situation would be to have the results of a survey done at exactly the same time, in which the same questions were asked, but with a sample drawn randomly from the general population. Had such a survey been conducted that night using the same questions asked of the *America on the Line* phone-in sample, we could assess just how representative that 314,786-viewer sample might have been.

In fact, exactly such a random sample was drawn. Concurrent with its phone-in poll, CBS also commissioned a survey that asked a randomly chosen sample of 1,234 Americans exactly the same questions as the phone-in sample. Table 5.3 shows the questions that were asked and the collective responses of both the randomly chosen sample and the much larger phone-in sample. Monette, Sullivan, and DeJong (1994) note that, given the size of the random sample ($N = 1,234$), we can compute that the degree of error involved is probably around plus or minus 3 percent. Thus, any

TABLE 5.3 ● Is Bigger Always Better? Comparing Simultaneously Drawn Probabilistic and Nonprobabilistic Samples

Question	Alternatives	Viewer Call-In (N = 314,786)	CBS Formal Poll (N = 1,234)
Are you better off now than 4 years ago?	(a) Better	29%	24%
	(b) Worse	54	32
	(c) Same	17	44
Are you worried about job loss this year?	(a) Yes	64%	48%
	(b) No	36	52
Would you pay more taxes for free healthcare?	(a) Yes	58%	46%
	(b) No	42	53
Does the president understand the middle class?	(a) Yes	30%	43%
	(b) No	70	57
Are media exaggerating how bad economic conditions are?	(a) Yes	39%	35%
	(b) No	51	64
Future of America's children? Will it be... ?	(a) Better	21%	24%
	(b) Worse	57	36
	(c) Same	22	39

Source: Adapted from Monette, Sullivan, and DeJong (1994).

difference between the random sample and the phone-in sample that was larger than 3 percent is unlikely to be due to chance variation alone and more likely due to something else—probably the different sampling methods used. As Table 5.3 reveals, only one comparison stayed within the range of 3 percent; the other 13 ranged from 4 percent to as much as 27 percent, with an average difference of approximately 14 percentage points between the two techniques.

Even more disconcerting is the fact that the two sets of results differ not only in *magnitude* but also in *kind*. The call-in results seem more pessimistic and critical. Those who phoned in reported feeling *worse* off than they had 4 years previously; were *worried* about job loss; wanted *free* healthcare access paid for by taxes; felt that the middle class was *misunderstood*; believed that "America's children" faced an even more *dismal* future; and believed that media portrayals of bad economic times were *not* exaggerated. In contrast, the representative sample of Americans reported feeling that things were pretty much the *same* as they'd been 4 years earlier; were *not* worried about job loss; were *not* willing to pay more taxes to cover free healthcare for all; and expected *similar* futures for America's children. They agreed with the phone-in sample that the president didn't understand the middle class and that the media weren't exaggerating when they depicted times as tough.

As these results help reaffirm, anyone who claims to have generated a representative sampling of opinion without having used a probabilistic sampling technique is skating on thin ice. Yet such claims appear in the mainstream media all the time. Radio phone-in shows, lobbyists who generate letter-writing campaigns, and newspapers that encourage readers to clip a coupon and send it to some local official often argue that the sheer volume of replies allows them to legitimately claim they represent public opinion. Obviously, any issue that can stimulate 100,000 people to send postcards of complaint to their local member of Congress must be more intensely felt and broadly contested than one that generates only 100 cards. But while those 100,000 cards may well indicate that an issue has captured public attention, it's sheer folly to say that the 100,000 people who sent in those cards somehow "represent" public opinion.

DISTINGUISHING REPRESENTATIVENESS AND GENERALIZABILITY

When a researcher has a well-defined population and the research question(s) and objective require that they be able to generalize results back to the broader population, then probabilistic methods clearly are the methods of choice and anything else is second best. But there are many other situations—and we would argue that these "other" scenarios comprise *most* of what social and health scientists do—when probabilistic methods are unnecessary, irrelevant, and clearly the poorer choice.

Representative samples aren't useless—far from it. When our research objectives are *descriptive*, that is, when we want to know something like "how Americans feel about changes to the healthcare system," "how Berkeley students feel about the prospect of tuition increases," or "how Montanans feel about their state government's education policies," representative sampling is clearly the route to take. But social and health scientists are rarely content with description alone. Our goal is generally theory and understanding, and we can't think of one theory that aspires merely to describe some singular state of affairs. Theories deal with variable*s* (note the plural) and the inter-relationships among them. So if a theory posits that a relationship should exist between variable *A* and variable *B*, all we *really* need in order to test that theory is a sample whose members are heterogeneous with respect to those two variables.

Cook and Campbell (1979) also encourage us to ask what we end up with when we acquire a formally representative sample. They point out that even if we acquire a representative sample and use it to generate results that can be generalized to the population as a whole, those results won't necessarily also hold for all subgroups within the population. For example, even if we find out the overall distribution of attitudes among Americans about environmental regulation, there are no guarantees that the same distribution would characterize people of different religious or political persuasions, or with different education background or income levels, or in different parts of the country. And of course, differences in attitudes among different subgroups of the population are often of greater interest to us than mere description of the population as a whole.

Thus, Cook and Campbell (1979) argue that we ought to distinguish between generalizing *to* populations of interest and generalizing *across* subgroups of interest. Ultimately, they maintain, the researcher who samples various "unrepresentative" (i.e., unique) groups of interest and then either demonstrates that the same results hold across all these groups or shows that—and perhaps explains why—results *differ* across groups is in a much more powerful theoretical position than is the researcher who can only describe the overall status of a variable in a population of interest.

Other researchers view the emphasis on representative sampling as simply misplaced. Researchers undertaking qualitative research have been the most vocal in this regard. Huberman and Miles (1994), for example, note that

> *[S]ampling choices within and across cases are powerfully determinative of just which data will be considered and used in analysis. Quantitative researchers often*

think randomly, statistically, and in terms of context-stripped case selections. Qualitative researchers must characteristically think purposively and conceptually about sampling. (p. 441)

Researchers who practice only one or the other of these approaches sometimes seem unable to relate to research approaches other than their own. Seeing all sampling situations as equivalent to the marbles-in-a-bag problem leads to researchers believing that the only way to achieve generalizability of results is by having a formally representative sample. Smaller samples and samples drawn using purposive sampling strategies are sometimes dismissed as "unrepresentative and thus nongeneralizable." We reject that view. Representativeness and generalizability are independent issues. While it is true that the findings from a randomly drawn sample allow you to generalize those results back to the population with confidence (with some degree of sampling error), just because a sample is *not* drawn to be formally representative of the population does not inherently mean that the results it produces cannot be generalized. They might or might not, and it will be up to us to determine which is the case by doing further research of our own and/or connecting with the literature to see how our results compare with the results of similar studies conducted with other samples in other places at other times (see Chapter 6, where we discuss external validity).

Finally, remember also the different role that theory plays in deductive and inductive research; these differences have implications for how we look at sampling issues. With more deductive approaches, you *begin* with theory, and the parameters of the theory tell us which samples and sites are relevant to look at because they are "covered" by the theory. The trick for sampling is to identify samples and sites that will be representative of the universe to which we wish to generalize. In contrast, remember that more inductively driven approaches aspire to *develop* theory. Thus, instead of the universe to which we wish to generalize being defined ahead of time, the challenge for the inductive researcher is to *figure out* what the universe of generalizability is for whatever concepts emerged in the initial study.

In sum, when we get to the end of a more deductive study that involved looking at the way that nurses in a hospital changed their behavior in response to a change in hospital policy, more deductive researchers will ask, "I wonder whether results will generalize to all nurses and all hospitals?" In contrast, the more inductive researcher is more likely to look at the results that emerged from their study of changes in nurse behavior after a policy change and start asking, "I wonder to whom and what these results would generalize?" This is a much broader question than just nurses and hospitals that encourages us to look at other situations where people are governed by policy directives—professors and students in universities, government employees, food suppliers—to see whether similar processes occur there. The preferred sampling strategy here is often not to look for another place where similar results might apply, but rather to try and think of places where the same results might well *not* occur; while positive results help broaden a theory's range, negative results are just as informative by helping us determine the boundaries of that range.

After noting that "sampling" is something that researchers engaged in both qualitative and quantitative research typically do, Morgan (2008) cautions that,

Beyond that similarity, however, the very different goals of qualitative and quantitative research lead to equally different procedures for selecting data sources from a larger population. It is thus important to understand the difference between the logic of purposively selecting a small number of sources for intense analysis in qualitative research, as opposed to the emphasis on randomly selecting large samples for statistical analysis in quantitative research. (p. 799)

We have already discussed the logic of probabilistic research and the sorts of situations in which they are ideal. Morgan's quote encourages us to understand purposive techniques available to us not as secondary choices to look at when a probabilistic technique is not available, but rather a separate set of sampling alternatives with their own logic and different objectives they serve.

FINDING THE RIGHT PEOPLE: PURPOSIVE, STRATEGIC, OR TARGET SAMPLING

While probabilistic sampling procedures are fine when you have a well-defined population and you want to ensure that you can generalize back from sample to population, we don't always have a "well-defined population." Sometimes it is unclear exactly who or what the population is. For example, consider the problem of trying to define the population of "musicians." Does this only include professionals who have made recordings or any professional who makes their living playing music? But how about the hobby accordionist who is an accountant by day and plays weddings and bar mitzvahs on the weekend or your father when he sings "happy birthday" to you? If a "musician" is simply someone who makes music, then surely the latter are "musicians," too.

Other times it may be clearer who the population is, but there has never been any formal enumeration of the members, which means there is no sampling frame from which to sample. In some situations it might be feasible for the researcher to go in and create one, but in many other situations, constructing one would be impossible or impractical. A list of "all people in Chicago who were sexually abused during their adolescence," for example, is impossible to construct, as is a list of "all people in Wyoming who are consumers of pornography." The same is true of lists of people who participate in cosplay, sex trade workers, corporate executives, university students who smoke cannabis, and people who like lemon in their tea. For many groups (or other units of analysis), sampling must occur without a sampling frame. Especially in the case of individuals who engage in behavior that is criminal or otherwise stigmatized or those who are very rich or powerful, we may have to work very hard just to find enough people willing to speak with us, which will encourage us when we get to the end of our study to ask questions about where our sample fits in the universe we are trying to understand.

And finally, the focus of our research is not always defined by a population. Much social and health science research begins not with an interest in testing a particular theory or in taking a sample of some well-defined population in order to generalize back to that broader group, but in scrutinizing a particular group of people (e.g., gang members, politicians, nurses), particular sites (e.g., online dating sites, public waiting rooms, a hospital emergency room), social artifacts (e.g., film portrayals, court decisions, policies, patient records, or social media posts), or behaviors (e.g., quitting smoking, voting, finding a mate, or cyberbullying). On some occasions it may be important to us to try and ensure we have a representative sample of whatever units interest us, but more often our interest is in simply better getting to know those people, or that site, or those artifacts or behaviors.

Given the above, you should not be surprised to hear that some of the most common sampling strategies employed in the social and health sciences are **purposive or strategic sampling** procedures (Palys, 2008). Of course, sampling is always "purposive" to some degree, since identifying a target population invariably expresses the researcher's interests and objectives. Some of the strategies that can be employed to serve different research objectives that have been noted by Bailey (2007), Morse (1994), and Palys (2008) are discussed below.

Stakeholder Sampling

This approach—which is particularly useful in evaluation research, policy analysis, and participatory action research—involves identifying and interviewing the key stakeholders who are involved in designing, delivering, receiving, or administering the program or service being evaluated. For example, when Ted did a study evaluating the impact of one of the early mobile computing systems that gave police officers access to offender databases from computer terminals in their cars (Palys, Boyanowsky, & Dutton, 1984), there were a number of stakeholders within the police department who were affected by the change including the patrol officers who had new freedom to run checks on people and vehicles outside the gaze of the department, the dispatchers who were now no longer the gateway to information the officers needed, and the senior administrators in the department who now had to identify and manage a whole new range of policy issues that arose because of implementation of the system.

Depending on research objectives and available resources, the range of stakeholders that Ted spoke with could have been expanded even further to include members of the community, individuals involved in the development of the system, and/or members of civil liberties groups concerned with possible human rights violations when police seek private information without a warrant or having to show reasonable cause. When done properly, stakeholder sampling ensures that all relevant views are represented and that "all voices have been heard." Sampling done in this way may form the basis for a consensual resolution on how to move forward and/or may simply provide the basis for understanding both disagreements and shared positions as well as the dynamics underlying interactions between the varying groups.

Extreme or Deviant Case Sampling

Sometimes extreme cases are of interest because they represent the purest or most clear-cut instance of a phenomenon we are interested in. For example, if we are interested in studying management styles, it might be most interesting to study an organization that did exceptionally well and/or another that had high expectations but did exceptionally poorly or that took a given business or discipline in an unprecedented new direction. A favorite study here would be something like the one that resulted in *Moneyball*—a book (also later made into a film) about the decision by Billy Bean, manager of the perennially low-budget Major League Baseball team the Oakland A's, to break all the rules by letting empirically derived statistical prediction guide their choice of players moreso than scouting reports and traditional wisdom. Although written by a journalist rather than an academic, the book is a fascinating study of the resistance that creative managers can face when they try to deviate from practices that are simply "common sense" to an existing culture of expertise that dominates a field.

Intensity Sampling

This involves sampling people whose interests or vocation makes them "experiential experts" because of their frequent or ongoing exposure to a phenomenon. For example, when the American Psychological Association (APA) set out to develop its first set of ethical guidelines back in the 1960s, the first thing they did was to identify and interview certain "high exposure" people such as journal editors, who review many manuscripts and thus would be seeing a broad range of research and the ethical issues different studies triggered. Two other samples included members of university ethical review boards that were operating at that time, who would have been exposed to a wide range of ethics issues, and authors of ethics texts, who would have opinions about the range of fundamental principles that should appear in any disciplinary-based code. Similarly, if you want to study techniques of persuasion, the logic of intensity sampling would suggest that you sample people who make persuasion their business, such as lawyers, sales reps, and advertisers. Note, however, that intensity sampling presupposes that you already know something about the target population in order to be able to distinguish prospective participants who qualify as "experiential experts" in the first place (see Patton, 1990, pp. 169–186).

Typical Case Sampling

Sometimes we are interested in cases simply because they are *not* unusual in any way. For example, When Howard Becker and some of his colleagues sought to do research on the socialization into the medical profession that happens to students during medical school, they decided they would not go to a famous medical school like Johns Hopkins in Baltimore or Stanford Medical School in Palo Alto. Instead, they went to the University of Kansas Medical School—a competent but not highly prestigious medical school—exactly *because* it was a run-of-the-mill medical school that would be typical of most budding doctors' medical school experience.

Maximum Variation Sampling

Many survey studies that are done to investigate relations between variables of interest do not necessarily need a representative sample of the population on which to test those relations. In many cases, a sample that is diverse will suffice. One example of this occurred a couple of years ago when Ted and his teaching assistant at that time, Aaren Ivers, offered an undergraduate methods course. The class research project for that semester was a survey on privacy and surveillance issues to which all the students contributed. The central focus was on how people use social media and their attention to privacy and surveillance issues when using the internet, and the students were active in suggesting questions for the survey, suggesting items for a scale that would assess how much privacy considerations governed their behavior, and analyzing some part of the data for their term research paper.

A random sample of the population would have been overkill for this demonstration project that simply needed a good diverse population. There were about 60 students in the class, and after Ted and Aaren worked with the class to draft an online survey everyone was happy with, each of the 60 students then was asked to solicit the participation of 10 people in their lives, preferably from a range of ages and education levels and with differing levels of concern about internet privacy. There was already a fair amount of diversity in the class in terms of cultural identity, and the hope was that this would lead to similar diversity among the sample. In the end, it proved a great way to acquire a sample of almost 600 people very quickly, which served the purpose for this particular project.

Indeed, many survey researchers do much the same thing when they just need a big diverse sample and approach a company that offers researchers access to online panels such as Qualtrics and OvationMR.[2] The companies vary considerably in the types of samples they can give access to, but when all you need is "a bunch of people," they are a quick and efficient source. We will mention these again in Chapter 9 on surveys. Suffice it to say for now that anyone interested in using these panels would be well-advised to see the *AAPOR Report on Online Panels* commissioned by the American Association for Public Opinion Research (Baker et al., 2010).

Criterion Sampling

This involves searching for cases or individuals who meet a certain criterion, e.g., they have a certain disease, meet specific age or language requirements, or have had a particular life experience. For example, the research that Chris has done with people involved in the sale and purchase of sexual services would be considered criterion sampling since, to have been eligible to participate in his research, respondents had to have been English or French speaking (Canada's two official languages), over the age of 19, a resident of Canada, and sold or purchased sexual services on one or more occasions during the previous 12 months.

Companies that offer online panels for survey researchers often allow for a type of sampling they refer to as "river sampling" that accomplishes what we refer to here as criterion sampling. Such organizations typically have huge pools of people who have

---

[2]For a more extensive list, see https://www.greenbook.org/market-research-firms/online-panels.

registered with them to participate in surveys in return for some incentive such as a small fee per survey. Although the way these pools are constructed differs between organizations, some emphasizing more probabilistic procedures while others simply offer large numbers of people who have registered with them, most offer the possibility of floating a criterion question in "the river," i.e., what we have called the participant pool. Any person who says "yes," i.e., indicating they meet the criterion, is immediately invited to participate in that survey.

Critical Case Sampling

Here the researcher might be looking for a "decisive" case that would help make a decision about which of several different explanations is most plausible or is one that is identified by experts as being a particularly useful site because of the generalizations it allows. Chris administers a program of research on the influence of community systems on human early learning and development. In one of their research projects the team was interested in understanding the impact of a newly created government-funded program designed to promote improved access to services for families with small children. In order to assess impact, the team decided to conduct in-depth community case studies in four communities. Each case was selected on the basis of the community's early development vulnerability score, with two communities representing critical cases of high vulnerability and two communities representing critical cases of low vulnerability.

A recent analysis by Ted and colleague David MacAlister would fit into this category as well (Palys & MacAlister, 2016). Although there had been previous legal challenges to research confidentiality in Canada, in 2012, the Ontario Supreme Court heard a case in which the police executed a search warrant to obtain the tape and transcript of an interview that had been done several years earlier with a former sex worker who was now accused of murder. The researchers argued that a researcher–participant privilege should be recognized and the search warrant quashed, and the court agreed. The case could be considered "critical" because it was the first time a significant court in Canada had ever ruled on the question of whether communications between a researcher and a research participant should be protected, which meant that there were lessons to be learned about how the court would evaluate the evidence, how the legal principles involved in making this sort of decision would be applied, and how researchers in future might best prepare for such challenges.

Disconfirming or Negative Case Sampling

This strategy demands that we deliberately seek out cases that are in some way atypical or different from the cases that comprise the rest of our sample to ensure that all sides of an issue are represented or that the picture that emerges from our data is not distorted toward one perspective. Here the researcher is looking to extend their analysis by looking for cases that will disconfirm it, both to test theory and simply because it is often from our failures that we learn the most. The general principle here is, "If you think your results are not generalizable or the existence of a particular kind of case will undermine all that you 'know' to be true about a phenomenon, then look for that kind of case." Becker (1998) sees this as a fundamental strategy for qualitative research; the core principle is that you always should look for the toughest test of your developing theories because they are the ones that are most likely to cause you to rethink what you think you know and are thus by far the most interesting.

For example, for many years, people studying the sex industry focused their attention almost exclusively on female street-based sex workers. As a result, the theories that were developed about the sex industry painted a picture of drug addiction, mental health issues, sexual abuse, coercion, violence, and general despair. This picture dominated the theoretical landscape of the social and health science literatures on the topic until such time as researchers began to employ negative case sampling strategies. The picture that emerged from these efforts revealed not only that many people working in the sex industry do not fit the "desperation typology" but also that men and trans* people also sell sexual services and that the majority of sexual service-for-money exchanges occur in or through a wide array of venues or spaces that are far removed from the streets (e.g., escort agencies, massage parlors, dungeons, online webcam sites, etc.). Findings from this research have led many to rethink what it is that we "know" about the sex industry.

Representative Sampling

Although we have dealt separately with the issue of sampling for representativeness through probabilistic techniques, we also include it here by virtue of it being one of the many purposive strategies a researcher might employ. Although the particular research site we visit may be purposively chosen guided by any of the sampling strategies shown here, once we get to that site, we may well want to ensure that the sample of employees or clients or patients or files or whatever are representative of the population at that site. For example, an organization that wants to determine how employees are responding to a recent structural reorganization might poll a representative sample of employees to ensure that the views of a complete cross section of the organization are recognized.

The Thoughtful Respondent

In any field-based inquiry, researchers soon realize that prospective interviewees are *not* created equal; some are incredibly informative or provocative, others are unwilling to talk, still others can talk for hours without saying anything interesting. Many researchers would trade one thoughtful, insightful, and articulate respondent for a randomly chosen 50 any time. Although the thoughtful respondent might show up anywhere, two classes of respondents are often particularly helpful.

One group is the newbs … people who are new to a site … the new employees, the person just assigned there, and the recent graduate. To understand why, think back to the first week or two when you came to the university or college you are studying at now. Everything was brand new, fresh, and exciting, and if you were like both of us, you felt a bit like a stranger in a strange land. If you are an undergraduate, instead of the hundreds who attended your high school, now there are thousands and maybe even tens of thousands who attend your college. You have to figure out every-thing—how to get the courses you want; where the cafeterias and washrooms are; how to survive in a class of 300; where the sorts of people who will become your friends hang out—and it's because everything is new to you that you notice all sorts of things that someone who has been there for a few years already will by now be taking for granted. Similarly, if you are in a graduate program, you are now in that new limbo of professionalism where you are starting to move from "student" to "colleague" and taking on new responsibilities as you begin to learn more of that role.

The second group who often can offer some interesting insights are those at the opposite end of the spectrum, i.e., the veterans who have been around for quite a while and have observed people come and go, problems come and go, managers and fellow employees come and go, and stayed with the organization through good times and bad. Alternatively, it might be someone who has worked or studied in several different places. Both of these sets of individuals are in a good position to talk about change over time, how this place differs from others, and can put what you are finding as you speak with them now in perspective.

Snowball Sampling

Snowball sampling, sometimes referred to as network, chain referral, respondent-driven, or multiplicity sampling, takes its name from the experience of starting with a small snowball and, after rolling it down a hill or around in some damp snow, ending up with a huge ball that can serve as the base for a humanoid snow figure. By starting very small, you can still end up with something very big. In the sampling realm, snowball sampling involves starting with one or two people and then using their connections, and their connections' connections, to generate a large sample. This technique is especially useful if your target population is a deviant, marginalized, or "closet" population or isn't particularly well-defined or accessible.

Edna Salamon (1984) used the snowball procedure to good effect in her doctoral research on "kept women." Salamon wanted a sample of women who had received apartments, cars, trips, maintenance money, and so on in exchange for their camaraderie and involvement in an intimate relationship. But how and where can you acquire such a sample? There's obviously no sampling frame available. And there are no "kept woman clubs" to approach. Salamon was lamenting this problem to her hairdresser one day when he said "I know a few; I'll introduce you." He introduced her to a few kept women, each of whom introduced her to other kept women, who introduced her to others, until she had acquired a sizable sample of women.

The main danger in using this procedure is that your first snowball or participant may well influence the shape of the snow figure or wider sample or network of participants that results. Executives who went through Harvard Business School probably best know other executives who also went through Harvard Business School; street-based sex workers are probably more likely to know other street-based sex workers than they are to know escorts or independent companions, who travel in more exclusive company. In general, people are more likely to know people who are similar to them; in other words, our network of friends and colleagues tend to be more homogeneous than heterogeneous. Indeed, this social dynamic makes snowball samples possible in the first place. You must either remain cautious in generalizing results or try to start several different snowballs or network samples in several different niches or locations.

One extra thing to note with this sampling procedure is that institutional research ethics boards typically have strong preferences for how this is done. Years ago you simply would have asked someone at the end of an interview if they know of anyone else who might be relevant to the study and potentially interested in participating. The participant would have given us some contact information and we would go and ask that person whether they would like to take part. These days, institutional review boards see that approach as problematic in at least two respects. First is that they are concerned that the second person may feel inordinate pressure to participate, something along the lines of "Your friend participated so you should, too." Second is that they are concerned about violations of confidentiality because you are the one revealing to the second person that their friend participated ("Your friend Louise said that you might be interested in taking part"). Instead, institutional review boards now suggest that you ask the person who did participate in the study to pass along your contact information to anyone else they know who might like to take part. This places no inordinate pressure on the second person to take part, and it means that it is the first participant who chooses to reveal to the second that they took part rather than you being the one who does so.

COMPUTER NETWORKS AS A SAMPLING SITE

Just as the proliferation of the telephone in the 1930s and thereafter changed communication patterns and offered new ways to conduct social and health research, bourgeoning use and advances in information communications technologies (ICTs) such as mobile broadband cellular networks and the ever-expanding "Internet of Things" narrow the boundary between "real" and "virtual" worlds and make many different kinds of network-assisted research possible. Perhaps the most commonly cited advantage of using ICT and network technologies for acquiring samples is that they offer what is perhaps the most effective method for sampling participants from larger and more demographically and geographically diverse populations (Barry, 2001). Moreover, researchers have found that networked environments afford a unique opportunity to access difficult, deviant, hard-to-reach, or stigmatized populations (Atchison, 1996, 1998; Barry, 2001; Bungay, Oliffe, & Atchison, 2016; Fox, Murray, & Warm, 2003; Kolar & Atchison, 2013). Finally, they also have been useful for conducting research with elite groups (Bauman, Airey, & Atak, 1998) and with physically handicapped, shy, and disorganized individuals (Gosling, Vazire, Srivastava, & John, 2004) who are notoriously difficult to involve in research using other methods.

While ICTs and network technologies play a central role in the lives of many Americans, achieving success in computer-assisted social research requires us to understand who is and isn't using these technologies. According to the American Community Survey (ACS), in 2016, 89 percent of American households had a computer (which includes smartphones) and 81 percent had a broadband Internet subscription (Ryan, 2017). Moreover, the US Census Bureau reported that in 2016, nearly half of all the US households had a laptop or desktop computer, a smartphone, a tablet, *and* a broadband Internet connection. These "highly connected" (Ryan, 2017) households tend to be younger people/families that are more affluent and educated and are more likely to be found in metropolitan areas. Less-connected households (e.g., those reporting a smartphone as their sole internet-connected device) are more likely to be headed by older individuals (i.e., over 65), lower income, and located in nonmetropolitan areas. When we compare ICT usage from national surveys over time, we see it is constantly rising as more and more people integrate ICTs into their lives in an ever-greater variety of ways. Although there is still at this point a "digital divide," the disparity is less and less with time, in large part because the highest user groups are close to the ceiling (91–97 percent) while the lowest user groups keep rising.

SOLICITING RESPONSES AND PARTICIPATION

Regardless how we eventually decide to go about sampling, once we have decided on the most appropriate strategy and located prospective participants—or the places or things we wish to study—we are faced with the next challenge, which is to convince them to participate or grant us access to the things we want to study. Increasingly, it is not enough to simply approach, text, email, or phone a prospective participant or gatekeeper and say "I'm a researcher from State University, will you participate in my research or give me access to this space?" While participation rates vary by age, sex, geographical area, and research design, researchers from around the world have noted a steady decline over the years (Blumberg, Luke, & Cynamon, 2006; Mindell et al., 2015). The steady growth of the commercial research industry and the often invasive, unethical, and/or simply annoying tactics that market researchers have used to secure participants has made many members of the general public distrustful of research in general and unwilling to contribute their time (Blumberg, Luke, & Cynamon, 2006; Kaye & Johnson, 1999; Sheehan & Hoy, 1999). Additionally, the growing prevalence of call-screening devices (Tuckel & O'Neill, 2002) accompanied by rising cell phone use has all contributed to this observed steady decline in participation rates. This has meant that social and health researchers have had to develop a wide range of traditional and innovative strategies for "advertising" our research and soliciting responses.

Unless we are already personally acquainted with someone from the population we are interested in accessing (e.g., insiders or informants), we most likely will have to make a direct appeal to members of the population by placing an advertisement in newspapers, magazines, radio, or television programs or by distributing flyers, poster-ads, or business cards in areas where prospective participants might see our appeal. For example, when Chris wanted to contact sex buyers, he started by placing advertisements in specific adult newspapers, magazines, and trade papers that he had reason to believe were read by people who paid for sex. He also ran ads in local newspapers, magazines, and daily free papers and distributed posters, pamphlets, and business cards to STD/STI clinics, dance clubs and bars, and novelty shops throughout the cities and surrounding areas in which he was conducting research. Spreading his advertisements across multiple media sources and venues allowed him to get information about his research to a wide cross section of the population. While placing ads in newspapers and magazines or on local television has been a staple of participant recruitment in the social and health sciences for many years, readership and viewership in these traditional media have been declining steadily with the continued growth of the Internet. Since 2000, newspapers in the United States have faced a cumulative 25.6 percent loss in daily circulation; magazines and local television news also have faced steep audience declines (Pew Research Centre, 2010).

In response to the changing media landscape, many researchers have begun to make greater use of ICTs and other network methods for contacting and soliciting research participants. Some of the most popular ways of using technology to solicit participants include sending out bulk email, paying search providers such as Google to advertise your research website, posting notices on a social networking site or service such as Twitter, Instagram, or Facebook, and placing advertisements in online discussion boards where "communities" of people who share similar interests or experiences connect with one another (see Temple & Brown, 2011).

It is important to keep in mind that these are just a subset of available techniques. As networked environments continually change, there undoubtedly will be an increasing number of ways that Internets, intranets, and cellular networks can be used to contact and solicit research participants. For example, in one of his recent studies of the sex industry, Chris employed a solicitation strategy that leveraged the power of social networking applications and the structure of online "communities" in order to maximize the distribution of information about his research to a wide population of potential respondents. This approach—which he refers to as "viral recruitment" (Kolar & Atchison, 2013)—combines elements of traditional network sampling techniques with viral marketing, a form of word-of-mouth advertising that exploits the unique characteristics of computerized communications networks to aid the transmission of a message across multiple members of a social network (Kirby & Marsden, 2006). As the message (in this case, an infographic that conveyed the importance of research for the development of evidence-based social and health policy) was passed from one sex worker or sex buyer to the next, the message's exposure and influence grew exponentially (i.e., it "went viral"). Employing this approach helped to generate close to 900 participants from his target population.

A controversial issue that arises in relation to many types of research is whether respondents should be paid for their participation. One set of arguments—in articles that tend to focus on health-related research and especially research involving pharmaceutical companies engaged in clinical trials—focuses on the relationship between an individual researcher and individual participant. The big question in that area, where research participants are often exposed to substantial risks that cannot be fully predicted ahead of time, is whether the injection of money into the equation creates an "undue influence" for people to participate in situations that are against their better interests. Fry, Hall, Ritter, and Jenkinson (2006) found three main positions evident in the literature: (1) that payment creates an inherently "undue influence" and thus should not be allowed; (2) that payments are a justifiable incentive to participation that can raise recruitment levels without crossing the ethical line into undue influence; and (3) that payment to participants comprise a fair and equitable recognition of the effort and trust they extend and thus should be encouraged, if not required. Articles in the latter tradition distinguish different approaches to payment and argue about whether amounts offered should involve simple reimbursement of any expenses incurred, or wage-based approaches that treat participation as a part-time job, or follow a simple supply and demand logic where a project sponsor offers whatever it takes to acquire the number of bodies required for a proper statistical analysis of effects (e.g., Draper, Wilson, Flanagan, & Ives, 2009; Fry et al., 2006; Ripley, 2006; Stones & McMillan, 2010).

Along with these arguments is another set that poses larger questions about the relationship between the research community and participants and the social factors that play out on the ground when money is introduced into the equation. The tradition we were raised in was that participation in research should be voluntary. The idea was that committed field researchers should concentrate on building rapport with communities of interest and building credibility by showing that they would be nonjudgmental and fair in the treatment of their sample and the social groupings that led them to be of interest. If you did so, those you work with would be glad to participate because of a shared interest in your topic and a desire to contribute to knowledge in a safe and respectful environment. Money was viewed cynically as the substitute that bought access to vulnerable populations (e.g., sex workers, the drug addicted, the homeless, and the poor) for researchers who had no tradition in field work or the time or interest to get connected and establish credibility. Universities—who lionize those who get massive grants for the recognition it gets them in the academic community—are complicit in that transition.

The issue that concerns us is the extent to which those who work with marginalized communities have bought into the payment regime. In Vancouver, for example, those who live in the city's downtown east side (DES)—sometimes referred to as the poorest postal code in Canada and replete with individuals with significant problems including poverty, homelessness, drug and alcohol addictions, and mental health issues—have collaborated with researchers from Ted's university to produce a "Manifesto for ethical research" (Boilevin et al., 2019). While the report contains many excellent points about working with the DES community and includes calls for greater transparency by researchers as to their sources of funding and prospective implications (both positive and negative) for members of the community, it also takes the stance that participation in research should be seen as "work" for which participants should be paid:

> *Honour our ongoing work of survival and don't shy away from necessary, though sometimes uncomfortable, conversations about money. Pay us fairly and promptly for our work on your project. Don't assume that we have nothing better to do or that it's not a sacrifice to spend time working with you on a research project. Don't assume we owe you something because of your 'concern' for our community. Don't expect us to work for free. ALL of the time we spend with you working on your project needs to be compensated. Hustling for survival takes time, and if you take our time and don't pay us we might need to hustle in ways that put us at more risk. Paying us cash is best too. We don't ask what you do with your money, so don't try and police what we do with our money either (i.e. please no more gift cards!). (p. 18)*

Debates about the implications of paying participants continue. Does it ultimately end up favoring funded research and undermine those who self-fund in order to remain independent? Is the prospect of money an irresistible incentive that takes precedence over other interests (such as health, confidentiality) for someone who is poor, drug addicted, and/or homeless? Does it enhance validity by broadening the range of people who participate in research? Does it undermine validity by offering incentives for people to lie in order to participate and get the money (e.g., by saying they meet screening criteria when they don't)? If challenges to research confidentiality were to arise, would the courts protect research participants who engage in a cash-based transaction they themselves describe as "work" with the same degree of respect they have treated participants who have volunteered (see Palys & Lowman, 2014)?

While researchers working for large corporations may find it necessary to offer gifts or money because their research offers little direct benefit to people or society, much of the research we do in the social and health sciences is not motivated by profit or corporate interests. Social and health researchers might be more successful in soliciting participants if we took the time to fully illustrate to participants the intrinsic and practical benefits of participating in our research and how these benefits extend far beyond those they would get from the nominal amount of money we could offer them.

One final issue to consider, especially as you read through the chapters in this book that outline the specific techniques we can employ for making observations and collecting data, is the importance of participation options in helping you solicit people to take part in your research. The specific format of the research instrument greatly influences a potential respondent's willingness and ability to participate (Hampton & Wellman, 1999). Again, part of the success that Chris has had in securing participants from populations who are generally considered difficult to access can be attributed to his providing prospective participants with multiple participation options, thereby making participation easier and getting rid of at least one reason why someone might refuse. The inherent flexibility of computerized observation and data instruments has been instrumental in this respect. It is a relatively simple task for researchers to design shorter, simplified, and less obtrusive data collection instruments in order to improve response rates (Crawford, Couper, & Lamias, 2001). Additionally, designing the instrument so that less experienced users can respond using their mouse, keyboard, touchscreen, or voice activation is an increasingly realistic option.

SUMMING UP AND LOOKING AHEAD

Consistent with the theme developed elsewhere in this book, this chapter argues that there is no one "best" sampling procedure. Rather, deciding which is "best" depends once again on your research objectives, the nature of the phenomenon being studied, and pragmatic considerations related to your choice of site and sample. And of course, sampling strategies apply both to people and any other unit of analysis that we might wish to scrutinize, including objects (e.g., the products of a particular manufacturer, types of films) or a particular type of situation (e.g., marriage proposals, casual drug use, career decisions, emergency triage).

The chapter discusses a range of probabilistic, quasi-probabilistic, and purposive techniques, outlining the sorts of situations and research objectives for which each is suitable. Probabilistic techniques are the techniques of choice when acquiring a representative sample is crucial; quasi-probabilistic techniques can be a useful alternative when a random sample is not possible but the researcher nonetheless seeks a sample that is at least unbiased; and purposive techniques are the techniques of choice for more field-based situations where persons in the setting are not interchangeable and where position, point of view, access to particular information, and insight and ability to articulate are the more important criteria to maximize. Multifaceted research questions that frequently form the basis of mixed methods research designs often require that you use multiple and diverse sampling techniques.

The chapter then highlighted how increasing access to and use of ICTs has narrowed the boundary between "real" and "virtual" worlds and made it easier for social and health researchers to study a broader range of people and things. While there is still a digital divide that separates the digital "haves" from the "have nots," that divide is rapidly shrinking.

Finally, the chapter concluded with a discussion of how to go about getting people to participate or getting access to the groups, organizations, or artifacts that will provide you with the information you need to answer your research questions and achieve your objectives. Here we discussed the increasing challenges that social and health researchers are having soliciting responses and participation. While participation rates vary by age, sex, geographical area, and research design, researchers from around the world have noted a steady decline over the years. To address the challenges of securing participants, we argued that social and health researchers need to be wary of the issues that emerge from simply paying people to participate and called for greater creativity in drawing from, and often combining, a range of traditional and technology facilitated solicitation strategies.

We're at the point now in the research process where we have a topic; have found relevant literature; have identified a specific research question to pursue or hypothesis to test; have reviewed the ethics issues that need to be considered when dealing with human participants; and have discussed some options regarding where, when, and with whom we will focus. The next three chapters will take us into the realm of overall research design, where you will learn how you can structure or adapt to the research situation to in such a way to maximize clarity of inference about causes and effects through experimental, quasi-experimental, and case study designs.

Key Concepts

Criterion sampling 187
Critical case sampling 188
Disproportional stratified
  random sample 173
Extreme or deviant case
  sampling 185
Generalizability 153
Multistage cluster
  sampling 174
Negative case sampling 189
Population 160
Probabilistic sampling 163

Proportional stratified random
  sampling 172
Purposive or strategic
  sampling 184
Quasi-probabilistic sampling 174
Quota sampling 175
Random 153
Random error 166
Representative 155
River sampling 187
Sample 152
Sampling error 166

Sampling frame 165
Sampling ratio 170
Simple random sampling 166
Snowball sampling 190
Stakeholder sampling 185
Stratified random sample 170
Systematic error 166
Systematic sample with random
  start 170
Units of analysis 164
Universe 164

STUDY QUESTIONS

1. "Any study that doesn't use a representative sample will inevitably produce findings that are not generalizable." Discuss this statement.

2. What does it mean to say that a sample is representative of some larger population?

3. What criteria have to be met for a sample to be considered a random sample? Why would you want a random sample?

4. Gwen wants to acquire a random sample of people who attend a very controversial film. Which of the following procedures would give her a random sample? (1) She rolls a dice and a "3" turns up. Gwen approaches the 3rd person in line and every 10th person thereafter; (2) Gwen goes down the line and arbitrarily picks people by whim; (3) Gwen's favorite color is green, so she decides to interview every person who shows up wearing something green.

5. What is the relationship between universe, population, and sample?

6. Prepare a summary table of the sampling techniques discussed in this chapter. Begin by drawing four columns on a sheet of paper. Title the first column "Techniques"; in that column, list all the techniques covered in the chapter. Title the second column "Procedures"; in that column, describe in your own words the procedures involved in executing each technique. Title the third and fourth columns "Strengths" and "Weaknesses," respectively; in these columns, list situations for which each technique would be useful, along with the technique's advantages and limitations.

7. Alison wants to interview a representative sample of people who live in apartments in New York's high-rise haven, Manhattan. Unfortunately, no sampling frame is available, and it would be impossible to construct one. What sampling procedure would you recommend that she use? Why?

8. How does quota sampling differ from stratified random sampling?

9. Can an unrepresentative sample still be useful? If so, explain how.

10. You plan to study the department you're majoring in at your college or university. In particular, you want to examine the undergraduate curriculum to ascertain both how it came about and how it might be improved. You want to gather data via interviews. How do you decide whom to sample? Discuss some of your alternatives, describing their respective advantages and limitations.

11. This year's student council is evenly divided on whether the student-run cafeteria should be run on a not-for-profit basis (in order to minimize the cost of meals to students) or on a for-profit basis (with all the profits going to the student society's bursary program). Riaz decides to do a survey to determine the attitudes of the current student body toward these alternatives. He goes to the cafeteria at noon on a Thursday, numbers all the tables (from 1 to 250), randomly samples 50 of the tables, and interviews all the people sitting at those tables. He finds that 57 percent of the students interviewed prefer the for-profit alternative. How confident can Riaz be that this result is representative of the opinions of the student body? Could he be more confident in the representativeness of his results if he had interviewed people from 100 randomly chosen tables?

12. Chris takes a different approach to the problem outlined in Study Question 11. She approaches the college registrar for a list of all students who are currently enrolled; using a table of random numbers, she chooses one student from that list. When interviewed, that student expresses an opinion in favor of the for-profit alternative. Is that one student's opinion theoretically representative of the opinions of the entire student body? Explain why or why not.

13. Pat wants to do an interview study of "basketball fans." Suggest two probabilistic and two purposive techniques that might, under certain conditions (which you should specify), allow her to acquire such a sample. Discuss the advantages and limitations of using each of those techniques.

14. Identify a population of people that you are interested in knowing more about and devise a way to sample and solicit them that uses computer technology. Once you have devised your strategy, explain how you think your strategy is an improvement over more conventional approaches that you could have used.

15. Some people suggest that research participants should be paid for their participation, while others believe that it should be voluntary. What are some of the pros and cons of paying participants?

ELIMINATING RIVAL PLAUSIBLE EXPLANATIONS: THE EXPERIMENT

We've discussed general approaches to science as well as some of the ethical and sampling issues involved in doing research thus far. The next question we need to consider is how we can structure or take advantage of an existing situation so that our inferences about "what's going on" are both reasonable and justifiable. In that regard, many of our explanations and objectives are causal ones in the sense that we are often trying to understand how one thing—a situation, a set of attitudes, a program, a certain life experience, a new policy or law—affects some other class of things. The central challenge for us as researchers is to do our research in such a way that, when we get to the end of our study, we can say with some reasonable degree of confidence that a relationship proposed by some theory does appear to exist, that our intervention was successful, that the program created change, or that what we did had some impact. Equally important is knowing the processes through which those changes came about. These issues of inference are addressed in a group of research approaches that include the classic experiment, quasi-experimentation, and case study analysis. In this chapter we explain how the three share a common underlying logic that involves eliminating *rival plausible explanations* to make reasonable inferences about "causes" and other processes, but vary in the degree of predetermined structure each involves and the particular way they allow you to rule out competing explanations.

ISOLATING CAUSES: THE CONTROLLED EXPERIMENT

It seems we are always making attributions about causes and effects in the world around us, sometimes with good reasoning and sometimes with bad. We attribute the gulf that has been developing in the relationship with our partner to the fact that they are spending too much time with their friends, or have lost interest, or are going through one of "those" times, or are simply no longer the person we thought them to be. Much superstitious behavior comes from causal attributions we make that may make us feel better but are unlikely to have any real causal effect: we wear a certain hat to our final exam and do well, and from then on we "always" wear our "lucky hat" to exams. But as fallible as we are, it is probably a good thing and perhaps even a uniquely human thing that we can solve a problem at a high level of abstraction and broad scope—and thereby were able to figure out where babies come from, learned which plants would poison us and which made good eating, and discovered that leaving a plot of ground fallow every once in a while would help future harvests.

But how can we ensure we do it well? Methodologists and philosophers have given considerable thought to the way we draw inferences from what we observe.

Historically in the social and health sciences, experimentation, and laboratory experimentation in particular, has been seen by many as *the* route to the generation of reliable and dependable knowledge. Although research embodying experimentalist principles was being conducted long before our current canons of research were formulated (e.g., see Cook & Campbell, 1979; Shadish, Cook, & Campbell, 2001), our major contemporary debt in this realm is to John Stuart Mill, who said that, before we could say that one event or person "caused" some other effect, we had to demonstrate that three criteria (Mills's 3 criteria) held:

1. ***Temporal precedence***, i.e., because we believe that causes always come *before* effects, the first criterion requires us to show that the thing we think is a cause occurred *prior* to any changes or differences that we think might have been produced by it. Thus, if a light goes on and *then* we flip a light switch, our flipping of the switch cannot be the reason the light went on. Only if we flip the switch and *then* the light goes on can we continue to believe that the flipping of the switch *might* be the cause of the light going on.

2. ***Association or relationship***, i.e., if the alleged cause does indeed act to produce a given effect, then the second criterion requires we show that changes in the putative cause covaries in some reliable way with its alleged effect. To continue the light switch example, we would have to show that whenever we flip the switch, the light goes on, and conversely, whenever we don't flip the switch, the light does not go on. Of course the light switch is a very physical and deterministic example. In the social and health sciences, where causes and effects usually are not so mechanistic and many other variables can intervene, we do not expect a certain cause will necessarily happen *every* time the alleged effect is present, but we do expect it to happen "often," where "often" is typically defined as "more frequently than you would expect on the basis of chance alone."

3. ***Elimination of rival plausible explanations***, i.e., we are obliged to demonstrate that it is the putative cause per se that is responsible for changes in the dependent measure, rather than related variables, nuisance variables, artifacts, or other potential causal agents that might have been present.

Part of the reason that the classic laboratory experiment is so revered is because it does such a splendid job of addressing these criteria.

THE TERMINOLOGY AND LOGIC OF EXPERIMENTATION

Experimentation begins when we recognize or create a situation that includes the phenomenon of interest to us and embodies parameters suggested by theory or includes the intervention whose impact we wish to address. The situation or intervention does not need to exist in the real world; the lab affords us the ability to deal not only with realities that exist but also to consider *possible* realities that *might* exist if our particular intervention was implemented or if the world were arranged in the manner imagined by us or our theories.

You should see how the experiment makes it possible to meet Mill's first two criteria. Because the laboratory experiment is conducted on our turf, as we arrange it, and when we want it to happen, we have the luxury of causing the putative cause to occur at our convenience, enabling us to be there with measurement instruments in hand (whether that be an observational schedule, or interview, or questionnaire), waiting to catch the anticipated effects when and if they occur. The **temporal precedence** criterion is met because of the manipulative control that we impose on the timing of events. The *association* or *relationship* criterion is met by seeing the extent to which change has occurred and using statistics to assess whether the change observed is beyond what we would expect on the basis of chance variation alone.

The trick is the third criterion (see Palys, 1989). The problem is twofold. First is the truism that you probably have already heard about, which is that "correlation does not necessarily equal causation" (**correlation ≠ causation**). Just because two things happen to go together does not mean that one is necessarily the cause of the other. A famous example concerns fire trucks and fire damage: the more fire trucks there are at a fire, the more likely it is that the buildings they are trying to save will burn to the ground, but that does not mean that the fire trucks are causing the damage. Some consequences of assuming the two are the same is shown in Figure 6.1.

A second problem is that isolating causes can be a tricky process because so many different variables intervene between cause and effect, and so many others are often occurring at the same time. We may isolate one variable as a possible cause—and are often encouraged to do so because of our other beliefs and philosophies that predispose us to accept a particular explanation as plausible—but that may say more about us than it does about the world we are trying to understand. What is the source of America's financial troubles? For Republicans, the "causes" are a government that has grown too large and is paying for too many services for too many Americans who do not really need it. For Democrats, the cause is the great divide in wealth that sees

FIGURE 6.1 ● Implications of Confusing Correlation and Causation

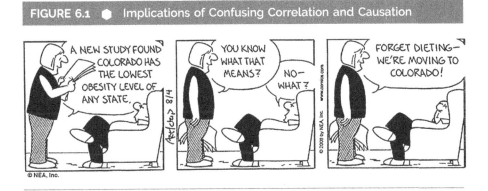

the rich get richer while the middle class and poor pay taxes with far too much spent on fighter jets, submarines, policing, and prisons instead of social programs that will build community and prevent crime. And none of them knows for sure because the American economy is far too complex, driven by far too many factors, and subject to far too many external influences to isolate any particular cause.

But now let's move to more of a social science example; we'll start with a very simple design and build from there. Suppose we want to know whether watching a series of films about immigrants' contributions to American culture will influence people's attitudes toward immigration policies and current immigration levels. Assuming that we have a reliable and valid measure of this attitude, one way to assess the impact of exposure to the films would be to measure the preliminary attitudes of a group of individuals regarding current immigration levels; show this group of people the series of films; and measure the group's attitudes once again afterward, in order to see whether any change in attitude had occurred. This process is illustrated in Figure 6.2.

FIGURE 6.2 ● Diagram of One Way to Access Change in Attitudes (One-Group Pretest/Posttest Design)

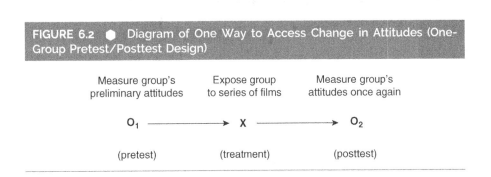

Independent and Dependent Variables

Our hypothetical study has two key variables. The first variable is the one whose impact we want to assess, namely, the exposure to a series of films. Note that the choice of which variable to impose or manipulate (i.e., exposure to the films) represents a decision we make *independent* of the actual execution of our study. This variable whose impact we are trying to assess is known appropriately enough as the independent variable, predictor, or treatment variable.

The second variable is the one we measure in order to see whether any effect has occurred, which, in our hypothetical study, is attitudes toward current immigration levels. What level or values will they take on in the study? We can't really answer that question until we actually do the study, since the values that variable takes on will *depend* on who is in our subject sample, what their attitudes are, and how potent or effective the independent variable actually is in causing change. Rather than being independent of the actual execution of the study (as was the case with the films), the values that the attitude variable takes on are very much *dependent* on what happens during the actual execution of the study. This variable is known as the dependent variable or outcome variable.

Internal Validity

Suppose that we do the study and find that, following exposure to the films, there *is* a change in our dependent measure. What can we conclude from that observation? We might *like* to conclude that the change we observed was attributable to the independent variable of interest (i.e., the film series). But how confident can we be in drawing that inference?

It's time to introduce a major concept: the internal validity of a study. This term, coined by Campbell and Stanley (1963), refers to *the extent to which differences observed in the study can be* unambiguously *attributed to the experimental treatment itself, rather than to other factors*. In other words, to what extent can we be confident that the differences we observe are caused by the independent variable per se, rather than by other rival plausible explanations? In the current example, how confident can we be that it was the film series that caused the change? Or could it have been something else?

But what else could it have been? After defining the term, Campbell and Stanley (1963) delineate a number of classes of "threats" (i.e., concerns or rival plausible explanations) to keep in mind when assessing internal validity. A number of these are relevant to our hypothetical research design.

History

The first potential threat to internal validity is **history**, which refers in pretest/posttest designs to the *specific events occurring between the first and second measurement in addition to the independent variable.* In other words, what other events might have occurred during the study that might also account for the results that we observed? In our hypothetical study, various events other than the film series might have occurred that also could have led our respondents to change their attitudes. They might have seen newspaper articles or TV shows about immigration successes or have been exposed to classroom materials dealing with immigration policies. How do we know it wasn't one of those *other* factors or variables that caused a change in attitude, rather than the films we showed? In the research design we have right now, there's no way we can tell for sure.

Maturation

A second threat to internal validity noted by Campbell and Stanley (1963) is **maturation**, defined as *processes within the research participants themselves that change as a function of time* per se (i.e., not specific to particular events), such as growing older, more tired, more hungry, and so on. This threat draws our attention to the fact that sometimes changes occur merely because of biological processes that happen over time, and we must be careful to recognize those processes and their effects when we're assessing the effects of other independent variables.

For example, suppose we come to you with a pill and suggest it will help children learn to walk. In order to demonstrate the effectiveness of this pill, we first acquire a sample of six-month-old children, none of whom can walk. We give each of the children (or their parents) a box of the pills, with the instruction that the children are to take one pill a month for a year. One year later, we come back and find that every single one of the children (now one-and-a-half years old) knows how to walk. The design would be like that depicted in Figure 6.3. Were the pills effective? Maybe. But

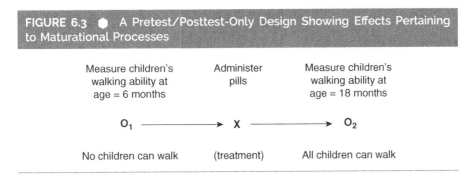

FIGURE 6.3 ● A Pretest/Posttest-Only Design Showing Effects Pertaining to Maturational Processes

Measure children's walking ability at age = 6 months   Administer pills   Measure children's walking ability at age = 18 months

$O_1 \longrightarrow X \longrightarrow O_2$

No children can walk   (treatment)   All children can walk a rather compelling rival plausible explanation would be that it wasn't the *pills* that caused the change, but rather maturational changes within the children (i.e., physical processes like bone development, physical competence, coordination) that now allowed them to walk. In other words, they probably would have learned to walk anyway, with or without the pills.

The above example may seem fairly obvious, but it shows how maturational processes can threaten internal validity. Sometimes, though, the effects of maturational processes are more subtle and, consequently, ignored. Returning to our immigration example, suppose we start by giving a questionnaire in the morning about immigration policies (i.e., our pretest), spend a solid 8 hours showing various films to our research participants and end the day by again giving the questionnaire on current immigration policies (the posttest). In the end, we find that our participants show more hostile attitudes and appear to be more critical of immigrants. Can we conclude that exposure to the films caused the change in attitude?

The films *may* have caused the change. And historical factors wouldn't be a threat to that conclusion, since our participants have been insulated from other events (e.g., news media reports). But look what we've done. We've required our participants to put in a long day, given them no opportunity to have lunch, and kept them busy doing our questionnaire and viewing our films. What happens to people in that type of situation? Many people get tired and hungry; over the course of a long, demanding day, they may also become more impatient, terse, and "hangry." Because of these physiologically based "maturational" changes, in other words, we might expect that by the time of the posttest, participants will have become slightly more hostile in their responses to our questions. Can we therefore conclude that the *films* caused the change to more critical attitudes? Although we might like to do so (given our interests), we also would have to consider (as a rival plausible explanation) that maturational changes may have caused the change.

Testing

A third threat to internal validity is **testing**, specifically, *the effects of taking a test on scores in the second testing*. Such effects can operate in several different ways. Having taken a test, you may become sensitized to the issue involved in a way that you wouldn't have been otherwise. Suppose somebody gives you a questionnaire regarding your attitudes about current immigration levels. The mere fact that you were administered the questionnaire may lead you to be more sensitive to, or more likely to pay attention to, related material that's presented online, on TV, on the radio, or in your classes. When you then receive the posttest after the administration of the independent variable, and it turns out your attitudes have changed, researchers can't be sure whether the change was produced by the independent variable or by the greater sensitization to issues induced by the pretest. Consequently, this phenomenon, known as **pretest sensitization**, is a threat to internal validity. Why? Because it offers a rival plausible explanation for the source of change.

Another way in which testing can threaten internal validity is through **practice effects**. If we were trying to assess your abilities, for example, it would be difficult to know in the posttest situation whether you had improved purely because of the practice the pretest gave you or because of the independent variable we had imposed on you. It is not unusual, for example, for students who take SAT or LSAT exams to do better the second time they take it. Why? In some cases it may be that an intervention occurred that caused them to do better—they hired a tutor, for example—but it may simply be because they now know more of what to expect, are less anxious, and/or now understand how to better allocate their time.

Regression Toward the Mean

A related yet very different threat to internal validity is known as statistical regression or **regression toward the mean**. Recall that, with testing, we were talking about *real* change occurring between pretest and posttest (e.g., because of practice, sensitization to issues, or greater motivation); in such a situation, the threat to internal validity relates to uncertainty about whether the independent variable or the testing effect was the source of the change.

With statistical regression, we also observe a change, but in this instance, the change is more illusory than real. We know that any measuring we do is subject to a certain amount of random error, no matter how many precautions we take to minimize it. Many (if not most) times, these positive and negative chance influences will be distributed equally across a group, or across time for a particular individual, so that in the long run, the *average* score of a particular individual or group will be a good indication of their "true" score. But on any given occasion, chance events may "stack up" in a positive or negative direction. Also known as regression toward the mean, statistical regression refers to *the propensity of extreme scorers on the first testing to score closer to the mean (average) of the group on the second testing*. This phenomenon occurs because chance events are unlikely ever to stack up to precisely the same degree on two successive occasions.

Let's take Kawhi Leonard as an example. In case you haven't heard of him, Leonard plays for the Los Angeles Clippers, a National Basketball Association (NBA) team. One of the game's elite players, he has already won championships with two different teams and dominates a game in the manner of a Michael Jordan or a Lebron James, averaging roughly 30 points a game. But even Kawhi Leonard has good games and bad games. Basketball fans know that Leonard is a great basketball player because they observe his performance over the course of a whole season year after year. But in the social and health sciences, we rarely have the luxury of such extended observation. Instead, our situation is often more like that of the person who goes to only one basketball game in which Leonard happens to be playing.

Suppose this person goes to a basketball game to assess how good a basketball player Kawhi Leonard is. And suppose Leonard has a great night: he can't do anything wrong, and he ends up scoring 50 points. If, on the basis of that single assessment, our observer concludes that "Kawhi Leonard is amazing; he gets 50 points a game," basketball fans know that the observer is *overestimating* Leonard's "true" ability. But (and here's the important part) what if the same observer goes to see Kawhi Leonard play in a *second* basketball game later in the same season? The last time they saw him, he scored 50 points, but his *average* is about 30 points a game. Now, if you were a betting person, would you bet that on this second occasion Leonard will (1) do even *better* than he did last time and score more than 50 points this time, (2) do the *same* as he did last time and score exactly 50 points, or (3) do more *poorly* than he did last time and score fewer than 50 points?

If you picked (1) or (2), please send us your name and address: we could use the money. Leonard *may* get 50 points or more in this second game, but the likelihood is much higher that he will perform more in keeping with his average or typical performance and get something closer to 30 points. This is true *not* because Leonard has changed or because of anything special that might have happened between the two games, but purely because the first performance was atypically high due to chance factors—one of those magical nights when all the bounces went his way. This phenomenon—the tendency of extreme scores to move ("regress" is the technical term) closer to the mean on a subsequent testing—is known as *statistical regression* or *regression toward the mean*. The more extreme the first score—whether unusually high or unusually low—the greater this propensity.

Regression toward the mean threatens internal validity whenever a group is picked *because* of the extremity of their scores on a pretest. For example, suppose that in the study concerning attitudes about current immigration levels, we decide to administer our immigration questionnaire to 100 people and then pick the 20 people from that group who were apparently *least* in favor of current immigration levels (i.e., the 20 people with the lowest scores on the pretest) to see whether exposing them to our film series will lead them to temper their attitudes somewhat. Although we're confident

FIGURE 6.4 ● The Different Propensity of Scores From Three Areas of the Normal Distribution for Regression Toward the Mean

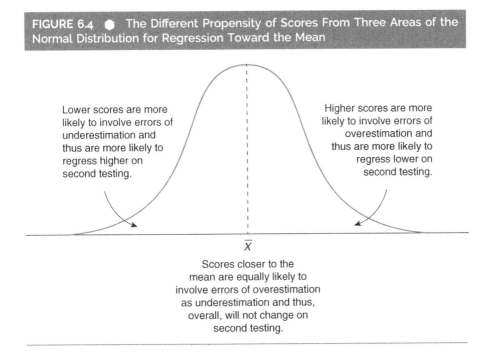

Lower scores are more likely to involve errors of underestimation and thus are more likely to regress higher on second testing.

Higher scores are more likely to involve errors of overestimation and thus are more likely to regress lower on second testing.

$\overline{X}$

Scores closer to the mean are equally likely to involve errors of overestimation as underestimation and thus, overall, will not change on second testing.

about the reliability and validity of our scale, no test is perfect so there will *always* be *some* degree of error in the scores. And as argued above, the odds are high that to the extent that we've erred in assessing our group's attitudes toward current immigration levels, the errors among the *lowest* scorers likely will be errors of *underestimation* (e.g., see Figure 6.4). Since on a second testing, the *chance* errors that contributed to the extremity of those low scores are unlikely to stack up to the same degree as before, the scores on the second testing will be less extreme (i.e., closer to the mean of the group). Thus, it will *look* as though there's been attitude change (because the average score changes), but all we've *really* witnessed is that phenomenon known as regression toward the mean. And we'll be uncertain as to what extent the change we observe is attributable to the independent variable (i.e., the film series) or to the regression artifact. The same would have been true, but in the opposite direction, if we had started with the 20 highest scorers on the pretest; they, too, would have moved closer to the mean, which would have given the appearance of their attitudes becoming more negative. As Cook and Campbell (1979) explain,

[S]tatistical regression (1) operates to increase obtained pretest-posttest gain scores among low pretest scores, since this group's pretest scores are more likely to have been

depressed by error; (2) operates to decrease obtained change scores among persons with high pretest scores since their pretest scores are likely to have been inflated by error; and (3) does not affect obtained change scores among scorers at the center of the pretest distribution since the group is likely to contain as many units whose pretest scores are inflated by error as units whose pretest scores are deflated by it. (pp. 52–53)

History, maturation, testing, and statistical regression are the only threats to internal validity we will deal with at this time. But keep in mind that **selection** biases (discussed later in this chapter; see also discussion of sampling in Chapter 5) and **instrumentation** changes (see discussion of archival methods in Chapter 12) may also threaten internal validity. Those interested in further reading should consult Cook and Campbell (1979) or the revised edition by Shadish et al. (2001).

The main point here is that, in any study, you always should ask *why* a particular result was observed. Did the independent variable produce the result, or could it have been produced by something else, i.e., some rival plausible explanation? In our hypothetical study, how confident are we that the changes in attitudes regarding current immigration levels were produced (caused) by the film series and not by something else? Given the *one-group pretest/posttest design* we have so far, we can't be very confident at all that the film series caused the change; in other words, we have low internal validity. Somehow we have to overcome that problem.

Controlling for Rival Plausible Explanations
Control/Comparison Groups

While the one-group pretest/posttest design did an admirable job of addressing the first two of Mill's criteria—we saw that a change happened and that it came *after* the putative cause we were testing—it failed miserably on the third. There were just too many *rival plausible explanations* that might also account for the observed result. The most common way to deal with that problem is to incorporate a second group into our design—known as a **control group or comparison group**. The control group starts off the same as our first group (the experimental group) and is treated identically to the experimental group in *all* respects except the control group *doesn't* receive the independent variable. This gives us the design shown in Figure 6.5: the *pretest/posttest control group design.* In our hypothetical study, our control group would receive the pretest and the posttest at the same times as the experimental group, but *wouldn't* be exposed to the film series. Instead, the control group might quietly sit and wait, watch a travelogue about a surfing contest on Hawaii's Northern Shore, or

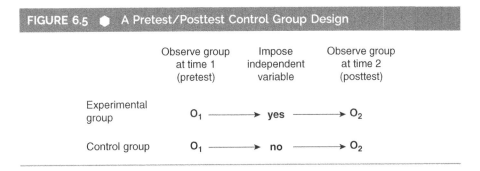

FIGURE 6.5 ● A Pretest/Posttest Control Group Design

	Observe group at time 1 (pretest)	Impose independent variable	Observe group at time 2 (posttest)
Experimental group	O_1 ⟶	yes ⟶	O_2
Control group	O_1 ⟶	no ⟶	O_2

do something else that keeps them busy for the same amount of time and at the same type of activity as the experimental group but that isn't directly related to attitudes regarding immigrants or immigration policies.

Suppose we do this study and obtain the results shown in Table 6.1. The control group's scores have changed slightly, but nowhere near as much as those of the experimental group. Now can we confidently assert that the changes in attitudes in the experimental group were a function of the film series rather than of rival plausible explanations?

Our internal validity in this case is actually fairly high. The best way to see this is to *try out* some rival plausible explanations to see what happens. Could the experimental group's attitudes have changed because of *history?* Maybe, but probably not. Why? Because the control group (as a group) was subject to those same historical factors, and their scores didn't change much at all. Could *maturation* have entered in? Maybe, but the control group had the same time delay between pretest and posttest, and it didn't cause them to change. Well, how about the effects of *testing?* Once again, pretest sensitization can't account for the results, because it would have had an equivalent effect on the control group, and they didn't change at all. So why did the experimental group change their attitudes? Given that the experimental and control

TABLE 6.1 ● Hypothetical Results for the Pretest/Posttest Control Group Design in Figure 6.5

	Pretest Scores	Impose Independent Variable	Posttest Scores
Experimental group	Average score = 43.6	→ Yes →	Average score = 58.6
Control group	Average score = 44.1	→ No →	Average score = 46.8

groups were equal to begin with (as shown by their similar pretest scores), and given that they were treated alike in every respect except for the imposition of the independent variable, the most likely explanation is that any change in the experimental group that wasn't observed in the control group must have been a function of the one element on which they differed: the film series.

The control group doesn't always have to be a "do nothing" group. *Control* groups are simply *comparison* groups that help us isolate and assess the impact or influence of particular variables. Accordingly, the nature of a control group will depend on what you're trying to assess, within the constraint of ethical considerations. Let's take two examples.

In the first example, imagine that you want to assess the effects that viewing explicitly sexual films has on those who view them. Your experimental group thus will comprise people to whom you show a sexually explicit film. In order to assess the effects of the film *per se*, you must choose an appropriate comparison group, a group that's similar to the experimental group in all respects, except that this group doesn't view a film with sexually explicit content. Let's say that the sexually explicit film you're showing is 30 minutes long. The procedures require that you welcome your experimental group to the lab, explain the nature of their participation, answer any questions, take them to the viewing room, and then give them a posttest measure. What would be an appropriate control group?

One possibility is simply to have a control group of people who come in, complete a pretest, sit around for 30 minutes, and then complete a posttest. But that creates more differences between the experimental and control groups than mere exposure to a sexually explicit film. Those who watch the explicit film have a whole range of experiences besides watching the film itself; for example, they receive the degree of attention (including instructions and explanations) accorded to people who are central to the research, and their attention is focused by a TV or film screen that they've been asked to watch.

A control group that comes in and does nothing, therefore, not only doesn't see the sexually explicit material. They also don't receive the same degree of attention from the experimenter and don't have their attention monopolized by a screen. Thus, when you come to the end of the study and want to evaluate internal validity, you can't tell for sure whether any differences between the two groups are due to the film, the attention paid to people, diverting their attention to a screen, or some combination thereof. A better procedure would involve giving everyone in the control group the same attention you give those in the experimental group and showing them a film, too, but ensuring that it contains absolutely no sexual content. In that way, you duplicate all aspects of the experimental group's experience except for the one element whose effects you wish to test: that is, the effects of viewing a sexually explicit film.

As a second example, consider someone who has developed a new counseling approach that is used to treat people experiencing depression. At the moment, suppose that these people receive "Don't Worry, Be Happy" (DWBH) counseling (a name we made up) that focuses on the counterproductiveness of compulsive worrying. People who use that method have a decent success rate, but you think that your program may be better, so you set out to evaluate its effectiveness. Your experimental group thus will comprise people who receive your new program. But what is an appropriate control group here?

A "do nothing" control group would be problematic in two ways. First, it would be a problem for the same reason noted in the preceding paragraph regarding the assessment of the effects of the sexually explicit film, that is, "attending a counseling program" and "doing nothing" differ on many more variables than just the content of the therapy. To counteract that, you might have the control group come in for equal periods of time and engage in some other form of interactive activity (e.g., playing a board game for an equivalent time period).

But ethical issues arise whenever you engage in research with people in need. "Doing nothing" may be a violation of your ethical obligation to ensure, to the best of your ability, the well-being of people under your care. Because of this, researchers in this situation will often use the "best known treatment" or "usual treatment" (the DWBH counseling, in this instance) as their basis of comparison.

The research question then changes from "Does the new program *work*?" (a question that implies a comparison between giving the program and doing nothing) to "Does the new program work *any better* than what we do already?" (a question that implies a comparison between giving the new program and retaining the old one). Often in such instances, the evaluation will measure many more variables than simple "treatment success," thereby allowing comparisons on other dimensions. It might be found, for example, that the new treatment is no different from the existing treatment in terms of success of treatment, but that it achieves that success at significant cost savings, allows clients to go home more quickly, has fewer side effects, or is less intrusive.

As the above discussion reveals, the logic of experimental design goes like this: *if* you have two (or more) groups who are equal to begin with and *if* you treat them identically in all respects *except* one (that being exposure versus nonexposure to the independent variable), any subsequent differences between the groups must be attributable to the one variable on which the groups differed. *Control* and *comparison groups* play a valuable function in empirical research by allowing you to isolate a particular reason behind any change that is observed. They're called "control" groups because they help control for rival plausible explanations.

Ensuring Pretest Equivalence

One point was glossed over in the preceding discussion that pertains to yet another possible threat to internal validity: **selection**. Thus far, we've said that *if we can assume our experimental and control groups were equal to begin with* and if we use appropriate controls, high internal validity will result. The italicized phrase refers to the assumption of **pretest equivalence**. But it includes a very big "if." How reasonable is the assumption that our groups are, in fact, equal to begin with?

In some instances, the assumption of pretest equivalence can't be made at all. This is typically the case in many *existing groups'* situations. For example, suppose we want to evaluate whether jail or the imposition of a fine is more effective in reducing the likelihood that people will reoffend. To do this, we get a sample of 1,000 people who have been sentenced to jail and 1,000 people who have been fined and then see how many in each group commit another offense during a two-year follow-up period. Would comparing these two rates tell us the relative effectiveness of the two sanctions in reducing recidivism? No. Why not? Because the two groups likely differed on many attributes other than type of sanction; that is, they probably also differed in terms of offense committed, prior record, or other variables that are also plausible alternative influences on our dependent variable.

The same is true whenever groups are formed on something other than a chance basis. Allowing self-selection or volunteer selection (i.e., letting people choose the groups in which they want to be), for example, can be problematic. Suppose we want to evaluate the effectiveness of a "defensive driving" course. We offer such a course to 16-year-olds at a local high school; some students sign up for it, while others do not. Two years after the course is completed, we compare accident records for all those students who received a license and find that those who took the course have been involved in significantly fewer accidents than those who didn't. Was the course effective? Well, maybe. But it's also possible that there was a selection bias because the two groups were not equal to begin with. Those who "self-selected" themselves into the course may have done so because of a greater concern over safe driving and, hence, might have been expected to have fewer accidents whether or not they took the course.

The opposite might happen when membership in the experimental group is *mandatory,* for example, where people charged with impaired or dangerous driving are sentenced by the courts to take a safe driving course. In this instance, we might well find that the "experimental" group does more *poorly* than a control group of other drivers picked at random—not because the course is poor, but because the process of group assignment created an experimental group that included those with poorer driving records and less skill and/or less motivation to drive carefully.

In either case, differences in motivation or concern that people bring to the study may be the "cause" of any subsequent differences in accident rates, rather than the driving course per se. Selection biases threaten internal validity by making the source of the observed change more ambiguous (i.e., increasing rather than reducing the number of rival plausible explanations).

In sum, selection biases form another possible threat to the internal validity of experimental research. So how can we ensure that our assumption of pretest equivalence is tenable, thereby enhancing internal validity? There are two major ways to do so: *random assignment* and *matching.*

Random Assignment. Given that you have a group of people ready to participate in your research, **random assignment** is achieved by letting "chance" be the *sole* determinant of which group (i.e., experimental or control) any given person is a member of. You might, for example, cut a deck of cards before each person comes to see you, with a red card indicating that the next person will go into the control group and a black card meaning they will go into the experimental group. Or you might flip a coin or use a random number generator. *Any* purely chance process is fine. Any procedure that's *not* a chance process (e.g., using existing groups, letting participants choose the group in which they want to be, putting the neediest or the first to arrive in the experimental group) is inferentially problematic.

Random assignment, coupled with adequate group sizes (e.g., ideally 30 or more per group), allows you to assume, with a reasonable degree of confidence, that the two (or more) groups, on average, are fairly equal on all pre-experimental variables on everything from their "average" attitude about nuclear disarmament to their average shoe size. Another way of looking at it is to assert that you have no reason *not* to assume that the groups are equal to begin with. And if they're similar overall in all respects, those variables have been equalized (or "held constant across groups") and hence can't threaten internal validity.

We have found that there is a common misunderstanding that novice researchers have about threats to internal validity that warrants explanation here. Let's take the example we used earlier that involved seeing whether exposure to a certain film series might change people's attitudes about appropriate levels of immigration. To do so, we randomly assign a large number of people to one of the two groups: the experimental group views a film series that shows some of the many immigration successes we see in this country; a control group, in contrast, sees a film series dealing with traffic safety (i.e., a topic that has nothing to do with immigration issues). In the end, we find that the group who viewed the immigration film series expresses significantly more positive attitudes toward immigration than the group who watched the unrelated films. When we use this example in our classes, we invite criticism of the design; more than one student has said, "But what if there are a few recent immigrants in the experimental group; wouldn't they be more positively disposed to immigration anyway?" or "What if there's someone in there who had a recent negative experience with an immigrant; wouldn't that bias the results?"

While such people certainly exist and may well find their way into our study, random assignment allows you to assume that these people will be *equally distributed* across all the groups in the study. Thus, while the experimental group may have some relatively recent immigrants in it, random assignment allows you to assume that there are probably just as many recent immigrants in the control group. Similarly, the two groups also will be equal, on average, in terms of the overall positivity or negativity of their experiences with immigrants.

Thus, even though we can think of lots of possible "contaminants" that might threaten the internal validity of our design, the question is always whether, overall, we have any reason to expect that such people will be *differentially* assigned to either of the two groups. No matter how many such contaminants we can think of, as long as the two (or more) groups are equally affected by their presence, then the two groups remain "equal overall to begin with," and internal validity is not threatened, at least not on the basis of selection.

Note that the power of random assignment allows an alternative to the pretest/posttest control group design. This new design, which is called the *posttest-only control group design*, is illustrated in Figure 6.6. The pretest is considered redundant in this design, since random assignment allows you to *assume* that the groups are equal to begin with. An added bonus is that this design circumvents any problems that might be associated with pretest sensitization, which cannot occur if there is no pretest.

In sum, random assignment is a very powerful research procedure that directly addresses the crucial experimental assumption that your experimental and control

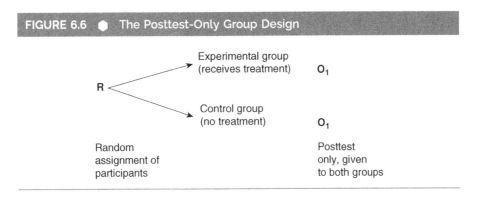

FIGURE 6.6 ● The Posttest-Only Group Design

groups are equal on average in all respects *before* you impose or administer your independent variable—the assumption of pretest equivalence. But random assignment has some limitations. Chance does occasionally play little tricks on us. Even though you flip a "fair" coin 10 times, and it *should* come down heads about half the time, and it usually does follow that pattern (or close to it), it may well happen that heads comes up every time—or never. Similarly, if we randomly assign people to groups, we assume that the groups are equal in all respects, but occasionally it might not work out that way. Thus, if we rely on random assignment, we'll generally be in fine shape but occasionally may be surprised.

The likelihood of being surprised in that way, however, is strongly related to group size. If our group size is small (i.e., fewer than 30 per group, and especially 10 or fewer per group), the chances rise of our getting an uneven distribution of characteristics between groups. Thus, researchers who rely on random assignment to create equivalent groups with small sample sizes are playing with fire, although even in that case it is noteworthy that the researcher is letting nothing other than chance influence assignment to groups and thereby creating a "fair" test and avoiding "stacking the deck" in one direction or the other. But what can you do if you have no choice but to use small samples and/or if you're unwilling to put your faith in chance? A second technique for ensuring group equivalence is known as *matching*.

Matching. While random assignment allows you to *assume* pretest equivalence, the **matching** process intentionally *creates* equivalence. In our study regarding attitudes toward immigration policies, for example, we may choose to match the groups on their pretest scores *or* (more typically) on some variable(s) we know to be related to attitudes regarding immigration policies (e.g., political conservatism, attitudes toward minority groups, authoritarianism). To show you how this would be done, let's use the example of matching groups on political affiliation.

To begin with, we have a bit of a procedural problem, because we obviously first need to know all our research participants' expressed political preferences. If we can get this information, we can look for matched pairs of individuals (e.g., two Democrats, two Republicans, two independents, etc.). For each pair, we might flip a coin to randomly assign one individual to the experimental group and the other to the control group. In this way, we'd be guaranteed groups that are constituted equally with respect to political affiliation and hence (since political affiliation is related to views regarding immigration policies) on pretest attitudes regarding immigration policies as well.

While the strength of matching lies in the fact that using this technique *ensures* pretest equivalence, its main weakness lies in the pragmatics of using it. Good matching technique requires that we identify "good" variables on which to match and that the information on which we're basing our matching is available. Achieving both of these conditions is often easier said than done.

In addition, matching very quickly gets out of hand if you try to match participants on more than one variable. For example, suppose we want to match respondents on sex, education, religion, political preference, and income. In order to create matched pairs on all five variables, we might have to find two "male Protestants with less than grade 10 education who vote Republican and make between $20,000 and $30,000 per year," two "female Catholics with some university education who vote Democrat and made more than $30,000 last year," and so on, depending on the particular people in our sample. Needless to say, this becomes a very complex and difficult task.

Random assignment, in contrast, is easy. Theoretically, you can use random assignment to create groups whose average units are essentially equivalent with respect to sex, age, political affiliation, attitudes regarding immigration policies, how they feel about their mothers, authoritarianism, height, how long it has been since their last bath, and all other variables, both interesting and mundane. In sum, matching (at least within the controlled experiment) hardly seems worth the effort and might be justified only when the number of participants per group is small. Although random assignment would still leave you being able to claim there was no systematic bias in assigning participants to groups, real equivalence becomes a bit more risky, in which case creating matched pairs on a relevant variable and then randomly assigning one member of each pair to treatment and control would be the safer course.

External Validity

Our focus so far has been entirely on *internal validity:* the extent to which *differences between groups* can be unambiguously attributed to the experimental treatment. But there are three other types of validity on which any given study can be evaluated: external validity, ecological validity, and **statistical conclusion validity**. (Note that there are numerous other types of validity we haven't yet considered; some will be addressed later in this book in relation to other methods, while others are included in more specialized texts.)

External validity refers to the *generalizability of results beyond the specifics of the study* (e.g., see Cook, 2000; Shadish et al., 2001). As you now know, doing research involves applying relatively abstract, theoretical concerns to very concrete situations. Suppose our theoretical interest is in assessing the relationship between "anxiety" and "performance." Following the literature in this area, we might say that there is a curvilinear relationship between these two concepts (see Figure 6.7): performance is optimal when anxiety is at a moderate level and poorest when anxiety is either very high *or* very low.

Our *theoretical* interest lies in the relationship between *all* types of anxiety and *all* types of performance in *all* situations and across *all* people. But we obviously can't be everywhere and do everything at once. Rather, we must become very concrete in how

FIGURE 6.7 ● The Theoretical Relationship Between Anxiety and Performance, According to the Yerkes-Dodson (1908) Law

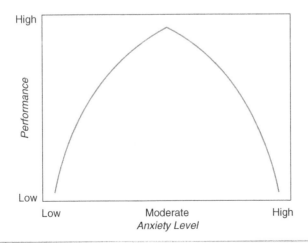

we assess these variables. For "anxiety," we might choose to focus on the anxiety that some students feel when they write exams, and we might operationalize "anxiety" as the response people give when asked "Please rate how anxious you feel right now, on a 10-point scale," as they sit down to write their final exam in this research methods course. For "performance," we might decide to look at the grade the students receive on that final exam. Our sample of research participants might include all students taking your research methods course this semester.

Suppose that, having done the study just described, we do indeed find the curvilinear relationship between "anxiety" and "performance" we hypothesized. What have we found? In a literal sense, all we have found is that when one class of this semester's research methods students sat down to write the final exam, their self-reported levels of anxiety were curvilinearly related to their grades on the final exam. But, ultimately (theoretically), that's not what we're interested in; our study was just one of the many possible studies we could have done to assess the *theoretical* anxiety–performance relationship in which we're interested. Thus, we'd want to know whether the results we observed were obtained merely because of the specifics of our study or whether they reflect a more general relationship between anxiety and performance.

In sum, we are interested in the *generalizability* of our results to other people, situations, measures, and times. Would we have obtained the same results if we'd done the study with other students? In other courses? In other semesters? If we'd taken physiological rather than self-report measures of anxiety? If we'd looked at anxiety in a job interview or before giving a speech rather than in an exam situation? Or if we'd used a measure of performance other than grades? These are obviously all empirical questions that can be addressed in future research and/or that may have been found by other researchers and reported in the literature. In the interim, they suggest that we'd be wise to consider the limitations of what we've achieved and to be cautious in how far we extrapolate.

Ecological Validity

While *external validity* refers to the generalizability of results to other persons, setting, and times, there's another type of validity—ecological validity—that can be considered a type of external validity, since it also addresses issues of representativeness and generalizability, although it does so in a slightly different way. First used by Brunswik (1955), *ecological validity* refers to the representativeness of the treatments and measures you use in relation to the particular milieu to which you wish to generalize. Devlin (2018) helps us understand the difference between external and ecological validity thus:

External validity needs to be distinguished from ecological validity. In ecological validity, the emphasis is on the degree of verisimilitude (i.e., lifelikeness) of the research to the events and characteristics of real life. The two concepts overlap in that both relate to situations beyond the immediate research setting, but ecological validity specifically emphasizes the realism or degree to which the situation reflects real life, which is not necessarily the case for external validity. (p. 71)

For example, let's return to the anxiety–performance study described above. We were interested in the *theoretical* connection between anxiety and performance, with the particular experiment we did being one of the many studies that could have been done that embodied the key constructs specified by the theory. Our external validity concerns were over whether the results could be generalized to other persons, settings, and times.

But suppose we now want to take a more *applied* approach and are interested in studying anxiety and performance in the classroom. We might very well end up designing the very same study—one that looks at the relationship between pre-exam anxiety and exam performance—but our analysis of it would be quite different. Here, instead of asking how well the experiment's conditions represent the theoretical universe, our question becomes how well the situation represents the kinds of situations to which we're interested in generalizing, that is, how well does the experiment represent the *social ecology* of our situation of interest?

In this classroom-based example, ecological validity would be fairly high, since we're using real students who are experiencing real anxiety of a type that commonly occurs in classrooms and who are engaged in an ecologically relevant task (their final exam) with real consequences (their final grade) on the line. But it's easy to imagine other studies that aren't so clearly connected to their real-world counterparts.

For example, consider one line of research that focused on how we form our impressions of people. Typical studies in that area investigate how we combine information about people, how we resolve conflicting information about people, and how different aspects of our history or character affect the impressions people have of us. One series of studies investigated the way that wearing glasses can affect impressions. In study after study, the experiments demonstrate that if you show photos of people either wearing glasses or not wearing glasses to the typical sample of volunteer undergraduate research participants and ask them to rate the people in the pictures on myriad different dimensions (like intelligence, sincerity, and honesty), participants will quite reliably rate people with glasses more highly on those dimensions than people who aren't wearing them (e.g., Manz & Lueck, 1968; Thornton, 1943, 1944).

The nice thing about using an experiment to test this effect is that taking that approach offers tremendous control over the situation: you can actually have participants rate the *same people* by using similarly composed pictures of them with and without glasses, thus controlling for other differences, such as attractiveness. Now, if you wear glasses as well as contact lenses, does this mean you should wear your glasses to job interviews to get an edge over all those people with 20:20 eyesight?

At first glance it would seem so. The results of those studies, in addition to being *internally* valid, were also very high in *external* validity: different researchers in different settings at different times using different subject groups have produced the same result again and again and again. However, the experiment isn't particularly *ecologically* valid. Recall that we're trying to learn about how people really form impressions about others. But how often do we really make judgments on the basis of just a picture alone? When we meet people at parties, are introduced by good friends, or learn about them in job interviews, we also can talk to the person, hear about their attitudes and values, glean more information from the way they dress, act, and talk about themselves, and so on.

Thus, while the "glasses" experiments may have high *internal* and *external* validity, they appear to have poor *ecological* validity, because the experiments fail to simulate the kinds of situations we're most interested in understanding. That state of affairs creates a certain irony: it becomes possible to create knowledge that's true in *theory* but misleading in *practice*. The results of the glasses experiment show that glasses *can* make a difference, but whether they *do* make a difference in a real-world evaluative situation is another issue entirely.

Indeed, some years later, Michael Argyle of Oxford University—a primarily laboratory-based experimental social psychologist who was beginning to consider the role of context in experimentation—extended the basic "glasses effect" research in an interesting way. Instead of making "glasses versus no glasses" the *only* piece of information that raters knew about a person, Argyle *began* by gathering the "first impression" data, which showed that he could replicate the well-known "glasses effect," but then simply let the scene run further: the people in the pictures started talking about their interests, values, and experiences. The end result? Not surprisingly, under those conditions there was *no* "glasses effect." In sum, the "glasses effect" is "true" in the sense that it can be reliably replicated by any experimenter who wants to perform the study, but it's true *only in particular circumstances* within the strict confines of the laboratory, that is, when "glasses versus no glasses" is the *only* information people have on which to base their judgments. As soon as they have access to other information they can use, the "glasses effect" no longer occurs; what previously seemed like such an important variable (when it was the only variable under consideration) faded into nothing. Because of this, many authors (e.g., Manicas & Secord, 1983; Palys & Lowman, 1984) suggest that while the purely theoretical "can" questions are eminently suitable to experimental analysis, an experiment may *not* be a particularly useful launching point for the "does" questions unless ecological validity—how well our research conditions represent the important elements of the context to which we wish to generalize (e.g., see Palys, 1978; Palys & Lowman, 1984)—is explicitly considered.

Statistical Conclusion Validity

Suppose you watch someone who has a 25-cent coin. They flip it once and get tails. They flip it again … and get tails. Once again … and it's tails. Another flip, another tail. Another flip, another tail. If they continue flipping the coin and continue getting tails, at some point you'd probably begin to suspect that the coin is rigged, that the person is not reporting truthfully, or that they are not flipping correctly. Ted has in fact done just this in his undergraduate research methods classes on a few occasions. Students usually start voicing suspicions after the fourth or fifth tail in a row. Why do you think that happens?

From experience, we "know" that there are two possible outcomes when we flip a coin: heads or tails. The probability of getting tails on any given flip of the coin is 1 out of 2. The joint probability of getting tails twice in a row is 1 out of 4. For three in a row, it's 1 in 8. The event "four tails in a row" has a joint probability of 1 in 16. And the joint probability of getting five tails in a row is 1 out of 32.

When Ted starts flipping a 25-cent coin in his class, people seem to assume that he's flipping a "fair" coin and that he's accurately reporting what he sees. There's nothing unusual about a coin coming up tails when you flip it. Nor is there anything especially atypical about getting two tails in a row. Three in a row might be worth a chuckle, but still represent no particular problem. But four in a row? Suddenly people start to wonder. That *is* a fair coin, isn't it? Five in a row? What's going on? Note that we *start* by supposing that "nothing special" is going on, that chance alone is operating, and that the rules of probability theory apply. When what we see deviates only slightly from what we'd expect by chance alone, we might find the oddity interesting or cute, but strange things do sometimes happen, so we likely don't question our assumptions. There comes a point, though, when what we observe is a little *too* atypical; that's when we start to question whether it's really chance alone that's operating or whether "something else" is going on.

Researchers in the social and health sciences go through much the same sort of process when they come to the end of a piece of research. Suppose we did the "attitudes about immigration policies" study described earlier. Suppose further that at the end of the research, we want to compare the attitudes of those who were exposed to the film series to the attitudes of those who were not. What are the alternatives? One alternative is that there's no difference between the experimental and control groups. If that happens, we'd probably say that there was no evidence that the film series had any effect.

But we shouldn't be too surprised if the average scores of the two groups aren't *exactly* the same, since we might expect a certain amount of variation just by chance alone. In other words, the average scores in the two groups might not be 4.64 and 4.64, but they might be 4.64 and 4.65. That does not seem like much. How about 4.64 and 4.70? 4.64 and 4.90? 4.64 and 5.34? At what point are we no longer prepared to write off the difference as mere chance variation? At what point, in other words, do we decide that the difference is sufficiently large that chance variation *alone* can't account for it and that "something else" must therefore be going on? Where do we draw the line?

Social and health scientists rely on elementary probability theory to help them make this decision. Many statistical tests (e.g., t-tests, chi-square, analysis of variance) are designed to tell us the exact probability of obtaining the results we observe *if* chance alone is operating. For social and health scientists, this information is crucial, since the central issue is not the mere magnitude of differences between groups but the probability of observing that magnitude of difference if chance alone is what's operating.

Recall that the students in Ted's classes tend to get suspicious about his coin flipping after 4–5 flips when the probabilities reach in the neighborhood of 1 in 16 (.06) or 1 in 32 (.03). In the social and health sciences, researchers agree that the odds must be at least 1 in 20 (i.e., .05) or *less* (e.g., .02, .01) before we can say that something other than chance must have been operating to produce the observed results. Only at that point, in other words, are researchers prepared to say that a difference they've observed is *statistically significant*.

Why .05? Why not .10 or .01 or some other level? Although Sir Ronald Fisher (1925) is generally credited with fixing .05 as the required probability for considering a difference statistically significant, Cowles and Davis (1982) identify Karl Pearson as having played an important role with his development of the chi-square "goodness of fit" test in the 1890s, since this test was the first to allow the computation of the exact probability that observed deviations from expected (theoretical) distributions could be attributed to chance variation. Pearson and his contemporaries exchanged views concerning what value to use as a cutoff for **statistical significance**. Articles by various authors in the first two decades of the 20th century gradually honed in on .05 as the consensus choice. Fisher (1925), whose significant contributions in research design and in developing the Analysis of Variance earned him senior academic status, may thus be seen as having given his blessing to a well-established tradition. Ultimately, the choice of .05 was relatively arbitrary; it simply represents the consensus of turn-of-the-20th-century academics.

The subjective appeal for this choice is certainly reaffirmed in Ted's experiences with the coin-flipping exercise. Students quite reliably get suspicious after about four or five successive "tails" flips — the joint probabilities of which are .06 and .03, respectively—suggesting that the .05 level *does* correspond reasonably well to people's intuitive sense of when a given observation is sufficiently "special" or "atypical" or "unusual" to get excited about. And while the choice of .05 per se is merely a tradition or convention, its value rests in the very fact that it *is* a tradition, generally considered to be beyond the control of the experimenter/researcher. As such, .05 is an independent arbiter that impartially distinguishes between observations that are statistically significant (and hence deserve further scrutiny) and those that aren't (and hence can be written off to chance variation).

In this sense, statistical significance is an all-or-none event; either a result is statistically significant or it isn't. Basketball provides a useful analogy here: when Stephen Currie of the Golden State Warriors dribbles down the court, "success" is defined as shooting the ball into the opposing team's basket. Either the ball goes through the hoop or it doesn't; if it *doesn't*, it doesn't particularly matter whether the shot hits the rim or is a complete air ball, although our hearts may flutter a bit more in the former instance, because neither is a basket. Similarly, observations that have a probability of occurrence of .05 or less are considered statistically significant; if the probability level is any higher (regardless of whether the observed probability level "hits the rim" at $p = .06$ or is an "air ball" at $p = .20$), the results are still considered within the range of what you can expect on the basis of chance variation alone.

What, then, does it mean to say that your data are statistically significant? All it means is that if chance alone was operating, the probability of obtaining the results you did is equal to or less than 5 in 100 (i.e., $p \leq .05$). In other words, your results are sufficiently rare or atypical to suggest that chance alone cannot account for them. And if chance alone cannot account for the results, "something else" must be going on. Statistical significance does *not* imply that what you've found is important. Nor does it imply that your study is internally valid, since the statistics are blind to the adequacy of your design (at least in terms of its internal validity). Importance and internal validity are both separate issues; neither is indicated by statistical significance alone.

AN EXAMPLE: ASSESSING THE EFFECTS OF VIOLENT PORNOGRAPHY

In order to see how the concepts we've talked about "work," we'll now take a step back and take a close look at one particular study from a highly controversial program of primarily experimental research that sought to assess the effects of viewing violent pornography. Writing a textbook like this one involves doing more than explaining concepts; it also involves finding just the right example to illustrate those concepts. Although the experiment that we want to describe to you is already a few decades old, we've picked it as the one we want to take apart for you for several reasons. First, the issue of violence against women is as important now as it was in the 1980s when this research was first done, and violent pornography has been cited by various theorists as one of the many factors that exacerbate that phenomenon. Second, the experimental research that was done in this area, primarily by Ed Donnerstein of the University of Arizona and Neil Malamuth of the University of California at Los Angeles (UCLA), adheres particularly well to experimental principles. Third, these researchers and their research became quite influential in the social policy arena. Donnerstein and Malamuth have served as expert witnesses in courts where they testified about the effects of viewing violent pornography, and both also have testified before federal commissions in the United States and Canada that looked into whether and to what extent pornographic materials should be the subject of legal censure, suggesting that they and the commissions saw direct policy relevance to their laboratory-based research.

The research also played a role in the Canadian court case of *Little Sister's* v. *The Queen,* which went all the way to the Supreme Court. "Little Sister's" is short for Little Sister's Book and Art Emporium, a retail establishment in downtown Vancouver that sells primarily sexually oriented material (mostly books and magazines) to a largely gay and lesbian clientele. The case arose because materials destined for Little Sister's from other countries were often impounded at the border by Canada Customs officials, who would then notify Little Sister's, who then had to go through an extensive legal and bureaucratic process in an attempt to have the material released. Indeed, seizures happened so often, and so much *more* often than they happened to bookstores and video outlets that dealt primarily in heterosexual material, that Little

Sister's decided to take Canada Customs (and the federal government) to court, alleging that the store was a victim of homophobic harassment and that this process of prior restraint was inexcusably contrary to the Canadian *Charter of Rights and Freedoms*. The federal government acknowledged that its procedures *were* contrary to the *Charter* but argued that such procedures were necessary to prevent the harms that would result from the proliferation of such material.

This large, complex case occupied considerable court time. One issue that had to be considered centered on the question of whether exposure to gay sexual material, especially violent gay sexual material, creates harms, in particular, by somehow promoting sexual violence. The federal government hired Neil Malamuth, one of the foremost experimental researchers in the field, to make it's case, a task that he tackled by relying almost exclusively on the experimental evidence that he and his colleagues had generated over the previous decade or so. Ted offered to help Little Sister's (which had a shoestring budget and relied extensively on volunteer help) by writing an opinion on Malamuth's opinion (see Palys, 1994).

The way Ted approached that task was *not* to question Malamuth's qualifications or the quality of the research that he and his colleagues had done. Malamuth is clearly well-respected in the field of experimental social psychology, and his research is exemplary within that tradition. Indeed, a large part of Ted's written opinion involved showing how carefully constructed the research was. At the same time, Ted expressed concerns about how Malamuth and his colleagues interpreted the results of their research. Ted reexamined their work using the various concepts we've discussed in this chapter (although so far at a largely theoretical level), as well as posing questions about the meanings we attribute to our research.

Isolating and Operationalizing the Variables

The laboratory experimenter's challenge is to create a situation where the effects of a single variable can be isolated and observed without changing the very nature of what is being looked at. As we've seen, experimental social and health scientists approach this problem in much the same way that physicists or chemists might seek to observe a single electron or observe a chemical reaction in a contrived situation ostensibly free of worldly contaminants. Implicit in this view is the idea that the thing being observed may be changed in *magnitude* by its removal and relocation into the laboratory, but not in *character*.

People who want to ban (or strictly regulate the distribution of) violent video pornography have argued that allowing it to be available creates social harms, primarily by increasing the likelihood that those who are exposed to it will themselves engage in sexually violent behavior. Looking at such behavior directly, either in the lab or anywhere else, would clearly be unethical. Researchers who wanted to test this hypothesis thus had to look at other kinds of aggressive behavior, propelled by the belief that although the behavior investigated in the lab—the act of giving small electric shocks to a stranger—is far removed from the brutality of a sexual assault, it is nonetheless comparable to such an assault in its essence: both behaviors are manifestations of the concept "aggression"; and the two behaviors differ only in magnitude, not in kind. The primary *dependent variable* in the "effects" research area is thus the average level of electric shock that one person is prepared to deliver to another person.

The key "causal" variable (or *independent variable*) of interest in the effects literature is exposure to pornography, especially violent pornography. In order to assess pornography's effects on the *dependent variable* (the level of aggression exhibited against a stranger), the logic of the experiment requires the researcher to create two conditions (in the simplest case) that are identical in all respects except one: the presence or absence of the variable whose effects you wish to assess. Most of the effects literature involves more complicated designs, but the fundamental principle that drives such studies involves comparing two or more groups that are equivalent in all respects, on average, on every variable except one.

The Sample

The research participants in Donnerstein and Berkowitz (1981) were all male, undergraduate, introductory psychology student volunteers, as is true of most studies in this area. Eighty males took part in this study. When each participant showed up for his appointment at the lab, he was told that another person (always a woman) also had an appointment and that the two of them would be participating in the study together.

Procedures and Design

Following introductions, the experimenter turned on a tape recorder. The taped instructions revealed that one of the two participants would be a "learner," whose job would be to try to remember certain word pairs, while the other participant would assist the experimenter. An apparently random draw was then held to determine who would play each role. We say "apparently" because unbeknownst to the male participant, the draw was actually rigged: the woman always became the learner, while the man always became the experimenter's assistant. The woman, as you may suspect, was actually an employee of the experimenter who was trained to respond in the same preprogrammed manner each time the experiment was run.

With the pair's roles determined, the experimenter next stated that the woman would be given some time to study the word pairs before she would be tested. The man, in the interim, was to spend his time writing a brief essay about the possible legalization of marijuana (which was illegal throughout the United States at that time). When he finished, the woman was brought back into the setting, where she was supposed to evaluate the essay. She remained on the other side of a partition, however, and wasn't supposed to communicate directly with the man. Instead, she communicated *indirectly*, by written note and through the delivery of some electric shocks via finger electrodes placed on the man's hand. Her evaluation of the essay was unambiguous; her written evaluation stated that the essay was terrible, and when faced with the choice of how many electric shocks to deliver to the man, she delivered 9 out of a possible maximum of 10.

This little interchange served two experimental goals. First, it helped reaffirm the "reality" of the electric shocks to the male participant. This was important, because the man would soon have an opportunity to deliver electric shocks to the woman, and the experimenter needed the man to believe that any shocks he delivered were real. Second, this interchange—known among effects researchers as the *anger manipulation*—has become a virtual requirement of effects testing, since it seems that unless the woman first angers the man, no effects of exposure to violent pornography are observed.

After the anger manipulation is performed, the woman is allowed further time to study. Noting that this studying will take some time and that the male participant now has nothing to do, the experimenter says something along the lines of "By the way, a friend of mine down the hall is preparing some film clips for another experiment, and he needs people to make some ratings of them. Since we have some time to kill, would you be interested in going down the hall and helping him out for a few minutes?" Virtually all participants agree to do so.

At this point the manipulation of the independent variable occurs. Participants are *randomly assigned* to one of the four experimental conditions; the only difference between the conditions is the type of film clip to which participants are exposed. In Donnerstein and Berkowitz (1981), two of these clips portrayed (1) a *nonsexual and nonviolent* clip of a talk show and (2) a *sexually explicit but nonviolent* depiction of a man and a woman engaging in mutually consenting intercourse. Each video segment was about 5 minutes long. The other two clips were of similar length; both involved a scene in which three people—a woman and two men—are studying together when the men begin to make sexual advances toward the woman. She resists but is raped. The difference between the third and fourth films was not in their visual content (which was identical), but in the voice soundtrack: in one version (3), the woman protests at first, but soon begins to enjoy the process (a rape myth depiction; the "*sexually violent/positive outcome*" condition); in the other (4), the woman resists at first and throughout the process, experiencing all the horror of a sexual assault she is powerless to stop (the "*sexually violent/negative outcome*" condition).

Note, by the way, that sending the participant down the hall to help another experimenter achieved at least two other important experimental objectives. To explain what it achieved, imagine first that the experimenter in their study did *not* send the person down the hall, but instead showed one of the films themselves. One worry would be that this would make it very obvious that the film was part of the experiment and that the researchers were wondering what its effects might be. Experimental psychologists tend to believe that participants should be naïve about what an experiment like this is "really" all about (from the experimenter's perspective) so that their behavior is more "natural" and often use deception to ensure that naiveté. By creating the impression that the films had nothing to do with the experiment and was simply a favor that would kill some time, presumably the participants did not make any connection between the two.

Note also that sending the participant down the hall to some other experimenter creates what is referred to as a **blind condition** for the first experimenter where they have no idea which film the participant actually sees. A program of research conducted by Robert Rosenthal regarding "experimenter effects" (e.g., Rosenthal & Rosnow, 1969) had shown that when researchers know what results they expect and know what groups research participants are in, they can unintentionally influence the results by providing certain verbal and nonverbal cues that even they may not know they are giving. By ensuring they do not know to what condition the participant has been assigned, they preclude the possibility of creating that effect.

To reassert the study's design using some of the terminology you have been learning, the *independent variable* in the study was the "exposure to a film" at one of the four "levels," one corresponding to each of the four conditions above. The *dependent variable* was the average level of shock delivered by participants from each of the four groups. Technically speaking, this design is a *randomized nonpretested comparison group design*, as is represented in Figure 6.8.

After viewing one of the four film clips and completing a few rating scales (consistent with the cover story that was offered), the male participant returns to the first

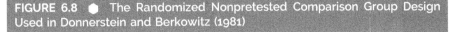

FIGURE 6.8 ● The Randomized Nonpretested Comparison Group Design Used in Donnerstein and Berkowitz (1981)

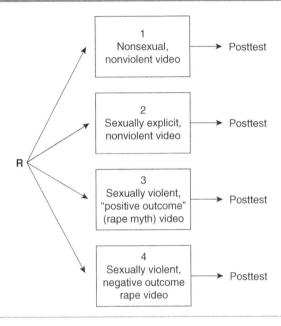

experimenter, who is now ready to receive him. By this time, the woman has ostensibly completed her studying and has had some electrodes attached to her fingers. The man, adopting his assigned role of assistant to the experimenter, begins assessing whether the woman remembers the word pairs she has been studying. Whenever she makes a mistake—and recall that each of these mistakes is programmed to occur at exactly the same time for each session—the male participant's job is to determine how many electric shocks she should receive and then deliver them. Of particular interest to the experimenters was the average number of electric shocks that the male participants would deliver (i.e., the *dependent variable*) and how (if at all) that number would vary depending on the type of film clip the participant had viewed.

Were the Differences Significant?

Recall the basic logic of experimentation: *if* the groups are all equal to begin with, any subsequent differences in the dependent variable (here, the average shock level) among the groups must be due to the one variable on which their experience varied (here, the type of film to which they were exposed). We must first, therefore, try to find out whether there are in fact any "differences" to worry about. If there are no differences among the groups, then there's nothing further to explain.

Donnerstein and Berkowitz (1981) found that after being exposed to the anger manipulation, the two groups who viewed the sexually violent film clip, regardless whether it was accompanied by a "positive outcome" or by a "negative outcome" soundtrack, administered a significantly higher average level of shock than did either the group of participants who viewed the sexually explicit but nonviolent depiction or the group who viewed the nonsexual and nonviolent talk show clip (see the graph of these results in Figure 6.9).

FIGURE 6.9 ● Graphed Results From Donnerstein and Berkowitz (1981) Showing Mean Shock Level Administered by Each Group

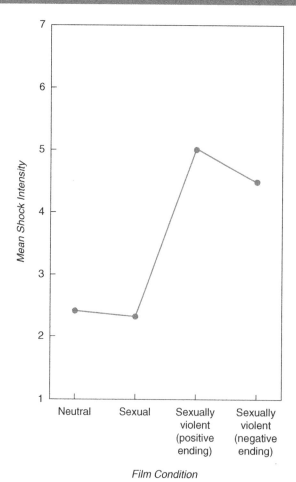

Assessing Internal Validity

Remember that a result's statistical significance does not imply anything about that result's importance. Nor does it necessarily imply that the independent variable had an effect. It means only that the degree of difference between the two groups is greater than we would expect on the basis of chance variation alone. If chance alone cannot fully account for the difference, clearly something else must be going on. But what might the "something else" be?

After reading Donnerstein and Berkowitz (1981), we might like to suggest that the differences between the groups are a reflection of the effects of viewing the films. But we must assess the study's internal validity before taking our best guess in that regard. Let's consider the various threats to internal validity that were explained earlier in the chapter to see how well Donnerstein and Berkowitz (1981) controlled for them.

If the Two Groups Are Equal to Begin With...

A first possible threat is *selection*. This threat would strike right at the heart of the design, since it undermines a fundamental element of experimental logic: the assumption that the two groups are equal to begin with. If the groups are not equal to begin with, any after-the-fact differences may merely reflect the before-the-fact differences.

We can indeed assume that the four groups in Donnerstein and Berkowitz (1981) were equal on average to begin with. Why? Since participants were assigned on a purely *random* basis to one of the four conditions, we have no reason to believe that, before viewing the videos, one group (overall) was any different from any other group (overall). People who have more or less proclivity to violence, more or less experience with having viewed video pornography, more negative or more positive attitudes toward sexual material, or whatever other individual difference variable that we can think of all will have been equally distributed across the groups. We might feel more comfortable if the researchers had assigned 30 or more participants per group rather than 20, but there's still no reason to assume that the deck has been stacked in favor of one group any more than any other. So selection doesn't seem to be a threat to the internal validity of this design.

... And Are Treated Identically in All Respects...

Several other threats also can be ruled out. *History* cannot be a threat, because every effort was made to treat everyone identically in all respects except for the level of the independent variable they received. They all came to the same lab, met the same female confederate and the same experimenter, heard exactly the same tape-recorded instructions, and received the same evaluation of their essay by the confederate, all according to the script laid out by the researchers. Even the four levels of the independent variable were administered in similar ways: all four groups were asked to do "a favor," all four groups had to go down the hall to meet another experimenter in another room, all four groups saw a video of similar length (with only the content varying), and all four groups completed a series of rating scales after they saw the film.

The whole experience occurred within an hour for each participant, so *maturation* seems unlikely to have entered in as a threat. In any event, to the extent that there *were* any maturational influences, such as the participants' getting more tired as the experiment progressed, these would have been equal, overall, across all groups.

Testing couldn't have been a threat, because there was no pretest. Similarly, *statistical regression (regression toward the mean)* couldn't have been a threat, because neither group was selected on the basis of any sort of extreme score.

Taken together, the preceding paragraphs suggest that the internal validity of the Donnerstein and Berkowitz (1981) study is quite high. Although we cannot be positive, because there might have been some threats we haven't considered, it seems that the only difference between the four groups was in the content of the film they viewed. And if that's so, it must be because of the content of the films that they reacted differently to the confederate when given an opportunity to administer electric shocks.

Assessing External Validity

Although their theoretical interests are in how exposure to violent pornography affects "people," Donnerstein and Berkowitz (1981) conducted this study, as is the case with most of the experimental research in this area, using a specific type of research participant: male, undergraduate, introductory psychology students who volunteered to take part in the study. Because such a group is obviously anything but a "representative sample" of the general population, many critics of the effects literature (e.g., Byrne & Kelley, 1989; Fisher, 1986) question the *external validity* (generalizability) of the research results. Can *any* result obtained with such a sample be generalized to the broader population of interest (i.e., all people, or even all males)?

We do *not* see that criticism as particularly relevant here. Even if we acknowledge that male introductory psychology students are *not* typical of all people, so that the question of who is sampled becomes an important one, a criticism based on their being "unrepresentative" is empty unless we identify the nature of the sampling bias that exists and then consider the possible implications of that bias for the results the researchers obtained.

In that regard, we can expect several differences between male, undergraduate, introductory psychology students, and the general male population. Not only have such students received more extensive formal education than the average population member, but also we might speculate that they might be less likely to use "physical" means to solve conflicts or achieve goals, and perhaps be more introspective about their behavior and the motives underlying it, for example. But if that's so, it might be argued that these people may be even *less* likely than the general population to engage in aggressive and assaultive behavior.

Of course there is an opposite argument to be made as well. Sexual assault happens on university campuses just as it does elsewhere in society, and it is noteworthy that most male introductory college students are in the 18–25 years age range that is most strongly associated with criminal involvement. Indeed, this may be exactly the right population to look at in some ways, while the upshot of the sample's "unrepresentativeness" is that if it can be demonstrated that even such a relatively well-educated and literate group can be affected by exposure to violent pornography, then this study's results may well be, if anything, a *conservative* estimate of the extent to which such effects will exist in the population as a whole. Malamuth (1989, p. 183) makes a similar argument.

And recall that generalizability refers not just to generalizability of results across people. Other dimensions of external validity can be considered as well. For example, in different times—these days of #metoo, for example—would the results be the same? Or have young adult men in general become more attuned to and sensitive about aggression toward women? Would the results be the same in other societies where crime rates are higher or lower or where the role of women vis-à-vis men is more or less egalitarian? Would we find the same enhanced aggression in same-sex pairs as Malamuth found with opposite-sex pairs? Would the results be the same for films other than those shown in the study? What if "aggression" was defined in some way other than electrical shocks? Ultimately, these are all empirical questions that we can address through further research or by seeing how those variables have fared in the literature, but for the moment they encourage us to be cautious about the limitations of our work and how far we can extrapolate from the results.

Assessing Ecological Validity

The laboratory experiment involves creating a contrived setting designed to provide a "pure" test of a theoretical proposition among a designated sample of research participants. This contrived setting can pose a problem when researchers engage in experimental research that is later used to influence social policy. The problem arises when, in the interests of experimental purity, researchers (1) create situations that are related only obliquely to situations in the world that the researchers are ostensibly trying to help us understand and (2) create misleading results because of the way in which they virtually *create* the very effects they're allegedly trying to *test*. These considerations have been embellished in greater detail elsewhere (see Palys, 1989; Palys & Lowman, 1984) but also deserve some attention here.

Laboratory experimentalists are taught several basic principles for use in designing an experiment. Two of these, both rooted in the *F*-ratio (the statistic typically used to compare groups), are (1) the principle of *maximizing between-groups variation* (i.e., the degree of difference between experimental and control groups), to make as clear a differentiation between conditions as possible, and (2) the principle of *minimizing within-groups variation* (i.e., the degree of "natural" and "random" variation that exists within the groups being tested), to make as "sensitive" a test of the hypothesis as possible.

In studies like the one being considered here, researchers push the groups as far apart as possible by choosing the most gruesome "violent pornography" they can find, choosing sexually explicit material that is extremely explicit and not at all violent, and making the "neutral" material as devoid of sexual and violent content as they can. They minimize the amount of variability within the group by using relatively homogeneous populations of respondents, who in this case were male, undergraduate, introductory psychology student volunteers, i.e., a small subset of the larger male population. This is supplemented by efforts to exert experimenter control over the situation to standardize conditions as much as possible. For example, tape-recorded instructions mean that every participant is hearing exactly the same voice read exactly the same words in exactly the same way, and having the woman confederate send her insulting statement about the male participant's essay via written note meant that there would be no possibility of variation in the interchange as might happen in a human interaction, so that the message every participant gets remains exactly constant across all tested groups.

A third principle of experimentation advises experimenters to *control all available response alternatives* so that any impetus to behavior that is created by the conditions of the experiment is harnessed in the service of the dependent variable. Underlying this view is something of a "hydraulic" model of human behavior: the belief is that if a stimulus can effectively energize a behavioral response, the astute experimenter will "dam up" all behavioral alternatives but one, so that the magnitude of all behavioral impulses will be visible in the chosen place. In the context of the effects literature, where the interest has been in determining aggressive impulses, this has meant that participants have been given only one way to express themselves: by delivering electric shocks to the woman on the other side of the partition.

All of these principles have been employed in the studies described in the effects literature produced by Donnerstein, Berkowitz, Malamuth, and their colleagues. Indeed, they are widely represented as principles of "good experimentation" (e.g., Aronson & Carlsmith, 1968; Festinger & Katz, 1953; Kerlinger, 1973; Rosenthal & Rosnow, 1984), and they do make great sense *if* you are addressing a purely theoretical question of interest, where the central issue for the researcher is whether a theoretically hypothesized relationship *can* be given empirical life.

But when we make decisions about cases in court or try to develop social policy, we're interested not *solely* in questions of theory but also in their implications for practice. The interest of the court, for example, in *Little Sister's* v. *The Queen*, as Ted understood it, was not in the answer to the question "*Can* exposure to aggressive pornography increase the likelihood of subsequent harm?" but rather, "*Does* it do so?" Those are two very different questions. The first is more purely theoretical. To ask whether something *can* happen is to ask simply whether a particular phenomenon can be generated, that is, whether there is any evidence that a specified theoretical linkage can occur. The second is a more contextualized and applied question; it asks whether, in the real world, the conditions exist in which the phenomenon of interest occurs. Think back to the studies reviewed earlier in this chapter about the effects of wearing glasses. The early experimental research showed that wearing glasses *can* affect the impressions that other people derive of you. But later research showed that it generally *doesn't*, unless that's the only piece of information that people have of you, a condition that rarely applies outside laboratory experiments. In sum, it's not inconsistent or implausible for the answers to those two questions to be "Yes, it *can*" but "No, it *doesn't.*"

Donnerstein and Berkowitz (1981) clearly show that, under certain conditions, viewing violent pornography *can* affect the likelihood that people will engage in aggressive behavior. But in order to address the question of whether it *does* have such an effect, we must consider the study's **ecological validity**, asking how well the experiment's conditions approximate or represent the actual conditions in the world in which pornography is consumed. Stated another way, we must ask whether, in the interest of living up to experimentalist ideals, Donnerstein and Berkowitz have made the situation into something *other than* that which they set out to investigate. For example,

1. While the aggressive behavior that's of interest to us is *severe* (e.g., violence in the form of sexual assault and other sexual abuses), ethical requirements constrain laboratory investigation to behavior that's relatively *trivial* (small electric shocks that cause minimal pain and no long-term trauma or damage) and hence may well result in an overestimate of the extent to which people are prepared to engage in the more severe forms of such behavior.

2. While aggressive behavior is *discouraged* in society (e.g., people are subject to arrest and imprisonment for behavior such as sexual assault), the experiment requires it to be *encouraged* in the experimental setting by an experimenter who, as an authority figure, represents the interests of legitimate science. Indeed, the whole rationale given to participants explains that they are actually *helping* the experimenter by being the person who delivers the electric shocks.

3. While in the real world we have many *alternatives* about how to respond when we're angered (e.g., by withdrawing from the situation, by talking to the person who has angered us), the effects researchers offer their research participants *only one way* to communicate any displeasure they may feel: by delivering an electric shock to the fingertips of the woman on the other side of the partition.

At least two studies have investigated the impact of some of the above factors. Regarding caveat 3, for example, Fisher and Grenier (1994) wondered what would happen if research participants were given a broader array of response alternatives than just delivering shocks. They discovered that when response alternatives were given, the vast majority of respondents—no matter which film they'd been exposed to—chose to *talk* to the woman who had angered them, rather than to deliver electric shocks.

Regarding caveat 2, relevant evidence has been supplied by Malamuth (1978). He describes this research in a later publication (1984) as follows:

> *Following exposure to these [visual] stimuli, all subjects were insulted by a female confederate and then were placed in a situation where they could aggress against her via the ostensible delivery of electric shocks under one of two assessment conditions. Half of the subjects were assigned to read a communication that suggested it was "permissible" to behave as aggressively as they wished (disinhibitory communication); the other half were given a communication designed to make*

them somewhat self-conscious about aggressing (inhibitory communication) ... The results revealed no significant differences in aggression following the inhibitory communication. (p. 35)

In sum, as soon as conditions in the experiment start to better approximate those in the real world, that is, when people have alternative ways of responding and when aggressive responses are discouraged, the findings of the laboratory-based research appear to vanish, and no effects are found.

At the same time, by creating a set of conditions under which effects of viewing violent pornography *were* observed, Donnerstein and Berkowitz (1981) *have* helped to show some of the parameters that might affect the likelihood of aggressive behavior in the world, for example:

1. One element of their research was that students were, by the nature of the situation, actually *encouraged* to aggress. This should attune us to the need to ensure that people are discouraged from believing that aggression is a legitimate way to respond to provocations and frustrations in the world.

2. Similarly, Donnerstein and Berkowitz created a situation where respondents experienced *no consequences* for their aggression, either to themselves (in the form of punishment) or to their victims (in the form of pain and trauma). This suggests that those who see sexual assault and violence against women as behaviors they can engage in with impunity may be more likely to engage in such behavior. This in turn should sensitize us to the need for competent investigation and prosecution of assaultive behavior, so as to maximize deterrence. Similarly, it suggests that greater emphasis should be placed on educating people about the experience of assault victims, particularly in terms of the pain and suffering that they endure.

3. Further, the Donnerstein and Berkowitz (1981) study, coupled with Fisher and Grenier (1994), shows that aggression is more likely to occur when there are no behavioral alternatives available or when none are *perceived* to be available. This should sensitize us to the need to encourage people to recognize that there are a variety of ways to deal with frustration and anger other than through aggression.

In sum, this analysis suggests that looking for effects of certain images per se is probably a fruitless task. Instead, it appears that any effects are mitigated by other variables, such as the meanings that are attached to our behaviors and the context in which those behaviors occur.

The Fragility of Media Influence Effects

It seems fairly clear from the literature that any "media effects" that can be attributed to the message or content of violent pornography per se are, in the grander scheme of things, a fairly trivial influence. Even Malamuth (1989), who built much of his reputation on demonstrating these effects, recognized that the media may not even be a particularly important element in the behavioral equation:

> *As with many behaviors, it is apparent that antisocial behavior against women is a function of many interacting causal factors. It is very difficult to gauge the relative influence, if any, of media exposure alone. However, by itself, it is likely to exert a small influence, if any. (p. 198)*

Context, Meanings, and Behavior

The experimental paradigm is typically silent with respect to variables of the sort that people doing qualitative social and health research cherish most dearly, for example, the *meaning* of images to people and the role that culture and individual differences can play in the generation and interpretation of images.

In this regard, Abramson and Hayashi (1984) offer a comparative analysis of Japanese and American pornography, attitudes about sex, the role of sex in the media, and so forth. They note, for example, that Japanese laws and mores completely prohibit images that many North Americans would find relatively tame (e.g., neither pubic hair nor adult genitalia may be shown), while at the same time allowing a variety of images that many North Americans would find horrendous (e.g., the admonition against showing pubic hair has resulted in the proliferation of sexualized images of prepubescent girls).

Given these differences, if it were in fact the case that sexually violent themes and images in and of themselves somehow "cause" greater aggressiveness, sexual aggression would be rampant in Japan—and at higher levels than in the United States. But despite the pervasiveness of such material, rates of sexual assault and other forms of sexual abuse in Japan appear to be far lower than those in Western countries.

These observations about the importance of culture in the rules of sexual practice and the interpretation of sexual and sexually violent images are particularly germane to the court case involving Little Sister's. Since the store caters primarily to the homosexual community, another question of interest in considering this case concerns whether any of the findings reported in the effects literature are applicable to that community.

External Validity Revisited: Generalizing to the Gay Community

All the experimental effects research has involved mixed-sex dyads. Would the effects observed among mixed-sex dyads also be seen if same-sex dyads were involved? This question clearly concerns the *external validity* of the research. Malamuth was asked by the Department of Justice to comment on that issue with respect to the Little Sister's trial.

Malamuth's opinion was that any effects that were observed for heterosexual pornography among members of the heterosexual community would in all likelihood be the same for homosexual pornography among members of the gay and lesbian community. Although he acknowledged having no data that bore directly on this issue, he based his speculation on the answers to three questions: (1) Are the messages in homosexual pornography basically the same as those in heterosexual pornography? (2) Are the minds of homosexuals basically the same as the minds of heterosexuals? (3) Are there problems of sexual conflict within the homosexual community? In all three cases he answers yes and, on that basis, concludes that the same processes prevail among the homosexual community as among the heterosexual one.

The difficulty we have with Malamuth's responses is his tenacious belief in the objective qualities of messages. When he asks whether homosexual pornography and heterosexual pornography are basically the same, Malamuth is led by his belief in the "objective," observable content of messages to answer yes. To Malamuth, the question "Are homosexual minds and heterosexual minds basically the same?" seems to involve knowing only whether the basic physiological material and information processing capacities of homosexuals and heterosexuals are the same; he concludes that, at that level, there are no differences between the homosexual mind and the heterosexual mind. And, of course, he's right.

But Malamuth misses the point. Although the superficial content that appears in some heterosexual pornography and some homosexual pornography may be similar, the *meanings* associated with those images, and hence their relationship with behavior, may well be considerably different. In this regard, we must remember that the historical experience of homosexuals and heterosexuals has been very different. While heterosexuals have enjoyed feeling "normal" about their sexuality, the gay community has endured many years of being considered "deviant" and/or "unnatural," and it is not even that long ago that it was actually illegal. Because being homosexual has been an unwarranted source of stigma for many years, and persecution of gay people still exists in many quarters, many gay people still feel reluctant to "come out of the closet." Given homosexuality's historical status as an oppressed lifestyle (e.g., through institutional harassment and hate crimes such as "gay-bashing"), we might anticipate that gays' marginalized status would have left a greater sense of shared community and interdependence among homosexuals than among heterosexuals. Some authors also have argued that, when it comes to matters of sexual violence, the situation in homosexual relations is unique in the sense that it might be more inherently egalitarian because of the gender similarity of the two people involved (e.g., see Brock & Kinsman, 1986).

Taken together, all these differences between homosexuals' and heterosexuals' life experience would leave us surprised if the two communities did *not* attach different meanings to sexual practices and sexual images. There's clearly a need for more research in that area, particularly by LGBTQIA researchers who are part of those communities, to articulate these issues. In the interim, the safer course would be to assume, on the basis of LGBTQIA people's significantly different social history, that differences in meaning do exist.

A third element considered by Malamuth was whether there is any evidence of violence in the gay community; to this question he also answers yes. And indeed, the gay community, like any other community, is not immune to sexual violence. But to assume that the same dynamics must therefore characterize both homosexual violence and heterosexual violence seems inconsistent with the feminist literature that Malamuth suggests informs his analysis. For example, to the extent that sexual violence between men and women involves not only violence but also *gender* violence, embedded in a history of patriarchal relations, how could patterns of sexual violence among same-sex partners (who are equal in overt gender status) be a product of the same dynamic? Overall, the biggest threats to homosexuals involving violence probably involve people from *outside* the gay community (harassment—and worse—from the intolerant and from gay bashers) more than people from *inside* it.

THE EXPERIMENT IN PERSPECTIVE

In offering the preceding detailed analysis of the Donnerstein and Berkowitz (1981) study, we have several aims: we hope we've shown how analyzing and critiquing a piece of research involves considering it in the light of the concepts (e.g., statistical conclusion validity, internal validity, external validity, ecological validity) introduced in more abstract form in the earlier part of this chapter. You should now be able to go through any example of experimental research and do the same.

You also should consider experimental research in the terms introduced much earlier in the text, particularly in terms of notions of engagement. As we've noted several times before, doing a piece of research involves *engaging* a phenomenon of interest, and the results that we acquire will bear the imprint of the tools we use to engage them. The "truth" that emerges from each method of engagement is no more and no less true than any other; each just gives its unique glimpse into the phenomena we study. We can engage phenomena by observing them, interviewing people about them, gathering archival information about them, or experimenting with them. Seen in this way, the experiment, as a way of understanding, is no more right or wrong than any other means of gathering data; it has unique strengths and weaknesses that the thoughtful researcher will consider when interpreting an experiment's results.

The experiment represents a powerful venue in which to develop a certain kind of dependable knowledge. The lab offers maximal manipulative control over the experimental situation and is ideally suited to situations where creating or simulating the phenomenon of interest is conceptually defensible and causal inference and precision are the highest priorities. In the lab, we can randomly assign our participants to the various experimental and control groups and hence ensure that the crucial experimental assumption of pretest equivalence is met. Since we create these groups, we can construct situations ideally suited to the research questions we wish to answer. And of course, because these experiments occur on our own turf, when we want them to, we are best prepared to measure the dependent variable with instruments of demonstrated reliability and validity.

This creative power has other benefits as well. In the laboratory, situations can be created that do not yet exist in the world, as can situations that we hope will not exist. As an example of the former, we might use the lab to do preliminary testing of emergent technologies or different organizational structures before they're foisted on users in the field. As for the latter, we wouldn't intentionally make a real airplane carrying real people crash, but we can use lab simulations to assess and/or train those who might have to deal with such events (e.g., Palys, 1978).

Finally, the laboratory experiment is ideally suited in many ways for addressing strictly theoretical questions, perhaps more so than practical or applied research questions. Given that various authors have affirmed that theory is *the* goal of science (as opposed to "truth" or "knowledge" or "facts" per se), this suggests that the lab plays an important role in social and health science. Note also that much theorizing is of the *ceteris paribus* variety (implying that theories assert the relationships among variables of interest, all else being equal), and laboratory experimentation is one manifestation of that logic. If a theory suggests that variable *A* should or might have a certain effect on variable *B*, for example, then you can observe variable *B* in a lab situation where all variables except variable *A* are held constant or otherwise equalized across groups (e.g., by random assignment to groups). Variable *A*, of course, would be present in one group (the experimental group) but not the other (the control group). By doing so, you would have investigated the effects of variable *A* on variable *B*, *ceteris paribus*.

As long as our interests are purely theoretical, and as long as we limit our interpretation to this generic *ceteris paribus* situation, the laboratory can serve a useful role. But if we're more interested in contextualized behavior in that open system we call the real world, the lab's role may be more limited (e.g., see Manicas & Secord, 1983). Researchers who extrapolate answers to applied questions from their theory-based lab research may be on tenuous ground, since all else is never equal in the real world; every setting embodies its own unique context (e.g., see Palys & Lowman, 1984).

Many social and health scientists believe that the controlled lab situation allows a "pure" test of the relationships among variables in a vacuous, context-free situation (e.g., see Festinger, 1953). But in the early 1970s, various European authors began to challenge this view (e.g., see Israel & Tajfel, 1972). They asserted that since all behavior occurs within a context and since "laboratory behavior" is still "behavior," attention is warranted to the context within which lab behavior occurs and to the relationship between the lab context and the context of the "real world" (see especially Tajfel, 1972).

Argyris (1975) and Brandt (1975) were among those to agree that the laboratory does indeed embody a social context, but both authors suggest that in many ways that context is the "wrong" one. They depict the experiment as embodying the most imperialist of tendencies—a centralized authority (the experimenter) defines the game and decides the rules, participants are often kept in the dark as to the experimenter's full motives and methods, the role of "subject" is to accept the experimenter's definition of the situation and respond within those constraints, and the preferred epistemology underlying the experiment is one that embraces the utility of manipulative control. The criticisms? Too centralized; too controlling; too hierarchical; too secretive; too minimizing of participants' views and interpretations. The authors remind us of our social responsibilities and suggest that such control-oriented methods encourage control-oriented policy (see also Latour, 1987); instead of empowering, such methods and policies are arguably exploitative.

Manicas and Secord (1983) subsequently took up the torch in their articulation of the contemporary critical realist perspective in social science. They agree with those who assert that the laboratory is a place to test theory (e.g., Kerlinger, 1973; Mook, 1983), since it's a closed system in which basic structures of individual human behavior (e.g., competencies, abilities, powers) can be investigated. But there's a bigger question: Do our interests lie exclusively with the concoction of theories of lab behavior per se, or are we also interested in theorizing about life in its broader context? If the latter, then Manicas and Secord assert that it's a whole new ball game. In sum, they argue that traditional experimentalists are accurate in their analysis (as it pertains to lab behavior), but myopic (because the conditions they study exist only in the lab).

As this summary suggests, some of the major questions about laboratory research revolve around the notion of exactly what lab behavior means. But the lab has even more clear-cut limitations. Not the least of these is that there are many phenomena that we would prefer to attend to *in vivo* (a Latin phrase meaning, literally, "in life"). Not all phenomena can be transported into the lab, nor can all be scrutinized conveniently in the typical hour-long laboratory session (e.g., the aging process, the development of criminal careers, observations of social change, the impact of deinstitutionalization, etc.). And when the mountain can't come to us, then we must go to the mountain.

SUMMING UP AND LOOKING AHEAD

When people construct an experiment, they're usually doing so because they're interested in assessing the causal impact of one variable (the independent or treatment variable) on another variable (the dependent or outcome variable). Philosophically, the criteria governing when you can legitimately infer that a causal relationship has occurred are delineated by John Stuart Mill (1843/1965). Mill states that one must meet three criteria:

1. temporal precedence (i.e., since we believe that causes come before effects, we must demonstrate that change in the variable we think is a cause did indeed come before its alleged effect);

2. existence of a relationship (i.e., if the alleged cause really is a cause, changes in it should be associated with subsequent changes in its alleged effect); and

3. elimination of rival plausible explanations (i.e., one must rule out the influence of all possible variables other than the one being considered as a source of causal influence).

The traditional experiment elegantly addresses these three criteria. Inherent in the traditional conception of the experiment is the idea that the experiment happens because and when you want it to happen. This allows you to prepare suitably reliable and valid measures of your dependent variable and can measure it at appropriate times. In the same vein, you make the experiment happen by manipulating the independent variable and assessing its effects. The temporal precedence criterion is addressed: because you "cause" the cause to occur, you are able to assess whether the level of the dependent (effect) measure is different only after the imposition of the independent variable.

Of course, we'd expect to observe a certain amount of variation (i.e., change) in the dependent variable over time purely as a function of chance. The first question of interest to us after completing a study, therefore, is whether any change we observed is greater than we would have expected on the basis of chance alone. This question concerns the statistical significance of the results. If the change we observe is statistically significant, we will have demonstrated the relationship criterion that Mill espoused: we will have demonstrated that a change in the independent variable is associated with a change in the dependent variable and that the latter change is greater than might be anticipated on the basis of chance variation alone.

Remember, though, that finding statistical significance in our results doesn't immediately allow us to say that the independent variable caused the change. All we know at this point is that chance alone wasn't the cause of the change. But what was? That's an internal validity question. We must consider rival plausible explanations as well, such as history, maturation, testing, and other threats to internal validity. According to the logic of experimentation, if two groups are equal to begin with and if they are treated identically in all respects except for the presence or absence of the independent variable, any subsequent differences between those groups can be accounted for only by the influence of the independent variable. And while control groups exist to ensure that the groups are "treated identically" in all respects, recall that either random assignment or matching allows us to ensure that the groups were indeed equal to begin with.

Even if we can meet Mill's criteria, we face the question of whether the results we've observed are generalizable beyond the specifics of the study. Can the results be generalized across time, people, and settings? This, of course, is a question of external validity. And finally, the concept of ecological validity raises questions about how well an experiment captures or represents the setting to which we wish to generalize. It's an important element for considering whether theoretical processes that can happen actually do.

The last part of this chapter analyzed a particular example of experimental research—Donnerstein and Berkowitz's (1981) experiment to assess the effects of viewing violent pornography on its viewers—in order to show how the abstract concepts described earlier in the chapter can be used to design, analyze, and critique a particular piece of research. The case is also made that, far from being a "privileged" mode of creating knowledge, the experiment, like any other method, is a tool that engages phenomena in a particular manner, with unique strengths and weaknesses in the way that it does so.

Wouldn't it be a good thing if we could take this experimentalist logic and move it out into the field to assess the effects of social change or law and policy changes? Donald T. Campbell was one of the people who thought so, encouraging us to be more of an "experimenting society" where we created and implemented social programs and policies on the basis of evidence of their effectiveness instead of sheer political power and ideology? His answer came in the form of suggestions for quasi-experimentation, which we will explain in the next chapter.

Key Concepts

Blind condition 232
Ceteris paribus 246
Control group or comparison
    group 212
Correlation ≠ causation
    204–205
Dependent variable 206
Ecological validity 222
External validity 221

History 207
Independent variable 206
Instrumentation 212
Internal validity 206
Matching 219
Maturation 207
Mill's three causal criteria 203
Practice effects 209
Pretest equivalence 216

Pretest sensitization 209
Random assignment 217
Regression toward the mean 209
Selection 212
Statistical conclusion validity 221
Statistical significance 227
Temporal precedence 204
Testing 208

STUDY QUESTIONS

1. Yasmin feels she has developed a cure for the common cold and wants to test it out. Fifty cold sufferers come to her office one Monday; each receives her treatment. A week later, they all come back, and Yasmin finds that 44 of them (88 percent) no longer have colds. She concludes that her cure is indeed very effective and cites an 88 percent cure rate. Would you agree with her conclusion? What *rival plausible explanations* would you entertain? How might you *control* for these?

2. Bill is a cautious fellow who wants to buy a safe car. He reads some published statistics that compare all the various models of cars in terms of the frequency with which they are involved in accidents. On learning that the BMW 735i sedan (a very expensive car) has the lowest number of accidents and the lowest number of fatalities, he goes out and buys one, believing that he will be safer. From an empirical perspective, would you agree with the logic underlying his decision? Why or why not?

3. Students who take our undergraduate research methods courses receive tutorials (small group "help" sessions where attendance is optional) in addition to the weekly lecture. Since we have often wondered how helpful the tutorials are to students, we have constructed an evaluation to find out. All semester long, attendance is taken at the tutorials. At the end of the semester, we use the attendance reports to construct three groups: those who always or almost always came to tutorial (e.g., missed no more than two tutorials over the semester); those who never or almost never came to tutorials (e.g., came to two or fewer tutorials over the semester); and those who fell in between (i.e., came sometimes). We then compare the average final grades in the course for the three groups. Suppose that this semester, we find that those who always or almost always came to the tutorials had the highest average grade, those who came part of the time had the next-highest average grade, and those who never or almost never came received the lowest average grade. Suppose further that the differences between the groups are statistically significant.

    a. Name the *independent variable* in this study.

    b. Name the *dependent variable* in this study.

    c. What does it mean to say that the differences between groups are *statistically significant?*

    d. Evaluate the study's *internal validity*, identify what threat(s) to internal validity you believe might be present, and state how you might redesign the study to control for those threats.

    e. Show that you understand the concept of *external validity* by identifying our external validity concerns in this study.

    f. Evaluate the study's *ecological validity.*

4. Jill intends to perform an experiment in which she will compare whether "factual" appeals or "emotional" appeals are more effective in changing people's attitudes regarding nuclear disarmament. About 100 people have volunteered to participate in her study, and she wonders whether *random assignment* or *matching* would be the better procedure to use in assigning participants to groups. Compare the relative advantages of these techniques in Jill's situation, state which you would recommend, and explain how you would do it.

5. Why are control groups called *control* groups, that is, what do they *control for?*

6. People are different from one another. In what sense, then, can random assignment or matching be said to *equalize* groups?

7. Jerry reads the Donnerstein and Berkowitz (1981) study regarding the effects of viewing pornography on aggression and says, "Yeah, but I'll bet some of the people in the control group were consumers of pornography *before* they participated in the study. Wouldn't that undermine differences between the groups and mess up their conclusions?" How would you respond?

8. LeBron, the head coach for Little League, has developed a series of clinics to teach the kids the essentials of base running. A total of 60 kids end up playing on league teams. Always seeking a challenge, LeBron identifies the 20 kids who had the slowest times during the tryouts and makes them the "experimental" group, which is then exposed to his base running expertise. Another 20 kids are randomly chosen to be the "control" group, that is, they are not given any particular instruction in base running. In order to equalize the amount of attention the two groups receive, however, the control group is given extra practice at bunting, a skill that has no relation to base running speed. After two weeks, the kids are assessed again. LeBron finds that the base running times of those in the experimental group have improved significantly, while times of the control group have remained unchanged. He concludes that the techniques utilized in his base running clinics are indeed effective.

    a. Name the *independent variable* in LeBron's study.

    b. Name the *dependent variable* in LeBron's study.

    c. Indicate what *threat(s) to internal validity* LeBron should be concerned with here.

    d. Indicate what LeBron's *external validity* concerns might be in this situation.

    e. Differentiate between *random selection* and *random assignment.* Which is more relevant to internal validity and which to external validity? Explain.

9. Just because an experiment shows that a phenomenon *can* occur in the lab does not mean that it *does* occur in the world. Would you agree or disagree with that statement? Explain.

10. What are some of the strengths of experimentation as a method? What are some of its limitations?

11. Although the initial conceptualization of the experiment was something along the lines of what a test tube is in chemistry or a vacuum in physics—a clean and "pure" setting apart from the rest of life that allows testing under controlled conditions—some researchers disagreed. They argued that all behavior occurs in context and that the laboratory was no exception. So how would you characterize the context in which experimental behavior occurs?

FROM MANIPULATIVE TO ANALYTIC CONTROL: QUASI-EXPERIMENTATION

Discussing the logic of experimentation was a convenient way to introduce and apply some very basic empirical concepts (e.g., operationalization, internal validity, external validity, statistical significance) that are relevant to all experimental and experimentalist inferential research. But not all interesting phenomena can be recreated and/or observed in the laboratory. Nor would we necessarily *want* to spend all our time in the lab. But is it possible to maintain the intellectual and inferential rigor of the experiment in the field? And would we want to if we could?

DONALD T. CAMPBELL AND QUASI-EXPERIMENTATION

Not even 50 years ago, most researchers in the social and health sciences felt that leaving the lab and entering the real world meant that we had to throw principles of experimentation, and opportunities for causal inference, out the window. Only in the lab could you gather "clean" data in well-controlled situations created at the whim of the experimenter; the field necessarily involved "dirty" data subject to too many uncontrolled influences. Aspects of the experimental method that were seen as integral to experimentation—random assignment to groups, for example—were seen as impossible to duplicate to any significant degree outside the lab. "Evaluation research" (i.e., studies that attempt to assess the effects of a particular program or the impact of policy or legislative changes) was seen as a necessarily subjective and error-prone task. There was a clear hierarchy of methods, with the experiment at the top and case study methods at the bottom.

The individual who played the most significant role in encouraging us to reconsider that view was the late Donald T. Campbell. His classic article "Reforms as Experiments" (1969b) was the one to break the ice, although its themes had been the subject of discussion for some years before it was published (e.g., see Campbell, 1957; Campbell & Stanley, 1963). Campbell's contributions were twofold. First, he supplied a vocabulary and a set of dimensions on which research might be evaluated. Almost all of the terms you learned about in the previous chapter—e.g., "internal validity," "external validity," and all the various threats —are due to him. Second, he argued that researchers should not confuse the trappings of experimentation with its underlying logic.

Recall the three criteria of causality that John Stuart Mill (1843/1965) said must be satisfied in order to identify a "causal" relationship:

1. *Temporal precedence*: the presumed cause (X) must come *before*
   (i.e., is "temporally precedent" to) the effect (Y);

2. *Relationship*: the presumed cause and effect are indeed related to each other (i.e., the presence or absence of X is associated with an increased likelihood of the presence or absence of Y); and

3. *Elimination of rival plausible explanations*: the relationship between X and Y is not explained by the presence of other plausible causal agents.

We saw in Chapter 6 how these criteria are addressed in traditional experimental design. The temporal precedence criterion is met by the fact that the researcher manipulates the presumed causal variable (i.e., the researcher "causes" the presumed "cause" to occur) and is there waiting to measure changes that occur afterward in the dependent (or "effect" or "outcome") variable. The existence of a relationship is demonstrated by an observed difference between the "experimental" or "treatment" group and the "control" group beyond what would be expected on the basis of chance variation alone. The final criterion—the absence of rival plausible explanations—is addressed by the concept of internal validity which, in the context of the traditional experiment, is accomplished by (1) manipulation of the independent variable; (2) the creation of experimental and control groups; and (3) random assignment to groups. These directly and elegantly address Mill's criteria. Surely proceeding without them would be like trying to fly without wings.

But Campbell (1969b) encouraged us to take experimentalist logic a step further. He recognized the importance of being able to do research in the "real world," arguing that we'd all be a lot better off if we could somehow evaluate the effects of legal reforms and other social changes—that is, become more of an "experimenting society" rather than operating chiefly on the basis of intuition and subjective self-interest (see Campbell, 1991). To do so, he suggested, we first would have to stop confusing the *trappings* of experimentation with its *logic*. To quote one of his former colleagues at Northwestern:

> The assumption of [quasi-experimental design] is that the experimental method has much broader application than its laboratory version suggests. …What is important is not [the] ability to manipulate and assign randomly, but the ends these procedures serve… The problem then becomes one of providing the proper translation rules to get the social scientist out of the lab and into the "real world," while retaining some of the strong inference characteristic of the laboratory setting. (Caporaso, 1973, pp. 6–7; our emphasis)

In other words, if manipulation of the independent variable and random assignment to groups become difficult to accomplish in field settings, we should not resign ourselves to the feeling that causal inference is thus impossible, but rather should look to the underlying logic of experimentation for alternative procedures that will fulfill these same experimental objectives. According to Campbell (e.g., 1969b), the temporal precedence criterion of causality (i.e., cause before effect) is relatively easily dealt with in many field situations by the acquisition of time-series data. With respect to the inability to randomly assign participants to groups, Campbell (1969b) notes that

> *the advocated strategy in quasi-experimentation is not to throw up one's hands and refuse to use the evidence because of this lack of control, but rather to generate by informed criticism as many appropriate rival hypotheses as possible, and then to do the supplementary research... which would reflect on these rival hypotheses. (p. 413)*

THE LOGIC OF QUASI-EXPERIMENTATION

One of the first places that Campbell demonstrated the logic he was advocating in quasi-experimentation was in his analysis of the effects of a crackdown on speeding that occurred in the state of Connecticut in the 1950s. The crackdown was implemented following a year in which a record number of people died on Connecticut highways. Like many others, Governor Abraham Ribicoff believed that excess speed was a major cause of traffic fatalities and that the point system that had been in effect in Connecticut until that time was ineffective in keeping speeders in check. In its place, Governor Ribicoff announced that from that day forward, all people convicted of speeding on the highways would have their licenses suspended. There would be a 30-day suspension for the first offence, a 60-day suspension for a second offence, and an indefinite suspension, the exact duration of which would be the subject of a hearing after 90 days, for a third.

There were, in fact, fewer deaths on the highways of Connecticut the following year: 284 persons died, which was 40 fewer than had been killed on the highways in the previous year. Ribicoff was very pleased with this decrease, arguing that the saving of 40 lives was well worth the inconvenience to individuals who had been guilty of speeding. The Connecticut crackdown was the subject of considerable national attention because of its apparent success, and Governor Ribicoff proudly accepted awards from agencies such as the National Safety Council for his efforts.

Campbell and Ross (1968) did not question Governor Ribicoff's statements that the saving of 40 lives was "worth it," since the relative worth of 40 lives versus inconvenience to speeders is obviously not an empirical question, but rather one of value and philosophy. Instead, the two researchers addressed the question of whether Ribicoff was correct in identifying the crackdown *per se* as the causal agent in the change that was observed, or whether some other rival plausible explanation(s) might account for the results.

In traditional laboratory experimentation, we simultaneously eliminate numerous rival plausible explanations by randomly assigning participants to groups (thereby ensuring pretest equivalence) and by creating a control group that is equivalent to the experimental group in all respects except for the introduction of the independent variable. But that luxury obviously isn't available to us here; you can't randomly assign laws to some states and not others, or randomly assign some drivers to be suspended while others are not. So what can we do?

Was the Independent Variable Really Manipulated?

The first thing you'd want to establish is whether a speeding crackdown really did occur, as Governor Ribicoff said it did. Is there evidence that the independent (treatment) variable of interest really *was* manipulated? If it wasn't, then you could hardly argue that *that* was the source of any change that occurred. This may sound somewhat obvious, but much of politics is theatre, and it's not uncommon for politicians to say something will happen when in fact it doesn't. On some occasions this failure occurs at the political level, for example, when the proposed change doesn't make it to or doesn't survive the legislative process. On other occasions, people on the front lines in the institutions or bureaucracies that are supposed to carry out the change in policy can be quite inventive in finding ways *not* to do so (e.g., by finding loopholes in the policy, giving the matter low priority, or moving discretion to another bureaucratic level).

The evidence from Connecticut generally supports the notion that a crackdown really did occur, just as Governor Ribicoff had said it would. To ensure compliance among judges, Ribicoff went on public record to state that judges who did not follow his directive of suspending speeders would find that they wouldn't be reappointed next time their positions came up for renewal. The most direct evidence on this point would be an increase in the number of license suspensions, and Campbell found that in the first six months of the year the number of suspensions did indeed increase dramatically, from 231 in 1955 to 5,398 in 1956 (an increase of more than 2,000 percent). Figure 7.1 shows the significance and abruptness of this change.

But there also appear to have been some changes in how speeders were treated by both the police and the courts. Figure 7.2 shows there was a noticeable decrease in speeding violations expressed as a percentage of all traffic violations. This decline may

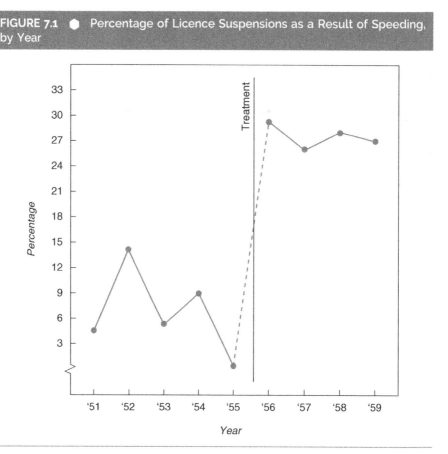

FIGURE 7.1 ⬤ Percentage of Licence Suspensions as a Result of Speeding, by Year

Source: Campbell, D. T., & Ross, L. H. (1968). The Connecticut crackdown on speeding: Time-series data in quasi-experimental analysis. *Law and Society Review, 3,* 48. Reprinted by permission of the Law and Society Association, University of Massachusetts.

indicate that the crackdown was effective and fewer people were speeding. It also could mean that police officers had become less likely to ticket speeders, knowing that the inevitable punishment for the ticket would be a licence suspension (i.e., they may have given a larger "grace" region before actually giving a ticket) and/or had become more likely to give speeders a ticket for something other than speeding (e.g., showing undue care) that would lead to a fine but not cause them to lose their license.

Similarly, Figure 7.3 reveals a noticeable increase in the percentage of speeding violations that were ultimately judged "not guilty." Perhaps alleged speeders became more likely to fight their tickets in court, since avoiding a license suspension is worth taking up time for. Another possibility is that judges may have

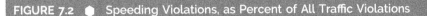

FIGURE 7.2 ● Speeding Violations, as Percent of All Traffic Violations

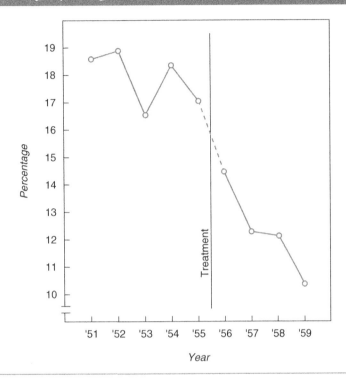

Source: Campbell, D. T., & Ross, L. H. (1968). The Connecticut crackdown on speeding: Time-series data in quasi-experimental analysis. *Law and Society Review, 3,* 48. Reprinted by permission of the Law and Society Association, University of Massachusetts.

become more likely to dismiss charges on minor technicalities, given the harsh punishment they'd otherwise be obliged to bestow.

There also was some evidence that the harsh sanctions imposed in the crackdown had the unintended effect of creating even greater violation of the law by people continuing to drive despite their licenses being suspended. As Figure 7.4 indicates, before the crackdown it was literally unheard of for Connecticut drivers to be caught driving with a suspended license. After the crackdown, with suspensions going through the roof (recall Figure 7.1), the percentage of new suspensions caused by driving while suspended suddenly rose to more than 4 percent and as much as 7 percent.

Although these unintended effects are interesting for what they reveal when an extremely harsh policy is put into place—mechanisms are triggered to ameliorate its

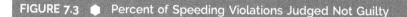

FIGURE 7.3 ● Percent of Speeding Violations Judged Not Guilty

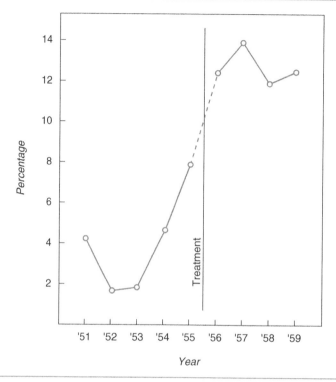

Source: Campbell, D. T., & Ross, L. H. (1968). The Connecticut crackdown on speeding: Time-series data in quasi-experimental analysis. *Law and Society Review, 3*, 51. Reprinted by permission of the Law and Society Association, University of Massachusetts.

more unjust impacts—the huge size of the crackdown (Figure 7.1) compared to the relatively minor shifts observed in Figures 7.2 and 7.3 nonetheless convinced Campbell and Ross (1968) that the independent variable really was manipulated quite dramatically.

Was There a Change in the Dependent Variable?

So we know there really was a crackdown. The second question to ask is whether there is any evidence at all that the crackdown was effective. The answer to that one is fairly obvious, since we've already noted there were 40 fewer deaths after the change than in the year before. So change did occur, and it was in the predicted direction (i.e., fewer rather than more deaths). This is immediately evident in the simple before–after "gee whiz" graph (see Huff, 1993) shown in Figure 7.5.

FIGURE 7.4 ● Percentage of New Suspensions Caused by Driving While Suspended

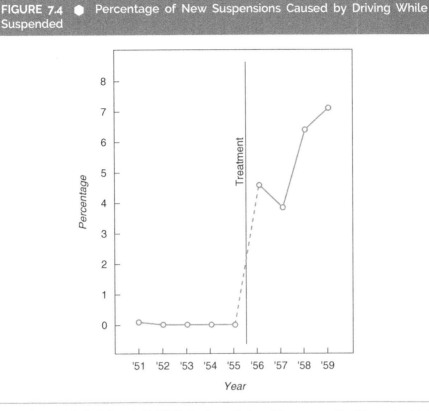

Source: Campbell, D. T., & Ross, L. H. (1968). The Connecticut crackdown on speeding: Time-series data in quasi-experimental analysis. *Law and Society Review, 3*, 50. Reprinted by permission of the Law and Society Association, University of Massachusetts.

So what do we know at this point? First, we know that the independent variable really was manipulated. Second, we know an attendant change in the dependent variable occurred *after* the independent variable was manipulated; that is, a decrease in deaths was observed *after* the speeding crackdown came into effect. In investigating the question, "Did the Connecticut crackdown on speeding cause a substantial decrease in the highway death toll?" two of Mill's criteria have thus been established: (1) the presumed "cause" *did* precede the alleged "effect" and (2) the introduction of the change in law was accompanied by a change in the dependent variable (i.e., the number of deaths). It is Mill's *third* criterion that's missing at this point: we haven't yet demonstrated that the observed change in the dependent variable was not caused by some plausible factor(s) *other than* the crackdown. And of course *that's* the tough part!

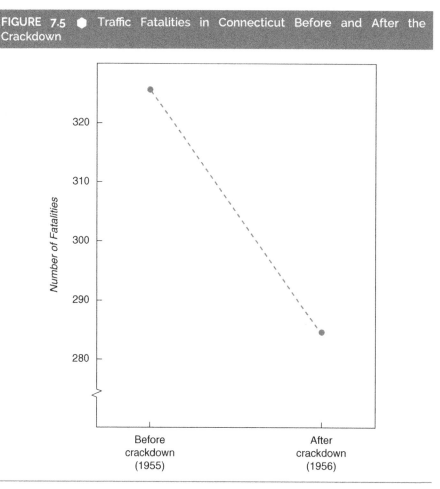

FIGURE 7.5 ⬠ Traffic Fatalities in Connecticut Before and After the Crackdown

Source: Campbell, D. T., & Ross, L. H. (1968). The Connecticut crackdown on speeding: Time-series data in quasi-experimental analysis. *Law and Society Review, 3*, 38. Reprinted by permission from Blackwell Publishing.

Eliminating Rival Plausible Explanations

A Plausible Alternative? Check It Out!

At this point, Campbell (1969b) encourages us to make a cognitive shift in our approach to experimentation. What is our objective in this situation? We want to rule out rival plausible explanations. But how do we do that here? By starting off with the assumption, on the basis of the data shown in Figure 7.5, that the prevailing evidence suggests the crackdown *was* effective, and then systematically deriving, and then testing, all the rival plausible explanations we can think of.

In other words, Figure 7.5 can be viewed as the result of a one-group pretest/posttest research design that shows that there was an effect associated with the change in the independent variable. But what might have caused that change? The crackdown *may* have caused it. But are there other possibilities as well? This is where our list of potential threats to internal validity comes into play. The advocated strategy is not to be an armchair quarterback and say, "Oh, too bad there's such poor internal validity because this or that threat was not controlled" and leave it at that, but to say "Let's try and figure out what threats might actually be plausible in this situation, and see whether we can find the data we need to address each one." As Campbell (1969b) explained,

> *This is evaluation, not rejection, for it often turns out that for a specific design in a specific setting the threat is implausible, or that there are supplementary data that can help rule it out even where randomization is impossible. The general ethic, here advocated for public administrators as well as social scientists, is to use the very best method possible, aiming at 'true experiments' with random control groups. But where randomized treatments are not possible, a self-critical use of quasi-experimental designs is advocated. We must do the best we can with what is available to us.*
>
> *Our posture vis-à-vis perfectionist critics from laboratory experimentation is more militant than this: the only threats to validity that we will allow to invalidate an experiment are those that admit of the status of empirical laws more dependable and more plausible than the law involving the treatment. The mere possibility of some alternative explanation is not enough—it is only the plausible rival hypotheses that are invalidating. (p. 411)*

At the top of the list is *history*. What events might have occurred between the pretest and the posttest other than the speed crackdown that might have caused the decrease in deaths? Well, we know that weather conditions can make a difference to accident rates, so one possibility is that the year before the crackdown might have been particularly wet or snow-filled and/or that the year after the crackdown was particularly dry and/or snow-free. Meteorological records speak to this issue, so Campbell and Ross tracked down the appropriate records, and it turned out that in neither year was the amount of rainfall or snowfall exceptional in any way. Okay… one rival plausible explanation shot down.

What other possibilities are there? Well, road quality could make a difference. Did Connecticut make any significant improvements in the roads after the crackdown?

Road improvement budgets speak to that possibility, so Campbell and Ross went to check them, and it turned out there were no unusual expenditures for roads before and after the crackdown. Another rival plausible explanation eliminated.

Car safety perhaps? Did car manufacturers come up with some new technological development that would make new cars safer? Or were seatbelt laws or some other law changed that also could be expected to reduce the number of highway deaths? Once again the answers were "no" and "no." Two more rival plausible explanations go down in flames.

You've probably caught the general drift by now. The emphasis is on *informed critique* as a source for generating rival *plausible* explanations; your job is to be your own best critic, to anticipate as many rival plausible explanations as possible, and then to test systematically the plausibility of each one by gathering whatever data are appropriate. If the relevant data are not available to you, they may have been available in some other context for someone else, so another place to check will be the literature to see whether the influence of the factor has been tested elsewhere. Unlike the classic experiment where random assignment acts like pixie dust to allow you to simultaneously dismiss several otherwise plausible threats, quasi-experimentation place more onus on the researcher both to recognize potential rival explanations that are actually plausible and to identify the sorts of data that will address those possibilities. You probably wouldn't want to put too much trust in Ray, for example, the character depicted in Figure 7.6.

The resulting analysis will leave us with either (1) *no* rival plausible explanations remaining, in which case we conclude that the crackdown itself is the most compelling explanation we are left with or (2) *some* (or many) rival plausible explanations remaining, in which case we can do no more than list what these might be. Your challenge is to make a comprehensive inventory of these and to look for relevant data to test them out as thoroughly as possible, and/or to look to other research where the plausibility of an explanation was assessed. The relatively simple comparisons we've noted above also can be supplemented with more elaborate quasi-experimental designs, depending on the types of rival plausible explanations you are attempting to assess and/or on the specifics of the situation. A relatively exhaustive inventory and delineation of these designs can be seen in Cook and Campbell (1979) or its updated version by Shadish, Cook, and Campbell (2001). Our discussion here will continue with discussion of a class of techniques known as **interrupted time-series designs**.

FIGURE 7.6 ● Techniques Involving Analytic as Opposed to Manipulative Control—Such as Quasi-Experimentation and Qualitative Case Study Analysis—Are a Challenge to Do Well

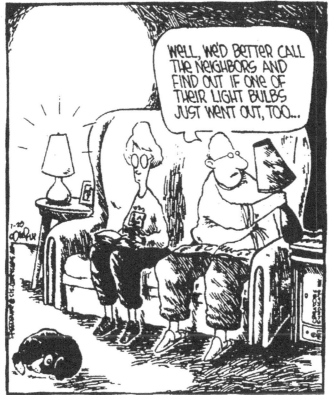

Time-Series Designs

One rival plausible explanation that deserves special note when we talk about quasi-experimentation, particularly in the evaluation research context, is *statistical regression*, or *regression toward the mean*. Remember how we said in the previous chapter that the situation in which you most need to worry about regression artifacts is when the members of your "treatment" group are chosen *because of* the extremity of their scores? The political climate that contributes to many programs coming into existence in the first place makes statistical regression a threat you must always worry about when evaluating the effects of social and health-related programs. Campbell (1969b) makes the point well in his facetious advice to "trapped" administrators: to look good, all you have to do is pick the worst administrative unit under your control as the target for your "experimental" program, and then wait for a year; there's a high probability that their performance will improve just because of regression toward the mean (but you, of course, take all the credit).

Even when such an approach isn't being taken by administrators for self-serving reasons, "extreme circumstances" often give birth to programs at short notice. When the media headlines scream "Worst Crime Wave Ever!," or "Hospital Emergency Wait Times at All-Time High!," politicians and civil servants may use their discretionary funding to show that they're doing something and to reassure the public that everything is under control. Of course, it's exactly such circumstances that are most often associated with regression artifacts, in which case the situation in all likelihood will improve by next year, whether or not anything is done.

One of our concerns with the Connecticut speeding crackdown data thus should be the question, "How typical was 1955?" An intervention or "treatment" as severe as the Connecticut speed crackdown most likely would arise in the kind of extreme conditions most conducive to regression artifacts, and we were told that 1955 involved a "record high" number of highway traffic deaths. How can we address that threat to internal validity? The answer: by gathering time-series data that show the maturational trend of the data. These are shown in Figure 7.7. You can see where the 1955–1956 pre–post comparison "gee whiz" graph (Figure 7.5) fits into the picture. It reveals that regression to the mean is indeed a plausible concern; 1955 *was* an atypically high year, and so it should be no surprise that there would be a decrease in 1956.

Multiple Time-Series Designs

To delve further into that issue, we can extend the *single* time-series design noted above into a *multiple* time-series design. Recall that part of what makes the classic experiment the uncontested choice for maximizing internal validity is the ability to randomly assign participants into treatment and control groups. That possibility is (by definition) missing when it comes to quasi-experimentation, which is often the method you are using when evaluating the impacts and effects of social and health programs. Why? Because when you are dealing with changes in law or health policy and it is real people with real problems who are involved, random assignment of people or other units (families, teams, states, neighborhoods) is often not possible because it would be unethical, unfair, or simply not procedurally manageable.

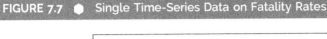

FIGURE 7.7 ●   Single Time-Series Data on Fatality Rates

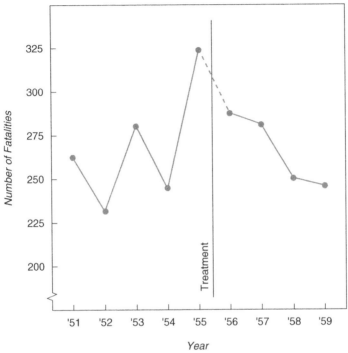

Source: Campbell, D. T., & Ross, L. H. (1968). The Connecticut crackdown on speeding: Time-series data in quasi-experimental analysis. *Law and Society Review, 3,* 42. Reprinted by permission from Blackwell Publishing.

Remember, however, the attitude that Donald Campbell wanted you to be guided by: "We must do the best we can with what is available to us" (1969b, p. 411). When you can't do things like randomly assign, consider what it is that random assignment accomplishes, and look for other ways to achieve that objective. In the experiment, the main thing random assignment accomplishes is the goal of ensuring that the two (or more) groups are equal on average prior to the introduction of the independent variable—the assumption of pretest equivalence. If the groups are essentially similar at the pretest, and thereafter treated identically in all respects but one—the treatment group receives the independent variable while any control or comparison groups do not—then we can feel assured that any difference we see at the end is due to the independent variable.

When we are in that situation where we cannot randomly assign people to groups, or laws to states, or policies to hospitals, then Campbell encouraged us to start looking for "nonequivalent" controls that would allow us to at least make some reasonable guesses about the plausibility of different rival plausible explanations. The term "nonequivalent" at first blush may make this strategy seem a bit useless—an admission that the principle of equivalence at the pretest is untenable—but you should see it simply as a recognition that equivalence is not automatic (as it would be if you randomly assigned), and instead will need to be thought through and justified.

One example that Cook and Campbell (1979) discuss is the situation where you have more people than a service provider can offer at any one time so that waitlists are created. The possibility this creates is to use people on the waitlist as your control group. These waitlist controls are subject to the same selection processes as the group that is receiving the treatment now, so differences between groups are minimized, and the ethical problem of holding some people back from receiving the service is bypassed because they will be receiving the service in due course. Because they will be entering the program or receiving the service, it may even mean that you have descriptive information about both those on the waitlist and the group currently receiving treatment, which may allow you to actually test how equivalent the groups are by comparing them on service-relevant variables. All you are doing is using the opportunity the existence of a waitlist allows.

That example would not work with the Connecticut speed crackdown, but what sorts of comparisons would give a reasonable basis for comparison? Campbell and Ross (1968) decided to put together a composite of four neighboring states, explaining it thus:

> [I]t is in the spirit of quasi-experimental analysis to make use of all *available data that could help to rule out or confirm any plausible rival hypothesis. In a setting such as this, no randomly assigned control group is available. But in quasi-experimentation, even a nonequivalent control group is helpful. It provides the only control for history (for those extraneous change agents that would be expected to affect both the experimental and control group), and assists in controlling maturation, testing, and instrumentation. For Connecticut, it was judged that a pool of adjacent and similar states—New York, New Jersey, Rhode Island and Massachusetts—provided a meaningful comparison.* (p. 43; emphasis in original)

You can see these data in Figure 7.8. Note that while they are looking at other states that are "nonequivalent" in the sense that every state has its own unique characteristics (as the proud residents of every state will tell you), it is not just *any* other states they are including, but four states that are matched as closely as possible with

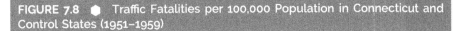

FIGURE 7.8 ● Traffic Fatalities per 100,000 Population in Connecticut and Control States (1951–1959)

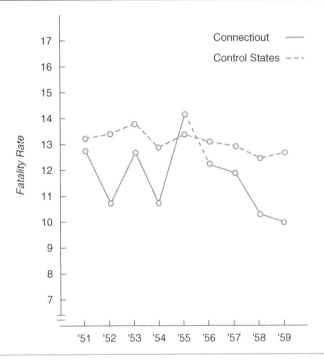

Source: Campbell, D. T., & Ross, L. H. (1968). The Connecticut crackdown on speeding: Time-series data in quasi-experimental analysis. *Law and Society Review, 3*, 44. Reprinted by permission of the Law and Society Association, University of Massachusetts.

Connecticut and thus allow for a "meaningful comparison." In this case they chose the four states that neighbor Connecticut and thus would have roughly similar topography, road conditions, and perhaps even citizenry (New Englanders). Clearly this is a much better choice than comparing Connecticut with Texas, Arizona, California, and Nevada, for example, where weather conditions would be very different, and the land itself would create very different driving conditions (e.g., treed versus desert; flat and straight versus hilly and winding).

The smoothness of the control series, by the way, is accounted for largely by the aggregation of four states, such that chance deviations on a state-to-state basis tend to cancel one another out. Note also that Figure 7.8 provides a bit of support for *both* the "regression" *and* the "crackdown" explanations. As Campbell and Ross (1968) explain it,

While in general these data confirm the single time-series analysis, the differences between Connecticut and the control states show a pattern supporting the hypothesis that the crackdown made a difference. In the pretest years, Connecticut's rate is parallel or rising relative to the control, exceeding it in 1955. In the posttest years, Connecticut's rate drops faster than does the control, steadily increasing the gap. While the regression argument applies to the high point of 1955 and to the subsequent departure in 1956, it does not plausibly explain the steadily increasing gap in 1957, 1958, and 1959.

In sum, 1955 *was* quite an atypical year; however, the trend in the control states is for relatively flat or slightly increasing numbers of traffic deaths over time, while the Connecticut trend following the crackdown is for a decrease that continues dropping beyond 1956.

Besides providing some degree of control over history threats (e.g., given sufficient proximity, to control for weather changes), **multiple time-series** may also (in some circumstances) control for *instrumentation* threats (i.e., changes in the measurement instrument or in the data-gathering procedure). This is not the case in the present data, since each state keeps its own books, but might be relevant in situations where all the control units (e.g., states) share the same recordkeeping procedures (e.g., UCR crime rate statistics) and all make a change in procedure at the same time.

The final data Campbell and Ross (1968) share with us (in Figure 7.9) deaggregate the control series of Figure 7.8 into separate states. Once again, the evidence is mixed, but it offers some support for a real effect over and above a regression artifact. The trend in most states is for a continuation of or even a slight increase in the number of highway deaths. The most similar profiles came from Massachusetts and Rhode Island. In both cases (and particularly with Rhode Island), increases in 1954–1955 are followed by decreases in 1955–1956. But in both cases, the trend rises again shortly thereafter. In contrast, the Connecticut trend is for a continuing decrease, leading Campbell and Ross (1968) to argue that while *some* of the change in the dependent measure is probably attributable to regression toward the mean, there's also evidence to suggest that the crackdown did indeed have some effect.

By way of conclusion, the authors assert that the Connecticut speed crackdown was indeed a crackdown of epic and harsh proportion, with some degree of effect over and above the regression artifacts. Of perhaps even greater interest to future evaluators were the indications of how a system—the justice system in this instance—responds when asked to invoke an extreme sanction. The police start calling the behavior something else to avoid an outcome they see as too extreme, while judges start to look

FIGURE 7.9 ● Traffic Fatalities for Connecticut, New York, New Jersey, Rhode Island, and Massachusetts (per 100,000 Persons)

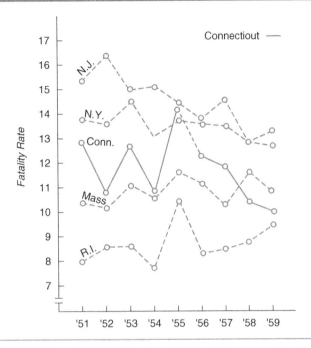

Source: Campbell, D. T., & Ross, L. H. (1968). The Connecticut crackdown on speeding: Time-series data in quasi-experimental analysis. *Law and Society Review, 3,* 45. Reprinted by permission of the Law and Society Association, University of Massachusetts.

for reasons to find people not guilty. And in a state where driving for many is essential, whether for employment or simply taking the kids to soccer practice, there was evidence many people were willing to risk even more severe sanctions for driving while suspended, thereby undermining the rule of law.

REVIEWING THE LOGIC OF QUASI-EXPERIMENTATION

Although the substantive aspects of the speed crackdown are interesting, the authors remind us that the bigger lessons from the study and the purpose of the analysis were to offer an illustration of how to implement a quasi-experimental approach. In that regard, there are several steps to follow in executing a quasi-experimental design. First, ask yourself whether there really was a change in the independent (treatment) variable. Campbell and Ross (1968) started in that way by looking to see whether there was any evidence that a "crackdown" on speeders had indeed occurred. If there really was a manipulation of the independent variable—then the next question to address is whether there is any evidence of a change in the dependent (outcome) variable—and if so, whether that change occurred after implementation of the independent variable. For example, Campbell and Ross (1968) compared the number of traffic deaths in 1955 and 1956 and found that there was indeed a decrease.

If the answer to either of these first two questions is "no," there's little sense in going further. But if both answers are "yes," you then move to the third criterion. A relationship evidently exists between the putative causal (independent or treatment) variable and the effect (dependent or outcome) variable, but *what factors other than the independent variable might also have accounted for the observed relationship?* Here, Campbell and Ross (1968) affirm, you must be your own best critic—if you aren't, you can be certain someone else will be. You must identify *plausible* alternative explanations and doggedly pursue the relevant data that will allow you to test each of those alternatives. As Campbell and Ross explain,

> *A final note on the treatment of uncontrolled variables is in order. On the one extreme there is that attitude often unwittingly inculcated in courses on experimental design, which looks askance at all efforts to make inferences where some variables have been left uncontrolled or where randomization has not taken place. In contrast, the quasi-experimental approach takes a radically different posture: any experiment is valid until proven invalid. The only invalidation comes from plausible rival explanations of the specific outcome. Regression effects and test-retest effects are such in many settings. An absence of randomization may in some specific way plausibly explain the obtained results. But unless one can specify such a hypothesis and the direction of its effects, it should not be regarded as invalidating. Subsequent consideration may uncover plausible rival hypotheses which have been overlooked, but such transitory validity is often the fate of laboratory experiments too. (p. 53)*

This approach is not intended as a license for laziness, or permission to assert your favorite causal explanation in the absence of a diligent effort to generate and address rival plausible explanations. "The quasi-experimentalist is obliged to search out and consider the available plausible rival hypotheses with all the vigilance at [their] command" (Campbell & Ross, 1968, p. 53).

If you follow these steps, in the end you will be able to formulate a reasonably good answer to such questions as "Did the new legislation have some effect?" or "Did the program cause a change?" or "Does the new policy make a difference?" And while this approach lacks the simplicity and elegance of the "true" experimental design and its almost formulaic ability to control for rival plausible explanations, certainly the importance of such a task makes it worth doing anyway.

New Threats to Internal Validity

The **time-series design** that the analysis of the Connecticut speed crackdown is based on is not the only way to proceed in the field. Campbell and his colleagues have come up with many different types of quasi-experimental designs, far more than we can cover in this book. Those interested in more advanced treatment of the topic should consult the classic reference by Cook and Campbell (1979) or its newer incarnation by Shadish et al. (2001).

The important turn that Campbell took us through was the idea that **manipulative control** (the ability to create situations at whim and randomly assign people to this or that group) was not the be all and end all of experimentalist research, and that **analytic control** (using our heads to anticipate and address all rival plausible explanations) could accomplish the same ends. Part of the trick then is to understand the kinds of rival plausible explanations that should be considered. Campbell had supplied a number of categories in relation to laboratory experimentation that we considered in Chapter 6—history, selection, statistical regression, and so on. While these threats are equally relevant to quasi-experimental research, several other classes of threats to internal validity are more likely to appear in evaluative settings in the field. We will discuss five of these: diffusion of treatment, compensatory equalization, compensatory rivalry, resentful demoralization, and mortality.

Diffusion or Imitation of Treatments

Within the confines of the laboratory, it's generally fairly easy to isolate experimental and control groups from each other. Even when participants know that there are other groups, they probably won't know much, if anything, about how their own experience differs from others. Their participation is usually short-lived, and lines of communication between participants in different groups are rare or nonexistent. From the experimental perspective, this is as it should be, since clear inference benefits from clear isolation of groups.

In the field, however, it's not unusual to be faced with intact groups that can't be isolated from one another. Instead of having two (or more) comparison groups that are clearly different on the independent variable being considered, we may find that the boundaries between the groups are or become somewhat blurred. For example, if the groups are differentiated by their access to varying sets of information, any communication between groups about the nature of this information will make each group a little more like the other(s). This **diffusion of treatment** (sometimes called **imitation of treatment**) will act to minimize the groups' separation and heighten their similarity. The independent variable, in other words, doesn't have a real opportunity to "work." If this occurs, you might be left concluding—perhaps erroneously—that the treatment variable is ineffective, when in fact it might have been quite effective had it just been given a reasonable opportunity and if the difference between groups was more clearly defined (i.e., a false negative).

Diffusion is actually the one down side that Campbell and Ross mention with respect to their choice of comparison states. Recall that part of the reason for choosing New York, New Jersey, Rhode Island, and Massachusetts as control states was because they were nearby and roughly similar in road and weather characteristics. As Campbell and Ross (1968) explain,

> *The list of plausible rival hypotheses should include factors disguising experimental effects as well as factors producing pseudo-effects. Thus, to the list should be added* diffusion, *the tendency for the experimental effect to modify not only the experimental group, but also the control group. Thus the crackdown on speeding in Connecticut might well have reduced traffic speed and fatalities in neighboring states. ...If highly similar remote states were available, these would make better controls, but for matters of either weather or culture adjacency and similarity are apt to be strongly associated. (p. 46)*

The problem for them was that they could not find comparison states that were both topographically/climactically similar *and* far enough away that they would be unlikely to hear about policies just across their state border. It was one or the other—choose more distant states to ensure there would be no influence from diffusion, or go for more similar states that are close by but more likely to be affected by diffusion—with the authors choosing the latter to maximize comparability.

Compensatory Equalization

Another threat that may act to obscure differences between groups is **compensatory equalization of treatments**. Cook and Campbell (1979) explain that this problem arises when the treatment being evaluated involves goods and/or services deemed desirable, and where there is a large disparity between groups. Administrators, those charged with implementing the treatment, or some of the recipients may reroute some goods or provide access to services among some or all members of the disadvantaged group in an effort to alleviate disparity. This in most cases will be well meaning and well intended by those involved; they see their colleagues disadvantaged and want to slide some resources under the table to reduce some of the inequity. However, doing so plays havoc with our ability to evaluate a program. The more compensatory equalization occurs, the more it will tend to equalize the groups, which means you will be less likely to find a difference between treatment and comparison groups because the boundary between them has become less and less clear, leading to an erroneous finding of "no difference" (i.e., a false negative).

Compensatory Rivalry

New programs and legislative changes are often much more public than experiments occurring in laboratories. If it's known that an evaluation is in progress, another threat for you to be on the lookout for is compensatory rivalry by those who are receiving the less desirable treatment(s). This occurs when people know they are in the disadvantaged group and this spurs a competitive spirit to overcome adversity and perform well. This is particularly likely to be the case in situations where the group already perceives itself as a group (e.g., work teams, crews, classes) and members have a lot to lose if a difference is revealed.

This threat to internal validity has also been dubbed the John Henry effect (see Cook & Campbell, 1979), after the legendary individual who, when he learned that his performance was to be compared to that of a steam drill, worked so hard that he outperformed the drill but died in the process. As a threat to internal validity, compensatory rivalry obscures "real" differences between groups, potentially leading you to conclude "no difference" when, under more normal circumstances, a difference would have been found (i.e., a false negative).

Resentful Demoralization

An obvious inequity between the treatment and control groups also sometimes can produce the opposite effect. While compensatory rivalry sees the disadvantaged group take up the challenge and rise to the occasion, if those in the control group perceive the result as adverse and inevitable, resentful demoralization may occur. Members of the comparison group may not even try to compete, and may even intentionally reduce their performance. In this instance, the researcher may *overestimate* the actual potency of a treatment (i.e., a false or exaggerated positive).

Mortality

Although mortality is a threat to be considered in laboratory research and was featured even in earlier treatments of internal validity (e.g., Campbell & Stanley, 1963), we left it for this chapter as it is a threat more likely to occur in field research. Mortality, in the present context, refers to a situation in which some individuals drop out of the research before it's completed. Single-session, short-term laboratory experimentation virtually precludes mortality as a problem. But in the field, where time-series data and a succession of follow-ups are more likely, the mortality problem increases in relevance. Some individuals who are recorded as participants at the beginning of the study do not return to receive the dependent measure at follow-up; for example, they drop out of therapy, choose to withdraw from the group, move to another jurisdiction, are released from care, join another club, get lost, or die.

To illustrate the problem, let's say that a "March for Millions" is being held in your city—a walk or run in which people register to walk for 25 miles for a particular charity and the farther they walk, the more money they raise. We won't get into the details of it, but a theory such as cognitive dissonance theory would suggest that the farther you walk, the more you will believe in the legitimacy of the cause you are walking for. The prediction arises from your alleged need to rationalize to yourself why you are expending so much energy: the longer you walk, and the more tired you get, the stronger your need to rationalize, and hence the more fervent you will become about the cause in order to justify to yourself why you didn't stop 5 miles ago when the blisters started appearing on your feet.

In order to test the theory, a researcher goes to each 5-mile marker along the route and asks people to provide a number of ratings about how important they think the cause is that they are walking for. The findings are as predicted: at the 5-mile mark, the average rating is that the cause is "pretty important"; by the 15-mile mark the average rating is that the cause is "very important"; and by the end of the walk, the average rating is that the cause is "extremely important." The researcher concludes that the theory is supported. Would you accept that conclusion?

The problem, as we hope you can see, is one of *selection bias* that creeps in because of participant mortality. To the extent that there are differences between those who depart and those who remain, it spoils our ability to conclude that it is the independent variable per se (the walk in this instance) that is causing a change in attitude. The problem arises because each group at each 5-mile marker is comprised of a different subset of people from the one preceding it, and the group that finishes is not the same as the group that began. Consequently we do not know whether the people who continue walking are becoming more and more enthusiastic about the cause, as the theory would predict, or whether attitudes are not changing at all, but it only looks that way because the people who care less about the cause are dropping out along the way while those who care the most are the ones who continue walking.

This threat is particularly problematic in situations where you have treatment and control groups (e.g., when evaluating a new therapy or other clinical treatment) when there is differential mortality between groups. Such a situation happens often, since those in the control group have the least reason to return and are often participating only as a favor. Even if people were randomly assigned to groups in what was hoped would be a true experimental design, the assumption of pretest equivalence may be violated if there is differential mortality. Whenever mortality occurs, you must question not only the representativeness of those who remain but also people's reasons for leaving: (1) Who are those that drop out? (2) In what ways, if any, do they differ from the remaining individuals in the group? (3) What is the relationship between (a) the variables on which those who drop out and those who remain differ and (b) the dependent measure? The trick in this situation is to anticipate this possibility from the outset and to gather sufficient pretest information to deal with this eventuality.

Can you think of a way that you could deal with these issues in the "March for Millions" example? One possibility—not the only one—would be to ask a few questions of every participant when they register for the walk, including some measure about how important they believe the cause to be. That way, when we ask those questions of the people who show up at each 5-mile mark, we can determine where those who drop out and those who keep walking fit in the group as a whole.

As the above discussion suggests, many new challenges await you in the field. But why do these things happen? Some are simply the product of the social interaction that is a part of everyday life that experimenters work so hard to control and preclude in the lab. On some occasions, the vagaries of chance just seem to stack up against you, and Murphy's Law rules the day. But much also happens because of the human motives and emotions that are awakened by the particular topic of study. Welcome to the politics of evaluation research.

THE POLITICS OF EVALUATION RESEARCH

As you may have surmised from the examples we have used in this chapter, as well as the attention we have drawn to Campbell's vision of an "experimenting society," quasi-experimental approaches are very commonly used in evaluation research where the impact of some treatment variable—a new therapy, program, policy, or other initiative—is being assessed. We were even tempted to include "evaluation research" as part of the chapter title because of that close relationship between the two. The problem, however, is that while quasi-experimental approaches are used extensively in evaluation research, it is by no means synonymous with it. Quasi-experimental designs are commonly used in evaluation research, but not all evaluation research involves quasi-experimental designs. Evaluations can involve true experiments, case study designs, and include single or mixed methods, and we highlight such examples throughout this book.

That said, when we were deciding on where to include a discussion of the real-world dynamic that you encounter when you go to do research in the field, the common relationship between quasi-experimental approaches and evaluation, and the fact most quasi-experimental research is done in the field, led us to include that discussion here. Field research is more blatantly a part of the phenomenon it investigates than laboratory-based research. Certainly, the negotiation of design and measurement techniques required for research in the field is an interpersonal as well as a cognitive process, and the consequences of your decisions and findings may be more visible. For these and other reasons, field research is a different kind of animal.

In Chapter 4 we discussed some of the ethical and moral decisions that researchers face when negotiating the terms under which a study will be conducted. Here, we'll discuss evaluative research within a political context, attempting to make explicit some of the roles researchers play within that process. In keeping with this book's general theme, the emphasis is less on telling you what to do than on articulating the decisions you will face, and which most certainly should be made as a result of conscious choice rather than out of habit or naiveté.

Programs Are Political Creatures

In an article that has become a classic in the evaluation research literature, Weiss (1975) identifies three major areas in which evaluation researchers should be aware of political considerations. The first she notes is that programs aren't the result of some anonymous individual exclaiming, "Gee, why don't we give *this* a try?" Quite the contrary: "they [have typically] emerged from the rough-and-tumble world of political support, opposition and bargaining; and attached to them are the reputations of legislative sponsors, the careers of administrators, the jobs of program staff, and the expectations of clients" (p. 14). In sum, many, if not all, *programs are political creatures.*

This reality has several implications. First, researchers should realize that the program's official goals are not necessarily a reasonable statement of its initiators' actual goals. In an effort to appease various stakeholders and to sell the desirability of program implementation, legislators and policymakers often make inflated and even grandiose claims that go beyond the capacity of any given program. A basic goal of public housing, for example, is to provide decent accommodation to those who might otherwise be disenfranchised. Yet what we hear in the news is that "public housing will not only provide decent living space; it will also improve health, reduce crime, and lead to improved school performance" (Weiss, 1975, p. 16).

At the same time, public articulation of goals and objectives may also *omit* mention of many other goals that were considered when the program was formulated. These might include the desire to avoid layoffs of bureaucratic personnel, a desire to extend political power and influence, and/or the need to be perceived by the public as *doing something* about some area of social concern. Researchers also must realize that the perception of project goals will not necessarily be consistent throughout all levels of program implementation. As Weiss (1975) notes, "what the [government] writes into legislation as program objectives are not necessarily what the secretary's office or the director of the program see as their mission, nor what the state or local project managers or the operating staff actually try to accomplish" (p. 16).

Thus, evaluation researchers must appreciate that there *are* political dynamics to the process of program development and implementation, and they must make sure that their evaluations and reports *speak* to the various constituencies. This is not to say that researchers should become coopted by political considerations, whether by coercion (e.g., you will only be given the opportunity if you show that you will deliver a positive evaluation) or voluntary zeal (e.g., the researcher takes an advocacy role and is willfully blind to potential problems). In our view the best evaluator is someone who respects the objectives of the program, understands that different factions will view it differently, and seeks to be an *independent* evaluator who *realistically* examines the program or phenomenon from the perspective of multiple constituencies. If the objectives are worthwhile, then you and policymakers both should want to know whether and to what extent those objectives are being achieved.

The Politics of the Decision-Making Process

A second way that Weiss (1975) notes that politics enter the evaluation research process requires an appreciation for the *politics of higher-echelon decision-making*. To begin with, the funds that pay for evaluation research rarely come from the particular program being evaluated. More frequently, these funds originate from more senior bureaucratic levels, who are less concerned with program and organizational survival than those on the front lines. You might think that senior decision-makers would be more likely to consider the research evidence more dispassionately, but they have their own constituencies to whom they're accountable.

In sum, the decisions of senior decision-makers ostensibly go beyond considerations of program effectiveness per se:

> *Their decisions are rooted in all the complexities of the democratic decision-making process, the allocation of power and authority, the development of coalitions, the trade-offs with interest groups, professional guilds, and salient publics … [The research evidence] will not be the sole basis for a decision, and legitimately so: other information and other values inevitably enter a democratic policy process. (Weiss, 1975, p. 17)*

The researcher, in other words, *can* make some reasonable statements about how things *are*, but affirmations about how things *should be* enter moral and ideological rather than empirical grounds. Researchers can expose fallacious belief, and they can unearth some historical or contemporary consequences of particular strategies of action. But in arguing over the desirability of different social futures, they are just one of many voices in the democratic decision-making process.

The Political Stance of the Evaluation Itself

As Weiss (1975) points out, the third major way politics intrudes into evaluation research is in the stance of the evaluation itself:

> *Social scientists tend to see evaluation research, like all research, as objective, unbiased, nonpolitical, a corrective for the special pleading and selfish interests of program operators and policy-makers alike. Evaluation produces hard evidence of actual outcomes, but it incorporates as well a series of assumptions; and many researchers are unaware of the political nature of the assumptions they make and the role they play. (p. 19)*

As noted earlier, one of the differences between the laboratory and the field is that the latter is a more interpersonal and visibly consequential process. Although you rarely see evaluation research on the evening news, it *is* a matter of some significance in the milieu under consideration. The researcher is a professional, but often an outsider, brought in to evaluate. Their mere presence on the scene has several implications.

It suggests that the researcher accepts the legitimacy of the goals and objectives being pursued. It also implies that the rationale underlying the program is a reasonable one. If it wasn't, why bother to evaluate the program? The researcher's presence alone gives an aura of legitimacy. Furthermore, the money to do the evaluation will probably have come from an "establishment" source, and those to whom the researcher will have access and who will read the report are most likely to be members of that group. All the above suggests a status quo orientation.

Typical design considerations also often promote a status quo view. Researchers should be aware that, when they limit their selection of independent variables to a particular set, they're implicitly stating that other variables are irrelevant or unchangeable. It's no accident that biogeneticists offer genetic solutions, economists see economic solutions, and lawyers offer legal solutions. Obviously, you must limit your choice of variables in order to actually *do* a finite piece of research. But most evaluations limit their comparisons to those who receive the program and those who don't, ignoring (both in the design and in the final report) the social–structural conditions within which the program operates—and thus implying that these conditions are a constant.

Researchers also have been employed as the heavy; they were particularly useful (and used) in the conservative climate of recessionist restraint and fiscal retrenchment in the late 1970s and early 1980s. Most programs that have been evaluated show little or no direct effect in the social areas they have been designed to address (Weiss, 1975). For example, consider a study like Campbell and Ross's (1968) classic evaluation of the Connecticut speeding crackdown. Campbell clearly selected that program as the one to write about because it allowed him to illustrate principles of quasi-experimental design. Governor Ribicoff conveniently made his pronouncement at the end of the calendar year, thus affording an easier year-to-year comparison. The change he introduced was implemented swiftly, intensely, and pervasively. And even in that situation, the picture *could* have been more clear-cut, since regression artifacts were never completely dispensed with as a rival plausible explanation.

So how much *can* be expected of any more modest program? One more hour of counseling isn't going to eliminate crime, and one more housing development is not going to eliminate poverty. Nor is one more program of any kind going to alleviate all our social ills. So why are some programs picked for evaluation and others not? "The evaluation researcher—now that somebody was paying attention to findings—was cast in the role of political hatchet man" (Weiss, 1975, p. 23). Evaluations of particular programs have often been treated as synonymous with evaluations of the *objectives* that underlie them. Rather than leading us to seek alternative ways of pursuing worthy social goals, evaluations often lead decision-makers to cut funding for certain programs as a class and hence for the goals that those aim to reach. The political dilemma has been a real one for many researchers, who feel uncomfortable seeing programs that address important social objectives being terminated without replacement.

So What Can a Person Do?

Weiss (1975) offers three pieces of advice for dealing with this array of potential pitfalls and complexities. First, she suggests that program goals be put "in sensible perspective," a task that requires attention to the plurality of goals represented by multiple constituencies. If you are going to believe in the virtues of heterogeneity and tolerance, then you must tolerate heterogeneity of perspectives and address these in the context of your research design. Certainly it seems advisable to consider alternative models of social justice to the utilitarian one that so pervasively guides evaluation research (e.g., see House, 1976; Pepinsky, 1987; Rawls, 1971).

Weiss's (1975) second piece of advice is "to evaluate a particularly strong version of the program before, or along with, the evaluation of the ordinary levels at which it functions" (p. 23). Clearly, such an approach would represent a fairer test of the efficacy of any given piece of social tinkering at its best. It is also consistent with Campbell's (1969b) notion of the "experimenting society," where we essentially adopt a local "pilot policy" approach to assess the prospective large-scale effect of policy alternatives. The articulation (and hence greater accountability) of social objectives that such a society would require might promote a welcome dialogue. But in practice, this advice brings us back to the status quo orientation inherent in the evaluation process when researchers limit themselves to the perspective of the funding agency. As Henry (1987) argues, even when you are critical of or attempt to set yourself apart from some other group, any discussion in that group's terms serves only to reaffirm its perspective—and hence its power.

This brings us to Weiss's (1975) third admonition, which is to do something *other than* evaluation research. She may be overly narrow in her implied definition of evaluation research as in-house evaluation bound by the perspective of the funding agency. But we concur with her statement that too often,

> ...*we concentrate attention on changing the attitudes and behavior of target groups without concomitant attention to the institutional structures and social*

arrangements that tend to keep them "target groups." ...There may be greater
potential in doing research on the processes that give rise to social problems, the
institutional structures that contribute to their origin and persistence, the social
arrangements that overwhelm efforts to eradicate them, and the points at which they
are vulnerable to societal intervention. (p. 24)

You will see more of these themes in Chapter 11 when we talk about critical
ethnography and participatory action research.

More recently, Weiss (1993) has written a reflective article that she describes as
"mellower" than the statement she wrote in the 1970s. Although she reaffirmed her
belief in the need to understand the political climate in which evaluations are conducted, she also felt that evaluation itself had matured in the intervening years and, as
a result, had become both more useful and more credible. In particular, she notes
that,

In part, the successes are the result of using more realistic standards for evaluating
success. Evaluations are generally not holding programs up to the inflated and
unreasonable expectations that prevailed in the past. In part, too, the happier
messages have come through because evaluation has widened its purview. Instead of
concentrating solely on the outcomes of programs, evaluations now examine the
whole context in which programs operate: from the initial definition of problems,
through the development of program models, to the operation of programs in their
settings. With this broader orientation, evaluations learn much that enriches our
understanding of social needs, interventions, implementation, and community
response.

Evaluations are also making effective use of a wider array of methods and
techniques. Perhaps the most notable difference from earlier days is the more
frequent use of qualitative methods of study. Evaluators today engage in intensive
interviewing, observation, review of documents, and other such techniques. They
often spend enough time on site to observe changes in environment, program, and
participants and to develop insights about conditions associated with beneficial
change. They have more to say about the "how" of programs and the "why" of
consequences. (p. 108)

In a subsequent book that compiled reflections by many of Donald Campbell's
former students and admirers of his legacy, Weiss (2000) reaffirms not only the
importance of understanding the political context in which the evaluator operates but

also reminds us of the limitations of the role of evaluators and evaluations. She lists four conclusions for the would-be evaluator:

1. *Avoid evaluation imperialism*. Although many researchers seem to take it as a given that the world would be a better place if it were run by empirically driven evaluators whose results would determine what happens next, Weiss urges us to see ourselves as only one piece of a bigger democratic process, and that it is the democratic institutions that bring together different perspectives, including those of researchers and the communities we work with, that we should support most strongly.

2. *Study actual uses of evaluation*. Rather than seeing the evaluation as an end in itself, Weiss suggests we should also study the process of evaluation implementation as part of better understanding how we can produce evaluations that people actually find useful enough to implement.

3. *Recognize that evaluation cannot be insulated from politics*. Rather than avoiding the politics, Weiss suggests we should embrace them, in part simply to be wiser about the arena that will now digest our results. This includes understanding both how evaluation findings might be used to buttress the positions of some, and how the results can be "distorted, neglected or undermined" (p. 299) by others. Accordingly, she acknowledges evaluation is itself a political act—evaluating a program involves making tacit assumptions that the goals of the program are worthy ones, expresses values in the choice of questions to address and measures to incorporate, and the evaluation itself may advantage some and disadvantage others both in how it is formulated and the results it produces. To use a phrase you will see at various times in this book—any piece of research tells us something about the world *and* about the researcher.

4. *Make evaluations more valid and interpretable*. There is a place for evaluation researchers in the political processes and issues that accompany evaluations, but Weiss reminds us that the unique expertise and contribution we can bring to the exercise is our understanding about methods, data, and analysis, and that delivering on that expectation is a prerequisite to having any impact at all. At the same time, she encourages us to accept that there is no one correct method of evaluation nor one correct set of interpretations from any given set of data. As she explains, "Evaluators should recognize the political cast of these choices and understand that other readings of the situation are possible and legitimate. They cannot assume that they have

produced the single and total truth" (p. 300), which leaves open the possibility that different evaluators might proceed in different ways and come up with different conclusions. She urges transparency and an ongoing willingness to disseminate and explain what we have done.

We agree in general with her conclusions. While evaluation began as a very centrally controlled enterprise dominated by funder definitions and seeking to impose the desiderata of experimental and quasi-experimental design on "bottom line" evaluations of effectiveness, the biggest developments in evaluation research in the two decades since Weiss's article have been in (a) the broader range of perspectives that are recognized as requiring inclusion in any comprehensive evaluation; (b) the growth in respect for the unique contributions that qualitative approaches and mixed-method designs bring to evaluation and the greater light they shed on process as opposed to a more simple bottom line; and (c) the wisdom of utilizing more collaborative approaches, such as those integral to participatory action research, that make for more culturally sensitive and more inclusive designs (see Samuels & Ryan, 2011) that "speak" to those most directly affected. In order to more fully appreciate these developments we need to extend our articulation of experimentalist logic by taking the next step to qualitative case study analysis.

SUMMING UP AND LOOKING AHEAD

The previous chapter showed the logic underlying traditional laboratory experimentation; the current chapter encourages you to consider the principles underlying the inference process and to translate those to the investigation of behavior in the world through quasi-experimentation. In each case the challenge is in how best to eliminate rival plausible explanations, with the difference between them residing in the extent to which each uses manipulative and/or analytic control to accomplish that.

In contrast to laboratory experimentation where the researcher creates the situation and uses techniques such as random assignment to exert manipulative control for the elimination of rival plausible explanations, quasi-experimentation emphasizes analytic control for those same ends. Doing so involves being your own best critic and brainstorming with those who have strong local knowledge about what those rival plausible explanations might be, and then either (ideally) gathering the data that allow you to address those possibilities, or searching the literature to see if the factor has been assessed elsewhere in a way that allows you to consider its plausibility in the specific context you are investigating. The social dynamic attendant to many field situations led us to discuss some of the unique categories of rival plausible explanations that can arise there and hence must be addressed. Ideally, you will be able to eliminate all but one of the rival possibilities, in which case the one remaining is the most plausible explanation.

Quasi-experimentation was developed in part because of Donald T. Campbell's dream of us becoming an "experimenting society" where researchers did not make societal decisions, but instead used systematic field-based methods to inform political leaders and the citizenry about how well socially important goals were being met, and what strategies worked best in achieving them. The major limitation of using quasi-experimental methods is that they work best when asked to inform about whether the bottom line is being met, i.e., purely outcome-oriented.

A review of Carolyn Weiss's series of articles on the politics of evaluation research argued that researchers who do such work need to ensure they are aware of the broader context in which they are operating, and how better to ensure that the result of their efforts takes its place in the democratic process. Weiss also notes how mixed-methods strategies that now more commonly bring in the qualitative case study component are creating more comprehensive and contextualized evaluations that go beyond the bottom line to consider why those bottom-line effects might have occurred.

Chapter 6 outlined the vocabulary and logic of experimental design and the manipulative control it embodies. Chapter 7 has shown how that same underlying logic could incorporate analytical control in field research situations that have proven especially useful in evaluation research that contributes to rational decision-making in an experimenting society. In the next chapter we consider how that same underlying logic and analytic control can be extended to the case study context.

Key Concepts

Analytic control 273
Compensatory equalization of
    treatments 274
Compensatory rivalry 275
Diffusion (or imitation) of
    treatment 274

Evaluation imperialism 284
Interrupted time-series
    designs 264
John Henry effect 275
Manipulative control 273
Mortality 276

Multiple time-series 270
Nonequivalent controls 268
Resentful demoralization 275
Time series design 273
Waitlist controls 268

STUDY QUESTIONS

1. What are some advantages and disadvantages of laboratory experimentation?

2. In traditional laboratory experimentation, internal validity is maximized by randomly assigning participants to groups and by creating control groups that are equivalent to the experimental group(s) in all respects *except* for the independent variable. But those luxuries are frequently not available in field settings. What substitutes for them in quasi-experimental research, and how do those alternatives address the elimination of rival plausible explanations?

3. What is the difference between *manipulative* control and *analytic* control? What are their similarities?

4. According to Donald T. Campbell, why must researchers always be *particularly* vigilant about checking for *regression toward the mean* (otherwise known as *statistical regression*) when evaluating the effectiveness of social programs?

5. Field researchers often face evaluation research situations in which they must deal with intact groups who know about and can share information regarding the evaluation. What new threats to internal validity arise from this state of affairs? Explain how these *are* threats to internal validity, and in each case suggest how the researcher can prepare for or deal with those problems.

6. Your state government decides to introduce photo radar in order to control speeding, which your state Governor believes is getting out of hand. They do so in July. In the first month after it is introduced more than 49,000 speeding tickets are sent out to speeders caught by photo radar. Danielle and Sanjeeta undertook a study to determine whether the advent of photo radar was indeed effective in reducing the number of accidents on provincial roads as the police suggested. They approach the state government for relevant accident data and are given accident records for August of the previous and current year for 10 regions of the state (areas around the state's 10 largest business centers) in which photo radar was used in the first month of operation. These data revealed that, in every one of the 10 jurisdictions, there were fewer accidents after the introduction of photo radar than in the same month the previous yea. Danielle and Sanjeeta did the appropriate statistical test on the data and found that, overall, the reduction in accidents was statistically significant.

a. What is the *independent variable* in Danielle and Sanjeeta's research?

b. *What is the dependent variable?*

c. What are two *rival plausible explanations* (RPEs) that you believe may threaten the internal validity of their research? What data you would ask for/obtain to address those RPEs?

d. What is *external validity*? Give two specific concerns Danielle and Sanjeeta might have regarding the external validity of their study.

e. Would *time-series data* be useful for Danielle and Sanjeeta? What advantages might if offer them?

7. In what sense is evaluation research part of a political process? What are some things a researcher can do to avoid being or becoming a mere pawn in that process?

8. According to Weiss, in what way has the incorporation of more qualitative methods to create more mixed-method research designs added to the quality of evaluation research?

8

CASE STUDY APPROACHES

ANALYTIC CONTROL IN THE CASE STUDY CONTEXT

We began our chapters on research design by telling you about John Stuart Mill's three criteria for establishing the existence of a causal relationship and explained how elegantly those criteria were met by the classic experiment. It was also an opportunity to introduce you to the vocabulary of experimentation articulated by Donald T. Campbell (see Campbell, 1957; Campbell & Stanley, 1963) that allowed us to be able to talk about the internal dynamics of the experiment, to understand its strengths and limitations, and to compare different designs and different studies in terms of their ability to provide us with reasonable inferences about whether particular treatments led to particular outcomes. A key aspect of the classic experiment is the manipulative control that it incorporates in order to achieve control over a number of different rival plausible explanations. When (1) individuals are randomly assigned to treatment and control groups; (2) the two groups are treated the same in all respects except for the presence or absence of the independent variable; and (3) we use appropriate statistical tests to see whether any differences we observe are greater than we would expect on the basis of chance variation alone, the situation is ideal for maximizing internal validity and leaving us confident in our inferences about what does or doesn't cause what.

Of course all is not roses for the experiment. With its strengths come limitations. While it is an effective vehicle for telling us whether something *can* happen, that does not necessarily mean that it *does* happen out there in the real world. Why? Because while the classic experiment tells you whether a variable has an effect with all other variables held constant (ceteris paribus)—a kind of theoretical netherworld isolated from the vagaries of life—in the real world, *ceteris* (all else) is never *paribus* (equal) because all those other variables are operative as well, providing a specific context in which our variable of interest unfolds. In that sense, the experiment's greatest strength is also its biggest limitation. While theoretical knowledge is important, ultimately we generate and test theories because we want to figure out how the world works and not just how laboratories work. Nonetheless, for much of the 20th century, the idea that the classic experiment was the only way to generate dependable knowledge was taken as a self-evident truth, with any other methods seen to pale in comparison to the experiment, which was thought to epitomize a scientific approach to knowledge production.

While never doubting that the experiment was the premiere route to dependable knowledge, it was the same Donald T. Campbell who encouraged us to give our heads a shake when it came to doing research in the world. Wouldn't it be wonderful, he mused, if we could take this model of experimentation and apply it out there in the world and be a truly experimenting society? Doing so would allow us to evaluate our successes and failures in achieving important social goals through the programs, policies, and laws we create. The important turn he took us through was to encourage us to think not about the specific procedures that are used in the classic experiment, but rather the ends that these serve, and then to look for other means by which to achieve them. Instead of *manipulative control*, quasi-experiments emphasize *analytic control*; instead of *creating* the experimental environment, in quasi-experimentation, the researcher *adapts* to an existing environment, looking for reasonably equivalent control groups wherever possible and accessing whatever data might be available that allow you to address the plausibility of potential rival explanations.

But for many years that was where Campbell drew the line between research that met scientific standards and those that didn't make the grade. In his earlier writings, Campbell even referred to case studies as "prescientific" and "of little inferential value." For example, in his influential monograph with Julian Stanley (Campbell & Stanley, 1963), Campbell caustically noted that,

> [A]s has been pointed out, such [case] studies have such a total absence of control as to be of almost no scientific value…. Such studies often involve tedious collection of specific detail, careful observation, testing, and the like, and in such instances involve the error of *misplaced precision*…. It seems well-nigh unethical at the present time to allow, as theses or dissertations… case studies of this nature. (pp. 6–7)

As Palys (1989) explained in an article that sought to extend Campbell's "rival plausible explanations" logic into the realm of case study analysis, the main problem Campbell saw was that there were too many possible explanations and too few observations against which to assess the veracity of those explanations. We heard the classic example of this problem on a recent radio news program, which contained a story about a British gentleman who was celebrating his 111th birthday. As is usual in such interviews, the man was asked to what he attributed his longevity. Such a situation is problematic to the social and health scientist, in that it presents only one observation (i.e., the man is 111) while there are a lifetime full of explanatory variables that could potentially account for that outcome. As Campbell (1979a) later explained:

> The caricature of the single case study approach which I have had in mind consists of an observer who notes a single striking characteristic of a culture, and then has available all of the other differences on all other variables to search through in finding an explanation…. That he will find an "explanation" that seems to fit perfectly is inevitable, through his total lack of "degrees of freedom." (It is as though he were trying to fit two points of observation with a formula including a thousand

adjustable terms, whereas in good science, we must have fewer terms in our formula than our data points). (p. 54)

Campbell was not the only one to be stuck on that notion that experiments, quasi-experiments, and other techniques that rely on standardized data that can be compiled, averaged, correlated, and regressed somehow inherently involve "many cases" while case studies are "$n = 1$." But as Ragin (1992) argues, every research project represents a "case" because research is not done in the abstract—any research project is a concrete event bound in time and place. For example, a demographic analysis of the way Americans vote in the 2020 presidential election may involve 161 million "cases" (i.e., voters in this instance), but it is still only one election out of any number of federal and other elections that could have been scrutinized. Any "analysis of the 2020 election," regardless of whether the data gathered to understand it come from qualitative, quantitative or mixed methods sources, is at some level a "case study" no matter how we slice it. Further,

> *The view that quantitative researchers look at many cases, while qualitative researchers look at only one or a small number of cases, can be maintained only by allowing considerable slippage in what is meant by "case." The ethnographer who interviews the employees of a firm to uncover its informal organization has at least as much empirical data as the researcher who uses these same interviews to construct a data set appropriate for quantitative assessment of variation among employees in job satisfaction. Both have data on the employees and on the firm, and both produce findings specific in time and place in the firm. Further, both researchers make sense of their findings by connecting them to studies of other firms. Yet the ethnographer is said to have but one case and to be conducting a case study, while the quantitative researcher is seen as having many cases. (pp. 3–4)*

As Ragin (1992) explained, experimental, quasi-experimental and other more quantitative research approaches pay much greater conceptual attention to "variables," which are assessed in some standardized and structured way. Every person is asked the same questions; every article or file is content analyzed using the same coding scheme; every observation is made using the same category checklist. It is this structured consistency that allows each person or file or observation to be considered a "case"—one unit of whatever is being sampled. In contrast, case studies are far more likely to involve purposive sampling where particular units—individuals or other sources within the case—are sought in a more strategic way and the information sought from each of those individual sources may involve a different part of the overall picture. The emphasis is on understanding the case as a whole, and this is done by gathering whatever data will contribute to that understanding. But that case study encapsulates far more than one observation.

Much to his credit for the open-mindedness it showed, Campbell later understood his dismissal of case studies to be based on an undeserved stereotype and acknowledged his shortsightedness. He *had* seen the case study as *one* (collective) observation, as you would from the perspective of aggregate statistics. Later, he acknowledged that *myriad* observations are possible within the context of a given case study:

> *While it is probable that many case studies professing or implying interpretation or explanation, or relating the case to theory, are guilty of [the faults he had outlined], it now seems to me clear that not all are, or need be, and that I have overlooked a major source of discipline...*
>
> *In a case study done by an alert social scientist who has thorough location acquaintance, the theory he uses to explain the focal difference also generates predictions or expectations on dozens of other aspects of the culture, and he does not retain the theory unless most of these are also confirmed. In some sense, he has tested the theory with degrees of freedom coming from the multiple implications of any one theory. The process is a kind of pattern matching... in which there are many aspects of the pattern demanded by theory that are available for matching with his observations on the local setting. (Campbell, 1978, p. 57)*

In sum, just about *any* theory or explanation can account for a *single* observation. The trick is to evaluate and develop the theory by looking at the *multiple* observations it implies and by constantly considering rival, plausible explanations that might account equally well for some or all of these observations. Campbell also was struck by a state of affairs that should not exist if he were correct: if case studies are so easily supportive of whatever explanation a researcher brings to the situation, why do so many qualitative researchers report being surprised, changing their beliefs, and revising their theories (see, for example, Becker, 1970; Campbell, 1978, 1979a)?

> *In past writings... I have spoken harshly of the single-occasion, single-setting (one shot) case study, not on the ground of its qualitative nature, but because it combined such a fewness of points of observation, and such a plethora of available causal concepts, that a spuriously perfect fit was almost certain. Recently, in a quixotic and ambivalent article (1975), I have recanted, reminding myself that such studies*

regularly contradict the prior expectations of the authors, and are convincing and informative to skeptics like me to a degree which my simple-minded rejection [did] not allow for. (Campbell, 1978, p. 201)

The process Campbell envisioned is one in which a rigorous and self-critical scholar uses whatever sources of information are available as a vehicle for generating or evaluating the multiple implications of theory. To the extent that the scientist is attuned to such multiple implications and systematic and forthright in evaluating the consistency of any given theory,

[S]cience is much better than ignorance and, on many topics, better than traditional wisdom. Our problem as methodologists is to define our course between the extremes of inert skepticism and naive credulity. When a scientist argues that a given body of data corroborate a theory, invalidation of that claim comes in fact only from equally plausible or better explanations of those data. (Campbell, 1978, p. 185; emphasis in original)

Understanding in any given situation is thus a potential battle of rival plausible explanations. We are led to the picture of science as a community of disputatious, questioning truth-seekers where the role of every new generation of scholars is to marry a critical approach with an anticipation and consideration of rival plausible explanations.

Campbell is arguing for what Palys (1989) dubbed "the quasi-experimentation of everyday life" and suggesting that "good" case studies are those that expend the effort to achieve thorough local knowledge, draw inferences through the process of offering explanations to account for observations, and eliminate rival plausible explanations. He further suggests that engaging local knowledge is essential to that task:

When we get down to our own practical work, a plausible-rival-hypothesis approach is absolutely essential, and must for the most part be implemented by common-sense, humanistic, qualitative approaches. In program evaluation, the details of program implementation history, the site-specific wisdom, and the gossip about where the bodies are buried are all essential to interpreting the quantitative *data.*

Qualitative knowing is absolutely essential as a prerequisite foundation for quantification in science. Without competence at the qualitative level, one's computer printout is misleading or meaningless.

To rule out plausible rival hypotheses we need situation-specific wisdom. The lack of this knowledge (whether it be called ethnography, or program history, or gossip) makes us incompetent estimators of program impacts, turning out conclusions that are not only wrong, but are often wrong in socially destructive ways. (Campbell, 1984, pp. 30–34)

Instead of the traditional hierarchy of empirical "goodness" that tautologically reaffirms the desirability of manipulative control and thus places experiments at the top and case studies at the bottom, the argument here puts the continuum on its side and acknowledges that experimentation, quasi-experimentation, and case study analysis each employ some mixture of manipulative and analytic control in seeking possibilities for inference.

The trick, of course, is to ensure that we have the analytic acumen to do that job well. Yin (2018) suggests this is in fact one of the great challenges of case study research, i.e., that the lack of formulaic procedures such as random assignment or a standardized interview schedule requires a highly skilled investigator to accomplish well:

[T] he demands of a case study on your intellect, ego, and emotions are far greater than those of any other research method. This is because the data collection procedures are not routinized. In laboratory experiments or in surveys, for instance, the data collection phase of a research project can be largely, if not wholly, conducted by one (or more) research assistant(s). The assistant(s) will carry out the data collection with a minimum of discretionary behavior. In this sense, the activity is routinized—and analytically boring.

Conducting case studies offers no such parallel. Rather, a well-trained and experienced researcher is needed to conduct a high-quality case study because of the continuous interaction between the issues being studied and the data being collected. Mediating this interaction will require delicate judgment calls. They can involve technical aspects of the data collection but also ethical dilemmas, such as dealing with the sharing of private information or coping with unexpected field conflicts. Only an alert researcher will be able to take advantage of unexpected opportunities rather than being trapped by them. (p. 81)

Unlike the classic experiment, where rival plausible explanations are addressed by creating and manipulating the situation using such techniques as random assignment and equivalent control groups, case study analysis extends the quasi-experimental plunge into analytic control where the researcher has to understand the logic of experimentalist inquiry and the phenomenon under study so well that a reasonable inventory of rival plausible explanations can be generated and the data that will address those rival plausible explanations are sought. As Campbell (1978) suggests, collaborating with individuals who have "thorough local acquaintance" will be invaluable for generating and addressing those rival plausible explanations that should be considered.

WHAT IS A CASE?

For a concept that is so central to the notion of case study analysis, it is interesting to see variation in the social and health sciences regarding what a case is. To avoid becoming too mired in the nuance of these debates, we accept Stake's (2003) minimalist definition of a **case** as any "bounded system," that is, a focus of study bounded in space and time. Stated another way, it is "one among others" (p. 135). As such, a case can be a person, an organization, an event, a place, a file, a country, or just about any other entity we can clearly demarcate as a focus of study. Stake differentiates between three different types of case study analysis.

The first type of case study Stake describes is **intrinsic case study**, where the entire focus is on the one case and nothing else. Your interest at that time is not theory building or understanding the case as an exemplar of some larger class; the first and last interest is in understanding that case. He suggests that such cases often are the ones that fall in your lap as a professional whose job is to apply knowledge of the phenomenon of interest to the analysis of some particular case. Examples in the professional world of cases studies would include the following:

1. The coroner must ascertain the cause of death for each individual deceased.

2. The physician, in order to prescribe an effective treatment, must diagnose why that rash appeared on your forearm.

3. A plane crashes and all on board are killed. The Federal Aviation Administration investigates to determine its cause.

4. An engineering troubleshooter is brought in to determine why a certain bridge fell down during a recent flood.

5. A young adult is arrested at a public park for having an open can of beer. He is taken back to the station. Three hours later he is dead from a gunshot wound and the police interrogator claims he shot the man in self-defence. An inquest is called to determine what happened.

6. The mechanic must figure out why your car doesn't start.

7. The detective seeks to determine "whodunnit."

The list above illustrates well the idea that the focus during these case studies is on that particular case in all its uniqueness, trying to understand it on its own terms, for its own sake. However, Stake is correct when he says that the greater interest in academe is typically with his second category—the **instrumental case study**. In this type of case study, the analysis of the case is done because of the insights or generalizations it is hoped the case study will produce. Although the case continues to be the analytical focus, these studies are undertaken because the researcher thinks it will help them understand some bigger phenomenon or the broader set of cases of which the case is a part. The case may be "typical" of cases in its category or not—this relates to the purposive sampling strategies we discussed in Chapter 5—depending on the interests of the researcher and the objectives of the study.

Stake departs from many others who have written about case studies because of his strong commitment to intrinsic case study, which he sees as undervalued. We particularly appreciate his advice that you should start by treating any case study as an intrinsic case study, even if your eventual attention is to consider it more instrumentally. Why? Stake explains that focusing on the case as an intrinsic study means that you pay attention to the unique set of circumstances that came together in that case. When thinking in more instrumental terms, in contrast, out of analytic necessity you immediately start looking for dimensions that go across cases because those are the dimensions that allow you to compare and contrast cases. If you do that right from the start, says Stake, you do not allow yourself the opportunity to check out those unique elements that may well be the most important ones in that unique case, which you would have found if you had taken it on its own ground from the outset. By treating each case study as an intrinsic one, you get the best of both worlds by being true to the individual case, before looking for commonalities and differences with other cases in a process of theory development or generalization.

The third type of case study Stake (2003) discusses is the **multiple or collective case study**, which he describes as "instrumental study extended to several cases." The objective here in most cases would be to choose a set of cases that, in combination, will allow you to make comparison to consider the plausibility of rival explanations—comparing cases that have versus those that don't have some variable of interest, for example—or simply that have sufficient diversity that they facilitate theory development.

We will give examples of all of these types later in this chapter, but we'll also warn you now that the division between these three categories is clearer when written in a textbook that seeks to highlight their differences than it is in the research world where people make decisions on the basis of what works, and not because some textbook carved up the world in some particular way. Nor are the distinctions Stake makes the only way to distinguish between case studies; he is the first to remind us that other methodologists have sliced the case study pie in other ways.

WHEN IS A CASE STUDY APPROPRIATE?

For Yin (2018), a case study is called for when (1) you are asking a "how" or "why" question regarding some phenomenon of interest; (2) you have little or no control over what happens in the situation; and (3) the focus of your study is at least partly contemporary. We see this as somewhat restrictive and would agree more with Gray (2014), who adds that case studies can be done in a wide variety of situations and are compatible with a variety of epistemological approaches. For example,

> The case study method can be used for a wide variety of issues, including the evaluation of training programmes (a common subject), organizational performance, project design and implementation, policy analysis, and relationships between different sectors of an organization or between organizations. In terms of disciplines, case study research has been used extensively in health services research, political science, social work, architecture, operations research and business management.... The case study approach can be used as both a qualitative and quantitative method. (p. 266)

And, we would add, is completely compatible with mixed methods approaches as well.

CASE STUDY METHODS

If there is one word that describes the methodological attitude researchers are encouraged to bring with respect to case studies, it is *flexibility*, i.e., the willingness to go in and make some sense of a situation on its own terms, i.e., depending on what is available and what can be found or brought together to shed light on the case. Thomas (2016) emphasizes triangulation, which was discussed in Chapter 1, i.e., the idea that looking at the same situation from multiple perspectives and using multiple data sources can help give a more complete understanding as well as provide cross-checks on validity. Gray (2014) states simply that researchers should be ready to incorporate multiple sources of evidence. Yin (2018) also agrees researchers should use multiple data sources and triangulate whenever possible and in particular suggests that the trick is to set them up so that they converge on particular lines of inquiry as it is that convergence that gives triangulation its power. He mentions six different types of data that can be gathered in the case study context, as well as some of their respective strengths and weaknesses. We show our adaptation of his list for seven potential data sources (his list did not include surveys and questionnaires) in Table 8.1.

Table 8.1 ● Strengths and Weaknesses of Seven Different Data Sources in the Case Study Context		
Source of Evidence	**Possible Strengths**	**Possible Weaknesses**
Documentation	• Stable—can be viewed repeatedly • Unobtrusive—not created as a result of the study • Specific—can contain very detailed information about processes, involvement • Broad—can cover long time spans, many events	• Retrievability—can be difficult to find • Access—sometimes deliberately withheld • Selectivity—records created for reasons other than research and by people unknown to researcher, possible bias
Archival records	• [Same as those for documentation] • Precise and often organized by case	• [Same as those for documentation] • Access—may be problematic for privacy reasons
Surveys/questionnaires	• Targeted—can focus on case study issues and on purposive sample • Insightful—particularly regarding how attitudes and/or knowledge is distributed across the site	• Potential bias due to sampling procedures, constraints
Interviews	• [Same as those for surveys and questionnaires] • Insightful—allows people to explain their views; helps understand survey data	• [Same as those for surveys and questionnaires]

(Continued)

Table 8.1 *(Continued)*

Source of Evidence	Possible Strengths	Possible Weaknesses
Direct observations	• Immediacy—covers action in real time • Contextual—seeing behavior in the context in which it normally occurs	• Time-consuming • Selectivity—depending on site and number of observers, coverage may be limited • Reactivity—presence of observers may affect behavior of those observed
Participant observation	• [Same as those for direct observation] • Insightful in terms of interpersonal behavior and motives	• [Same as those for direct observation] • Participant observer must be careful not to unintentionally affect course of events
Physical artifacts	• Insightful into cultural features • Insightful regarding technical operations	• Selectivity • Availability

Source: Adapted from Yin (2018), p. 114.

We will be reviewing each of those data gathering methods in greater detail in subsequent chapters and include the list at this point—along with some of the strengths and weaknesses that can show up when using such data in the case study context—simply to make the point that the general tack to be taken in a case study is to descend on the site and pull together any and all data that will help understand the case within the parameters of our research objectives.

Knowing which sorts of data to acquire and what to do with them when you get them can be a challenge because of the ambiguity that awaits you when you get to your case study research site. There are no easy principles like random assignment that you can implement to simultaneously control most rival plausible explanations. We will talk more in later chapters about the kinds of considerations you need to worry about for each of the different methods, but suffice it to say for now that doing case study research well can be a challenge because so much must be decided on site. General statements about strengths and weaknesses of particular methods are not particularly useful; what is important is the ability to identify which strengths and weaknesses are relevant and actually apply *in that specific situation*. Similarly, although the generic list of rival plausible explanations that Campbell (e.g., 1963, 1978) gave us to apply to experimental and quasi-experimental study—selection, history, maturation, regression toward the mean, and so on—provides some useful dimensions for us to consider, ultimately that list, and the data needed to address them, will come from understanding methods well, benefitting from site-specific knowledge, and being skilled at understanding what methodological issues are crucial, and which are tangential or irrelevant, in that context.

Do Photographs Tell the Truth?

In a particular social or health science research situation, a specific list of rival plausible explanations to consider may or may not exist; if it does exist, it may or may not be well developed. The challenge to researchers is to take the general classes of threats Campbell identified and figure out how they might manifest themselves in the specific context you find yourself in. To date, however, little effort has been devoted to systematically articulating threats to case studies in the manner of Campbell.

A creative example to the contrary comes from Howard Becker. Besides his many other talents, Becker is also a photographer. He became curious about photo archives as a source of historical data, which in turn led to his writing an essay that considers the "truth value" of photographs, entitled "*Do Photographs Tell the Truth?*" (Becker, 1979).

At one level, Becker (1979) argues, *every* photograph is "true," insofar as any picture results from a purely mechanical/chemical process that occurs when rays of light reflect off the object in front of the camera and is recorded on film or as a digital image. But, Becker notes, you could equally well assert that every photograph is to some degree "false," since you easily could have taken a very different photograph of exactly the same scene, and that photo might have resulted in a totally different set of inferences being made. How can we decide which of those two characterizations is more appropriate for any given photograph?

Becker's (1979) discussion focuses chiefly on an explicit consideration of reasons why a particular photo might be *false:* (1) the photo was faked (e.g., retouched, contrived); (2) the photographer was more interested in æsthetic concerns (e.g., impact, genre) than in creating a historical record; (3) the photo inadequately samples events (e.g., focusing on unrepresentative parts of the action); and/or (4) censorship, whether externally or internally imposed, was involved. Each of these threats to the validity of an image has a parallel in interactive research: (1) data might be "fraudulent" in the sense that respondents may distort the representation of their beliefs or behavior; (2) researchers may give an unrepresentative edge to their work by limiting it to a particular ideological genre; (3) data may be sampled inadequately; and/or (4) censorship, whether self-imposed or externally imposed, may influence the range of inferences.

In telling you about Becker (1979), we are not aiming to encourage you to consider the truth value of photographs per se, although such a consideration might well be relevant to your case study, particularly with the emphasis these days on visual evidence and the ease with which images can be changed with Photoshop and similar image-editing software. Rather, we draw your attention to the *process* he followed, which parallels the process that any researcher should follow when examining their data. More specifically, you need to try to create an account that "explains" the data while also considering all the various reasons why that account might *not* be true. In qualitative data analysis, these requirements appear not only when considering the "truth value" to ascribe to any particular datum but also when engaged in negative case analysis in the context of **analytic induction**.

Analytic Induction

Although notions of inductive analysis have a lengthier history in philosophy, analytic induction was first described as a social science technique by Znaniecki (1934) and is now a standard inclusion when qualitative case study techniques are outlined (e.g., Denzin, 1989; Manning, 1991; Preissle, 2008; Silverman, 1985; Strauss, 1987; Vidich & Lyman, 1994). Denzin (1989) describes analytic induction as a procedural analogue to experimentation that borrows the notion of experimental and control groups to direct attention not only to instances of the phenomenon under study but also to noninstances, that is, occasions when the phenomenon does not occur. The technique is useful in cases involving what Stake (2003) referred to as multiple or collective case study. Vidich and Lyman (1994) explain that,

> [A]nalytic induction [is] a "non-experimental sociological method that employs an exhaustive examination of cases in order to prove universal, causal, generalizations." The case method was to be the critical foundation of a revitalized qualitative sociology. (p. 39)

Although some researchers would question the word "universal" in their formulation (e.g., see Ragin & Amoroso, 2018), and still others would quibble with "prove," the process begins when the researcher attempts to formulate inductively some generalization or theory to capture the data that were observed. Having formulated a theory, the investigator turns it back on the data in order to test systematically how well the theory actually accounts for the data. Contrary to the character portrayed in Figure 8.1, researchers engaged in qualitative case study analysis need to remain particularly open to and even go out of their way to search for **negative evidence**,

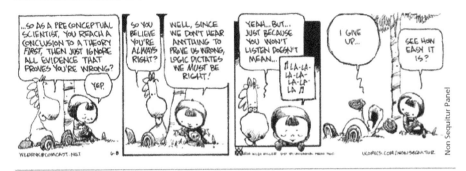

FIGURE 8.1 ● Unlike the Characters Depicted Here, Good Researchers Are Always on the Lookout for Evidence That Will Disprove Their Beliefs

since the times you're wrong can provide particularly rewarding information about how to improve your theory. Lindesmith (1952) describes this process:

> [T]he principle which governs the selection of cases to test a theory is that the chances of discovering a negative case should be maximized. The investigator who has a working hypothesis concerning his data becomes aware of certain areas of critical importance. If his theory is false or inadequate, he knows that its weaknesses will be more clearly and quickly exposed if he proceeds to the investigation of those critical areas. This involves going out of one's way to look for **negative evidence**. (p. 492)

We saw a wonderful illustration of the importance of looking for negative evidence in the YouTube video entitled, "Can you solve this?" that we described in Chapter 2. Recall that in that challenge, it was not until someone pushed the boundaries and guessed numbers they believed would *violate* the rule they had in mind that the challenge was solved. We appreciate the exercise because it shows the tendency we have to look for confirmation of our theories (called a "confirmation bias" by Kahneman, Slovic, and Tversky [1982], who have shown how pervasive it is), but even confirmation after confirmation is not enough because we may simply not have come across those instances that would disprove the theory. It is actually one of the challenges to our understanding that you can never really "prove" a theory true because complete proof would require you to have seen every instance in which a theory applies, which is clearly impossible. That is why in science an important quality of any theory is that it has to be disprovable—there has to be potential evidence in the world that would cause us to say "I guess we were wrong." A second element is that we always have to be actively trying to disprove our theories, giving them every opportunity to fail and going out of our way to look for negative evidence, because it is only by surviving those challenges that our confidence in the theory mounts, even though logically we can never actually "prove" it.

Consistent with that notion, Kidder (1981) explains analytic induction in terms of the underlying logic it shares with experimental and particularly quasi-experimental approaches. Her article "*Qualitative research and quasi-experimental frameworks*" reviews several classic studies that illuminate how the procedure can be understood in terms of an underlying quasi-experimental framework and vice versa. Our discussion below of Becker's (1963) famous study of marijuana users relies heavily on her analysis.

The basic challenge in analytic induction is to offer a general account, or theory, that accurately describes all known instances and noninstances of the phenomenon under study. It is particularly useful in a collective case study, which is how you might describe Becker's study of marijuana users in terms of Stake's (2003) typology that we discussed earlier. Among his many other talents, Howie Becker is a skilled jazz pianist. Many years ago when he was in graduate school, Becker would earn money by playing in bars. At that time—we're talking the 1950s here—marijuana consumption was still a more subcultural activity that many musicians engaged in before the drug started being consumed more widely during the musical and cultural changes that began in the 1960s. In one project, Becker (1963) sought to determine what distinguished those people who might try the drug once or twice and then abandon it from those who would try it and continue. Toward this end he interviewed people—ongoing consumers of marijuana as well as others who had tried it but decided not to continue—during breaks over the course of the evening. In the end, he concluded there were three prior conditions, *all* of which had to be present before an individual would become a regular marijuana user: (1) the person must learn the "proper" smoking techniques that allow an effect to be produced; (2) the person must learn to identify the relatively subtle effects that the drug produces; and (3) the individual must come to define those effects as enjoyable.

As Kidder (1981) describes it, the adequacy of that explanation was tested by assessing the extent to which all known cases (of regular marijuana use, and of noninterest in its use) could be fit into a cross-tabulation like that shown in Table 8.2.

Becker's (1963) analysis can be restated as a formula, where PC stands for "Prior Condition": PC1 + PC2 + PC3 = Regular User. Thus, in all cases where Becker found that a person was a regular marijuana user (i.e., phenomenon present), all three of those prior conditions were present (i.e., upper left-hand quadrant of Table 8.2). Further, in any case where a person was *not* a regular marijuana user

Table 8.2 ● Depiction of Classification of a "Successful" Analytic Induction		
	Phenomenon	
Prior Conditions	**Present**	**Absent**
Present	100%	0%
Absent	0%	100%

Source: Adapted from Kidder, L. H. (1981a). Qualitative research and quasi-experimental frameworks. In M. B. Brewer, & B. E. Collins (Eds.), *Scientific inquiry and the social sciences: A volume in honor of David T. Campbell* (pp. 226–256). San Francisco: Jossey-Boss. Used with permission of Louise Kidder.

(i.e., phenomenon absent), at least one of those prior conditions was missing (i.e., bottom right-hand quadrant of Table 8.2).

Also deserving of consideration are the remaining two cells of Table 8.2—both of which would be examples of *negative cases*—that is, where Becker's account didn't hold. The bottom left-hand corner would include instances of users (i.e., phenomenon present) who had *not* gone through all three phases specified by Becker. The top right-hand corner would include individuals who *had* gone through all three phases, but even so did not become regular marijuana users. Cases in these two cells would show the analysis to be inadequate or incomplete, since they'd reflect instances in which the theory was "wrong." As outlined by Kidder (1981), the analyst's task is thus to formulate progressively better explanations that will empty the cells of negative cases and fill the cells that are consistent with the theory. The final score, in other words, is supposed to be 100 to nothing, or it's back to the drawing board to try again.

More recent formulations of analytic induction step back from the notion that the researcher should be trying for 100% success. Ragin and Amoroso (2018), for example, say,

> *Rather than seeing analytic induction as a search for universals and one that is likely to fail, it is better to see it as a research strategy that directs investigators to pay close attention to evidence that challenges or disconfirms whatever images they are developing from their evidence. As researchers accumulate evidence, they compare incidents or cases that appear to be in the same general category with each other. These comparisons establish similarities and differences among incidents and thus help to define categories and concepts…. Evidence that challenges or refutes images the researcher is constructing from evidence provides important clues for how to alter concepts or shift categories. (p. 112)*

One reason for the departure from a search for universalism we have seen is that the revision process necessary to ensure that 100% of cases are successfully categorized can start to almost trivialize the result. A case in point is Cressey's (1953) theoretical analysis of embezzlement, which Kidder analyzes as another example of analytic induction beyond Becker's. Although it is an illuminating example as Cressey goes through five different iterations of his theory before he finally meets the 100–0 criterion, by the time he hits the third and fourth iteration, his revisions start to look like little more than the addition of caveats rather than true revision.

Cressey's research is also an interesting illustration of how sampling considerations can affect your theoretical conclusions; in his case it is noteworthy that only *convicted* embezzlers were included in his samples. This again reminds us that our conclusions are only as good as the samples they are based on, since it may well be that people who get away with embezzling differ in some way from Cressey's samples. It may be, for example, that our "commonsensical" conception of embezzlement as a financially motivated activity makes it more likely that individuals who embezzle for those reasons will get caught. If so, empirical scrutiny of only those who have been caught would simply reaffirm our original understanding about the phenomenon. People who embezzle for completely different reasons may be less likely to get caught because we don't treat them seriously as suspects; hence, they wouldn't end up in prison samples like Cressey's, posing a challenge to his theoretical formulations.

Although analytic induction as described by Kidder focuses on two research projects in which there literally were numerous "cases" you could look at in order to discern patterns that transcended those cases, the same logic can be applied to intrinsic or instrumental case studies in which the researcher does a detailed analysis of only one case that is likely to have numerous discrete sources of data that are not simply more of the same, but rather contribute unique information to an overall understanding of the case. In such situations, the emphasis is not on coming up with an explanation that fits all the cases, but rather on one that fits all the data.

AN INTRINSIC CASE STUDY: SHERLOCK HOLMES AND "THE ADVENTURE OF SILVER BLAZE"

Both the studies considered by Kidder in her articulation of analytic induction were multiple case studies, so we need to consider intrinsic and instrumental singular case studies as well. Although we soon will offer you examples of these from research we and others have done, it is difficult to find published studies that convey the richness and (dare we say) *thrill* of trying to figure out what is going on in any case study analysis. Such expositions are usually left to books because page constraints on journal articles encourage you to cut to the chase instead of focusing on the events leading up to it. Case studies represent research without the training wheels, and as such they can be exceptionally challenging and rewarding to undertake with nothing but your epistemological principles to guide you. Accordingly, we will begin this discussion by entering the world of fiction for an analysis that illustrates the ongoing interaction between theory and data, and induction and deduction, required for a comprehensive case study analysis. In this realm, we can do no better than to look at that master of sleuths, Sherlock Holmes. From Arthur Conan Doyle's many suitable stories, we've chosen to focus on *"The Adventure of Silver Blaze."*

The Phenomena: A Disappearance and a Murder

Silver Blaze is a racehorse, a particularly excellent one who has won many races and prizes for his owner, Colonel Ross. The adventure begins when we find that Silver Blaze has disappeared from his stables and that his trainer, John Straker, has been murdered. Although such a disappearance and murder likely would have been newsworthy in any event, they are particularly so for having occurred within a week of the running of the Wessex Cup, for which Silver Blaze was the favorite until his disappearance.

Holmes, along with many other Britons, has been reading about the case with interest in some of the daily papers. The story begins with his realizing that his preliminary working hypothesis has been refuted. As Holmes describes it,

> *I made a blunder, my dear Watson—which is, I am afraid, a more common occurrence than anyone would think who only knew me through your memoirs. The fact is that I could not believe it possible that the most remarkable horse in England could long remain concealed, especially in so sparsely inhabited a place as the north of Dartmoor. From hour to hour yesterday I expected to hear that he had been found, and that his abductor was the murderer of John Straker. (Doyle, 1986/1892, pp. 185–86)*

With two days having passed since the horse's abduction and Straker's murder, Holmes thus realizes that the case isn't as straightforward as it first appeared and, hence, that closer attention is warranted. The disappearance and the murder are thus the phenomena that await explanation, and Sherlock Holmes applies his investigative techniques to that end. Will he be successful in time for Silver Blaze to run in the Wessex Cup?

Gathering Preliminary Data

Holmes is often referred to as the master of *de*duction, but it's noteworthy that he begins his efforts at explanation in this case by following the *inductive* practice of gathering data first. His preliminary information regarding Silver Blaze has been based largely on archival sources, primarily the treatment of the case appearing in the daily newspapers. While such sources can be important, Holmes also recognizes their shortcomings:

> *The tragedy has been so uncommon and so complete, and of such personal importance to so many people that we are suffering from a plethora of surmise, conjecture and hypothesis. The difficulty is to detach the framework of fact—of absolute, undeniable fact—from the embellishments of theorists and reporters. Then, having established ourselves upon this sound basis, it is our duty to see what inferences may be drawn, and which are the special points upon which the whole mystery turns. (Doyle, 1986/1892, p. 185)*

Accordingly, Holmes also supplements his examination of newspaper accounts with direct communication with Colonel Ross, who has invited his involvement in the case, and Inspector Gregory, the member of the local constabulary to whom the case was assigned.

Two stables are approximately two miles apart in the otherwise minimally populated moor around Tavistock. Silver Blaze had been housed at King's Pyland. Desborough, his primary rival in the Wessex Cup, is kept at Mapleton Stables under the management of Silas Brown. Silver Blaze had clearly been the early betting favorite. Besides horse and trainer, Straker's wife, a maid, three stable boys, three other horses, and a dog all make their home at King's Pyland.

Security precautions had been taken as the race approached, with the three stable boys rotating through successive 8-hour shifts in the locked barn: while one was on duty, the other two slept in the loft above. The maid brought meals to the stable for the lads. On the night in question, she was carrying a dinner of curried mutton to the barn when a stranger, later identified as Fitzroy Simpson, suddenly emerged from the darkness. He offered a bribe to the maid and to Ned Hunter, the on-shift stable boy, apparently wishing to obtain inside information concerning Silver Blaze's fitness for the upcoming race. He fled when the two refused his money and Hunter set the dog on him. In response to a question from Holmes, the inspector notes that Hunter had locked the stable door behind him before giving chase and that the open window isn't large enough for a person to pass through. Note how Holmes's questioning is already being guided by thoughts of rival plausible explanations or clues. Might someone have gotten in the stable when the stable boy went running after Fitzroy Simpson? No. Was the window big enough for a person to fit through? No.

John Straker, the trainer, was described as having become rather excited when told about these events and must subsequently have had trouble sleeping: his wife saw him getting dressed and heading out to the barn at 1:00 AM, despite the rain. Mrs. Straker awoke at 7:00 AM to find that her husband had not returned. On going outside, she and the maid found the barn door open, Hunter in a drug-induced stupor, the other two boys still soundly asleep in the loft, and Silver Blaze gone. About a quarter of a mile away from the stables, John Straker's coat was found hanging from a tree branch, flapping in the breeze. Close to it lay the trainer's body.

> His head had been shattered by a savage blow from some heavy weapon, and he was wounded in the thigh, where there was a long, clean cut, inflicted evidently by some very sharp instrument… In his right hand he held a small knife, which was clotted with blood up to the handle, while in his left he grasped a red and black silk cravat, which was recognized by the maid as having been worn on the preceding evening by the stranger who had visited the stables. (Doyle, 1986/1892, p. 189)

When he regained his senses, Hunter agreed with the maid that the cravat was indeed the one worn by Simpson the night before. He also believed that the stranger must have drugged his food while distracting him with questions about Silver Blaze and the race. Analysis later revealed that his curried mutton was indeed laced with powdered opium, although the people in the house had eaten the same dish with no apparent effect. A check around the Tavistock area, including an examination of Mapleton Stables, showed Silver Blaze nowhere to be found. But "some gypsies" who had been seen camping in the area had apparently vanished the day after the crime became news.

Preliminary Induction

The gathering of preliminary data, as Scriven (1976) reminds us, is never done with "immaculate perception." The person who goes about gathering data will bring "commonsensical" or "informed" understandings to the situation, no doubt influenced by ideological and/or theoretical leanings. The data that are gathered, and the interpretations as to what those data mean, influence the range of alternative explanations considered. Preliminary induction involves drawing inferences from your data to create a plausible account of the causal agent(s) or sequence of events that "produce" the phenomenon.

For Inspector Gregory, suspicion fell immediately on Fitzroy Simpson, the stranger who had appeared on the night of the murder. Witnesses (the maid and stable boy) placed him at the scene of the crime, and his intentions appeared to be less than honorable. Hunter indicated that Simpson had had an opportunity to drug his curried mutton, and John Straker was found with Simpson's cravat in his hand.

Simpson was easily found in one of the villas near Tavistock the day after the crime, and new evidence seemed consistent with the idea that he might have committed the crimes. Apparently Simpson is "a man of excellent birth and education, who had squandered a fortune upon the turf, and lived now by doing a little quiet and genteel bookmaking in the sporting clubs of London. An examination of his betting book shows that bets to the amount of five thousand pounds had been registered by him against the favorite" (Doyle, 1986/1892, p. 189). Further, his clothes were wet from being in the rain the night before, his red and black cravat was indeed missing, and he was in possession of a lead-weighted walking stick, which might conceivably have caused the head injuries from which the trainer died.

Analytic Induction: A Dialectic of Theory and Data

Preliminary induction from the above data might be sufficient to generate the theory that Fitzroy Simpson was the murderer of John Straker and the abductor of Silver Blaze; however, the process of analytic induction requires that you pay attention to *all* relevant data, particularly to *negative* evidence that could serve to disconfirm your theory.

The inspector was sufficiently confident in his theory to arrest Fitzroy Simpson, but Sherlock Holmes's attention to the case brings with it a healthy air of skepticism. In explaining his thoughts on the matter to his colleague and biographer, Dr. Watson, Holmes states,

I am afraid that whatever theory we state has very grave objections to it… The police imagine, I take it, that this Fitzroy Simpson, having drugged the lad, and having in some way obtained a duplicate key, opened the stable door, and took out the horse, with the intention, apparently, of kidnapping him altogether. His bridle is missing, so that Simpson must have put this on. Then, having left the door open behind him, he was leading the horse away over the moor, when he was either met or overtaken by the trainer. A row naturally ensued, Simpson beat out the trainer's brains with his heavy stick without receiving any injury from the small knife which Straker used in self-defense, and then the thief either led the horse on to some secret hiding place, or else it may have bolted during the struggle, and be now wandering out on the moors. That is the case as it appears to the police, and improbable as it is, all other explanations are more improbable still. (Doyle, 1986/1892, pp. 189–190)

Holmes begins by questioning whether all evidence to date is indeed consistent with the theory that Fitzroy Simpson was the murderer, a reflection of proper negative case analysis. He wonders first why Straker's body was covered with considerable blood and bore a knife cut, suggesting a struggle, while Simpson's clothes had no bloodstains and showed no signs of struggle. As a possible explanation, Dr. Watson notes that the blows to the head might have caused involuntary convulsions, which in turn may have led Straker to have cut himself with his own knife. Holmes next notes that Silver Blaze is still missing; he asks how a stranger from London could know enough about the local area to keep a horse hidden on an apparently barren moor. The Inspector suggests that Simpson might have passed the horse over to the gypsies, who have now vanished, adding that Simpson was *not* a stranger to the area, having stayed there for significant periods during two prior summers. But Holmes isn't convinced. He suggests that the Inspector's case is still circumstantial, at best:

A clever counsel would tear it all to rags…. Why should he take the horse out of the stable? If he wished to injure it, why could he not do it there? Has a duplicate key been found in his possession? What chemist sold him the powdered opium? (Doyle, 1986/1892, p. 191)

The inspector responds to each query, but the responses are weak insofar as none has any sort of concrete manifestation. Perhaps he took the horse out so no one would hear the creature when the injury was done, or perhaps the motive was indeed abduction rather than injury. As for the key, perhaps it was acquired during one of his previous summer visits, and he probably threw it away once the crime was committed. The opium was probably bought in London, making it difficult to trace. All speculation devoid of concrete evidence.

Holmes becomes more skeptical than ever at this "shadow" evidence. He gives the *coup de grâce* by noting two events that, to him, make the current theory untenable and direct attention elsewhere. First, Holmes knows that opium powder has a very distinctive flavor, and he considers it too large a coincidence that the maid just happens to have served a curried mutton that night, a dish that would conveniently hide the taste of the opium. Clearly, Simpson could not have caused the particular choice of dinner that night; this suggested to Holmes that the perpetrator must be a person in the house who could make such a choice. Holmes also notes that although the dog barked loudly when Simpson paid his evening visit to the maid and the stable boy, it did *not* do so when the murderer/abductor arrived at the stable later that night. This fact suggested that the dog must have known the intruder, again focusing attention back on the members of the Straker household.

Another theory is clearly required, and with his attention now directed toward members of the household, Holmes refocuses his search for evidence. Holmes first turns his eye to the murder victim, John Straker, asking what objects were in his pockets on the night of the murder. These include numerous items, the most noteworthy of which are a candle, some papers, and the knife that had apparently caused Straker's leg wound. Curiously, the papers include a bill for a very expensive dress from a London milliner; the invoice is made out to a Mr. William Darbyshire. Holmes is informed that Darbyshire is apparently a friend of Straker's and that letters to him are occasionally received at the Straker home. As for the knife, closer inspection by Dr. Watson reveals that it is a very small, delicate, razor-sharp knife of a type used for cataract operations, leaving Holmes curious as to why Straker would have possessed such a knife and why he would have taken such a thing along as a weapon against an intruder, when larger kitchen knives—much more suitable for protection—were just as easily available.

Because the data that Holmes uncovers suggest that the murder/abduction was an "inside job," Holmes's attention turns to the Strakers, for only they could have chosen the menu that allowed the stable boy to be drugged. Although both may have been involved, only John Straker meets all the criteria of being able to determine the meal to disguise the opium, having a key to the stable, being able to handle the horse he trained, and being known to the dog so that it would not bark and wake the sleeping stable boys when he arrived to do something to the horse. But what was he intending to do? How? Why?

After identifying John Straker as having had less than honorable intentions, Holmes wonders whether Mrs. Straker also was involved; he looks for a motive for the crime. His inductive leap emerges from examining the invoice to William Darbyshire that is among Straker's personal effects. Why would Mr. Darbyshire have millinery bills delivered to the house of John Straker? Could John Straker and William Darbyshire be the same person? Or were Mr. and Mrs. Straker perhaps living beyond their means, using double identities, and led to crime by a need to meet debts created by an extravagant lifestyle?

To pursue this lead, Holmes employs a technique of indirect questioning to discover whether the dress billed to William Darbyshire was actually intended for Mrs. Straker:

> *"Surely I met you in Plymouth, at a garden party, some little time ago, Mrs. Straker," said Holmes.*
>
> *"No, sir; you are mistaken."*
>
> *"Dear me; why I could have sworn to it. You wore a costume of dove-colored silk, with ostrich feather trimming."*
>
> *"I never had such a dress, sir," answered the lady.*
>
> *"Ah; that quite settles it," said Holmes. (Doyle, 1986/1892, p. 192)*

And indeed it did. But if Mrs. Straker wasn't the woman for whom the dress was intended, then who was? If William Darbyshire was indeed John Straker, might there be *another* Mrs. Darbyshire/Straker? Or a mistress, perhaps?

The Master of Deduction

Holmes had arrived at a theory that was consistent with the evidence gathered to date. Certainly none of the evidence had yet been demonstrated to be *inconsistent* with the theory that John Straker, due to financial pressures from some possible parallel life he was leading, was involved in some despicable plot to abduct or injure Silver Blaze in order to gain funds, whether through bets or through bribery. But at this point Holmes goes beyond the domain of analytic induction alone: he now also starts including the deductive mode that so characteristically distinguishes him from most other fictional sleuths. More specifically, Holmes begins to hypothesize about data that *should* exist *if* his theory is true.

Straker's possession of a surgical knife leads Holmes to speculate that Straker may have been intending to somehow surreptitiously injure Silver Blaze temporarily so that the horse wouldn't be able to race. If that was so, Straker probably led Silver Blaze to the depression on the moor where the murder subsequently took place in order to ensure that any cries from Silver Blaze wouldn't wake the stable boys and to ensure that he wouldn't be seen perpetrating this deed. And if that was so, other evidence of that action should be found. Straker's coat, presumably removed in order to better perform the "operation," and an abundance of hoof and footprints in the vicinity of the body were certainly consistent with Holmes's theory, although not definitive. Recalling that candles were found in Straker's pocket, and surmising that he would have required a light of some sort in order to undertake an operation, Holmes hypothesizes that *if* his theory is correct, other evidence of candles or matches should be present at the scene. Neither Watson nor the Inspector is aware of Holmes's deductions as Holmes begins to closely scrutinize the area where the body was found:

Stretching himself upon his face and leaning his chin upon his hands, [Holmes] made a careful study of the trampled mud in front of him.

"Halloa!" said he, suddenly, "what's this?"

It was a wax vesta, half burned, which was so coated with mud that it looked at first like a little chip of wood.

"I cannot think how I came to overlook it," said the Inspector, with an expression of annoyance.

"It was invisible, buried in the mud. I only saw it because I was looking for it."

"What! You expected to find it?"

"I thought it not unlikely." (Doyle, 1986/1892, p. 193)

Holmes next turns his attention to Silver Blaze. If Straker abducted him but was then killed, Silver Blaze must have run off somewhere. But if so, why hadn't he been found? Holmes heard the inspector express the belief that the gypsies might have found and taken him, but views this idea as being based on a convenient but inaccurate stereotype. And even if they had done so, surely it would be absurd to believe that gypsies could have walked off with and sold the most famous and sought-after horse in England without anyone noticing. On the basis of his knowledge of horses, Holmes speculates with Watson on Silver Blaze's location:

The horse is a very gregarious creature. If left to himself his instincts would have been either to return to King's Pyland, or go over to Mapleton. Why should he run wild on the moor? He would surely have been seen by now.

Where is he, then?

> *I have already said that he must have gone to King's Pyland or to Mapleton. He is not at King's Pyland, therefore he is at Mapleton. Let us take that as a working hypothesis and see what it leads us to. (p. 193)*

But the inspector had already stated that he checked for 100 yards in all directions from the crime scene and was unable to find any further tracks. Still, acting on his theory and looking for indicators that could further test that theory, Holmes continues:

> *This part of the moor, as the Inspector remarked, is very hard and dry. But it falls away toward Mapleton, and you can see from here that there is a long hollow over yonder, which must have been very wet on Monday night. If our supposition is correct, then the horse must have crossed that, and there is the point where we should look for his tracks. (p. 193)*

Holmes brings along one of Silver Blaze's horseshoes, and evidence soon turns up that provides some support for Holmes's theory. Hoof tracks are indeed found, indicating that Silver Blaze did walk in the direction of Mapleton. In the process of following them, Watson chances upon a second pair of tracks—from a human's square-toed boots—that are seen to come from Mapleton and to intersect with the horse's hoofprints; horse and human travel in parallel toward King's Pyland for a short while, after which they reverse ground in tandem and head back to Mapleton.

On the basis of these new observations, Holmes infers that someone from Mapleton must have come on Silver Blaze as he wandered on the moor after running from Straker and, having begun to return Silver Blaze to King's Pyland, suddenly had a change of heart, succumbing to the temptation to take advantage of the act of fate that had brought Mapleton's main rival to its doorstep and to hide the horse in the Mapleton stables until after the Wessex Cup. The most likely candidate is Silas Brown, the trainer of Desborough and the manager of Mapleton Stables; only he would have known how to disguise or hide a horse, and only he would have the authority to bring a new horse in to the stables unchallenged.

If that theory is true, Brown would have to have been the first to rise that day. When they arrive at Mapleton, Holmes checks his reasoning indirectly, by querying a groom who, seeing Holmes and Watson coming, has directed them to leave the premises:

> *"I only wished to ask a question," said Holmes, with his finger and thumb in his waistcoat pocket. "Should I be too early to see your master, Mr. Silas Brown, if I were to call at five o'clock tomorrow morning?"*

"Bless you, sir, if anyone is about he will be, for he is always the first stirring. But here he is, sir, to answer your questions for himself." (p. 194)

Holmes's first hypothesis is thus supported, and a second is as well when Silas Brown strides toward him wearing square-toed boots that match the footprints Holmes and Watson observed on the moor.

Resistant at first, Brown admits to having hidden Silver Blaze after Holmes describes the events in such detail that Brown believes Holmes must have witnessed the entire scene. Empathizing with Brown's having succumbed to temptation without original criminal intent, Holmes provides Brown with a way to show his remorse: by promising to care for the horse and to ensure that the animal appears at the Wessex Cup on racing day.

Back at King's Pyland, feeling confident that his theory is most plausible but still wanting to ensure that all loose ends are covered, Holmes generates two further hypotheses that suggest two final tests of the theory. First, if Straker had been intending to administer a delicate but impairing incision to Silver Blaze, Holmes speculates that Straker probably would have practiced on other animals at the stables, and his eyes "[fall] upon the sheep." Accordingly, he questions one of the stable boys:

"You have a few sheep in the paddock," he said. "Who attends to them?"

"I do, sir."

"Have you noticed anything amiss with them of late?"

"Well, sir, not of much account; but three of them have gone lame, sir."

I could see that Holmes was extremely pleased, for he chuckled and rubbed his hands together.

"A long shot, Watson; a very long shot!" said he, pinching my arm. "[Inspector] Gregory, let me recommend to your attention this singular epidemic among the sheep. Drive on, coachman!" (p. 196)

With all but Holmes baffled at the meaning of that interchange, Holmes and Watson leave to test a further hypothesis. Promising Silver Blaze's owner that they'll see him and the horse on racing day, Holmes takes a photo of Straker along to London. The one portion of the theory that Holmes has not yet tested involves the question of motive. We do not yet know whether John Straker and William Darbyshire were indeed the same person, and whether Straker's extravagant lifestyle led him to attempt to solve his financial problems by fixing the Wessex Cup against Silver Blaze. Taking Straker's photograph to the milliner at the address on William Darbyshire's invoice confirms Holmes's suspicions.

A Satisfying Resolution

On the day of the Wessex Cup, Silver Blaze does indeed appear, and of course he wins the race. But with Silver Blaze safely found and returned, all of those present are still at a loss as to the identity of Straker's murderer. It is thus with no small sense of satisfaction that Holmes fills in the last piece of the puzzle: the murderer was none other than Silver Blaze!

> *"The horse!" cried both the Colonel and [Dr. Watson].*
>
> *"Yes, the horse. And it may lessen his guilt if I say that it was done in self-defense, and that John Straker was a man who was entirely unworthy of your confidence."* (p. 198)

Holmes continues with his litany, which is consistent with all the evidence, both inductively and deductively gathered. He recounts the evidence concerning Straker's double identity and the extravagance of his lifestyle. The choice of curried mutton to drug Hunter, the dog that didn't bark, and Straker's possession of the cataract knife are all explained. As for the trainer's death, Holmes describes the chain of events:

> *"Straker had led the horse to a hollow where his light would be invisible. Simpson, in his flight, had dropped his cravat, and Straker had picked it up with some idea, perhaps, that he might use it in securing the horse's leg. Once in the hollow he had got behind the horse, and had struck a light, but the creature, frightened at the glare, and with the strange instinct of animals feeling that some mischief was intended, had lashed out, and the steel shoe had struck Straker full on the forehead. He had already, in spite of the rain, taken off his overcoat in order to do his delicate task, and so, as he fell, his knife gashed his thigh. Do I make it clear?"*
>
> *"Wonderful!" cried the Colonel. "Wonderful! You might have been there."* (p. 200)

Dénouement

Although many people love Sherlock Holmes as a sleuth who makes insightful observations three steps beyond the rest of us, we especially love Holmes as a methodologist who is constantly moving back and forth between theory and data. The adventure of Silver Blaze shows Holmes at his methodological best. He gathers data—first from afar and then by visiting the site—and avoids premature conclusions that characterize his counterpart, Inspector Gregory. This open-mindedness is a key attribute for researchers to have that is paralleled in other occupations as well. The literature on wrongful convictions in the legal realm, for example, lists "premature closure" as a major contributing factor to innocent people ending up in prison (e.g., Godsey 2019). All eyes focus on one key suspect at the beginning of an investigation—just as Fitzroy Simpson was an early suspect in the case of Silver Blaze—and any subsequent evidence is interpreted based on an assumption of and in order to establish guilt rather than remaining open-minded about other possible suspects (rival plausible explanations) while evidence is being gathered. The same factor—premature closure and failure to adequately consider rival plausible explanations—is a major factor in medical misdiagnosis and malpractice as well (e.g., Groopman, 2008).

Holmes also is to be lauded for the variety of data sources that he brings to bear on his cases. He begins by reading the newspapers (an archival source) for the information those reports contain, but is much happier going to the site so that he can investigate for himself. At the site he observes the setting, which allows him to appreciate who was located where and the inter-relationships between all the people involved in the stable, all of which gives clues about what might have happened and more data that needs to be explained. He also interviews a purposive sample of individuals—those with any direct knowledge or experience with the crime—and inspects any physical evidence that he can find (items from Straker's pockets as well as at the murder site).

Holmes is also very creative in where he looks. While Inspector Gregory looked for tracks in a 100-yard radius around the murder site, Holmes noted that it was raining the night the murder occurred, hypothesized a direction the horse might have run—a splendid example of how inductive theorizing can lead to deductive hypotheses about what sorts of data *should* exist if the theory is correct—and looked in a low-lying area that would have been very wet and more likely to reveal tracks if any were to be found. Note also his use of indirect questioning in the case of Mrs. Straker, which allowed him to dismiss any possible involvement on her part while raising more questions about who Mr. Darbyshire might be and why his bills for expensive dresses would be coming to Mr. Straker.

More generally, there are two attributes of Holmes and his approach to determining who abducted Silver Blaze and killed Mr. Straker to which we attach special importance. First is that Holmes actually reality tests at various points along the way instead of inventing shadow evidence or simply speculating without looking for a way to test whether his speculations are on track. If Mr. Straker had taken Silver Blaze into the gully to ensure he would not be seen while nicking Silver Blaze's tendon, as the candle in his pocket suggested might be the case, then there must have been a match as well, which he gets on the ground to look for and finds. If Silver Blaze escaped this situation and ran to the rival stable across the moor, then Holmes hypothesizes there would be hoofprints in low-lying areas between the two stables. He goes to look for them and is rewarded. We even see some serendipity when Holmes also sees tracks from some square-toed boots, which offer a clue to the identity of the abductor. Finally, to test whether "Mr. Darbyshire" and Mr. Straker were one in the same person, Holmes takes a picture of Straker to the dressmaker in London to see if they can identify him. As a researcher you have to be ready to put your ideas to the test; the data have to matter.

A second attribute of Holmes and his approach we appreciate is that after gathering as much data as he can and being guided along the way by the new evidence he finds and the theorizing about who did the deed and why, in the end he is not satisfied until he determines a resolution to the case that accounts for *all* of the data. As a researcher you need to be sincerely curious about what you are looking into, cannot ignore evidence you don't like or that doesn't fit your early conceptualization of phenomena, and have to be willing to change your mind. But do case studies all play out so nicely and resolve themselves so completely in the real world?

CASE STUDY ANALYSIS IN THE REAL WORLD

Where Did That Equation Come From?

Social and health science case studies can be anything from small projects to book-length analyses. In the latter category, one of the most interesting books we have come across recently was a book by David Bodanis (2001) entitled $E = mc^2$, which, as you may know, is an equation advanced by Albert Einstein to reflect his theory of relativity: Energy (E) is equal to the mass of an object (m) times the speed of light (c) squared. The book is a case study in the sociology of knowledge, with each chapter focusing on a different element of the equation (including the equals sign), showing how each developed as a core construct. In the process, we come to appreciate the legions of people whose contributions to science were reflected one way or another in the evolution of those concepts, as well as the brilliance of

Einstein in drawing the threads together in so elegantly simple an equation that has had such profound implications.

How Were Those Decisions Made?

A more famous case study is the one that Irving Janis (1972) did of the decision-making of former President John F. Kennedy and his cabinet during both the Bay of Pigs invasion of 1961—which was widely recognized by many, including President Kennedy, as a colossal decision-making failure—and the Cuban Missile Crisis of 1962—which was broadly recognized as a decision-making success. Part of the problem with the first decision was that many cabinet members around the table held back on expressing reservations they had about the plot that was being hatched until after the fact when the decision was being reviewed. Kennedy subsequently put in place specific processes that encouraged debate and full consideration of alternatives before the Cuban Missile Crisis brought yet another important event to their table, leading to a more comprehensive discussion and a better decision. The fact that both decisions were produced by pretty much the same group of people created an interesting opportunity to compare the ways decisions were made with personalities essentially held constant.

Janis analyzed how the two decisions were made by examining declassified CIA documents. He offered the concept of "groupthink" to describe the process of decision-making that occurs when people value their membership in the group so highly they push quickly for unanimity. Hart (1991) summarizes its key points thus:

> *According to Janis, groupthink stands for an excessive form of concurrence-seeking among members of high prestige, tightly knit policy-making groups. It is excessive to the extent that the group members have come to value the group (and their being part of it) higher than anything else. This causes them to strive for a quick and painless unanimity on the issues that the group has to confront. To preserve the clubby atmosphere, group members suppress personal doubts, silence dissenters, and follow the group leader's suggestions. They have a strong belief in the inherent morality of the group, combined with a decidedly evil picture of the group's opponents. The results are devastating: a distorted view of reality, excessive optimism producing hasty and reckless policies, and a neglect of ethical issues. The combination of these deficiencies makes these groups particularly vulnerable to initiate or sustain projects that turn out to be policy fiascoes. (p. 247)*

The concept has proved useful in analyzing other conflicts that arose during the Cold War and since, thereby also showing how a case study analysis that was begun for intrinsic reasons—simply understanding that particular decision-making process—can also be instrumentally useful by providing concepts that help identify similar processes when they appear in relation to other decisions during crisis (Yin, 2018).

Where Did All the Referrals Go?

A more modest case study grew from a graduate class in research methods that Ted taught a few years ago. One of the areas in which he does research and teaches is Indigenous justice, which looks at relations between Native and settler peoples and Native and settler governments, particularly with respect to justice systems. Years ago, Native people in Vancouver, British Columbia (BC), had negotiated with the federal and provincial (state) government for the formation of an Indigenous justice program that would deal with offenders based on principles of healing and social responsibility (e.g., Palys, 1999). The agreement specified the circumstances under which Native people who had been charged in a British Columbia court could be transferred to the Native Justice Program, which involved members of the community meeting and deciding collectively on an appropriate resolution designed to identify and overcome the root of the problem, for the benefit of the offender, their family, and the community. The program continued for years and the number of referrals from the courts grew.

The provincial government subsequently decided to create a unique Downtown Community Court (DCC) that would deal with more minor offenses that arose in a particular part of the city where social needs were considerable because of the pervasiveness of drug addiction, alcoholism, poverty, and a wide range of mental health issues. The usual courts where these individuals would be processed were ill-suited to deal with people with varying connections to reality who often had completely forgotten about appearing because so much time had passed since whatever event brought them there, or who never received appearance notices because they were homeless and could not be found, and who often then became mired in even deeper legal trouble because of not following the rules. To address these problems, the DCC would process their cases more quickly, as well as aspiring to be a "problem-solving court" that would focus on helping offenders deal with the problems that were getting them in trouble in the first place, much like the Native program had already been doing for a decade.

The part of the city where the DCC would gain its clientele included many of the same people that the Native justice program was serving, and the choice of who would be referred to the Native justice program now fell largely to the personnel at the DCC, who had no prior connection with the Native justice program. The flow of cases going to the Native program slowed down to a trickle, to the point where it looked like the Native program might even have to shut down due to a lack of clients. Ted learned about the situation when the Executive Director of the program came to speak with Ted's students in a class he was giving.

Ted also knew the Executive Director of the DCC, who had obtained his Master's degree in Ted's department years previously. The possibility of a project came when two students in a graduate methods course that Ted was teaching—Richelle Shaefer and Yana Nuszdorfer—expressed interest in doing a case study of the DCC/justice program relationship. They decided that Richelle would interview personnel at the Native justice program while Yana would interview personnel at the DCC, and that Ted would join them in bringing the two sets of data together in a study that spoke not only to the question of why referrals stopped occurring but also addressed the broader question of how the relationship between these two entities reflected broader relations between the Canadian and Indigenous justice systems (see Palys, Schaefer, & Nuszdorfer, 2014).

Much of the case study proceeded relatively straightforwardly, but there were also several lessons that were learned in the process. One was a problem noted by both Gray (2014) and Yin (2018)—or at least a problem for researchers—which is that the world does not stay still when you are out there examining it. In this case study, Ted and the two grad students had two organizations who were both very willing to examine their internal processes and were interested in coming to some mutually agreeable resolution. However, both the DCC and the Native program began making changes as preliminary data were still being gathered. If this had been a study that was evaluating the outcomes of a treatment program or of the effectiveness of different sentencing options or comparing the two institutions' relative success in dealing with Indigenous offenders, then those changes may have been highly problematic with respect to internal validity, but because the project was focused primarily on the respective agencies' personnel's understandings of the two programs and the official and informal relationship between them, the changes being made did not adversely affect the results.

Another interesting element of the project was the separation of the two researchers who actually gathered the information on which the analysis was based. In part because the research was undertaken as part of a course exercise, the decision was made to keep Ted out of the data gathering portion of the exercise other than to make overall arrangements for the project with the heads of the two organizations and to split the interviewing so that Yana and Richelle each focused on one organization. Ted found it interesting how each of the researchers came to identify very strongly with the views of the organization they were researching. It was really only when the two sets of views were brought together in a final published report that a broader understanding of how the two sets of perspectives combined to create the situation they were now trying to resolve, and the broader lessons were drawn about how the Canadian and Indigenous systems of justice might co-exist (Palys et al., 2014).

How Does a Computerized Information System Affect Interaction?

As a final example of a case study, we present one that is somewhat more complex in terms of the number of different parts that were being scrutinized simultaneously by a team of researchers. This research harkens back to the 1980s—those dark days before there was an internet. Even personal computers, the ones we now know as desktops, were a relatively new development. The idea that you could put a keyboard and monitor in a car and have access to data was a big deal at that time, something that was not a part of anyone's experience. One profession who became quite interested in the possibility was the police. Until that point, whenever they wanted information, officers on patrol would have to radio in to a dispatch operator, waiting for their opportunity to occupy the air waves where all other officers in all other patrol vehicles were listening. Systems started appearing at various places in the world—France, the United States, and Britain initially—that engaged with radio networks to provide mobile terminals remote, direct access to databases housed on organizational servers. The police department in Vancouver became the home of what was then a state-of-the-art system in the early 1980s, and the federal government and the private contractor who developed the radio-based system wanted to do a full evaluation to understand how it performed, how it was received and used, and what implications might be associated with its development. Three evaluations were conducted.

The first was an engineering evaluation that examined the physical performance of the system under different conditions. A second evaluation was a cost-benefit analysis undertaken by some economists. Ted was asked to do the third evaluation, which was seen as a behavioral evaluation that would focus on evaluating how the system was used, the attitudes of members of the department toward it, and any implications that were evident either within the department or between the department and members of the public.

One of the things that made this project very interesting was the challenges that arose from a situation that was missing several elements that would have made the research team's inferential life easier. By the time Ted was asked to do the evaluation, the system had been in use for almost two years, so there was no way to put in place any "before" measures to monitor changes over time. There was also no opportunity to get any other police department to participate or provide records and act as a comparison or control department.

These deficiencies were more than made up for by the access to data he had through the cooperation of the police department. The main emphasis was placed on understanding the way the system was being used now, using a triangulated mixed method strategy that included (1) interviews with purposively chosen samples of individuals at the police department who were members of internal stakeholder groups (e.g., administration, dispatchers, IT personnel, patrol officers); (2) archival data supplied by the department that recorded every transaction over the system; (3) archival data from professional publications (such as *The Police Chief* and *The Sheriff's Star*) that circulated among police departments commenting on the possibilities that similar systems held for the future of policing; (4) more than 300 hours spent with officers on patrol to observe use of the system firsthand and interview officers as opportunities presented themselves; and (5) a self-administered survey that was completed by more than 200 members of the department. The priority for the survey was to obtain a diverse sample from throughout the department. They were volunteers comprising about 20% of all personnel; demographic questions in the survey showed that the sample's demographic structure mirrored the overall structure of the department.

Recall that at an early point in his career, Campbell had dismissed case study designs as pretty much useless and "prescientific." Although he would later change his mind and become very supportive of case study methods (as we discussed earlier in this chapter), the reason behind his dismissal was instructive.

Basic to scientific evidence (and to all knowledge-diagnostic processes including the retina of the eye) is the process of comparison, of recording differences, or of contrast. Any appearance of absolute knowledge, or intrinsic knowledge about singular isolated objects, is found to be illusory upon analysis. Securing scientific evidence involves making at least one comparison. For such a comparison to be useful, both sides of the comparison should be made with similar care and precision. (p. 6)

This is good advice to keep in mind. The comparisons do not necessarily need to be pre- and post intervention or between a treatment and a comparison group as experimentation and quasi-experimentation require in order to be informative. In Ted's evaluation of the computerized information system, there were numerous comparisons that started almost popping out of the woodwork. It turned out that cars sometimes were used by one patrol officer, and sometimes by two working together, which created different conditions for use of the system that revealed something about when the system "worked" and when it proved problematic. There was also variation among officers in how much experience they had with the system, the attitudes they held about technology and the "professionalization" of using a computer in their job symbolized to many (and particularly to younger officers), the sensitivity they had to rights issues, and how all of this fit into the way they conceived policing and their relation to the community. There was also huge variation in how officers used the system; in a 4-hour shift, some officers were seen to use the system a dozen times or less, while others used it hundreds of times, entering license plate after license plate into the system hoping to find a stolen car or an owner with outstanding warrants.

Building comparison into the surveys that were administered to a 20% sample of the department allowed the researchers to get into the time dimension as well. For example, the survey first asked about situations where they found the system particularly useful or problematic, which was followed by questions that asked how they would have dealt with that same situation in a radio-only car. This proved helpful in sensitizing the research team to the social changes that the system was creating, such as leaving the dispatchers feeling less important because they were no longer the exclusive information source for members on patrol or giving the patrol officers greater satisfaction because they could choose their own policing style instead of being subject to the norms of the group over radio. This also helped make clear there were things the officers missed, such as a feel for how the day was going that was conveyed by hearing how busy the network was and the nature of the requests being made and the sense of common mission this encouraged.

The study was also a splendid opportunity to experience the benefits of triangulation, which were evident in several ways. While the surveys allowed the research team to hear from more than 200 members of the department, spending several hundred hours in the cars with officers on shift allowed the researchers to see how what the officers *said* corresponded with what they *did*. And while the surveys with their more structured response options generated more summary-type information about how respondents felt about the system—how many respondents agreed or disagreed with different statements about the system—the interviews allowed the research team to find out why some people would feel that way and to talk about the implications that flowed from their point of view.

While riding with officers in patrol cars was seen as the best way to get a firsthand look at how officers used the system, one concern Ted had was over how the behavior of the officers might change when there was an observer in the car with them. There were aspects of the design of the study that were thought to help in this regard. For example, several of the observers/interviewers that Ted hired were graduate students in criminology who were interested in policing issues, and who it was felt would more easily develop a rapport with the officers and make them feel less scrutinized. Also, there is a lot to be said about simply spending time with people—4 hours per shift, and a total of 88 patrol officer shifts overall can help you become part of the woodwork and encourage officers to simply focus on the work ahead of them rather than with the person riding with them.

Particularly useful in this situation, however, was the fact the research team was given access to the data archive produced automatically by the system that recorded every single transaction. The basic structure of the system was that there were eight different "forms" that could be called up at any point, where each "form" had a certain function or gave access to a specific type of information. For example, one form might give access to license plate data, where officers could find out whether a car had been reported stolen and the name of the registered owner of the vehicle. Name information could be entered on another form to determine whether there were any wants or warrants out for that person. Access to this archive allowed the research team to compare how frequently the different forms were used in the department overall to how frequently they were used when the research team was in the cars. This comparison revealed that the distribution of use of forms when researchers were in the car was identical to when they were not, with one exception. The one exception was a form that was basically an early form of email or texting that allowed officers to send text messages to other specific cars or to everyone on the system. Knowing this, and because they had ongoing access to officers in the observational portion of the study, the research team was able to ask about this anomaly. Officers shared that the system was often used to send jokes and other remarks to each other that observers might find frivolous or offensive, and that they had been told in their morning meetings about the existence of the study, along with the admonition that, while the department and system were under the spotlight, they should minimize their frivolous uses of the system.

Readers interested in more of the findings can see them in Palys, Boyanowsky, and Dutton (1984). Ted reports that it was very instructive to him to find that what at that time was still considered a "prescientific" case study design unworthy of consideration could turn into one that remains one of the best examples he knows of an evaluation that lived up to its promise and provided a detailed understanding of the social and behavioral issues that played out when the system was introduced, and what it might mean to both the police and the citizenry.

SUMMING UP AND LOOKING AHEAD

Chapters 6 through 8 have outlined three different ways that researchers have approached the challenge of dealing with the third criterion—eliminating rival plausible explanations—with the difference between them residing in the extent to which each uses manipulative and/or analytic control to accomplish that objective.

As outlined in Chapter 6, the core of experimentalist logic is that if two or more groups are equal to begin with and are treated identically in all respects but one, then any differences that emerge between the groups must be the result of that one thing on which the groups differed. In the "true experiment," this involves exerting manipulative control in which you create whatever experimental and control groups you want and randomize the assignment of participants to groups in order to ensure that internal validity is maximized. External validity—the extent to which the results are generalizable across persons, settings, and times—often remains an empirical question, although the literature may shed light on that issue as well when similar hypotheses have been tested in other contexts at other times. Ecological validity—the extent to which the experimental situation corresponds to the real-world situation we are interested in understanding—is often the weakest element in at least the laboratory version of the true experiment. This can leave us knowing that a particular outcome *can* happen in the *ceteris paribus* situation that is the lab, but not knowing whether it *does* happen when the variable we are testing competes with all the other variables in the world that vie for attention.

In Chapter 7, we explained how Donald T. Campbell had urged us to consider the broader applicability of experimentalist approaches in the interest of developing more of an "experimenting society." He envisioned a time when programs, policies, and laws would be subject to empirical assessment in order to evaluate and hopefully improve our ability to achieve socially important objectives. Doing so required moving from an approach based on manipulative control to one based more so on analytic control—essentially adapting to situations instead of creating them. The trick was that we should not get too hung up on the specifics of experimental practice and go back instead to the first principles that the experiment was designed to address. When the manipulative alternative is not available, Campbell exhorted us not to throw our hands in the air in despair, but to look for other ways to achieve those objectives. For example, in the true experiment, participants would be randomly assigned to experimental and control groups in order to meet the assumption of pretest equivalence. In the quasi-experiment, identifying nonequivalent controls that are as similar to the treatment group as possible, incorporating those on waiting lists as a comparison, and implementing matching are three alternative ways to achieve the same objective.

In the current chapter we extended the logic even further into the realm of case study design, where comparisons between groups often are not available, and the comparisons necessary to start making sense of the situation arise through differences that exist within the situation—e.g., comparing what people do when a variable of interest is present versus how they behave when it is not—and/or by triangulating different sources of information in a multi-method project that helps address different rival plausible explanations. Doing so requires you to be your own best critic and brainstorming with those who have strong local knowledge about what those rival plausible explanations might be and then gathering the data that allow one to address those possibilities.

While case study approaches have much broader utility than evaluation research *per se*, one of their great advantages in the evaluation research context is the extent to which they help shed light on *process*—all those things that happen between inputs and outputs—and bring skill sets that have been found to be highly important in doing effective evaluation: adapting to emergent situations; establishing rapport with those in the setting being evaluated; familiarity in dealing with multiple sources of data; understanding the logic underlying purposive sampling; and so on. Negative cases are particularly sought; more data are gathered, and their (in)consistency with the theory is scrutinized.

We summarize some of the general strengths and challenges that each of these methods for dealing with rival plausible explanations brings in Table 8.3. The strong logical ties underlying the whole continuum from experimental study to case study analysis should be evident. Ultimately, the research task, whatever form it takes, is a dialectic process involving theory and data, where the goal is to generate and decide on the relative plausibility of prospective competing explanations.

What these three chapters gave you are principles to guide you in how to structure or adapt to the structure of the setting you are in. The next four chapters will address how to set up the means for gathering data once you are there.

Table 8.3 ● Three Different Approaches to Dealing With Rival Plausible Explanations			
	Experiments	**Quasi-Experiments**	**Case Studies**
Type of control	Manipulative control	Mixture of manipulative and analytic control depending on situation	Analytic control
Internal validity	Achieved through random assignment, creation of equivalent controls, and control over procedure to create standardized conditions	Achieved through "nonequivalent" control groups, identification of rival plausible explanations, and gathering data that address those possibilities	Achieved through internal comparison, triangulation of methods, gathering rich detailed data
External validity	May or may not be; ultimately an empirical question aided by connecting to literature to see where results generalize and where they don't	May or may not be; ultimately an empirical question aided by connecting to literature to see where results generalize and where they don't	May or may not be; ultimately an empirical question aided by connecting to literature to see where results generalize and where they don't
Ecological validity	Usually involves creating a simulation of a real-world situation with low ecological validity, but field experiments possible as well	Usually done in real-world contexts and with real tasks; thus ecological validity is often higher than in experiments	Typically involving real-world contexts and observing behavior where it usually happens with real life consequences, i.e., usually high ecological validity
Strengths	Best for answering theoretical questions involving causal relations; high internal validity; shows something "can" happen, all else being equal	Creates possibility for an "experimenting society" by showing tool for evaluating impacts of changes to law and policy	Serves many objectives. Involves looking at behavior among people in the contexts in which they normally do them. Wealth of data; ideal for looking at process
Challenges	Just because something "can" happen does not mean it "does" in the world. Generalizing to real-world contexts can be difficult	Researchers must adapt empirical principles to situations, but are subject to the caprice of available data and comparison groups	Often challenge to gain access to appropriate sample and settings and ability to triangulate data sources; investigator competence crucial

Key Concepts

Analytic induction 302
Case 296
Confirmation bias 303

Disprovable 303
Instrumental case study 297
Intrinsic case study 296

Multiple or collective case
study 297
Negative evidence 302

STUDY QUESTIONS

1. In traditional laboratory experimentation, internal validity is maximized by randomly assigning participants to groups and by creating control groups that are equivalent to the experimental group(s) in all respects *except* for the independent variable. But those luxuries are frequently not available in field settings. How are they dealt with in the context of case study analysis?

2. Explain the process of *analytic induction* in your own words.

3. Why did Donald T. Campbell think, in his earlier articles on experimentation (e.g., Campbell & Stanley, 1963), that "rigorous" case study analysis was impossible? How might Louise Kidder (1981) have tried to change his mind?

4. Experiments emphasize manipulative control; case study analysis emphasizes analytic control. Discuss the relative merits and demerits of the two approaches as routes to understanding.

5. Choose any of the Sherlock Holmes stories other than the one featured in this chapter, and consider Holmes's investigative process from the perspective of case study designs.

6. In the Adventure of Silver Blaze we have two sleuths—Sherlock Holmes and Inspector Gregory—trying to solve the same crime. Compare the two in terms of their methodological strengths and weaknesses.

7. We offered several examples of professionals who are required to engage in case study analysis (i.e., physicians, mechanics, coroners, engineering troubleshooters). Can you think of other occupations that make the same demand? If you know someone in any of those occupations, interview them about the way they try to isolate causes. Do they follow the logic outlined in this chapter? Explain.

8. Select an article from a recent issue of a newsmagazine that purports to be "analytical" about current events (e.g., *Time*, *Newsweek*, *Breitbart*), and consider the way the article's author develops their analysis. Is the logic of the analysis evident? Does the writer follow the steps required for rigorous case study analysis?

SURVEYS AND QUESTIONNAIRES

Surveys have been a popular way to gather large amounts of structured data to inform us not only about how different people or the citizenry as a whole feel about different social issues but also to inform us about niches of life we otherwise would know little to nothing about. Looked at from the outside, surveys look like the easiest thing in the world to construct. After all, what could be easier than creating a bunch of questions, throwing in some rating scales and there you have it … a survey? But while a survey is indeed the easiest thing in the world to construct, especially these days when all you have to do is go to **Survey Monkey or Qualtrics** to put one together in a few minutes, constructing a *good* one where every question is equally meaningful and understood by everyone who participates is an incredible challenge. The difficulty comes from the fact that when we create a questionnaire, we often do it based on our own understanding, where the words we use have certain meanings for us, and where what we are trying to find out seems so obvious. But other people are not us and they may well have a very different understanding and *way* of understanding the phenomenon we want to find out about. The two of us have been constructing surveys for decades and still run pilot studies to make sure others understand the words the way we do, and we are still surprised by our occasional blindness to how a question we thought was so clear could have been so misunderstood. In this chapter you will learn why constructing a quality survey is such a difficult thing to do, as well as some of the many principles you need to keep in mind when you construct one.

We will use the words "survey," "questionnaire," and "survey questionnaire" interchangeably in this chapter to refer to a fairly structured set of questions or other items that are finalized ahead of time and can be either self-administered or delivered by a researcher whose role is typically to stay focused on the questions and to keep interaction to a minimum. The specific questions can be of many different types that will range from highly structured to more open-ended, but a general characteristic is that all respondents normally will receive exactly the same set of questions worded in exactly the same way. An objective of such research typically will be to amass as large a sample as possible, and for data analysis to involve any of a variety of statistical techniques ranging from simple descriptive information regarding the distribution of responses (e.g., percentage breakdowns for each item, as you often see when opinion polls are published) to more complex statistical techniques designed to explore the data to explain variations in responding or to compare the responses of different groups. As this description suggests, surveys and questionnaires normally are considered more "quantitative" techniques for all the reasons that you should recall from Chapter 1.

Our use of the word "survey" also will include techniques that share the interactivity we usually associate with interviews—successive questions asked by a researcher who notes down the responses made by the respondent in a telephone survey, for example. The difference for us between the two sets of techniques is not in the presence or absence of direct interaction as much as it is in the degree of structure and closure involved in the responses that participants can make. What we think of as a "survey" may well include a few open-ended questions where people are given the opportunity to explain further—something we encourage for just about any survey—but for the most part response alternatives are limited to a finite number of categories from which respondents can choose. This standardization puts a huge onus on the survey designer to "get it right" by ensuring that the questions asked are meaningful ones, the order in which they are asked makes sense to all respondents, and the response alternatives that are provided cover the range of alternatives that respondents would have come up with if left to their own devices.

STRENGTHS AND LIMITATIONS OF SURVEYS

Surveys offer many strengths as an information gathering tool. You can ask questions about anything in every kind of survey, and there are many different question formats (reviewed later in this chapter) that are all equally easy to include. Questionnaires in most cases also make it easy to gather data anonymously, which may make it easier and more likely that participants will respond to sensitive questions they might otherwise avoid if they thought they could be identified. And although there are significant differences between the different media of survey administration, surveys also allow you to amass a fairly substantial amount of data quite quickly, particularly relative to the time it would take to amass a comparable number of interviews.

As we noted above, many survey data archives also now can be accessed via the internet where any researcher, and especially beginning researchers, can see how particular issues that are often common to many surveys (e.g., the way demographic information is sought) are addressed by respected survey agencies such as the Census Bureau in the United States, Statistics Canada in Canada, or the Home Office in Britain. Checking these archives to see how others have asked questions in your area of interest is a good way for newer researchers to benefit from what others have done and can enhance the comparability of results across surveys. Structured surveys also are highly appropriate for more deductive types of research where the phenomenon being scrutinized is already fairly well understood and/or where theoretical propositions are being tested, such that the "right" questions to ask are fairly clear. And of course the opposite is true as well; sometimes researchers will put all sorts of items into a preliminary survey on a topic in a more exploratory/inductive effort to see what sorts of distributions arise and what kinds of relationships appear to exist among variables that can be tested more systematically in a subsequent study.

The structure of surveys also is ideally suited for particular types of research questions. Because questions are standardized, comparisons between subgroups are possible by comparing average responses or the distribution of responses across response categories. Standardized data sets involving many cases also allow you to use a wide variety of powerful statistical techniques to both summarize and analyze the data. This also makes survey data ideal for hypothesis testing and thereby for theory development, particularly within the more hypothetico-deductive traditions.

As with any method, there are also some limitations to all forms of survey. First is that, in most cases, getting someone to complete a questionnaire requires them to be literate. The fact that most surveys are standardized instruments given to the entire sample also means that you have to make decisions about vocabulary to ensure that all questions will be understood by everyone, which can be a real challenge when the sample is highly diverse. Further, the data you get from surveys are limited to what the respondent places on the paper or indicates on a computer screen; at that point you can no longer ask the respondent to clarify or further embellish upon their response, and there are no nonverbal or contextual cues to help you interpret what the respondent has stated.

Surveys also can be hampered by low **response rates**, which can create generalizability issues if you are doing the research with a sample and had hoped to be able to generalize the result on a statistical basis to the broader population from which the sample was drawn. Recruitment is always an issue with surveys and, generally speaking, the longer the survey gets, the less likely people are to participate. Among those who do begin, the longer the survey, the more likely they are to abandon it before completion.

TYPES OF SURVEYS AND QUESTIONNAIRES

At least three different types of survey questionnaires can be distinguished, on the basis of the medium through which each is administered. They include (1) the pencil-and-paper questionnaire; (2) the telephone survey; and (3) the network-administered survey.

The Paper-and-Pencil Questionnaire

One way to administer a survey—a mainstay through much of the 20th century—is to place your questions on a piece of paper, to deliver these papers to prospective respondents by mailing them to their last known address or handing them over in person in an individual or group setting, and then simply to collect all that paper and begin processing the information the respondents have given you.

Although obviously very "old school," there are unique benefits to administering a survey in this way. In the case of a mail-out survey, the respondent can choose their own time to do the survey and return it, and if a sampling frame is available from which to randomly sample, or a multistage cluster sample can be identified on a geographical basis, a theoretically representative sample can be contacted. Paper is also reasonably portable, can be taken anywhere, and does not require electricity, a computer, or any computer skills to read. When distributed in person in group settings, paper-and-pencil surveys allow you to amass large amounts of data very quickly, which can be very handy if the sample you are targeting is one that meets or can be brought together in a specific locale (e.g., classrooms, meeting halls, hospitals, care facilities, a prison).

The fact that respondents answer questions on their own may not only enhance feelings of anonymity that will leave people more willing to respond to sensitive questions but also pose special constraints to consider. We've already noted issues of literacy and language and the need to anticipate possible ambiguities or mis-understandings. The questions themselves and the instructions to respondents must be clear, and the design of the survey itself must be kept simple enough that anyone can follow through without getting lost. **Contingency questions**, for example—the ones that say things like, "if you answer 'yes,' proceed to question 14; if 'no' go to question 17"—must be kept to a minimum or avoided entirely because too many people miss the instructions or have a difficult time following them and get lost.

An absent researcher cannot monitor other procedural aspects of the study. Except for obvious flippancy—e.g., the respondent who answers "Saturn" or "in a hospital" when asked about their place of birth—we cannot know whether respondents took the task seriously and gave their most comprehensive and candid responses. Such problems are thought to be relatively uncommon, since people who aren't interested in and/or serious about the topic of study are likely to simply ignore the questionnaire and fail to return it. But to the extent that such tendencies *do* exist, they make the data less valid.

And finally, paper-and-pencil surveys end up being very inefficient when it comes to the actual processing of the data. Someone must take the checkmarks and written comments from the piles of paper they are written on and digitize them so that they can be analyzed. This takes time, is incredibly boring to do, and ends up being an error-prone process that is best done twice in order to catch transcription errors and ensure you end up with a clean set of data.

The Telephone Survey

Although it was invented in the late 1800s, it was not until well into the 1900s that the telephone went from being a high-tech toy of the wealthy to an essential tool of life in the industrialized world. It did not take researchers long to see its potential for reaching broad samples of respondents quickly and efficiently. Initial concerns about the selection bias involved in contacting samples via telephone had all but vanished by the 1970s and 1980s. By the end of the 20th century, in countries such as the United States and Sweden, 94–99 percent of all households could be reached by phone. Although there was some variation between groups, particularly on variables associated with income, penetration rates were well above 90 percent in every income group; for example, in households with incomes above $75,000, the rate was 98.5 percent, while among those with incomes less than $20,000, a full 94.7 percent had phones (Federal Communications Commission, 2011).

Telephone surveys appealed to researchers for other reasons as well. The costs of administering a face-to-face survey were rising rapidly, and telephone surveys offered an inexpensive alternative with little or no loss in response rates. They are still less expensive than in-person interview studies, but are generally more expensive than online surveys. Personal safety also was becoming a concern, particularly in urban centers in the United States. The concern went both ways. Respondents were becoming increasingly reluctant to allow strange interviewers into their homes but remained willing to "let them in" by phone. Meanwhile, interviewers were becoming increasingly worried about their own safety as they walked the streets in some neighborhoods; contact by telephone was safer for them, too.

The centralization of telephone surveying also meant that research directors could take greater care in monitoring "quality control." Conversations between interviewers and respondents could be recorded or monitored and critically analyzed for training and "quality assurance" purposes. And instead of losing prospective respondents for whom English was not a first or preferred language, a group of interviewers could be amassed who, collectively, could handle a broad variety of language situations in one centralized location (e.g., see Gorden, 1980). The development of **random digit dialing (RDD)** techniques for a time made representative sampling a real possibility.

What made RDD possible was the direct tie that used to exist between phone number and location. If you wanted to sample people in Montana, for example, you knew that all their phone numbers would begin with area code 406. For Nebraska, there are three area codes—308, 402, and 531—which meant that researchers could even focus more specifically on certain parts of the state if they wanted to. The next three digits at one point would have been tied to a particular neighborhood. By knowing these connections between phone numbers and certain physical locations, you could randomly sample people in those locations by beginning with a known area code and using a random number generator to pick the next seven digits, or if you wanted to sample smaller neighborhoods, you could start with a stem of the area code and neighborhood exchange and then randomly generate the last four numbers. At a time when all phones were "landlines," RDD would give access to a random sample of households, so that survey researchers would then randomly select people from within each household.

Nowadays, however, the popularity of the telephone survey is dropping rapidly. RDD has become ineffective because phone numbers are no longer tied to a particular family or social unit in a particular place; phone companies now let subscribers carry their phone numbers within the same area code so that the connection between localized, identifiable neighborhoods, and phone exchanges is rapidly becoming a thing of the past. Phone plans that allow national calling have resulted in more and more people simply staying on the same plan and keeping their phone numbers as they move from state to state, thereby lessening even further the connection between area code and location. People also now have multiple phone numbers and multiple phones—there may be a cell phone for each member of the family as well as a landline, which makes any sort of probabilistic sampling difficult. Household numbers are also becoming increasingly less representative as more and more people abandon the idea of a home landline in favor of exclusive use of a cell phone. In 2010, 24 percent of US adults were living in cell phone–only households (Bernard, 2013); by 2017, that same number ranged from a low of 35.6 percent in New Jersey to a high of 65.6 percent in Idaho and 65.3 percent in Texas (National Centre for Health Statistics, 2017).

TABLE 9.1 ● Surveys Face Growing Difficulty Reaching, Persuading Potential Respondents	1997	2000	2003	2006	2009	2012
Contact rate (percent of households in which an adult was reached) (%)	90	77	79	73	72	62
Cooperation rate (percent of households contacted that yielded an interview) (%)	43	40	34	31	21	14
Response rate (percent of households sampled that yielded an interview) (%)	36	28	25	21	15	9

Source: The Pew Research Centre. (2012). *Assessing the representativeness of public opinion surveys.* Washington, DC: Pew Research Center. Retrieved from https://www.pewresearch.org/wp-content/uploads/sites/4/legacy-pdf/Assessing-the-Representativeness-of-Public-Opinion-Surveys.pdf.

In addition, far too many harassing phone calls from salespeople or market researchers phoning in the guise of a survey have made it more and more difficult for social and health researchers to distinguish themselves from entrepreneurs and scammers. Patience also wears thin quickly during telephone surveys; after about 15–20 minutes, people start to hang up (Bernard, 2013). Overall, it is becoming more and more difficult to contact people due to call screening, and of those who can be contacted, participation rates have been dropping steadily. Table 9.1 shows how contact rates, cooperation rates, and response rates all decreased steadily from 1997 to 2012. Although the official opinion of the Pew Research Center that compiled those numbers in 2012 was that representative samples could still be reached by phone at that time, that conclusion becomes increasingly more tenuous with each passing year.

Although telephone surveys are still conducted and still can be useful when a diverse sample is sought, for more serious polls where representativeness of the sample is crucial, telephone surveys are not something we would recommend. Thoughtful and forward-looking survey companies are hedging their bets and looking elsewhere, particularly to online techniques.

The Network-Administered Survey

Prior to the popularization of the internet, Kiesler and Sproull (1986) provided a roadmap for using networked computers to conduct social and health science research. While they were optimistic about the potential of computer technology, they felt that "until such time as computers and networks spread throughout society, the electronic survey will probably be infeasible" (p. 403). That time would seem to have arrived. The internet is expanding at an unprecedented rate; its growth has eclipsed all other technologies preceding it (Dahlen, 2002). Although its precursors extend back to the 1960s, the contemporary internet is generally considered to have begun in the early 1990s with creation of the first web page by Tim Berners-Lee. Between 1994 and 1998, 50 million people logged on to the internet worldwide (United Nations, 2004). In December 2005, one billion people worldwide were online (United Nations, 2004); by 2011, internet usage had passed *two* billion people; by 2019, we were at 4.5 billion out of a world population of 7.7 billion![1]

Notwithstanding this tremendous growth in access and usage, network-administered survey techniques still have much room for improvement (e.g., see Palys & Atchison, 2012). Only recently have we seen the broad availability of online survey creation software that allows you to go beyond creating a paper-and-pencil survey and placing it on a computer monitor. But the possibilities are far more than that.

One of the most cited practical benefits of computer-assisted survey research is the effect that implementing a computer-assisted design has on the speed and duration of the research process; **computer-assisted social research (CASR)** can be much faster than comparable traditional designs. In networked environments, the footwork of the design and administration process is done by network connections. Research teams can create, edit, and finalize the research instrument without the burden of scheduling and attending physical meetings, and the research team can administer the design without having to physically connect with the participant. Once in motion, CASR allows researchers to move from design to observation and from observation to analysis much more quickly than conventional survey designs. When research is conducted over wide area networks such as the internet, observations can be made and data collected 24 hours a day, 7 days a week.

Computer-administered observation and data collection instruments can enhance usability in three major ways: design, control, and accessibility. Design programs such as Adobe Dreamweaver and scripting languages and frameworks such as AJAX, JScript, and Bootstrap can be used to create attractive, interesting, and compelling research instruments (Fricker & Rand, 2002; Pettit, 2002; Schmidt, 2002). Those who are less computer-savvy have commercial do-it-yourself (DIY) options like Survey Monkey and Qualtrics. We often work with a graphic designer to ensure the look of any survey we prepare will be appealing to the audience we seek.

Computer-assisted surveys make a whole new way of asking questions possible through the integration of pictures, audio, and video media into the research

---

[1] See internet usage statistics at http://www.internetworldstats.com/stats.htm.

instrument. For example, researchers can include a short multimedia clip in a structured survey and ask questions related to that clip. Also, response formats can be made much more intuitive for participants. For example, instead of asking participants to rate their level of happiness using a nondescript numeric rating scale, it is possible to provide a series of detailed animations that change as the participant moves a slider up or down the scale.

The strategic use of interface design and scripting also allows researchers to incorporate **adaptive questioning** into the research instrument in a manner that is neither obvious nor disturbing to the research participant. With adaptive questioning, answers to specific questions influence which subsequent questions will be asked (Bauman, Airey, & Atak, 1998; Liu, Papathanasiou, & Hao, 2001). For example, an early question in a survey might ask which of eight different sporting activities an individual engages in on a regular basis. The responses to this question can then be used to determine which subsequent sections are asked. Someone who answers "none" will be skipped to the next section of the survey, while someone who checks off swimming, golf, and hockey will see only those subsequent questions that deal with swimming, golf, and hockey and never see the ones that deal with Ultimate Frisbee, rugby, or jogging. Individual respondents aren't bothered with irrelevant questions, and the complexity of the overall instrument is reduced for respondents since they no longer need to read and follow skip patterns and instruction sets.

In addition to enhancing the complexity of the data collection design, a well-constructed computerized instrument can help ensure that questions are completed and done accurately (Liu et al., 2001). Unlike a human researcher who may forget to ask a specific question, with computer-assisted surveys all questions are asked (unless adaptively programmed not to) because the computer always follows the programmed routine (Peiris, Gregor, & Alm, 2000). In less structured surveys, researchers can script in pop-up dialog boxes that automatically ask the respondent to elaborate a bit further if a certain number of keystrokes are not present in a particular answer. Computer-assisted surveys also allow researchers to build in programmed checks of the responses provided to ensure that all required questions have been answered and that the information provided corresponds to the expected format.

Perhaps one of the most promising possibilities that computerized instruments offer in the way of format and design comes in the form of improved access. Multimodal participant input devices can be created to facilitate the participation of people who have physical disabilities, limited reading or computer skills (Black & Ponirakis, 2000), and attention deficits. Additionally, instruments can be customized to adapt to language and cultural differences. For instance, participants can have the option of filling out forms in any of a number of different languages or the digital voice on a computer can be changed to one that the participant is more culturally familiar with (Black & Ponirakis, 2000). It is also possible to build in instructions or construct elaborate help or frequently asked questions (FAQ) sections that can be made available to a research participant at the click of a mouse (Karr, 2000). Finally, the instrument also can be set up to provide feedback or instructions to any respondent who has problems navigating, filling out questions, or submitting responses (Bauman et al. 1998; Woong Yun & Trumbo, 2000).

Computer-assisted surveys also allow you to control access to the survey itself—either leaving it open or creating password or other private access—and to collect precise data about the process of survey completion that can help inform better survey development. For example, you can get information about the types of operating systems and browsers that respondents are using, and their IP addresses will give some indication of where respondents are located. You also can track exactly how long it takes respondents to respond to each question, which allows you to identify spots where respondents tend to slow down (perhaps indicating that the content is overly complex or confusing and thus requires simplification) and also where they stop participation before completion, if at all.

On the down side, in some cases the initial design and administration of the research can be prohibitively time-consuming. When the research team is inexperienced with the use of technology or the technological infrastructure for the research is not already in place, extra training and the installation and testing of hardware and software may be necessary. Furthermore, researchers who are new to the technology are more likely to make errors during the administration and observation stages, which can result in even greater time delays in the research.

When it comes to the cost of materials and labor, there are several distinct differences between CASR and conventional research methods. The hardware, software, and scripting that is required for the observation and data collection portion of a CASR project can cost researchers thousands of dollars. However, researchers can offset the software and scripting costs by using freely available open-source software and scripts instead of high-priced commercial applications. Furthermore, while equipment and design costs can be high, these costs are generally recouped through savings on paper, postage, transcription, mileage, lodging, the renting of research venues, and repeated research. While it is uncommon to find hard-to-estimate human labor costs factored into discussions of many traditional data collection methods, the introduction of computer programmers and graphic and Web designers into the CASR design process has required many social and health science researchers to begin to account for the cost of labor. The rate that most programmers and designers charge can be well over $100 per hour. The result is that in some situations CASR can be a cost-effective solution for the North American researcher. This advantage does, however, depend on researchers having enough experience with technology that they can implement solutions that require specialized user and programming skills.

It also is important to recognize that there can be considerable startup material and personnel costs associated with CASR, but repeated research is less costly since much of the investment is saddled by the first project and the cost of upgrading vital research materials is much less than first-time expenditures. For research designs that are not dependent upon the physical presence of a researcher, network-based CASR facilitates the solicitation and recruitment of large, geographically, and demographically diverse samples (Fox, Murray, & Warm, 2003; Gosling, Vazire, & Srivastava, 2004). These larger samples make it possible to amass large amounts of data in a relatively short time. Additionally, with the increasing availability and affordability of handheld smartphones, tablet and laptop computers, and wireless networks, researchers can easily go mobile to collect and analyze data.

DESIGNING YOUR SURVEY

Who Are Your Respondents?

Once you've decided on the type of survey most appropriate for your topic and interests, you're ready to begin designing one. The first thing you need to do is to make some decisions about who you want to sample—the people who will be the source of your data—because who they are will have implications for the way you design your survey. Although it may seem obvious, it bears saying that the purpose of putting together a survey is to gather valid and reliable information about some people or some phenomenon of interest they know something about. A prerequisite for that is that respondents need to understand what you want to know. In our experience most people who agree to participate in a survey come into it with the intention of being a "good respondent" who is willing to share their opinions or some aspects of their lives with you, such that all you need to do is provide the means for them to do so. You want to feed and maintain that sense of good will by being transparent about your purpose, asking what you want to know in clear and understandable language, not violating any taboos, keeping a good flow, and not wasting their time.

There is no one perfect way of asking questions or creating a survey. It has to work on *this* topic you are interested in with *these* people you have access to. Wording is crucial, and the attributes of your sample will make a difference. How diverse or homogeneous is your sample? How old are they? What sort of educational range will they have? Will all participants be native English speakers or do you need to plan for additional languages? Are you approaching a more general citizenry or are they somehow specialized in a way that means they likely will have a unique vocabulary you need to know (e.g., gang members, hospital workers, real estate sales personnel)? Can literacy be assumed? Are people likely to have a smartphone, computer, or other network access? Each of these considerations will have implications for the types of questions you ask and the way that you ask them. We will not try and create an inventory here of all the different considerations that you need to have in mind as you formulate questions, but will make note of some places where it clearly makes a difference as we explain the different kinds of questions and give different survey examples later in this chapter.

The next thing you need going in is some sense of the content you want to include or address in your questions. Your challenge in designing a survey is to create an engaging encounter with the participant that reflects their understanding of whatever it is that you are asking about, but to do so in a way that taps into the information you are searching for. That said, a "survey" is more than a bunch of questions; the survey as a whole has to have an organization and flow to it that makes sense to the respondent, creates confidence that you are worthy of their candid responses and time, and helps you fulfill the objectives that brought you to create the survey in the first place.

Question Content

We can't begin to count the number of times we've read student research papers that feature a good introduction that contextualizes the issues well by summarizing relevant literature and identifying a reasonable research question, followed by a reasonable "methods" section that includes a copy of the research instrument—but where the two don't match! This situation leads to some very interesting "discussion" and "conclusion" sections: students end up going through some incredible verbal acrobatics trying to actually say something about their research question from their data. Asking the wrong questions and often being afraid to directly ask the "right" ones are two of the most common mistakes novice researchers make.

Examples in the Literature

Ideas for question content come from a variety of different places. Sometimes we just sit down and brainstorm possibilities of things we would like to include based on what we know and whatever else we are curious about. You may also go and check out the literature to see what sorts of issues people have addressed already and where gaps might exist that you can fill. The literature is also a good place to see the exact questions that others have used. There is a lot of borrowing that goes on in the survey world; one of the reasons for this is that people do learn what works as they do more and more surveys, such that seeing how others have worded common questions such as demographics can be helpful and save you some time in getting to a wording that people will respond to in meaningful ways. Using items from existing studies also helps to establish comparisons between findings. This can be helpful if you find differences between your study and someone else's because it gets rid of the rival plausible explanation that the difference is simply because you have asked a question in a different way.

Using Mixed Methods to Inform Questioning

Probably the biggest thing to remember when you go into designing a survey is that, while you are the one designing the survey for purposes that are meaningful to you, the survey itself is not about you, but about your participant. That is the person for whom the survey has to make sense. Ted has a quote taped to his office door due to author John Le Carré from his novel *Tinker Tailor Soldier Spy* that says, "A desk is a dangerous place from which to view the world." It seems particularly appropriate in this context. When you sit at your desk and brainstorm about what to ask, you are delving into an experience that may be helpful, but which also inevitably will be limited. At its worst, your understanding will come from stereotypes or "common sense" that you have in mind rather than any real encounter with the phenomenon as it actually exists in the world. But even if it is based on your own experience, that is still but one experience, which may or may not reflect the way others experience or perceive that same phenomenon.

One way to address this limitation and to make more meaningful surveys that reflect participant views is to use other methods to gather that information as part of the process of survey construction. In many cases, more field-based researchers already will have spent considerable time with the people they are now surveying as an ongoing career interest. When Ted does research with Indigenous communities or talks to research ethics board members or when Chris talks to people who provide sexual services for their clients, we bring at least some understanding of who these people are because of the decades that we have spent working in those areas. As a neophyte researcher, the first thing you need to consider is just how far you need to go in order to understand the language, culture, and perspectives of the people who will be participating in your research.

We are also an interesting example here because Ted is not Indigenous, nor does he sit on a research ethics board, and Chris has never been either a sexual service provider or client of one. Although some people engage in research where they are part of the group being researched, more often researchers are not part of the community and those they research are an "other." There are advantages and disadvantages to being insider or outsider that are beyond the scope of what we will be discussing in this chapter (but see Chapter 11). Suffice it to say that one of the great wonders of being a researcher is the willingness people have to share their lives with you if they trust you and feel you will treat them fairly and respectfully and take their interests and aspirations seriously.

Personally we do not understand people who do surveys who never do the complementary work of interviewing any of the people they presumably are trying to understand. Howie Becker (1996) tells of lessons he learned from Herbert Blumer:

> [A]ll social scientists, implicitly or explicitly, attribute a point of view and interpretations to the people whose actions we analyze. That is, we always describe how they interpret the events they participate in, so the only question is not whether we should, but how accurately we do it. … Blumer argued that if we don't find out from people what meanings they are actually giving to things, we will still talk about those meanings. In that case, we will, of necessity, invent them, reasoning that the people we are writing about must have meant this or that, or they would not have done the things they did. But it is inevitably epistemologically dangerous to guess at what could be observed directly. The danger is that we will guess wrong, that what looks reasonable to us will not be what looked reasonable to them. This happens all the time, largely because we are not those people and do not live in their circumstances. (p. 58)

An example of this phenomenon and an illustration of the merit of mixed-method inquiry occurred in a research methods class that Ted taught recently. One of the grad students in that class, Amanda Champion, is a talented survey researcher whose research interests include "Technology Facilitated Sexual Violence," as occurs when people are sexually harassed online or have been the victims of "revenge porn," i.e., when one individual, often the rejected person in a relationship, tries to embarrass and humiliate the other person in the former relationship by posting nude and/or explicit images of the other person online without their consent. Amanda's project involved a sequential multimethod design where she began by putting together a survey that (1) asked a criterion sample of people about their experience with different TSFVs; (2) included open-ended questions at the end of each section to provide an opportunity for further commentary in their own words; and (3) also provided an opportunity for respondents to indicate if they were interested/willing to be interviewed at greater length at a later date.

The survey she put together was based on the literature, and part of her interest was in determining what sorts of effects were associated with having been a victim of "revenge porn." The first version of her survey went online and responses started coming in. Several of the people who provided early returns indicated they were interested in being interviewed, which Amanda was eager to do while waiting for other completed surveys to arrive. As soon as she started talking to people, however, her understanding began to change and the shortcomings of her draft survey became apparent. For example, one area that she was interested in was the perceived impacts of the victimization on their lives, and she had included one question about that, as did most people who contributed to that literature. But Amanda's interview partic-ipants started telling her that any discussion about effects needed to take time into account because, although they had been mortified and thought their world was ending at the time of the victimization, over time most were able to deal with it and come to some resolution about it.

The experience led her to revise her survey in order to include more of a time element to the questions—asking about initial impacts and how things had gone afterward, how other people in their lives had provided support, and so on. Something that would have been completely missed now ended up being an interesting dimension that had not yet received any attention in the literature and thus was a significant contribution she could make. To the extent this also opened the door to seeing what sorts of strategies helped victims get beyond those initial feelings of humiliation and betrayal, or identified the helpful role that support people in our lives can play, other researchers with other interests—like those who do therapy, for example—can benefit by sharing these empirically derived strategies with their clients.

An Iterative Process Starting With General Objectives

Another useful technique for generating survey questions is to follow a systematic iterative approach to design that begins with your objectives that are then embellished further in a series of steps designed to take you from abstract aspirations to a concrete set of questions or other items that will address those objectives. A good example of this approach occurred during a study we told you about in Chapter 8 when we were discussing case study designs—the one that set out to evaluate the impacts of introducing an online computer-based information system in police patrol cars.

"Doing an evaluation" is a rather amorphous objective. The first thing the research team had to do was to develop a clearer understanding of what "doing an evaluation" would look like in this context. Discussion among the research group, as well as with stakeholders from the funding agency (the federal government department) and at the research site (the Vancouver Police Department – VPD), led to the identification of two key components they wanted to examine: (1) attitudes about the system and (2) how the system was used in the process of the organization's activities.

The next step was to begin moving from abstract "issues" or "phenomena" and to start considering how exactly these abstract concepts took on life with this system in this context. Attitudes about what aspects of the system and on what basis could you start to understand system use? A bit of exploratory research helped to identify salient issues. This included reading some of the relevant "trade" literature (i.e., policing magazines and journals that included articles discussing similar information systems); accompanying officers on patrol, both to see how they used the system and to have a chance to talk with them about it away from more formal meetings at headquarters; undertaking informal target and focus interviews with different people in the police department—patrol officers, administrative staff, dispatchers—to gain insight into their opinions about the system; and some final brainstorming among the research team members to identify issues of personal interest. The big issue they brought forward involved trying to understand the *implications* of what were then the first glimmerings of what would later become a permeation of computerized information systems throughout society.

You can see this process beginning to unfold in Figure 9.1, which shows the beginning objective (to evaluate the information system, known as the Mobile Radio Data System, or MRDS) followed by the three types of evaluations that were included (engineering; cost-benefit; social/behavioral) and the first iteration of the social behavioral evaluation that identified the three main issues to be addressed in the social/behavioral evaluation—system use, satisfaction, and implications. As Figure 9.1 shows, in the end the research team was able to undertake a multimethod evaluation that would give a comprehensive view of the system and those who used it.

Figure 9.2 shows how the three domains of interest were taken through further iterations to get to an eventual set of items. For the first area—attitudes—the research team found several different dimensions that seemed to contribute to the variety of attitudes that officers held about the system. These included effects of the system on job satisfaction (for some the system enhanced it; for others the system detracted from it); beliefs about impacts of the system on job effectiveness (some believed it helped them in their jobs; others believed it did nothing or detracted); beliefs about impacts of the system on officer safety (some believed it enhanced safety; others

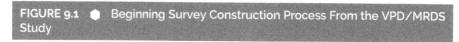

FIGURE 9.1 ● Beginning Survey Construction Process From the VPD/MRDS Study

	Engineering Study	
	Cost/Benefit Study	
Evaluate MRDS	Social/Behavioral Study	**Attitudes** • Self-administered survey 　• 207 officers • Structured observation 　• 88 ridealongs × 4 hours • Semi-structured interview schedule 　• Administered on ride-alongs
		Use/Behavior • Archival data supplied/generated by VPD 　• Memos from implementation 　• System use data • Exploratory interviews 　• VPD Admin 　• VPD Patrol 　• VPD Dispatchers 　• VPD Technical
		Implications • Other archival/professional literature 　• *The Police Chief* 　• *Sheriff's Star* 　• *Law and Order*

thought it undermined it); and so on. Note, by the way, that the reason these elements were identified is because they were aspects of the system on which there was variability—people had different views about these elements—and the exploratory research had given the research team reason to believe that they were important in understanding overall views of the system.

If you proceed to the next column of Figure 9.2, you'll see that the next step was simply to create items that reflected those various elements—in this case they created what are called **"Likert-type" items**, which involve statements (rather than questions) to which respondents indicate their level of agreement or disagreement.

The eventual survey was completed by more than 200 officers, and the results allowed the research team to report back to both the federal department and the local organization with answers to the questions they had posed. Why? Because each step of the iterative process was connected to the one preceding, which meant that the product at the end of this design process—the very specific and concrete items respondents reacted to—had a very clear and demonstrable connection to the objectives that started it all off.

FIGURE 9.2 ● Development of Items in Survey Construction Process From the VPD/MRDS Study

ATTITUDES	Job Satisfaction	MRDS has had a positive effect on my job satisfaction.
	Effectiveness	I think MRDS helps me be a more effective officer.
		MRDS produces so much information it makes me a less effective officer.
	Safety	I think MRDS makes policing a lot safer.
		MRDS can create a false sense of security with suspects.
	(In)dependence	I find that with MRDS I end up relying on the system more and more.
	Relations with Community	I find I check out a lot more people now than I did before MRDS.
	Overall	Overall I like MRDS.
USE/BEHAVIOR	Ease of data access	With MRDS I get information much more quickly than with radio only. I feel tied to my car with MRDS.
	Frequency of Access	With MRDS I probably investigate cars or people I otherwise wouldn't have bothered with.
	1-person vs. 2-person patrol	MRDS is of less use when I'm on patrol by myself than when I have a partner.
	(Non)Stressful Situations	MRDS is of less use in highly stressful situations.
	MRDS vs. Radio	I would rather work in a radio-only car.
		[Situational scenarios also addressed this element]
IMPLICATIONS	Implications for officers: • Professionalism • Man/Machine • Autonomy/Self-Def'n	[See "attitudes" sections; also arose in more depth interviews; big differences among officers in how they saw themselves and how they related to the machine; some viewed it as a duller of instincts and human connectedness, while others saw it as something that gave them autonomy, control, professionalism]
	Relations within VPD	MRDS makes me more independent of the dispatcher.
	Relations between police and community	Ultimately I think MRDS dehumanizes policing.

As you can see, you need to do much of your thinking *ahead of time* when it comes to designing a questionnaire or structured interview. That includes doing the literature review and exploratory research that will allow you to create an informed and useful research instrument. It's all time well spent because it ensures that your objectives are indeed addressed by the data you gather.

Having gone through these considerations so that we know what content we wish to include, we must next address how to ask those questions. The following section covers some of the variety of alternatives that are available.

Question Structure

The main types of questions are open-ended and closed or structured questions. **Open-ended questions** are those that give the greatest latitude for the respondent to answer. The expected answer might be as little as one word (e.g., Where were you born? What is your occupation?), a phrase, a sentence or two, or as much as paragraphs long. Examples of open-ended questions that call for a bit more than one-word responses might be, "What do you like most about this text?" or "How would you evaluate this course so far?" Even more open-ended might be a simple probe such as, "Tell me how you feel about the course so far."

With **closed or structured questions**, the respondent's options are limited to choosing from among response categories or rating scales that are supplied. Examples of closed questions about the text might include a categorical question like, "Which of the following attributes do you think is most important to include in a textbook: (1) cartoons; (2) examples; (3) citations to the literature; (4) study questions; (5) other. A question that asks for a rating might be, "Please rate this textbook on how useful you find it as a resource for your current research methods course on a 5-point scale running from 1 (not at all useful) to 5 (very useful)."

Open-Ended Questions

Strengths. As with virtually every other method described in this text, it is not possible to say that either open-ended or structured questions are better on some overall basis. We hope you are getting used to the idea that the correct answer to just about any question you ask about methods is "**It depends.**" Your job is to know what it depends on, and how those contingencies relate to different ways of answering your questions, because the advantages and limitations that any given method may have in general may or may not be relevant to the situation you are dealing with right now.

Open-ended questions are clearly superior if you are interested in hearing respondents' opinions in their own words. The words and concepts people use to talk about their lives is often exactly what researchers want to understand. Open-ended questions are also particularly useful in exploratory research where you don't yet know what range of responses can be anticipated. You don't want to ask a question only to discover when you go to analyze the data that the majority of respondents checked off "other."

In exploratory and pilot research for survey design, the responses to an open-ended question can be used to create the alternatives for structured questions in a later study with more focused objectives. This allows you to be guided by people who are similar to those who will be responding to your survey, which in all likelihood will be superior to what you might come up with on your own. Open-ended questions are also useful when you want to determine the salience or importance of opinions to people, since people tend to mention those matters that are most important to them first (see Kahneman, Slovic, & Tversky, 1982). In this sense, open-ended questions can also operate as "indirect" measures, generating answers that are minimally affected by external influence or by suggestion emerging from the structure of the research instrument itself.

Open-ended queries are suitable for larger-scale studies as well. Many respondents appreciate being offered at least a few chances to express matters in their own words; at the very least, a space should be designated at the end for "anything else you would care to add that hasn't been adequately addressed" or "any comments you might care to add about the survey." When interwoven within a structured questionnaire, open-ended items can alleviate the repetitiveness of checkmarks or clicks by providing more reflective moments that often provide a rich source of illustrative vignettes that can be included in a final report. Open-ended responses also can provide material that helps the researcher interpret responses, improve the survey, and/or better understand the limitations of their research.

Finally, open-ended questions are also useful when the choice otherwise would be to offer an extremely long list. There are at least several hundred different occupations, for example; it would be silly to try to compile a huge list of these for respondents and then expect them to hunt through the list for theirs. A far easier alternative is simply to ask "What is your occupation?" or "How would you describe your occupation?"

Limitations. Of course, open-ended questions also have disadvantages. One of the biggest is that you cannot include too many of them in a survey. Respondents have expectations of moving through surveys fairly quickly. If methods have a rhythm, then the rhythm of a survey is a quicker tempo with a solid beat. While the occasional open-ended question may provide a welcome change of pace, too many open-ended questions in a survey will start to feel slow and laborious, where something that was advertised as a questionnaire starts to feel like an essay exam. Unless you show indications you will be moving back to a quicker pace again, respondents will become more and more likely to abandon the questionnaire with each passing question. Robinson and Leonard (2019) suggest this is a good reason for making open-ended survey questions optional as an opportunity for additional comment. That way the participant can embellish if interested or just go on to the next section if they have no more to add.

Another drawback to open-ended questions is that the responses can become incredibly cumbersome for the researcher as your sample size and/or the number of questions increases. How do you *deal* with all these open-ended responses you've gathered? The uniqueness of each person's priorities, views, and means of expression can make it seem that you have as many different categories as you have respondents. Of course what one researcher sees as "laborious" is another researcher's "labor of love" that they can't wait to dive into. As you'll see when we talk about content coding in Chapter 13, coding respondents' open-ended narratives can be a very interesting process but is also a labor-intensive one.

Being able to make comparisons between different people, whether in the content or intensity or priority of the opinion they express, can become more challenging with open-ended responses than it is for closed questions, as we will discuss below. To code open-ended responses properly, content coding schemes must be developed, coders must be trained, and their ability to code reliably should be assessed. Because of these challenges, researchers, especially researchers engaged in studies with larger sample sizes, have tended to rely on more structured response alternatives that come "precoded." It's a much more efficient process. The challenge is to ensure that the structured device does justice to the opinions and feelings that lie behind people's responses.

Closed or Structured Questions

Closed or structured questions have their own advantages and disadvantages, as you might expect. Their biggest advantage is probably their efficiency. If you manage the pacing and look of the survey well, you can ask a *lot* of questions in a relatively short period of time. We will talk about overall design later in the chapter; suffice it to say for now that creating blocks of questions that use a consistent response style and flow smoothly from one subtopic to the next can make even very long surveys seem much shorter than they actually are.

While open-ended questions need to be content coded in order to establish whatever themes or patterns underlie the responses, another advantage of closed items is that they come essentially precoded, with respondents getting the choice of how they would like to categorize themselves. Given that this is ultimately what many researchers do with the raw data that they have anyway, i.e., content code it on dimensions on which respondents can be aggregated, compared, correlated, and so on, then having respondents self-code would seem a win-win as long as we provide them meaningful ways to do so.

Researchers also like closed items because of the standardized structure that ensures all responses follow a standard form (e.g., using the same set of categorical alternatives or the same rating scale), which makes comparability between respondents or groups of respondents easier. It also makes it possible to make a simple summary statement such as "64 percent of males compared to 37 percent of females agreed with the proposal" or that "males gave an average rating of 3.6 while females gave an average of 5.6 on the 7-point scale." Computerized scoring and analysis of data are also made easier. The big trick comes in whether the researcher has done a good job of considering the range of response alternatives that accurately and comprehensively reflect respondents' views.

Many research participants like closed items because they are clear and direct in terms of what information the researcher wants to know, are also clear in terms of what response categories are possible, and for those reasons require less mental energy to complete. Or at least that is true as long as you have designed the survey well, have included questions that are on topic and that make sense to the respondent for you to have asked, and the response alternatives you offer are ones where the respondent can find an alternative that satisfies them. It is also a good reason to always have an "other" category for categorical items to ensure your response options are exhaustive.

Combining Question Types

As you've seen, both closed and open-ended questions have advantages and limitations, and the particular mix you choose to incorporate into your own research will depend on where you are in the research process, the nature of your objectives, who your audience is, whether there is a well-established literature on the topic, and so on. Do you go for *breadth* (lots of questions but relatively superficial responses) or *depth* (fewer questions but more elaborate responses)?

Of course there are no rules that say you cannot have the best of both worlds. Just as mixed-methods research allows you to enjoy how the advantages of one method can overcome the limitations of another and vice versa, combining the structure and efficiency of closed questions with the informational and exploratory benefits of open-ended ones can offer a path to data that answers whatever direct questions you are ready to pose, while simultaneously opening doors to understanding and interpretations you may not yet have considered.

The Variety of Structured Questions

While the previous section discussed open-ended and closed or structured items in general terms, in this section we show you specific item formats you can use for the questions you want to pose.

Single-Response Items

One way to present a structured question is merely to ask it and provide respondents with an empty space in which to write their response. This type of question is called a **single-response item** and is the simplest type of open-ended question. The following three questions are of this type:

> In what year were you born? _____
>
> What was your total family income last year (before taxes)? $_____
>
> What is your official job title in this organization? _____

Each asks the respondent to supply a very specific piece of information.

One problem sometimes associated with this form is that people may be reluctant to provide an exact number or a one-word response, especially to questions about age and income or to those that would seem to warrant more complex responses. Respondents may therefore be more likely to skip the question or to give a simplistic response that doesn't really capture their opinion on an issue. You're left with missing data in the first instance and with incomplete or invalid data in the second. Moreover, if people don't have an exact response readily available (e.g., few people know their total family income down to the last dollar), a false sense of precision may result. The answers may *appear* very precise but may really be just "ballpark" guesses. If people *are* willing and able to provide the information, *single-response* items offer both precision and great flexibility in how responses will be aggregated across participants (e.g., they can be grouped by $5,000 increments, $10,000 increments, etc.). So if you *can* ask a single-response question, do so; if you suspect that people may be unwilling to respond or unable to give precise information, choose a *categorical response item* instead.

Categorical Response Items

Categorical response items refer generally to the closed items that we discussed in the previous section. However, there are many different categorical response item types. The simplest type of categorical question is the **dichotomous item**. As the prefix *di-* suggests, such questions have only two response alternatives. For example, the question, "If a referendum were held tomorrow for the reinstatement of capital punishment, would you vote for or against?" has only two alternatives: for or against. Although there are many "natural" dichotomies (e.g., sex is typically dichotomized into male and female, although this is beginning to change as greater gender diversity becomes recognized and respected), *any* continuum can be dichotomized. Attitudes about the death penalty, for example, can be seen as a continuum ranging from extreme support to complete rejection, or they might be dichotomized, as they were above, into "for" and "against." Whether you use a continuum or dichotomy would depend on your research purpose.

Such reduction inevitably means a loss of information and may distort the phenomenon under consideration. For example, there was considerable discussion in Canada in the 1980s about capital punishment. Ardent supporters of the death penalty unerringly pointed to opinion polls that showed that approximately 75 percent of Canadians expressed support when asked a dichotomous question on the subject. But a more detailed analysis (Palys & Williams, 1983) showed that most proponents were guarded in their enthusiasm, exhibiting considerable ambivalence about the death penalty's prospective application. The media image of Canada's collective run "back to the noose" was anything but accurate. Consistent with Palys and Williams's (1983) analysis, and in contrast to earlier media reports, a proposal on the issue was soundly defeated when it came before Parliament for a vote.

Other categorical items offer more than two categories. Here's an example:

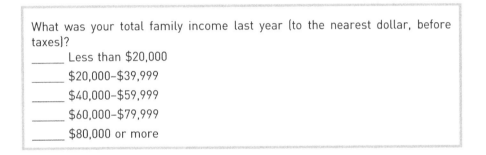

Categorical items offer several advantages. First, respondents often are more willing to place themselves into categories (especially with sensitive topics like income) than they are to give exact responses. Second, accuracy is less likely to be affected by ballpark guesses, since the question itself asks people to place themselves in a ballpark. The main disadvantage with categorical items is that they are considerably less flexible than single-response items; you can always aggregate categories together, but categories can never be taken apart. This problem may not affect a given study, since you choose category intervals appropriate to your particular needs and interests, but you might find it hard to compare the results of different studies (e.g., if you used $15,000 increments to code income, and another study used $20,000 increments).

There are two characteristics of categorical items you should concern yourself with. First, the categories must always be **exhaustive**, that is, they must cover all possible alternatives. Second, for most questions, the categories also should be **mutually exclusive**; there should be no overlap between categories, that is, there should be only *one* category per respondent that is appropriate. In sum, there should be an alternative, but usually only *one* alternative, for everybody. The "income" question we gave you earlier met both of these criteria: no matter what your total family income, there was a category—and only *one* category—into which you could place yourself. But consider the following question:

What was your age in years at your last birthday?

_____ (a) less than 20

_____ (b) 20–30

_____ (c) 30–40

_____ (d) 40–50

_____ (e) 50–60

These categories are *not* mutually exclusive: they overlap. A person who is 30 years old, for example, could legitimately check either "b" or "c." Nor are the categories exhaustive. Which alternative do 65-year-olds choose, for example? There's no place for them. If you understand the notions of exclusivity and exhaustiveness, you should be able to rewrite the question above so that it meets these criteria.

Although categorical questions are ideally always exhaustive, one type of categorical question, the **multiple-response item**, does *not* require the respondent to choose only one alternative. For example, you might ask a question like this one:

Which of the following have you done in the last month? (check all that apply)

____ gone out to dinner at a restaurant

____ seen a film at a cinema

____ seen a play at a theater

____ attended a professional sporting event

____ attended a concert or dance at which live music was played

____ read a book for pleasure

____ gone to an art gallery or museum

As always, the choice of issues to address will reflect your research objectives and/or theoretical curiosities, as will the content and range of alternatives offered. The above example might be appropriate for a marketing questionnaire or for a study of leisure preferences among members of some identified social groups.

A limitation of the response structures described thus far is that they look no further than simple dichotomies (did/did not; true/false; yes/no; no way/way) or category memberships (e.g., is or is not described by a given category). But in most situations, we are interested in embellished *continua* that are *scaled* by gradation.

Rating Scales

A third type of structured question is the *rating scale*, which is extremely pervasive in social and health science research. Several types of rating scales are shown in Figure 9.3 from the "quality of life" literature that focuses on the degree of satisfaction that people have with their lives. The "satisfaction" scale shown here is probably the most commonly used; it supplies verbal labels at either end of the scale, with numbers in between that the respondent would circle depending on the *direction* (or "valence") of their feelings (i.e., satisfied or unsatisfied) and on the *intensity* of those feelings (i.e., the number 7 expresses more intense satisfaction than the number 5).

There are many variations on this type of scale. Figure 9.3 shows a 1-to-7 scale, but there's nothing magical about 7-point scales. It's not unheard of to see 5-point, 10-point, or even 100-point scales. Some scales leave out the numbers entirely and merely present respondents with a line and adjectives or descriptors at the ends; the respondent puts a stroke through the line at whichever point best represents their opinion. "Scores" or "ratings" are produced by measuring the distance from one end of the scale to the place where the stroke intersects. When rating scales are administered through browser-based surveys, the equivalent would be simply to present respondents with a slide bar that allows them to use their mouse or fingertip to drag the slider up and down the bar, positioning it at a point on the continuum that reflects their point of view.

The ladder shown in Figure 9.3(b) is another type of rating scale, first used in an international survey regarding people's evaluations of their quality of life conducted by Hadley Cantril (1965). As a respondent, you first would have been asked to imagine and describe the *worst* possible situation in which you could see yourself. That situation would be considered a "1" on the scale. Next, you'd be asked to imagine and describe the *best* possible situation in which you could imagine yourself, one where all your dreams and aspirations were realized. That situation would be considered a "10." With the scale's ends thus defined, the next question was "Where on the scale would you say you are *right now*?" Cantril's scale is known as a

FIGURE 9.3 ● Three Samples of Rating Scales

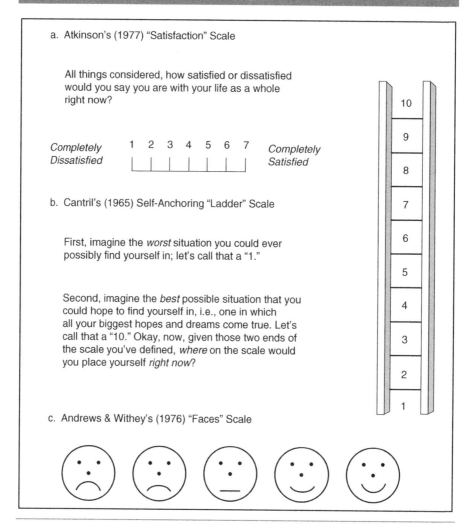

a. Atkinson's (1977) "Satisfaction" Scale

All things considered, how satisfied or dissatisfied would you say you are with your life as a whole right now?

Completely
Dissatisfied
1 2 3 4 5 6 7
Completely
Satisfied

b. Cantril's (1965) Self-Anchoring "Ladder" Scale

First, imagine the *worst* situation you could ever possibly find yourself in; let's call that a "1."

Second, imagine the *best* possible situation that you could hope to find yourself in, i.e., one in which all your biggest hopes and dreams come true. Let's call that a "10." Okay, now, given those two ends of the scale you've defined, *where* on the scale would you place yourself *right now*?

c. Andrews & Withey's (1976) "Faces" Scale

self-anchoring scale, since the end points are personally defined (i.e., your best aspirations and worst fears will undoubtedly be different from those of others).

A final example of a rating scale is the "faces" scale shown in Figure 9.3(c). Visual aids like these are particularly useful when dealing with children or with others whose literacy level might be questionable. The respondent is directed to "pick the face that best illustrates how you feel" about the attitude object in question; this scale is useful when the ratings being made are on a like-dislike or happy-sad type of continuum.

Note, however, that people other than young children may find the use of such a scale somewhat condescending.

And of course all of the examples shown in Figure 9.3 are very static, as they would be in any paper-based survey. The same questions and scales in any digitized context can be made more colorful and dynamic, e.g., by asking the respondent to move their finger up the ladder to indicate where they are on the scale or to adjust the smile on the faces so that it reflects their own like or dislike about whatever is being asked about.

Likert-Type Items

The fourth type of structured item is known as a "*Likert-type*" questionnaire item because its format is of the type included in an attitude scale developed originally by Rensis Likert (1932). Two attributes distinguish a "Likert-type" item. First, the item is a statement (rather than a question). Second, the respondent's task is to indicate the extent to which they agree or disagree with the statement. Typically, if **Likert-type items** are used, a number of them are given in succession on a questionnaire. Once respondents get used to using the agree-disagree format, which happens very quickly, they can go through many items quite quickly. The following is an example of a "Likert-type" item:

All things considered, I think we need more laws that restrict the availability of guns.

_____ disagree strongly

_____ disagree somewhat

_____ neither agree nor disagree

_____ agree somewhat

_____ agree strongly

The Likert-type item is useful if, instead of being interested in hearing the respondent's position in their own words, you're interested in the extent to which a person agrees or disagrees with a position you have formulated, or that has been asserted in the media, or that other sources of interest to you have expressed. In other circumstances—in an interview study or in a survey that is more of an exploratory venture, for example—a researcher might want to ask an open-ended question in order to have respondents explain their views. In a more structured survey, an item like the example above might be used simply to get a "bottom line" position, to see whether and to what extent the respondent will agree or disagree. Often this will be done because the researcher is interested in correlating views on one item with responses to other questions included in the survey. To continue our example, agreement or disagreement with an item about gun laws might be correlated with responses to questions dealing with positions on other social issues, support for different politicians or political parties, beliefs about the causes of violence, gun ownership, and so on. Doing so allows you to understand better the logic or belief system that underlies different positions or to distinguish between people who hold similar positions for different reasons.

Using Multiple Items to Create Scales

The reason we refer to items with the format above as "Likert-type" items rather than simply as "Likert" items is to distinguish single items that happen to follow the Likert format from the scaling procedures Likert made famous and are still used. His procedure is built on the idea that many items could be used in combination to create a more reliable measure than any single item can provide. It is not at all uncommon for survey researchers to include specific scales within their surveys if they are particularly interested in establishing a more valid and reliable measure of some core construct rather than leaving it to one single item.

As one example, we note there are a variety of "social desirability" scales available that allow researchers to assess the extent to which individuals will go out of their way to present themselves in a positive light. If your survey happens to deal with issues where some responses are more socially desirable than others or that asks respondents to talk about negative or stigmatizing behaviors they engage in, it might be desirable to include an independent assessment of how prone each respondent is to portraying themselves in a positive light. The Marlowe-Crowne Social Desirability Scale lists 33 different statements about personal behaviors that have a social desirability element to them, whether positively or negatively (see Crowne & Marlowe, 1960). Table 9.2 shows six items from the Marlowe-Crowne scale, three positively worded and three worded in the opposite direction. Respondents are supposed to indicate whether each statement applies to them ("True") or not ("False").

The "positively" worded items are considered so because the "socially desirable" response would be to agree with the item. The "negatively" worded items are considered that because *disagreement* with the statement would be the socially desirable response. If you were to say "true" to the positively worded items and "false" to the negatively worded items in Table 9.2, you would have 6 points toward your score on the scale. "But hey," you say, "I'm a nice person and I really do believe that I

TABLE 9.2 ● Six Items From the Marlowe-Crowne Social Desirability Scale	
Positively Worded Items	**Negatively Worded Items**
I never hesitate to go out of my way to help someone in trouble	I like to gossip at times
No matter who I'm talking to I'm always a good listener	I can remember "playing sick" to get out of something
I am always courteous, even to people who are disagreeable	I am sometimes irritated by people who ask favors of me

help people when I see they are in trouble. I said that because it's really true, not because I'm trying to impress you or look good!" That may well be the case. The scale is built on the notion that we all have positive and negative qualities, and there no doubt will be "socially desirable" responses you agree with because most of us are decent human beings who care about the world and people around us. The scale is used to identify people who go far beyond the norm, who are always or nearly always picking the "look good" response across the 33-item scale. The assumption here is that scorers at the extreme are either next in line for sainthood or are too good to be true, with the latter being the more likely alternative.

Hundreds of different types of scales have been developed over the years to assess a variety of attitudes, personality types, aptitudes and interests, and behavioral propensities, many of which find their way into surveys when they are a core concept in the research and the researcher wants a more reliable and valid measure of some concept than any single item or question can give.

Semantic Differential–Type Items

Another type of questionnaire item is the **semantic differential–type item**. As was the case with Likert, the designation of it as a "type" is meant to distinguish the general format of the items—which we offer here—from the original semantic differential scale, which has a very specific form and purpose. In this case the scale was developed by Osgood, Suci, and Tannenbaum (1957). Devised to assess the *meaning* associated with particular attitude objects, it involved a set of bipolar adjectives (or dimensions) upon which any given attitude object could be described. For example, you might see the words "this textbook" (or some other object of assessment) printed at the top of the page, and your task would be to rate "this textbook" on a list of bipolar adjectives such as those shown in Figure 9.4.

FIGURE 9.4 ● Items From the Original Semantic Differential

Please rate this textbook on the following dimensions:

Fair	: ___:___:___:___:___:___:	Unfair
Good	: ___:___:___:___:___:___:	Bad
Heavy	: ___:___:___:___:___:___:	Light
Fast	: ___:___:___:___:___:___:	Slow
Hot	: ___:___:___:___:___:___:	Cold

Although the original semantic differential still sees occasional use in attitude research, it's more typical to see its influence in the semantic differential–type response format. Respondents are asked to express their attitudes or feelings by providing ratings with respect to bipolar scales (i.e., opposing concepts, words, or phrases), where the two poles of the continuum are separated by some odd number of spaces (usually, but not necessarily, 5 or 7) separated by colons. Browser-based surveys also can be constructed in that way or as a series of sliding response scales.

For example, let's say we are interested in obtaining your evaluation of your local medical clinic. Instead of using the semantic differential (with its given adjectival pairs), we might decide to adapt the format to more relevant dimensions by asking you to rate the service provided by the medical staff at your local medical clinic on the dimensions depicted in Figure 9.5. Note that you can use any opposing words, phrases, or other concepts that are of interest. Note also that the presentation of dimensions has been varied (i.e., the continuum's "good" end is sometimes on the left, other times on the right) in order to inhibit response sets, where people get into a groove of positive or negative responding and start to pay less attention to the content of the items.

Some Advice About Response Categories

Although sometimes it seems most of our attention in survey construction focuses on the questions we ask, survey researchers are equally concerned about the response options we give our participants. Several issues dominate the discussion (see Robinson & Leonard, 2019 for an excellent chapter on response categories that goes beyond the dimensions we discuss here).

FIGURE 9.5 ● Items in the Adapted Semantic Differential

Please evaluate the level of service you receive from the medical staff at Everyperson's Medical Clinic on the following dimensions:		
Friendly	: ___:___:___:___:___:___:	Unfriendly
Efficient	: ___:___:___:___:___:___:	Inefficient
Can never get a quick appointment for urgent matters	: ___:___:___:___:___:___:	They always find a way to fit you in
Always in too much of a rush	: ___:___:___:___:___:___:	Always have time to talk and ask questions

---

How Many Categories?. Although this question has been debated for decades, there is really no other answer than "it depends." We do know that the number of response alternatives needs to be smaller when doing telephone surveys where the respondent has to keep all the alternatives in their head while the question is being read to them until they respond. With self-administered questionnaires and network-administered surveys where the text is visible in front of them, more alternatives can be offered.

The types of questions we are thinking of here are ones where respondents are asked to indicate their level of agreement or disagreement (Likert-type items), how frequently they engage in some behavior (e.g., once per day, a few times a week), and any other rating scales where verbal labels are given (e.g., degree of satisfaction, level of comfort, expressions of quantity). To take Likert-type items as an example, how many scale points should respondents be offered to express their level of agreement or disagreement with a statement? In this case, agreement-disagreement is a bipolar scale that makes sense to have a "neutral" or "neither one nor the other" option in the middle, ensuring it will have an odd number of response categories. But how many? 3? 5? 7? 21?

This is considered a question of **granularity**, and the Goldilocks solution—not too many and not too few—is what you are looking for. If you have too few categories, respondents are unable to make the sort of distinctions they would like to make. Dichotomous items, although useful in some circumstances, often limit how much we can say about a variable. But if you go to the other extreme and offer too many categories, respondents can no longer make the distinctions at the level of granularity you are presenting to them. When that happens people start "ballparking" it, which creates more sloppiness in the numbers and lower reliability of scores, i.e., something you would prefer to avoid. With respect to Likert items, the favored number among experienced survey researchers going back decades seems to be either 5 or 7. Most researchers agree there is little to be gained beyond 9 (Robinson & Leonard, 2019).

Response Symmetry. One of the things you are always trying to avoid in any survey is any appearance of bias in the types of responses you expect. Regardless of the number of response categories you offer respondents, in most cases researchers should strive for **response symmetry** as part of that effort to avoid the appearance of bias. Robinson and Leonard offer the example shown in Figure 9.6 from a client survey an airline might use.

Note how the response scale for the first two items are not in balance—there are three positive points (excellent, very good, and good) and only two more negative ones (fair, poor). This is what a response scale looks like when the authors of the scale are trying to push you in a positive direction. Notice also how the word at the positive end of the scale is very positive—"excellent"—while the label at the opposite end is not equally negative. Robinson and Leonard (2019) suggest a better balanced scale would feature the following alternatives: excellent, very good, average, poor, terrible.

As a contrast, note how the response scale for the second two questions is balanced. The two polar ends are mirror images of each other, one positive ("will") and one negative ("will not"). And there are two positive alternatives and two negative ones with a clearly neutral alternative in the middle.

FIGURE 9.6 ● Balanced and Unbalanced Response Options

Based on this flight, please rate this Airline on the following scale:					
	Excellent	Very Good	Good	Fair	Poor
Overall experience with this flight:	o	o	o	o	o
Value for fare paid:	o	o	o	o	o

How likely are you to:					
	Definitely will	Probably will	May or may not	Probably will not	Definitely will not
Recommend this airline to others:	o	o	o	o	o
Fly with this airline again:	o	o	o	o	o

Source: Robinson and Leonard (2019, Figure 5.3).

Did Somebody Change the Topic?. A final admonition we will include about response categories is how important it is for the labels for the various responses to reflect the categories that are contained in or implied by the question. The example in Figure 9.7 is taken from an actual survey by a major retail chain.

Note how the question asks about how "satisfied" the respondent is, while only one of the five alternatives focuses on satisfaction as a response. A better set of five categories might have gone from "Completely satisfied" to "Completely dissatisfied," with a neutral midpoint that said something like, "Neither satisfied nor dissatisfied."

Another place you see mismatched questions and response categories is when the survey designer decides to use one set of response categories across a large number of items. Sometimes doing so is more efficient by giving the respondent a consistent format. Other times it can be frustrating when the labels have at best a tangential relationship to what is supposedly being asked. Robinson and Leonard (2019) found the example in Figure 9.8 in a doctor's office follow-up survey.

This survey is so bad in so many different ways that Robinson and Leonard (2019) actually use it as a study exercise at the end of their chapter on response categories, as will we. For now, let us just point out how the response categories bear no connection whatsoever to the questions being asked. Many of the questions call for a yes/no response—e.g., "Were you greeted with a smile?—rather than a scale. Others are a mystery as to what they are asking in the first place. For example, after asking one question about rating the quality of care—one of the few questions where the response scale actually fits the question—respondents are asked to rate their "total visit time"? Is this asking about the duration of the appointment? Or the Muzak playing over the sound system? Or the quality of toilet paper in the washrooms? Presumably it is asking about all those things, but why? How is it in any sense informative for a physician who presumably is offering the survey to improve the quality of their clients' experience? By the time you get to the end of this chapter, you should be able to do a new version of this survey that actually makes sense.

FIGURE 9.7 ● Mismatched Question and Response Categories

Overall, how satisfied were you with the purchases you made today?				
Very Poor	Poor	Satisfactory	Good	Excellent
○	○	○	○	○

FIGURE 9.8 ● Mismatched Questions and Response Categories From a Doctor's Office Follow-Up Survey

Was the (health care facility name) staff friendly, knowledgeable, and helpful?	Excellent	Good	Fair	Poor	N/A
Front desk/reception	○	○	○	○	○
Technologist	○	○	○	○	○
Medical assistant	○	○	○	○	○
Were you able to make an appointment quickly and easily?	○	○	○	○	○
Were you greeted with a smile?	○	○	○	○	○
Upon arrival, was the registration quick and efficient?	○	○	○	○	○
How thoroughly was your procedure explained to you?	○	○	○	○	○
Do you feel your exam was performed professionally?	○	○	○	○	○
If you meet with a physician, was she/he polite and informative?	○	○	○	○	○
How would you rate the comfort and cleanliness of our facility?	○	○	○	○	○
Overall, how would you rate the quality of care you received?	○	○	○	○	○
How would you rate your total visit time?	○	○	○	○	○

Source: Robinson and Leonard (2019, p. 131).

Question Wording

Thus far, the discussion has emphasized determining both the general content and the structure of the questions. Another important aspect of the questionnaire (or interview) is the actual wording of the questions (e.g., see Bernard, 2013; Gray, 2014; Robinson & Leonard, 2019; Sudman & Bradburn, 1982).

A Rose by Any Other Name

One famous anecdote—so famous that its origins are now unknown—tells the story of two priests who argue about whether it is appropriate for someone to be smoking a cigarette and praying at the same time. No resolution is found, but the two clergymen agree that each will go and ask his respective Bishop for the "official" answer. The two go away and meet the next week and, to their surprise, find that they had received exact opposite answers from their respective Bishops. "But what did you ask?" queries each to the other. The first says, "I just asked, 'Is it acceptable to smoke while praying?' to which my Bishop said 'no' most emphatically and went on to give me a lecture about how sacrilegious it would be to sully such a sacred act with a cigarette." "Ah," said the other. "That explains it. What I asked my Bishop was, 'Is it acceptable to pray while smoking?' to which he replied, 'There is never an unacceptable time to pray.'"

The anecdote suggests that what can appear on the surface to be very minor changes in wording can have very big effects in terms of the results that are observed. But are real survey results so fragile? Researcher Donald Rugg (1941) originally posed this question many decades ago by asking another—Is there any difference to you between "forbidding" something and "not allowing" it? He went on to test this in a survey by asking the following two questions of two comparable national samples of respondents:

> Do you think the United States should forbid public speeches against democracy?
> Do you think the United States should allow public speeches against democracy?

The two questions seem to be addressing essentially the same thing, but one is positively worded and the other negatively worded. The percentage of people who *agree* with one item ought to be roughly equal to the number who *dis*agree with the other. That is, if 30 percent of the people say "yes" to the first item (that the United States should *forbid* such speeches), a similar percentage should say "no" to the second item (indicating that the United States should *not allow* them).

But in fact, while 54 percent said that the United States should *forbid* such speeches, a full 75 percent said that they should *not be allowed*. In hindsight, perhaps we can think about the two words and make some distinction between them, but who could have predicted such huge variation on the basis of what still seems little more than a difference of nuance? A swing of 21 percent on the basis of a small shift in wording makes any of the statements we always see about the sampling error's being "plus or minus 2.5 percent, 19 times out of 20" seem downright trivial, if not misleading. If such enormous swings can occur because of relatively small wording changes, then perhaps *wording* is the more important issue to attend to.

One of the few studies to directly and comprehensively look at the effects of variation in question wording was by Schuman and Presser (1981), who went beyond single examples like "forbid versus allow" to ask broader questions about general types of wording shifts. For example, the forbid/allow variant is subsumed under the general category "changes in the tone of the wording." Their general finding, consistent with the forbid/allow example, is that small differences in wording can produce substantial swings in results. Ironically, however, and contrary to the common wisdom, the most blatant examples of biased wording were the *least* effective in influencing results. Schuman and Presser explain that "respondents seem to recognize and discount the more obvious instances of bias."

The authors note that one implication of this finding is that when researchers want to examine changes in attitudes over time by comparing newly acquired data to old, it's very important to replicate the original wording exactly. For example, when they replicated the forbid/allow experiment almost 40 years after Rugg's (1941) study—they found the same 20 percent difference between the two different wordings. But when they compared the results of the two *matched* sets of wordings (i.e., comparing the 1941 "forbid" data to the 1981 "forbid" data, and the 1941 "allow" data to their 1981 "allow" data), each matched set revealed about a 30 percent change in the direction of a more tolerant response. The importance of keeping wording constant is made clear, though, when we consider what conclusions would have resulted had *mismatched* wordings been used:

The two possible *mismatched* replications of the question (comparing 1940 data from the "forbid" version to mid-1970s data from the "allow" version, and vice-versa) would yield two very different results: evidence of either a slight (less than 10 percent) increase in tolerance, or a whopping increase of 50 percent. (p. 2)

Clearly, then, question wording must be kept identical if you want to compare the results of two or more surveys. If a change of wording is necessary for some reason, you should include both wordings on at least one occasion, so that an explicit comparison can be made that will allow an assessment of the effect of the wording change.

Sample-Appropriate Wording

We've already mentioned that keeping your prospective research participants in mind is crucial when designing your survey. Age and education level are two important considerations, for example. A vocabulary that is appropriate for your university endeavors may not be a language that your respondents understand. The challenge to communicate effectively is yours.

You should be sensitive to local jargon and be able to use terms that have well-defined local meanings. For example, if doing research in a prison, instead of referring to "a prisoner who shares information with prison authorities," it would probably be appropriate simply to use the term "rat." Another technique involves first asking the people you interview what word *they* prefer to use for a given thing or behavior. In a survey on sexual behavior, you might begin by asking respondents what words they use to refer to two people engaging in sexual intercourse. If a respondent says "make love," you would then use that phrase in any question about that behavior: "Do you think it is acceptable for two people to make love on their first date together?" This is a place where the adaptive questioning that is possible in network-administered research can be very helpful. To continue the above example regarding sexual behavior, if the person responds that "make love" is the phrase they use to describe sexual intercourse, then that phrase can be programmed to appear in the remainder of the survey whenever a question includes reference to that behavior.

And finally, given the diverse multicultural makeup of North American culture, it is important to ensure you have adequate cultural information to create a survey that takes different languages and sensibilities into account. Robinson and Leonard (2019) discuss the issue as a matter of "cultural competence"—a skill that would-be researchers need to learn as much as how to build rapport, identify an appropriate sample, or implement an experimental design. The authors pose the challenge thus:

> *Cultural competence is about the ability to work across cultures. It's about conducting research in a manner that is respectful and responsive to all people, allowing us to understand, relate to, and learn from those involved. Cultural responsiveness extends the concept of competence, calling for researchers to adapt and respond appropriately to a given culture and context, effectively customizing their efforts. (p. 53)*

There are many dimensions to cultural competence that go beyond simply making the survey available in another language. It means being attuned to differences in power and avoiding comparisons that normalize one culture as the standard by which others are measured. It means paying attention to how and with whom any measurement scales have been validated and to understand that a scale validated with one group does not necessarily mean it will be valid with another. It also means understanding the other language well enough to go beyond the Google Translate version of a translation to understand its colloquialisms, sensitivities, and taboos.

Avoiding Ambiguity

Watch for ambiguities in the terms you use. Even though *you* may know what you mean, you must ensure that you and the respondent are talking about the same thing.

If we ask people whether they go skiing or have a drink "often," for example, "often" may well have different meanings for different people, or even for the same people for different behaviors. There are many other examples of ambiguous concepts. A question about "drug use," for example, is highly ambiguous. Do you mean Aspirin? Alcohol? Prescription drugs? Marijuana? Heroin? You must be very specific, or at least ensure that you and the respondent are on the same wavelength by, perhaps, describing what you are trying to find out about in a preamble. With network-administered surveys it is possible to indicate what a specific word or phrase means by highlighting the word as a link so that when the respondent rolls their mouse pointer over the word, a pop-up dialog box appears displaying the full definition. These issues are more problematic in a questionnaire than in an interview, since interviews allow for some clarification of ambiguities (assuming you catch them); in a questionnaire, they simply produce unreliability and inconsistency in responses.

Meaningless Responses

Avoid questions that can be answered by the respondent without any knowledge about the topic. For example, consider "Do you agree with the President's new foreign policy initiatives?" This question could be answered by someone who doesn't know who the President is, let alone anything about their foreign policy initiatives. Rubenstein (1995) reports that when surveys include questions that ask respondents to express their opinion on nonexistent laws (e.g., a nonexistent *Public Affairs Act*), 25–35 percent express an opinion anyway, while the rest (65–75 percent) will volunteer that they have never heard of the Act or say they have no opinion on it.

A good way to minimize the chances that a respondent answers a question on a topic they have no knowledge about is to simply include a preliminary question asking them if they are aware of the President's new foreign policy initiative (to continue the example above) or if they know enough about it to answer a few questions about it. If they are, you can then ask them how they feel about it; if they are not, you can have them skip to the next question. Of course in network-administered surveys, the skipping is done for the respondent and they will never see questions that do not apply to them.

Double-Barreled Items

Avoid **double-barreled items**, that is, two questions in one. For example, the question "Would you be upset if you found out that your 18-year-old son or daughter was smoking and selling marijuana?" is really asking about four things: smoking and selling and sons and daughters. The respondent might not feel the same way about all parts of the question. Low reliability of responding is the result as people pay more or less attention to one or the other alternative depending on how they are reading the question or what referent they have in mind on any given day.

Acronyms

Don't assume that people know acronyms, unless you're dealing with a very specialized audience and have done the preliminary exploratory work that allows you to feel confident that "everyone" in the setting is familiar with them. Otherwise, you should generally avoid questions like "What's your SSN?" or "Do you know anyone at LAPD?" or "Which of the following would you rather work for: HEW, NIH, the NIJ, or the AG's office?" Although this is a rather blatant example, the central message is simply to watch what you take for granted.

Survey Look, Organization, and Flow

So far, we've concentrated on the discrete elements of surveys and questionnaires: choosing content, considering different ways to word and structure individual questions. Now it's time to consider the research instrument as a whole. How do you put a sizable number of these individual questions together in a way that will make the experience of completing the survey as enjoyable and free of frustration as possible for respondents, while ensuring that your own objectives as a researcher—to maximize response rates, minimize error, and obtain candid responses—are also met?

For the most part, matters of general organization are similar in the preparation of both survey questionnaires and interviews, but some elements are also unique. In the discussion below, we focus primarily on questions of general organization that are applicable for surveys in keeping with the focus of this chapter.

Aesthetic Appeal

Many texts emphasize the creation of a questionnaire that is aesthetically inviting and easy to follow (e.g., Gray & Guppy, 1994), although most books that deal with aesthetics cite the extensive work on this topic by Don Dillman and his colleagues at the Washington State University survey research center (e.g., see Dillman, Smyth, & Christian, 2014). The general impression given by this literature is that if a questionnaire looks pretty and professional, is well laid out and easy to follow, doesn't include too many open-ended questions, and doesn't seem too big, you'll increase the likelihood of snagging a respondent. That view may be overly simplistic, but certainly if the converse is true—if your questionnaire is *not* well laid out, seems difficult to follow, has too many open-ended questions, and is big enough that it looks like it will take a sizable chunk of time to complete—only the most motivated of respondents will complete the questionnaire, and your response rates will suffer.

Dillman's research into the issue even gets down to the question of what color of paper to use—he recommends white—and that paper-and-pencil versions of a survey should be in booklet form on one side of the paper with nothing on the cover but an engaging title, the name of the survey's sponsor, and an "eye-catching" graphic design or photo that conveys something about the focus of the survey but does so in a very neutral way. He also advises that mailed surveys should never exceed 12 pages and 125 questions, noting that response rates start to drop dramatically after that point. For further advice, see Dillman et al. (2014), Bernard (2013), or Robinson and Leonard (2019).

A Formal Introduction

Your first task in a questionnaire should always be to introduce yourself with a brief statement about who you are and the purpose of your study. Any promises you're prepared to make—e.g., that a brief summary of results will be sent to participants following completion of the study if they're interested—also should be made here. In the case of a questionnaire, respondents should be told whether they should identify themselves or complete it anonymously. If respondents are identifiable either because you are compiling names or the amount or type of information you have might render them identifiable even without their names attached, you should specify clearly what steps you will take to safeguard their confidentiality. This all can be accomplished in a few sentences or a short paragraph, for example,

My name is Pat Wallace, and I'm a graduate student in sociology at State University. This questionnaire is part of my master's thesis, which deals with how different parents teach "appropriate behavior" to their children, so it includes a number of questions that ask about your parenting practices. The whole thing should take no more than about 20 minutes to complete. I hope you'll answer all the questions, but feel free to leave out any that you feel uncomfortable about. Finally, please note that responses to this questionnaire are intended to be anonymous. If you'd like to receive a brief summary of the results of the study after it is completed, please fill out the small card at the end of the questionnaire and submit it separately from your completed questionnaire. Thank you very much for agreeing to participate.

Notice how ethics-relevant statements are included here as well. In this example, prospective participants are told that the survey is being done anonymously, but that is not always the case. Three such situations come to mind. If you are doing a longitudinal study where you are hoping to interview the same people again at a future date, then you will need to include an identifier that will allow you to link successive surveys from the same people together. It could be their names, some other identifier such as a social security or student number, or a unique code that you create with your participants using bits of information only they would know. A second situation is where you are taking a mixed-method approach and want to give people the opportunity to be interviewed at greater depth, in which case you will need to identify them and/or get some contact information that will allow you to schedule the interview. The third situation is where you have so much data on people that even though it is "anonymous" in the sense that no names are given, the sheer volume of information you have may make them identifiable. In any of these cases, you would want people to be assured that they could never be identified and would explain the steps you were taking to ensure that was the case.

Getting to Know You

After the basic introduction, the first topic that's asked about is often relatively trite and superficial, devoted to acquiring preliminary information, for example, to ensure that the respondent is an eligible participant in the study and perhaps to ask about a few demographic details. There is actually some division of opinion with respect to demographics and where they should be located. Survey researchers like Dillman et al. (2014) suggest that your first questions should be nonthreatening, lightweight in content, but clearly connected to what you told the participants the survey was about. Perhaps because so many of us have been asked if we would take part in a survey for one purpose only to find out that the "real" purpose was to sell us a holiday or ask us to buy a membership in something, most survey researchers would suggest you get immediately into content questions that show the survey is about what you said it would be about and move on from there.

There is an argument to be made for locating some more demographic items early in the survey, however, particularly with online surveys. Two questions you often need to address in survey research, especially when the sample surveyed is intended to be a representative sample of your population of interest, are as follows: (1) who is your sample relative to the population from which they were drawn; and (2) of those who volunteered to participate, who actually completed the survey? Asking some demographic questions at the beginning can help you address both questions. If you have information about the population as a whole, then including demographic information in the survey allows you to compare your sample to the population, but that information could be anywhere in the survey. The way demographic information at the front end of the survey is most helpful is that it allows you to have an answer to the second question—who started the survey but dropped out, and are those who finished any different from those who started it?

Three concerns about including demographics at the beginning are as follows: (1) respondents may wonder why you are asking questions that are not on the topic you advertised and instead seem to be focusing on other details about them; (2) after just telling them that the survey was anonymous, respondents may wonder why are you asking questions that seemingly could be used to identify them; and (3) demographic questions can be very personal—especially if you are asking about "touchy" topics like income and age—and respondents may be more likely to leave those items blank at the beginning of the questionnaire than nearer the end, after they have already shared all sorts of information about themselves.

Clearly this is a situation where there are trade-offs in either direction so you will need to decide on the basis of your topic, your respondent population, and your own empirical needs on how to balance those concerns. Keep in mind that it need not be thought of as an all-or-none choice. A third option is to include some demographics earlier in the survey that are most essential for identifying any sample biases, while leaving more personal items until later in the survey. For example, in the study we've mentioned that Ted did regarding the computerized information system in patrol cars, some of the information he had about the population as a whole was the rank structure of the department and how long officers had been with the department. Questions about where they fit on these dimensions could well be asked early on both because they "make sense" to ask in a survey dealing with their on-the-job experience and, generally speaking, are not very "personal." We say "generally speaking" because occasions may arise where that would be problematic, which you need to recognize. For example, if there is only one recently promoted Inspector who has been with the department for less than a year, then asking about rank and time in the department would make that individual's data identifiable, so you will want to be extra careful about how you report that person's responses.

Anticipating a Conversation

Beyond the first impression, your next challenge is to organize the questionnaire and its constituent parts so that it follows a logical sequence and, ideally, reflects and anticipates a social conversation. Numerous principles can be used to guide the sequencing of questions. If a chronological sequence is involved in the phenomenon being addressed (e.g., the way information is processed in an organization, the development of a romantic relationship from first date to some state of mutual commitment, questions on child rearing that ask about sequential stages of child development), the questionnaire's sections can follow that chronology. Alternatively, questions can be arranged by topic, grouping together the ones that are thematically related, from general to specific, from most important to least important, and/or from least threatening to most threatening (Bernard, 2013; Robinson & Leonard, 2019).

The big trick with creating a questionnaire is to try to organize it in a way that mirrors a conversation you might have with a respondent, preferably with an emphasis on the way the respondent would probably organize things, and not your anticipated analysis or the way you think about the phenomenon. Data can always be reorganized when you start your analysis. Too many novice researchers let their perspective and interests dominate the questionnaire, instead of putting their own structures "on hold" and letting the respondent's schema organize the show. Of course, you'll want to ensure that all the questions that are important to you are addressed. But the order in which they are addressed should be governed by the respondent's convenience, not yours. Remember, it's not about you.

The same is true of the interview, of course, but the very nature of the interview means that you can adapt somewhat to the unique social dynamic that arises with each respondent; in contrast, once the questionnaire is photocopied, you're stuck with the standardized setup you've created. Network-administered surveys allow more opportunity to change after the fact. Preliminary exploratory work, through exploratory interviews, and/or focus group discussions can play a crucial role in helping us know how best to organize our research instruments, and a pilot study that includes pretesting or cognitive interviews of the research instrument with a sample similar to the one that will be involved in the research is invaluable.

Respondents also benefit when we give them signposts that tell them what we are doing and what will happen next, so it helps with the flow of the survey to present questions in thematic blocks and provide an ongoing roadmap by introducing each section (e.g., "First I need to ask just a few general questions so that we have a record of how many children you have and how long you've been a parent"). The same is true at the end of each section, both to keep the respondent informed and to provide a bit of a mental break before digging into the next thematic block. For example, a transition might be "That completes the first section regarding some of your early experiences as a parent; now we'd like to ask a few questions on how you handle different kinds of situations that can arise with young children."

Loose Ends and the Final Word

The final section of the questionnaire should tie up loose ends and leave some positive resolution. For example, the final section often will include whatever **demographic items** you did not ask earlier that would be useful to describe your sample and perhaps engage in subgroup analyses. Introducing it in exactly that way—that you are not interested in identifying people but merely wish to have some information to be able to convey who participated—is nonthreatening and understandable at that point in the questionnaire.

You also should endeavor to leave respondents with a good taste in their mouths. Every survey should conclude with a "thank you" and a final question that asks whether they have anything they wish to add to their responses or further comments to make about any aspect of the survey.

Pilot Studies and Cognitive Interviews

Once you've created your survey and revised it to a point you feel happy with, you should always do a brief **pilot study** or trial run before administering your survey "for real." There are always things you take for granted without recognizing, and there are always surprises you never even considered when constructing the questionnaire. The time to catch these difficulties is before you commit major resources to duplicating the questionnaire or go "live" with a network survey. Focus groups (discussed in Chapter 10) can be ideal venues for piloting a questionnaire.

One form of preliminary testing that seems particularly useful and offers yet another example of how mixed methods can complement one another is **cognitive interviewing** (e.g., Beatty & Willis, 2007; French, Cooke, McLean, Williams, & Sutton, 2007), otherwise known as the **think-aloud interview** (e.g., Bernard, 2013; Dillman, 2009). The technique involves asking a sample of people who are similar to those you intend to sample to go through your survey and read each question aloud and then literally to think out loud as they decide how they would respond to each item. To illustrate the process, when Dillman and his colleagues (Dillman, Smyth, & Christian, 2009) asked the question, "How many windows are in your house?," they found that different questions would come up as people tried to figure out an answer, like whether a sliding glass patio door counted as a door or a window. In contrast, when asked how many residences people had lived in their lifetime, people would use different strategies to come up with the answer—some would count the cities they lived in while others would count individual residences—but seemed to understand the question in much the same way and as the researchers intended. Although a trivial example, using that process can highlight where ambiguities exist in question wording, where wording can be sharpened to get more clearly at whatever your interest is and which questions are simply confusing and need a more complete overhaul.

As an example of the latter, French et al. (2007) included a partial transcript of a respondent who was looking at a negatively worded Likert-type item, which meant, as you know, that their task was to indicate how much they agreed or disagreed with each statement. The survey dealt with different aspects of physical activity and exercise and one item read, "Most people whose views I value would disapprove if I was more physically active in the next 12 months," to which one think-aloud interviewee responded,

> *Well they wouldn't disapprove so no, I disagree. Hang on. Do I disagree or am I agreeing? Hang on. Most people whose views I value would disapprove if I was more physically active in the next … I'd agree. Yes. They would … No. They wouldn't disapprove. Sorry. I've got myself confused now! You're right. They would disapprove. No. They wouldn't! God. What have I done? (p. 675)*

Clearly this is an item that needs to be reworked, though we note the problem it highlights—how to respond on an agree-disagree scale to negatively worded items—has been found to be a significant problem with Likert-type items generally (e.g., see Altemeyer, 1970, 1981).

The cognitive interview is also an appropriate technique to address one of the challenges we identified earlier, i.e., developing cross-cultural competence. Willis and Miller (2011) argue that doing cognitive interviews with participants who represent the range of cultures you intend to include in your eventual survey sample is an excellent way to ensure not only that questions are all understood by participants from different cultural backgrounds but also that the meaning and appropriateness of the questions is constant across groups.

Finally, Reeve et al. (2011) undertook a study in which they did cognitive interviewing with a multicultural sample regarding a 9-item scale designed to measure "everyday discrimination." An interesting twist was that they were able to compare the results they obtained via cognitive interviewing with the results of a psychometric analysis of the same scale that had been done with a national sample of more than 3,000 people who had self-identified as Asian American, Hispanic or Latino, Black or African American, American Indian/Alaska Native, or non-Hispanic white. Part of what made the study so interesting was that although the researchers recognized that the two forms of analysis produce very different products—cognitive interviewing produces verbal transcripts about how participants perceive items while psychometric analysis produces quantitative measures of psychometric quality—they conclude that the two sets also complement one another very well, with the qualitative think-aloud data being helpful in explaining why the psychometric measures turned out as they did.

THE MEANING OF SELF-REPORTS

The techniques described in this chapter reflect social and health scientists' desires to systematically unearth people's perceptions via self-report. Whether our items are open-ended or structured, at the heart of our efforts is the goal of acquiring whatever information people will tell us about their thoughts, feelings, beliefs, attitudes, opinions, or behaviors. Once we have our data, the temptation is to feel that we have unearthed some inherent truth(s). And perhaps we have.

And yet, self-report techniques are but one method and represent but one way of engaging truth(s). We must therefore try to contextualize these truths as we would any others. What exactly do we have when a respondent places a checkmark on a rating scale, answers "yes" to item 16, or embellishes in great detail when we ask an open-ended query? Although many different issues apply to self-report measures as a class, two will be considered here: the dangers of literalist fallacies and the relationship between self-reported attitudes and related behaviors.

The Naïveté of Literalism

As the preceding paragraph implies, we commit a major interpretive error when we give self-reports (or any other type of data) the status of *prima facie* or literal truth. Questions and rating scales are perhaps best seen as vehicles we create through which respondents can express their thoughts, feelings, and so on, making them visible to the researcher in the same way that smoke is used in wind tunnels to afford visibility to the air currents that exist but otherwise would go unseen. Two questions plague the researcher: what do those utterings and checkmarks mean and how useful are the individual and/or aggregate ratings for the research objectives at hand?

This is not to say that we cannot believe what people say, even though we must sometimes be cautious about that, too. As George Kelly (1955) once suggested, "If you want to know something about someone, *ask them*—they might just tell you." And as Kidder and Campbell (1970) confirmed, measures of reliability and validity are maximized when questioning is direct. By and large, our own experience tells us that people who participate in research generally don't set out to deceive you. They may package their information to show their best side, but in general, people seem motivated to put forth their views "truthfully" within the constraints you provide for their responses. Those who are not, assuming they have free choice about whether to participate, simply will choose not to take part.

Most respondents in social and health science research, particularly the typical university student or average member of the North American population, appear to understand the tasks we give them. They understand order and magnitude (i.e., that 2 is larger than 1 but not as large as 6) and appear able to deal with rating scales.

But a problem arises when we try to make comparisons among individuals. Does the fact that one person checked 5 while another checked 6 mean that one person's attitude is stronger or more extreme than the other's? Not necessarily. Researchers using quantitative techniques frequently assume that people's ratings really take on meaning only when they're aggregated (i.e., when we compile the responses of many different people together). The belief is that our various individual propensities—to avoid extreme categories or rely on them heavily, to be cautious or audacious in our responses, to underestimate or overestimate our perceptions—will cancel one another out overall in the population or will be equivalent overall in different groups we might wish to compare. This is the main reason that reliability and validity assessment almost uniformly relies on groups of individuals to assess or demonstrate their strengths; it is at that level that such power can be shown. Interpolating or extrapolating from aggregate to individual behavior is courting trouble.

Attitudes and Behavior

The question of meaning is not bypassed by focusing at the group level. Even when the attitudes or opinions of groups of individuals are assessed by interview or questionnaire methods, you must still consider what relation these measures, and people's responses, have to other indicators or measures of interest. One issue that has plagued researchers for years is the question of the relationship between what people *say* about their beliefs, attitudes, and/or opinions when you ask them and what they actually *do* when faced with real or simulated behavioral choices.

This area of inquiry was given a provocative initiation by LaPiere (1934), who performed a study in racist, ethnocentric Middle America during the Depression years. LaPiere was interested in studying prejudicial behavior toward minorities in real-world settings. Anticipating that there'd be a lot of it, he traveled around the United States with a young, foreign-born Chinese couple, carefully recording the number and nature of their interactions with the owners and employees of the hotels, autocamps, and restaurants they visited. He also varied the conditions of their approach (i.e., sometimes he did the talking, sometimes one of the couple did; sometimes he went in with them, sometimes they entered alone). In all, the trio traveled more than 10,000 miles, driving twice across the United States, stopping at 250 different establishments, and during all that time, they were refused service *once*.

That original finding would have been heartening, given their expectations, were it not for the follow-up study LaPiere undertook once he and the couple returned home. Six months after completing his original study, LaPiere sent questionnaires to each of the 250 establishments they'd visited on their trip. Recall that when they actually visited the places, LaPiere found that 249 out of 250 places (or 99.6 percent) welcomed them, while 1 (0.4 percent) did not. The 128 replies he received in response to his questionnaire from those same establishments revealed a very different story.

His questionnaire asked "Will you accept members of the Chinese race as guests in your establishment?" In response, 118 (or 92.2 percent) said "no," while 9 (7.0 percent) said "it depends," and only 1 (0.8 percent) said "yes." Rather surprised by these results, since they were so opposite to the trio's experience, LaPiere wondered whether their own visits to those establishments might have affected the responses. Accordingly, LaPiere then sent the same questionnaire to 128 similar places they had *not* visited—but the results were the same.

LaPiere felt that his study revealed severe limitations to questionnaire responses. He did see some utility to them (e.g., in asking about beliefs), but the huge inconsistency he observed between the questionnaire and behavioral data led him to distrust self-reports:

> *The questionnaire is cheap, easy, and mechanical. The study of human behavior is time-consuming, intellectually fatiguing, and depends for its success upon the ability of the investigator. The former method gives quantitative results, the latter mainly qualitative. Quantitative judgments are quantitatively accurate; qualitative evaluations are always subject to the errors of human judgment. Yet it would seem far more worthwhile to make a shrewd guess regarding that which is essential than to accurately measure that which is likely to prove quite irrelevant. (LaPiere, 1934, p. 237)*

Considering (In)Consistency

Although we agree with LaPiere's assertion that it's advisable to tackle what is most important rather than what is easiest, we question, as have others (e.g., see Oskamp, 1977), whether or in what ways LaPiere was justified in calling the results of his behavioral and questionnaire studies "inconsistent." Certainly, we assess people's attitudes not only because we're interested in their attitudes *per se* but also because we believe that knowing people's attitudes will help us understand and/or predict their behavior (e.g., see Fishbein, 1967; Oskamp, 1977; Zimbardo, Ebbesen, & Maslach, 1977). The relationship between the two is thus of interest to us and has been investigated extensively. The literature notes five considerations to keep in mind when assessing the correspondence between attitudinal and behavioral data, considerations that indirectly offer advice on how to assess attitudes.

Situational Thresholds. Consider the following scenario. You approach a woman at your local library as part of a study on attitudes about environmental issues and ask her first to rate her concern about climate change (i.e., an attitudinal measure) and then to tell you whether she attended last Saturday's "Walk for the Environment" (i.e., a behavioral measure). She indicates that she's "strongly" concerned about the environment but did *not* attend last Saturday's event. Is this an example of attitude-behavior inconsistency?

Campbell (1963) is among those who have suggested that situations like the above don't necessarily reflect inconsistency but, rather, may just indicate differences in situational thresholds. Expressing an attitude is much easier than doing a behavior (which invariably requires some level of time, effort, money, etc.). If people do the easier thing but not the harder thing, their apparent "inconsistency" in behavior may merely reflect the fact that they're prepared to go only so far; they surpass the first situational threshold but not the second. True inconsistency, according to Campbell, is evident only when a person exhibits the harder behavior (i.e., goes on the "Walk for the Environment") but fails to exhibit the easier one (i.e., does not express support for environmental issues). The literature reveals that such inconsistencies occur rarely (see Oskamp, 1977).

Different Stimuli. Returning to LaPiere's (1934) study, consider the two stimuli with which the hotel and restaurant managers were presented. The attitudinal measure asked whether they would allow "members of the Chinese race" as guests. In contrast, the behavioral measure, in effect, asked whether they would allow as guests the two specific people with whom LaPiere showed up. Were the attitudinal and behavioral responses made to the same stimulus? If not, then it hardly seems fair to draw a conclusion of inconsistency.

The evidence certainly suggests that the two stimuli were indeed *not* the same. LaPiere notes the stereotypical and prejudicial attitudes of Americans at that time to many ethnicities, including Chinese, and these are clearly reaffirmed in studies done during the same period by Bogardus (1925) and Katz and Braly (1933). But LaPiere's two Chinese traveling companions were "a young Chinese student and his wife," who were both "personable, charming, and quick to win the admiration and respect of those they had the opportunity to become intimate with." Further, although both were foreign-born, they spoke "unaccented English" (LaPiere, 1934). Researchers who wish to predict reactions to a particular behavioral criterion should ask about that criterion in their attitudinal measure.

Competing Motives. Questionnaire items often query attitudes in the abstract: respondents are asked how they feel, in general, toward environmental issues, tax increases, or immigrants from Slovenia. In contrast, behaviors take place in the context of everyday life, where we face many situational contingencies and choose among alternative actions. The question "To what extent are you concerned with environmental issues?" asks in general terms for an expression of concern for the environment. In contrast, the behavioral criterion of, say, whether the respondent attends a meeting that evening concerning a local development project involves many situational contingencies (e.g., free time, the availability of transportation to the meeting) and competing motives (e.g., concern with environment balanced against interest in development; time at the meeting balanced against desire to go bowling or spend time with family). From this perspective, being concerned about climate change but not going on the walk may merely reflect other priorities that were more compelling on that particular day rather than some inconsistency in their response to the general question.

Availability of Alternatives. Questions asked in the abstract also ignore the fact that the lack of behavioral alternatives may foster what would seem to be inconsistent behavior. You may not be particularly enamored of your local morning newspaper, for example, but may buy it anyway because it is the only morning paper with local news available. Similarly, some people watch television programs they don't like only because they have nothing better to do or because they find it a nonmedicinal way to relax and fall asleep at the end of a busy day.

"Normative" Prescriptions of Behavior. Many social situations prescribe particular ways of behaving as "appropriate"; individuals may suppress the

expression of some attitudes in certain contexts. We're taught, for example, to be polite to people even if we do not particularly like them; and, in the United States in the 21st century, we hope that expressions of racism or chauvinism are seen as offensive and tasteless. In 1930s America, however, the situation was quite the reverse; white hegemony dominated, and few thought it was inappropriate to express racist and prejudicial attitudes as the questionnaire respondents did to LaPiere (1934). But when faced with a particular stimulus (like the couple LaPiere traveled with), people felt similarly free to "make exceptions" if they chose to, perhaps depending on such considerations as how "white" and counterstereotypical the couple appeared to be.

Avoiding the Pitfalls

These five considerations suggest that overall, in the aggregate, there are many reasons *not* to expect a one-to-one correspondence between attitudinal measures and behavioral criteria, even if both are valid. At the same time, the existence of such pitfalls indirectly suggests precautions the attentive researcher can follow to avoid them.

General Interests? General Questions!

First, the evidence (see Fishbein & Azjen, 1975) suggests that correspondence between attitudinal and behavioral measures is generally weakest when a single-item attitudinal measure (e.g., "To what extent are you concerned with environmental issues?") is correlated with a single behavior (e.g., "Do you plan to attend Friday's meeting on environmental issues?"). Why? Partly because there's room for error in both. Psychometric studies show that the more times and the more different ways you express a question, the more reliable will be your characterization of the person on the issue at hand. The same is true in the behavioral domain.

Note that in each case we're looking at a general domain of interest to us (i.e., attitudes about the environment, behavioral manifestations of environmental concern), but sampling only one element of each. There are many different components to environmental attitudes, and there are many different ways for a person to express their environmental concern (or lack thereof) behaviorally. Just as we should be reluctant to generalize more broadly on the basis of a survey that samples only one person, we also should be reluctant to generalize about a person's attitudinal or behavioral leanings on the basis of one question or one behavior. To assess general proclivities, you must sample more broadly across both the attitudinal and behavioral domains.

Specific Interests? Specific Questions!

If a researcher is interested in predicting a very specific behavior, the situation warrants a very pointed question that simulates the criterion setting as closely as possible, either by varying the actual setting or by describing a specific hypothetical scenario in a preamble. Some of the most successful efforts at predicting actual behavior on the basis of attitude measures have been pollsters' astoundingly accurate election predictions. Part of their success is attributable to appropriate sampling for such a research objective, that is, by obtaining a representative sample of voters. But another factor is that respondents are asked a very specific question about their intentions regarding the behavior in question (i.e., "How would you vote if the election were held today?"). Further, efforts are often made to simulate actual voting conditions as much as possible (e.g., by providing respondents with some way to cast a "secret ballot" where only aggregate results can be known).

Considering Stereotyping/Prototypicality

Researchers should consider that people may hold many opinions about things with which they've had little experience. People do not refrain from having opinions about Guatemala even though they have never been there, have never met anyone who lives there, and know little about the country and its history. The stereotypes people hold about other social groups (or social objects or social policies) may or may not be accurate in general and are always inaccurate when they deny the possibility of exception. Yet people often use stereotypes as a departure point when we ask them about some social category "in general."

So researchers should consider the relationship between the stimulus they provide and the particular behavioral criterion they have in mind. For example, Ted's research experience regarding "pornography" shows that survey questions must be very carefully worded because of variation in what "pornography" means to different people. Asking whether "pornography" should be censored, classified, or left unregulated, for example, leads to trouble. Some respondents think the question refers to material that has some sexual content, whereas others assume the researcher is referring to sexual material that depicts violence, particularly toward women (see Palys, Olver, & Banks, 1983). The solution here is to (1) ask respondents to articulate their definition or sense of the term; (2) provide a definition for respondents; or (3) not even use the term but, rather, describe the scenario/stimulus you have in mind (e.g., video scenes involving female nudity; videos showing explicit sexual activity involving gay couples), since you're the one doing the research and hence have some objective in mind.

Assessing Contingencies

Finally, researchers can surmount the difficulties associated with "contextualizing" questionnaire responses by asking about the contingencies and competing motives that might intercede between attitude and behavior. Fishbein and Azjen (1975) show strong correspondence between the two with only three intervening variables considered.

SUMMING UP AND LOOKING AHEAD

This chapter reviews techniques that involve interaction between researcher and participant through survey questionnaires that may be administered by the researcher or self-administered and that can be delivered in person, by mail, over the telephone, or online. The advantages and disadvantages of each are discussed, and some of their similarities and differences noted. Considerable time is also spent outlining the various ways that questions can be phrased, some of the strategies and techniques used in the overall organization and implementation of a questionnaire or interview, and some of the obligations and responsibilities entailed in dealing with a respondent on a human-to-human basis.

A final section of the chapter examined the relationship between how we report our behavior on surveys and what we actually do. Various possible explanations for inconsistencies were discussed that showed that true inconsistency is actually quite rare, notwithstanding the provocative introduction to this area by LaPierre's (1934) finding of wildly inconsistent results between survey and behavioral measures of discrimination toward a visible minority group. Various lessons emerged for how questioning can be done more concisely and to avoid misunderstanding.

In the next chapter we will look to another mode of interacting with research participants that tends to be longer, more in-depth, and often involving a more targeted sample of respondents, i.e., the interview in its various forms.

Key Concepts

Adaptive questioning 340

Categorical response item 354

Closed or structured
   questions 350

Cognitive interviewing 376

Computer-assisted social
   research (CASR) 339

Contingency questions 335

Demographic items 376

Dichotomous item 354

Double-barrelled items 370

Exhaustive 355

Granularity 363

"It depends" 350

Likert-type items 359

Multiple-response item 356

Mutually exclusive 355

Open-ended questions 349

Pilot study 376

Random digit dialing (RDD) 337

Response rates 334

Response sets 362

Response symmetry 364

Self-anchoring scale 358

Semantic differential–type
   item 361

Single-response item 353

Think-aloud interview 376

STUDY QUESTIONS

1. The president of your university is interested in assessing the attitudes of people in this state regarding postsecondary education. Unsure whether to do the study using a telephone or a browser-based survey, they come to you for advice. What advantages and limitations do you see to each approach in this situation? How about if they wanted to do the survey with students and faculty at the university? Would the advantages and disadvantages be the same?

2. What advantages do browser-based online surveys bring to research relative to phone or in-person survey questionnaires?

3. What does CASR stand for and what advantages and difficulties does it bring to the research process?

4. What advantages does the internet offer as a place to conduct social and health research? What are some of its limitations?

5. Indicate the role that question wording and question context can play in the results obtained in a large-scale telephone survey. What is the magnitude of their effects, relative to the degree of sampling error that usually exists in most large-scale studies (which often have sampling error in the range of plus or minus 2.5 percent or 3 percent, 19 times out of 20)?

6. Is it okay to take questions that others have used on surveys that appear in the literature and use them in your survey? What advantages are there in doing so?

7. Look again at the section "Question Content" to see the steps involved in translating a general set of objectives into an inventory of concepts and then into specific questions that ask about those concepts. Form a study group with other people in your class and consider how you might follow through those steps if you wanted to put together a questionnaire that could be used at the end of any course offered in your department to evaluate student satisfaction with the course and with the effectiveness of its instructor.

8. Figure 9.8 shows what is discussed in the chapter as an example of a terrible survey that violates numerous principles of constructing a good survey. Go through the questions and (1) identify the problem, if any, with each question and (2) rewrite the question to improve the survey.

9. The president of your university or college wants to include both open-ended and structured items in the study described in Study Question 1. Which ones should be placed first? Why?

10. Create a small questionnaire on a topic of interest to you that includes one open-ended question and one of each of the types of structured items discussed in this chapter (i.e., a dichotomous item, a single-response item, etc.).

11. Leroy wants to include a question on income in his questionnaire. What are the relative merits of using a single-response item or a categorical response item to get this information?

12. Indicate what is obviously wrong with the wording of each of the following questions and then rewrite each question in an appropriate manner.

    a. How many times would you say you have purchased drugs within the last 6 months?

    b. Do you feel that pliobenthamiacine (PBM) should be made legal for over-the-counter purchase?

       _____ Yes

       _____ No

    c. Do you feel that the use of marijuana and cocaine should be decriminalized?

    d. How do you feel about the depraved individuals who use a dangerous drug like heroin?

    e. Finally, please indicate your age in years at your last birthday:

       _____ 20 years or less

       _____ 20–30 years

       _____ 30–40 years

       _____ 40–50 years

13. When asked what political party she prefers in the next election, a respondent indicates a preference but doesn't make a financial contribution to the party when asked to do so. Is this an example of attitude-behavior inconsistency? Suggest alternative interpretations.

10

INTERVIEWS

CHAPTER OUTLINE

COMPARING SURVEYS AND INTERVIEWS

In the previous chapter we began by saying that surveys and interviews are similar insofar as both are techniques where you make contact with a human respondent, present them with questions, and receive their responses in return. The primary distinction between them is in the degree of structure and closure involved in the responses participants can make.

With a survey or questionnaire, the questions are prepared ahead of time and standardized (i.e., everyone gets exactly the same questions). People have to be *very* interested in the topic under study to spend more than about 15 or 20 minutes on a survey. Accordingly, in the interests of both efficiency and the desire to amass as much data in as little time as possible, the responses that survey participants can give are pretty much limited to choosing which of several categories best reflects their views. Those design preferences make sense given that surveys are typically created with the idea of compiling responses from many people in order to compare the way different subgroups respond, or to look at relationships (and particularly to compute correlations) between the responses to different questions. Many (but not all) survey researchers also seek to obtain random samples of whatever population interests them so that they can generalize on a statistical basis, but even those who are not interested in statistical generalization typically want a diverse sample that produces a broad range of responses, which is optimal for statistical analysis.

Interviews are a different kettle of fish. Rather than restrict responses to a limited set of categories, interview studies usually involve more open-ended questions that allow respondents to answer at greater length in their own words. Rather than searching for random or diverse samples, interview studies also are more likely to involve purposive sampling strategies that target whoever you can learn the most from in relation to whatever site or group or phenomenon is being studied. The emphasis is less on breadth (responses to many questions from many people) and more on depth (more extensive questioning of a more targeted sample of people).

While well-designed surveys are an excellent way to gather information about how attitudes and attributes vary within and between populations, interviews allow researchers to probe more fully into *why* people might feel the way they do, *how* they came to feel that way, and the broader belief system and experiential base by which those attitudes make sense. The more fluid and open-ended nature of the interview—more of a protracted conversation than a multiitem personal quiz—also allows the interaction to go to places that were not originally anticipated by the researcher, and can be adapted as it happens to whatever revelations the interviewee decides to bring forward and that the interviewer decides to pursue. There often is less concern about ensuring questions are standardized and greater emphasis on making sure the interviewee understands the question and has an opportunity to explain their views at greater length and in greater depth.

Interviews also avoid other limitations that often haunt survey questionnaires. Participation rates among people approached for a face-to-face interview are typically much higher (often around 80 percent or even 90 percent) than they are for questionnaires, which means that volunteer bias can be less of a problem with interviews. The interaction of interviewer and respondent also offers benefits that can enhance the quality of the data gathered. For example, the interviewer can ensure that the appropriate person completes the interview, can clarify immediately any confusion about particular questions, and can use probes to encourage people who respond with only a few words or a one-sentence answer to elaborate further. Also, since the interviewer asks questions and records the responses, the respondent needn't be literate, although researcher and participant do need to share a common language. And although some participants may feel less anonymity in the personalized interview setting than with the impersonal questionnaire, skilled interviewers can often build sufficient rapport to alleviate such misgivings.

The major disadvantage to interviews historically has been the time and expense required to undertake an interview study of any proportion. Once your survey goes online you can amass hundreds if not thousands of responses within a week or two; with in-depth interviews a researcher is lucky to complete two or three in a day given the vagaries of scheduling and how mentally taxing it can be to do an interview well. The trade-off is breadth versus depth if you must choose one or the other; the ideal is a mixed-method strategy that allows you to benefit from the strengths of both methods.

There are far more variations of the basic interview than we can deal with in this chapter; it would be easy to write an entire book just on interviews, as many researchers have (e.g., King, Horrocks, & Brooks, 2019; Rubin & Rubin, 2012). In the sections below, we discuss three general classes of interviews that can serve a range of research objectives in the academic context and beyond: (1) the one-on-one interview; (2) focus group interviews; and (3) the oral history or narrative interview.

THE ONE-ON-ONE PERSONAL INTERVIEW

At its best, the one-on-one face-to-face interview is a wonderful opportunity for a researcher like you to discover the lifeworld of someone who is not you—a person willing to share what happens in their world and how they make sense of and find meaning in their experience. The flexibility of the method ensures it can be used with a wide variety of research objectives from exploratory to explanatory. It is one of the most direct ways to find out about a person's knowledge, values, preferences, attitudes, and experience. Hypotheses can be formulated and tested via the interview, and it is a method that can be used in combination with virtually any other methods we discuss in this book as part of a mixed-method inquiry (e.g., Gray, 2014; Rubin & Rubin, 2012).

That said, two strangers who sit down with one another do not normally just sit down and begin instantly divulging intimate and sensitive details about themselves. There is a social dynamic to the interview process and challenges to overcome. In the sections below, we take you through the various steps of undertaking an interview study from initial design to transcription to show some of the strengths and limitations of the method as well as indicating some of the range of alternatives you have available as you work your way through successive stages of design, execution, and analysis.

Before You Begin
Technology

Generally speaking, it is always better to record an interview than to take notes, although we advise you should always take notes, even when the interview is being recorded. There are several reasons for doing so. First, it is a way of staying engaged with and managing the interview. When people are talking, the last thing you want to do is interrupt (unless they stray far off topic or misunderstand your question). Taking notes allows you to continue listening while making notes about issues you would like to revisit later in the interview. Second, at least once in your research career, disaster will strike—your batteries will die prematurely, or your recording device will run out of space, or you will think you have pressed "record" when you have not—and as Murphy's Law dictates, it likely will come at the least convenient time. When that happens, your notes can serve as something of a backup if you write down each topic as it is discussed and perhaps a few key words or phrases in each interesting quote. Nothing is as good as a quality recording, but if disaster strikes and you have the outline of the interview in your notes, the first thing you should do after the interview is to sit down alone in some quiet place and embellish the notes with as much detail as you can while the interview is still fresh in your mind. Third, you never want to record an interview without the interviewee's permission, and some people will not want to be recorded, in which case you will need to be ready to take notes and write down choice quotes as close to verbatim as possible.

The "traditional" mode of recording, if we can call it that, involved researcher and interviewee sitting across a table from one another with a microphone pointed at the interviewee in between. Recording technology these days is much less intrusive and much more portable. For interviews that deal with topics that are not particularly sensitive, the smartphone that most of us carry will either come with a recording app or you can download one of the many available. After securing permission to record, you need only plunk it face down on the table, and assuming you have enough battery power and recording space remaining, can acquire a high-quality digital recording you can transfer to your computer for later transcription and analysis. We emphasize that this should be done only when the topic under discussion is not particularly sensitive. Smartphones are probably the least secure of digital technologies. Probably worse, and more likely, the interview file might even be stored automatically in the cloud with the owner of the app or operating system believing they have a proprietary interest in your interview according to the terms of service you said "yes" to without reading when you downloaded the app.

For more sensitive interviews where confidentiality is crucial, you want a stand-alone recording device that is not network-connected in any way, such that the recording is only made in that device via USB or memory card and the device is nonhackable and in your and only your possession. The recorders we use are smaller than a cell phone and can easily record more than 12 hours of interview, i.e., far more than we would ever use in one sitting. We also use a wireless transmitter that allows us to attach a small lavalier (lapel) microphone on the interviewee's clothing that has the added benefit of allowing us to record virtually anywhere quite unobtrusively, and does not even require us to remain in one place. Chris utilized this technique in his in-person interviews with clients of sex workers, which allowed him to conduct interviews in true conversational style in pool halls, moderately busy lounges or cafés, or while walking about busy city streets. Not having the visual distraction of the recording device present and not having to worry about being restricted spatially put participants at ease, which made it much easier to establish a trust and rapport that resulted in the typical interview lasting well over 2 hours. Participants often commented at the end of the session how enjoyable the conversation was and how much they appreciated being able to talk so openly and freely.

The mobility associated with this approach also allows for interviews to be conducted in the field where the behavior you are asking about usually occurs, which gives research participants visual cues they can use as they explain how particular events occurred and/or to explain their behavior or choices, which can enhance both the comprehensiveness of recall and its validity. For example, the two of us advised a publishing business in the health food industry that was undertaking in-house interview research with health food retailers regarding various aspects of the industry. Our advice included the suggestion that the interviews should be conducted in the actual store using wireless microphones while wandering about the venue. The feedback was highly positive. Retailers clearly felt more comfortable showing off and explaining "their" store, while the interviewer enjoyed having concrete referents to anchor what was being spoken about, and to be able to point to and ask about products, store features, and other issues that came to the interviewer's or retailer's attention.

Choosing an Appropriate Setting

A second decision you will make is in relation to where the interview will be held. The three main criteria you are trying to achieve here are comfort, privacy, and quiet (King et al., 2019). Comfort is important for putting the interviewee at ease. This normally means going on their turf, perhaps a room or meeting space in their organization or company where they can feel "at home," and of course their actual home is a possibility as well. One benefit of meeting a person in their home or office is that the setting itself can be a source of information about the person, and artifacts in the space—awards, photos, art—can be "icebreakers" in the chitchat that you will want to engage in as each of you gets settled and ready for the formal interview to begin, or something that might even provide a focus for part of the interview. Of course, the interviewer also has a right to feel safe and comfortable; you should never put yourself in a position where you might feel unsafe.

Sometimes the most public of settings can actually be quite private in terms of the ability to have a confidential conversation. There are no rules against conducting an interview in a coffee shop or restaurant or sitting on a park bench, although we caution that you also consider the acoustic qualities of the space and its implications for recording quality. Most microphones do not hear the same way that humans do, and those that do tend to be quite expensive. While most of us can be in a noisy restaurant and still hear the person we are with because our brain can distinguish their speech and relegate all the other conversations and noises to the background, most microphones make no such distinction. What your brain heard very clearly during the interview may be completely unintelligible afterward when you go to listen to the recording and find your interviewee's voice drowned out by neighboring conversations and clattering dishes.

Although the park bench may seem an idyllic alternative by providing a separation from all those walking by and offering both privacy and perhaps a beautiful view, the thing to keep in mind here is wind. Ted learned that one the hard way in a videotaped interview he did in Switzerland with a community organizer and social activist representing the Maasai people of Kenya at a UN meeting of Indigenous peoples. After completing several interviews with other delegates inside with no technical glitches, he and the Maasai delegate decided on a beautiful sunny day to hold their conversation on a bench on the grounds outside the meeting hall. The interview went smoothly and it was not until Ted later reviewed the video that he heard how the audio was spoiled by wind noises throughout the conversation. Fortunately, there are solutions to this sort of problem. He now knows to use a very simple screen that dissipates the wind, effectively breaking it up into many smaller gusts, and thereby reducing its power.[1]

Self-presentation

Who are you? Why are you interested in me/us as participants? And what are you bringing to the table in the way of background or expertise? Although much of this book speaks from a researcher's perspective—the research questions we want to ask, the research participants we would like to engage, and the analyses we would like to complete—prospective participants want to know about us as well. You will be doing some of that when you introduce yourself, but one of the things you also should expect these days is that as soon as your name is known to a pool of prospective participants, those you approach will be entering your name into their search engine of choice to see what they can find out about you. Do you have a particular agenda that is either consistent with or at odds with the group? In cases where a community shares some online forum, you can bet that your reputation will be discussed. For example, when Chris was doing a survey and interview study of clients of sex workers, one of the things he did was to monitor chat groups that operate in different cities where clients of sex providers share views about different agencies and those who work there, only to find that they were discussing him and judged him to be fair and reasonable. For example, one message stated,

> *I looked at the names of some of the people associated with the project (ain't Google wonderful!) and they have a number of legitimate research studies and analyses out*

---

[1]The noise problem and its solutions are discussed at https://www.shure.com/en-US/performance-production/louder/shure-tech-tip-methods-to-minimize-wind-noise.

> *there. As well, some have been involved in harm reduction strategies with the sex worker community and some have expertise in criminal justice issues. In a phrase, 'looks legit to me.'*

As we stated in another article, "The doors to the internet swing both ways" (Palys & Atchison, 2012), so understand going into your research that you will be both scrutinizer and scrutinized.

When you do approach prospective participants you should be ready to answer further questions as to what your study is about and why the particular people you approach are essential to your work, i.e., "Why me?" In most cases this will be a nonacademic audience who are less likely to be interested in your theoretical interests and more likely to want to understand why someone like you is interested in someone like them and what the implications might be for them. In Chris's case, he was all ready with a web page entitled "John's voice: Providing a safe space for sex buyers to be heard," which attempted to convey that this study simply wanted to hear what sex buyers—who in many forums were being vilified—might want to say and thereby to include them in the discussion. The web page set out what the research was about, who the research team comprised, why the research was being conducted, what methods would be involved, where they could see results of the study when it was done, and how they would ensure that responses for both the survey and interview portions of the study would remain confidential. For example, with respect to the focus of the research, the site said the following:

> *This research was designed in such a way that the results could be used to highlight the voices, experiences, issues and concerns of sex buyers. The topics that were covered and the questions that were asked were developed so that the data collected could be used to speak directly to current debates concerning the social, legal, political and health issues relating to the buying and selling of sex.*
>
> *One of our goals was to collect information that could be used to enlighten current policies, practices and understandings pertaining to prostitution by including one of the most valuable voices on issues surrounding commercial sex—those of clients!*

Researchers also should give thought to the level of expertise they bring to the interaction. Two possibilities that often come up are "the expert" and "the learner." Coming in as "the learner" is a useful approach in many cases because the person you are interviewing may well be the expert in their domain and odds are that you have a lot to learn. By coming forward as a naïve researcher who begins by asking, "Please explain how this place (or this phenomenon) works," you open the door to hearing each person's understandings of the place or process under scrutiny and hear explanations that people in the situation now take for granted. This approach is particularly useful when dealing with communities that you are not normally a part of, and where the people you are speaking with are directly engaged in the process you are trying to understand, or are the front-line people in whatever organization you might be interested in.

Coming in as something of an "expert" is particularly useful when you are trying to access people who occupy higher levels of an organization you are researching, who sometimes need to be shown that you are worthy of their time. If the information you seek is very basic, they will wonder why you do not simply read their brochure, or will pass you over to someone lower in the organizational hierarchy more involved in day-to-day operations. For example, in one recent study, Ted wanted to do a mixed-method study of institutional policies for the protection of research confidentiality, part of which would involve speaking with Chairs of Research Ethics Boards involving not only the policies but also the implications of having or not having one. The study was done in collaboration with graduate student Aaren Ivers, who contributed much as the study was being designed and later during the analysis of the data. However, they decided Ted was the better one to be doing the interviews because of his lengthy experience in that area. He was more likely to have a better sense of what questions and follow-ups to pursue, and Chairs, who tended to be senior faculty members at their respective institutions, would be more likely to open up to him as a senior faculty member and published author in that area. Had the study focused on research staff and perhaps been asking about how procedural decisions were made during ethics review, Aaren might have been the better one to do the interviewing, while someone like Ted might have been perceived as more threatening, or might have generated more awkwardness among respondents who would be wondering why someone with extensive experience was asking such basic questions.

Interviewing Online

Online interviews are a relatively new phenomenon that, until now, was limited by computer infrastructure and the availability of appropriate software. In the early days of the Internet, the best you could do was to text back and forth via e-mail or a chat program, which was often a long and arduous process. We were reminded of this fact when Chris had one interview participant in his research with the clients of sex workers who wanted to participate, but refused to do so through any medium but instant message exchanges. In contrast to his other interviews, which typically took 1–2 hours, Chris ended up spending more than 7 hours (!) with this one fellow over two evenings. The one redeeming feature of this technique was that, in the end, he was left with a ready-made and complete transcript of the conversation.

The door opened much wider for network administered interviewing with the development (in Estonia) of Skype, and especially by Skype's introduction of video conferencing in 2006. Further development is ensured by Microsoft's acquisition of Skype in 2011 and the proliferation of audio and video messaging and conferencing systems that have occurred since then. We have already seen its expansion to different operating systems (Windows, MAC, and Linux) and devices (desktop and laptop computers; tablets; smartphones). An added bonus is that some of these systems, such as WhatsApp and Signal, provide end-to-end encryption to ensure conversational privacy while at the same time being easily recordable by the actual participants in each call. We personally would avoid WhatsApp, which is owned by Facebook, because although the calls themselves are encrypted, Facebook retains all the meta-data about the call, and sells it as part of the surveillance economy that currently dominates the Internet.

A few researchers have found that the lack of physical presence in the research setting leaves them with less control over interactions with the participants or the setting (Epstein & Klinkenberg, 2001; Pettit, 2002). Accordingly, when conducting network-administered interviews or focus groups, differences among participants may be magnified and variations in the setting may be overlooked. It is also more difficult for both researcher and participant(s) to pick up on audio or visual cues that emerge during the interview or observational process, which would make it much more difficult to develop personal rapport in interview or focus group settings (Black & Ponirakis, 2000). Not being able to have physical connection with the participants and the currently limited ability to pick up on context significantly limits the type and range of data that are available to researchers. However, some researchers have found that in anonymous CASR environments participants are more likely to self-disclose (Epstein, Klinkenberg, Wiley, & Mckinley, 2001; Gravlee, 2002) and are thus more likely to take part in studies of reactive, socially taboo, or highly sensitive topics.

Doing the Interview
Getting Started

You always should go into an interview with a comfortable amount of time allotted not only for the interview itself but also for a bit of time before and after. You want time before the interview begins to ensure you are set up and any equipment you bring is working correctly (and make sure you bring spare batteries). Afterward you want to allow for 30–60 minutes of private time to complete your field notes by fleshing out all the cryptic comments you made to yourself during the interview, as well as any reflections on the interview as a whole, and any notes to yourself about things to pursue in the future that emerged during the interview (e.g., other individuals to approach, documentation to ask for, literature to check out). A nice way to show you are thinking about the interviewee's needs as well as your own is to bring along a bottle of water for each of you.

You also should allow some time for a bit of chitchat as you finish getting set up and the interviewee is getting settled. This helps break the ice, allows for an informal interchange about conversation pieces you see (pictures, awards, interesting collections) that is also a way of inviting the interviewee to be telling you stories, and get as far away as possible from one- or two-word answers. You want to make the interviewee as comfortable as possible not only by assuring them about the confidentiality of the interview but also by explaining how you will manage that confidentiality, who (if anyone other than you) will have access to their responses, and to what use the information will be put. Obviously, where possibilities for repercussions exist for the individual or to their group because of the results of the study or the sensitivity of the information, and especially if the researcher limits their pledge of confidentiality in any way, ethical practice requires that respondents be informed of that possibility and that researchers build in safeguards to the extent possible (e.g., Palys & Lowman, 2002). It is also a time to answer any last-minute questions they may have. You finish by reminding them that they do not need to answer any question they would prefer not to answer and can withdraw at any time, and asking two final questions: (1) do they consent to the interview? and (2) do you have their permission to record the interview?

Recording sometimes can be a touchy issue, although most people expect audio recording. If they wonder why, we explain it ensures that we get what they say right, and that it also frees us to focus on them rather than worrying about getting down what they are saying. We also tell them that if at any point during the interview they would prefer we turn off the recorder for a question or two, we are fine with that. We still take notes because doing so helps retain the flow of the interview. Most respondents expect you to write something down every so often, and notes give you a backup in case a technical foul-up renders the recording useless and you must regenerate the content of the interview from memory. Video-recorded interviews are also possible, but are much more intrusive and create a more identifiable record that cannot be anonymized easily. Ted has only done them on two occasions. One of these was in Switzerland when he was interviewing delegates to some UN meetings occurring there—people who were used to making public statements and being interviewed by filmmakers and TV news crews. The second was for an oral history that he did with a noted academic who was retiring that was intended for purely archival purposes, and over which the interviewee had complete control in terms of when and where it would be stored and potentially released.

Finally, we remind you that a big part of being a good interviewer is to come in with a nonjudgmental attitude with respect to whatever the respondent is willing to share with you, and to practice, practice, practice. Although you may be very intimidated by the prospect of your first interview, the more you do, the more comfortable you will become and the more amazed and grateful you will be at the range of things that interviewees will share with an interviewer who is a good listener who comes in simply wanting to understand. The big thing to remember is that it is not about you; it is about trying to understand why what the person in front of you does is perfectly logical and reasonable *to them* regardless of whether they are someone you personally admire or engage in behavior you find vile and loathsome.

What Do You Ask?

While the interpersonal, direct, and flexible interview method allows you to ask and discuss just about anything, King et al. (2019) identify six different types of questions that are appropriate for an interview:

- **Background/demographic questions**: These are straightforward questions that are useful in describing your sample and potentially also help you make distinctions within your sample that can be useful in your analysis, e.g., by helping distinguish points of view on the basis of position within an organization, or length of time on the job.

- **Experience/behavior questions**: These questions ask the interviewee to describe overt actions and events that you might have seen had you been there to observe it. Examples would be questions like, "What happened after you showed up at the doctor's office? And what happened after that?" or "How did you respond when they said that to you?"

- **Opinion/values questions**: These types of questions ask the respondent to reflect on the topic at hand in terms of their own values, goals, and priorities. For example, "What were you hoping to achieve by joining that group?" or "What do you think of the way the teacher responded to the class? How would you have responded?"

- **Knowledge questions**: King et al. (2019) point out that the distinction between these types of questions and opinion/value questions can be difficult to make, since the two often go hand in hand. The important consideration to keep in mind is that these questions refer to what the respondent considers to be the facts, which may or may not be what is literally true. Examples might be "What factors does your committee consider when deciding who will be admitted into your graduate program?" or "What do you think happened that led your partner to reevaluate your relationship together?"

- **Feeling questions**: These questions try and get at respondents' emotional responses to events or whatever phenomenon you are asking about. For example, "How did you feel about that?" or "What feelings did that reenactment stir in you?"

- **Sensory questions**: These deal with sensory experience as you might expect—what the participant saw, heard, touched, tasted, or smelled. King et al. (2019) immediately note that these may appear to overlap with experience/behavior questions, but suggest that questions that directly focus on the sensory dimension of our experience should be considered separately. Examples might be, "What was the first thing that caught your eye when you walked into the room?" or "The way you describe that scene makes me think it must have been complete chaos. What struck you first—the sounds? the sights? the smells?"

As these explanations suggest, distinctions between these question types sometimes can be hard to make, and there is certainly no requirement that you include questions of every type in every interview. Consider them simply as an inventory of the range of questions you might ask and hence that you might consider when you design your interview protocol.

How Structured?

One aspect on which interviews vary is on the degree of structure to the interview as a whole, as well as on the wording and ordering of questions. The three types you see in the literature are unstructured, semi-structured, and structured.

Unstructured interviewing involves the researcher asserting minimal control over the interview process and providing much leeway for the respondent to take the conversation in directions that are most meaningful to them. The epitome of this approach would probably be the oral history interview that we will discuss later in this chapter. Unstructured approaches are most useful when you are new to a setting, when you are still trying to figure out a research question, and you are still exploring the topic and don't yet know all the "right" questions to ask. They are also especially useful in situations where you cannot assume that all questions will be equally meaningful to all your respondents, such as in organizational case studies where different questions are relevant to different people depending on their location within the organization. The complete flexibility inherent to this approach will help you build rapport, will ensure you do not foreclose too early on your research focus, and gives you the most flexibility in adapting your questioning to the person in front of you.

At the other extreme, structured interviewing is most appropriate when you already have some experience with the phenomenon of interest and are familiar with the people and sites you are visiting, are confident that the questions you want to ask are the most meaningful in helping you understand the phenomenon or people under study, and can assume that the questions you want to pose are equally meaningful to all prospective respondents. The wording might shift slightly depending on the person to ensure they understand what you are after, but for this type of research you typically will begin with an interview schedule that you have designed that will be almost like a questionnaire in its consistency of structure, i.e., the same questions are asked in the same order, and relatively standardized probes are used to encourage more elaborate responses. Examples of when this approach would be useful are when interviewing employees on an assembly line who engage in basically the same task, or the nurses in a hospital who work in a particular ward, or all the students in your faculty who aspire to go to graduate school. Standardizing interview questions serves the same sort of purpose that structured questions serve in a survey—they allow you to aggregate responses to be able to make statements about the group as a whole (e.g., "75 percent of those interviewed thought unionization was a good idea"), or to make comparisons within the group (e.g., "While only 13 percent of the teachers at the elementary school level supported enhanced security measures, fully 60 percent of those who taught high school did so").

With the exception of those situations above where we mentioned that structured and unstructured approaches were exceptionally appropriate, the most common alternative for interview studies is semi-structured interviewing that incorporates a little bit of both. With semi-structured interviewing, there is typically a bit more emphasis on asking the same questions of everyone in order to have some degree of comparability, while the order in which they are asked and the way they are worded will vary from one participant to the next depending on the flow of the interview. You begin a semi-structured interview with a list of topics that you want to ask about, but would go with the flow of the interview in determining which order you do them in, and would remain open to new avenues of inquiry that come up in the interview that you hadn't anticipated.

Some advice we offer regardless of the degree of structure in your interview is that you begin with questions that are clearly on-topic and also that invite a lengthier response. By being directly on-topic, you reaffirm what you told the interviewee the interview would be all about, showing in a small way from the outset that you can be trusted to deliver what you promise, something that you will do again and again in the process of building rapport.

As for inviting a lengthier response, we think of interviews as having a rhythm associated with them that can be more staccato—Q-A-Q-A-Q-A—or, more desirably, a situation where a short question generates a lengthier response, more like Q-Aaaaaa-Q-Aaaaaa. Setting an appropriate rhythm begins very early as interviewees look for cues as to what you are after and the sort of responses you are looking for, particularly with respect to length. They start to respond and look at you after a sentence or two, as if to ask, "Is that enough? Do you want more? Or did I say too much?" Part of that is dealt with by the way you ask questions. For example, asking "How" invites the respondent to tell you a lengthier story, while asking "Why" seems to make respondents more defensive and tends to result in shorter justificatory responses. As an example, if I ask you "Why did you come to this institution to study?," a typical answer might be "Because it's closest to my home" or "Because I was accepted here" or "Because I could afford the tuition." In contrast, if I ask, "So how did you come to choose this institution for your studies?," it invites you to tell me your decision-making process, the different factors you took into account, and perhaps the programs available or other aspects of this campus that were appealing to you. Beyond asking questions in ways that invite lengthier responses, and particularly when dealing with people who tend to be more verbally stingy, the other way to establish a norm for lengthier responses is by using probes.

Probes

One of the great advantages to interviews over surveys is that the interaction allows you to encourage people to expand on their answers through **probes**, which are follow-up questions designed to encourage the respondent to dig a bit deeper and elaborate a bit further in their response. Although they can be particularly useful at the beginning of an interview to set an appropriate rhythm that involves lengthier responding (as we outlined above), they can be used at any point in the interview when you want to add more depth to an initial response. Bernard (2013) and Cresswell (2016) describe several different types of probes.

The silent probe. Sometimes, when a participant has given a preliminary response, the best response is to say nothing. Interestingly enough, for many people these are the hardest probes to do because they involve dead air space that we feel compelled to fill. Most simply, a response of silence shows the respondent that you are expecting more, and that the ball is still in their court. On other occasions, and we suggest this is particularly true of rookie interviewers, we can be our own worst enemy by jumping in when the pause was only because the respondent was thinking about where to take their answer next, or was mulling over which of a couple of examples they will give us. Doing so has two negative effects—we lose the information that the respondent would have shared with us; and we take the counter-productive step of encouraging shorter responses instead of longer ones. Of course, if the silence goes on too long, and the respondent had actually thought they had given enough, extending the silence may make it appear you are not listening, which of course should be avoided. In that case, we would move to another type of probe.

The echo probe. The echo probe involves simply repeating or paraphrasing the last thing the respondent said to you and then asking them to continue with their story. Used appropriately, it shows the respondent you are paying attention, reaffirms that they are providing helpful information, while also inviting them to expand further. For example, while telling you about the decision-making process that brought them to this institution, they bring you to the point where they have brought various information together on which to base their decision, and sit down to talk it over with their parents. A probe might say, "So at that point it seems you had all the information you felt you needed. What happened when you sat down to talk about it with your parents?" Like any other probes, this one should not be overused. Continually repeating what the respondent said may lead them to feel frustrated and wonder why you keep on repeating everything they say.

The tell-me-more probe. Although not formally a question, this probe is probably one of the most common, simply asking the respondent to go further in their explanation with wording such as, "Can you explain a bit more about how exactly that works?" or "And how did you feel when that happened?" Such probes are in keeping with the story you are being told, reaffirm you are listening, and simply encourage the respondent to keep going.

Probe for examples. Very often a respondent will make an assertion that expresses an opinion or value they hold dear, but leave it as something of an abstraction. For example, if you are interviewing salespeople about how they do their jobs, at one point you might hear, "At least that's what we do most of the time, unless you get a customer who's a real jerk and trashes the very product they are intending to buy in order to try and get a better deal." You might respond by asking, "I see. Can you maybe give me an example of someone who you felt was a real jerk and how you would respond to them differently?" In this case you are incorporating some of the "echo" probe by repeating the phrase "real jerk" that shows you are listening, while then asking them to take it a bit further by giving a concrete example of the concept they are using. You should not underestimate the importance of this type of probe because it is very often in the concrete details of these explanations that you learn much about how the person sees themselves and what they value in what they do.

Probe for clarification. It is not unusual for respondents to use jargon or simply site-specific vocabulary that you are not familiar with; clarification probes merely highlight one of these and ask the respondent to explain. Sometimes these are quite innocuous and you get a definition in return, but sometimes, along with the "give me an example" probe, these can open the door to far much more. One famous example occurred during the study of the socialization process that occurs in medical school that Howie Becker (1993) wrote about in an article about patients that the med students referred to as "crocks" that we described in Chapter 2. It was an offhand remark by one of the students that Becker happened to hear when he was joining the students in hospital rounds one day. Becker responded with the insightful question, "So what's a 'crock'?" The exchange went back and forth between Becker and the medical students for weeks as they tried to work out a definition, while in the process revealing much about what was considered "valuable" experience in medical school—the opportunity to see and hear real patients with real diseases—and what was a waste of time.

The examples above certainly do not exhaust all the types of probes you can make (see, for example, Bernard, 2013; Cresswell, 2016; King et al., 2019), nor all the different ways they can be distinguished. For example, Rubin and Rubin (2012) distinguish three types of probes they label as (1) attention probes, where you show you are paying attention while asking for more information; (2) conversational management probes, which you use to keep the respondent on topic, encourage them to clarify, and/or give you an example; and (3) credibility probes, which allow you to assess the credibility of the respondent by asking such things as how they came to that conclusion, or to determine whether the information they are offering is first- or secondhand, or to acquire an example.

Sensitive or Threatening Questions

Doing research in the social and health sciences takes you into many realms of human life including ones that are criminal, humiliating, stigmatized, embarrassing, depressing, and/or simply private and something we normally would consider "nobody else's business." Nonetheless, one of the best ways to understand those domains of life is to talk to people who have gone or are going through them, so we can find out more about how they got there, how they dealt (or deal) with it, and the implications it has had in their lives. However, people do not simply start telling you intimate things about their lives because you happen to be from a university or college and have a bona fide research project that has gone through ethics review. While it never ceases to amaze and humble us to see the extent to which people are willing to share these experiences with us, the privilege of being the recipient of such sharing is one that has to be earned, both during the interview and over the course of your career.

One of the biggest factors that plays into disclosure of sensitive information to an interviewer is timing. If you ask a sensitive question too soon, people will back off, become evasive, and may downplay or even lie about their involvement. So rule number 1 is that you need to be patient and build rapport—showing you are a good and caring listener who is just trying to understand how they see the world—before asking for intimate details. Rule number 2, however, is not to wait too long so that the sensitive questions come at the end and the interviewee is left hanging moments after having bared their soul to you.

Beyond that, however, researchers differ in the advice they give. Berg (2007), for example, offers what he refers to as a "dramaturgical analysis of the interview," analyzing in detail the different roles that interviewer and respondent occupy and the expectations that each commonly has of the other. He also discusses how the researcher can get maximal information with minimal defensiveness through sensitive attention to both verbal and nonverbal cues. Resistance in the respondent is thus a challenge to be overcome. For example, Berg spends considerable time discussing the "evasion tactics" enacted when we step over the line and ask about things that are too personal or painful.

> *Such evasion tactics may involve a word, phrase, or gesture that expresses to another participant that no further discussion of a particular issue (or in a particular area) is desired. Conversely, people also usually acquire the ability to recognize these evasion tactics and, in a natural conversational exchange, to respect them. (p. 84)*

But the interview isn't a "natural" encounter, and deferring to people's evasion tactics all the time would mean that much data of interest would be lost. Berg makes no bones about the mission:

This sort of deference [ceremony] simply cannot be permitted during the course of a research interview. In fact, the emergence of evasion tactics during the course of an interview is among the most serious obstacles to overcome—but overcome them you must! ... The interviewer must maneuver around a subject's avoidance rituals in a manner that neither overtly violates social norms associated with communication exchanges nor causes the subject to lie. (p. 84)

For Berg (2007), interviewers thus must recognize evasion tactics as they occur and respond to them with deference, but should also look for a chance to return to that sensitive area. The strategy thus mixes sensitivity with persistence. By deferring to the evasion tactic, interviewers show they are not insensitive to the respondent's feelings, earning "rapport points" by doing so. Berg suggests that the respondent now will be more likely to reply because the interviewer has shown they know when to back off.

Another way to approach sensitive questioning is to ask the question in such a way that it assumes the person has engaged in the behavior, rather than asking them whether they engage in it. This technique was made famous by Alfred Kinsey in his seminal research in the previously taboo area of human sexual behavior (e.g., Kinsey & Mart, 1948). One behavior that people are reluctant to admit to in interviews is masturbation. Rather than asking, "Do you masturbate?" and follow that with, "And how often would you say you do so?," Kinsey found people were more likely to admit to masturbation if he just assumed they did, so he would ask, "So how often do you masturbate?," thereby putting the onus on the respondent to correct the interviewer if the assumption was wrong. Assuming that the respondent engages in the behavior also conveys the idea that "everyone does it" and hence that admitting to it is really not that big a deal.

Bernard (2013), in contrast, advises interviewers to frame the question in a nonthreatening way. He encourages an extensive preamble at the point you ask the question, presumably to demonstrate that you are supportive and nonjudgmental, ready for whatever the participant might come up with. The example he gives involves asking about condom use: "We're interested in the various things that people do these days to keep from getting diseases when they have sex. Some people do different kinds of things, and some people do nothing special. Do you ever use condoms?" (p. 188)

Bernard also notes the findings of an interesting experiment by Dotinga et al. (2005) in the Netherlands. Their study focused on residents of Turk and Moroccan descent. Why Turks and Moroccans?

> *Because the religious and cultural background of Turks and Moroccans prescribes the abstinence of alcohol use, Turks and Moroccans can be expected to underreport their alcohol use to an even larger extent than the autochthonous population. Therefore, the assumption that higher alcohol reports constitute more accurate data is particularly tenable in research among Turks and Moroccans. (p. 243)*

Having located a sample of Turk and Moroccan participants, the researchers then created an experimental design by randomly assigning members of the sample to one of four conditions that included two independent variables: (1) the method of inquiry (mailed survey questionnaire versus in-person interview) and (2) among those interviewed, the ethnicity of the interviewer (Dutch interviewer versus Turk or Moroccan interviewer). The main dependent variable was the extent to which members of each group admitted to alcohol consumption.

Note the logic here. For Turks and Moroccans, questions about alcohol consumption would be considered a "sensitive question" that would require them to feel comfortable before they admitted to it. This is not to suggest that all Turks and Moroccans are secretly drinking, but rather to acknowledge that some proportion of any group will engage in behaviors that are officially proscribed or stigmatized within their culture or religion. If participants from those groups are randomly assigned to experimental conditions, then we would expect the proportion of people within each group who engage in those behaviors—consuming alcohol in this case—to be roughly the same in each experimental group. And if that is the case, then any differences in *reported* drinking behavior we observe between groups must reflect the independent variables we have varied.

With respect to the method of administration, Dotinga et al. (2005) found that those who were approached about an interview were more likely to participate in the research. However, participants who were sent the impersonal mailed questionnaire were significantly more likely to report alcohol consumption than those who were interviewed. These two findings are consistent with other literature that shows interview studies have higher participation rates than surveys, while the greater sense of anonymity people feel when completing surveys can lead to more extensive disclosure than occurs in face-to-face interviews (e.g., Gray, 2014; King et al., 2019; Rubin & Rubin, 2012).

As for the ethnicity of the interviewer, the experiment revealed that Turks and Moroccans were equally likely to participate in the research regardless of whether the interviewer was Dutch or the same culture/religion as them, but were significantly more likely to disclose alcohol consumption to Dutch interviewers than interviewers who shared their cultural and religious background. There was no reason to believe that the Dutch interviewers were any better interviewers than the ethnically matched interviewers. Bernard (2013) takes this as an indication that "people may be more willing to disclose undesirable behavior to interviewers who are not members of their own ethnic group." While that certainly may be true in some circumstances, our interpretation of the findings is closer to that offered by Dotinga et al. (2005), who suggest that it is not the mere fact that the Dutch interviewers were from a different group, but also that they were from a group with more liberal attitudes about alcohol consumption. This in turn can more generally be thought of as a reaffirmation of the principle that an interviewer who is nonjudgmental and focused on understanding the respondent's point of view is more likely to elicit disclosures of stigmatized or "deviant" behavior. What is not clear from the data is whether the difference is due to the Turk and Moroccan respondents being *more* likely to disclose alcohol consumption to a Dutch interviewer, or because they were *less* likely to disclose it to a Turk or Moroccan one, or both. This would require knowing how much they did actually consume, which was not investigated in that study.

Cultural Considerations

The Dotinga et al. (2005) study described above should alert us to the fact that an interaction as personal as a face-to-face interview can be influenced by similarities and differences in culture and group membership of the interviewer and interviewee. Unfortunately, there are no consistent findings that would allow us to say in some general way that similarity or difference is the better route. Instead, it appears highly situational, depending not only on interviewer–interviewee similarities but also on such factors as the topic under study, other relationships that might exist between interviewer and participant outside the study context, relations between the two cultures (whether harmonious or conflictful) and the particular culture being studied.

To the extent that similarity is preferred, the major advantages seem to come in studies (1) that are not particularly sensitive in the phenomenon being studied (in the sense that confidentiality would be crucially important); (2) where cultural barriers exist in terms of between-group interaction (e.g., in some cultures it would be quite inappropriate for a man to interview a woman on many topics, and vice versa); and (3) where similarity of culture implies shared cultural norms about appropriate behavior in such an interaction (e.g., how direct a question it is reasonable to ask, or whether it is appropriate to look someone directly in the eyes when speaking to them). Similarity is also preferred when it means that interviewer and interviewee have common cultural referents that come into play during the interview (e.g., cultural icons, significant historical events, language issues).

Methodologists also suggest that it is generally helpful for the interviewer and interviewee to be of similar ages, and that the interviewer dress professionally, where "professional" can take on different meanings with different groups (e.g., Bernard, 2013). For example, when interviewing judges or accountants you might wear some sort of suit, while interviews with jazz musicians or sex workers would call for something more casually dressy (e.g., collared shirt or blouse and clean jeans). As Bernard (2013) laments, there are no simple rules, "Here again, common sense goes a long way" (p. 194).

As to where *differences* between interviewer and interviewee are preferred, we look to places where connections between the two can be problematic. One such situation is where role conflicts can occur. For example, while it was once more common for government departments, agencies, and corporations to hire academic researchers as consultants, these days many have their own research departments or simply have people on hand who have some research experience and are given the responsibility for designing and executing an internal study. While such people can be perfectly capable of designing a study, the fact it is in-house can be problematic when the study is over and the people doing the study now have information about their colleagues that may show disgruntlement with the organization, how they are not following policy, and so on, i.e., information that could come back to haunt them if it were disclosed to managers or supervisors.

Particularly problematic are situations where norms that are very important to doing valid research conflict with norms and even regulations associated with the profession. For example, nurses will find themselves between a rock and a hard place when they find out information that pits the research obligation to provide strict confidentiality conflicts with their professional obligations to report unethical or otherwise poor practices. The same may be true of others with reporting obligations such as correctional officers, social workers, and physicians. Such situations should be considered before the study begins and the researcher should be clear about what they would do in such a situation. Our suggestion would be that the research obligation is paramount when doing research, and that those who are professionally unable to meet those standards would be better advised to look to an independent researcher in order to manage that conflict of roles.

Howie Becker (see Becker & Faulkner, 2008) has also written about "studying something you are a part of" and noted the awkwardness that can come from such situations because of the knowledge that interviewer and interviewee share. While an outsider is someone to whom you may find it easy to explain how things work in your agency or company, the same questions from someone you work with may leave you wondering why you are asking when you "must already know that," which can make your response feel artificial and contrived.

Bringing It Home

Whatever method(s) you are using, your last moments of contact with individual research participants and/or whatever research site you are visiting should leave them with a positive taste in their mouths about the experience. Interviews should finish with more innocuous questions to bring people back down to earth, particularly if the interview itself has been an intense and possibly emotional one, which is not unusual when more sensitive material, and the life stories that go with them, have been shared.

The interview may be a conversation, but it is unlike other conversations in your life. Part of why people will share things with you is the pledge of confidentiality you have given them and will now do everything in your power to honor, but part of it is also because, in most cases, you will now disappear from their lives, which means that what they shared can now go on to benefit others—as we believe knowledge does—without coming back to haunt them. Thank them for their participation, see if they have any last questions they would like to ask about you or the research, let them know if/when/how you will share findings with them, and see if it is possible to contact them again should you want to follow up or clarify anything they have said. The phrase you often hear is, "Don't spoil the field," i.e., think of yourself as an ambassador for the research community; leave people with a positive view of research and researchers and don't mess it up for everyone else.

After the Interview

That's a Wrap

Step 1 is to start packing up your microphones and recorder now that the interview is officially over. Those final moments can be fascinating ones, however, when you and the interviewee bask in the glow of a shared purposeful conversation now ended. Or has it? A good way to end is with some of the same chitchat with which you preceded the formal interview, but don't be surprised if this conversation wanders back and forth between things you discussed in the interview and perhaps some common interest the two of you discovered. This is also a time to pick up any documentation or whatever that the participant said during the interview they would provide you with or simply show you, such as memos, letters, pictures, and/or policy documents.

If you have done everything well, you may well be exhausted. The exhaustion is a cognitive one. When we refer to you ideally having done everything well, it is because you have managed the challenging job of juggling several different roles simultaneously. Part of you is devoted to being there for the person you are interviewing: making eye contact; listening attentively to what the interviewee is saying; giving nods of the head and occasional "uh-huh"s to show encouragement. Meanwhile, another part of you is almost watching yourself doing the interview and managing the process: Is the interview going well? Does the person seem engaged? Are they wandering too far off topic? Did their response to that last question tell you what you needed to know or should you follow with a probe? What will you ask next? Still another part of you is the technician: Is the recorder operating properly? Are the volume levels sufficient?

Before leaving, make sure you keep any notes to yourself about any promises you have made to the participant (e.g., documents or a reference you might have promised; summary of findings), and deliver on them at the earliest opportunity. You get bonus points for that because, with the interview done and in a file, the only thing compelling you to deliver to this stranger you have spoken with is your word, and the statement of integrity that goes with living up to it.

Transcribing

The labor intensiveness doesn't end when the interview is done. The next thing you will need to do is transcribe your interviews because text files are far easier to deal with than audio or video files. Individual digitally recorded interviews ideally should be transcribed as soon as possible, and in most cases will be anonymized in the process.

For many people, this can be the most tortuous part of the process; estimates of how long it takes to transcribe an interview accurately range from 5 hours per hour of interview to as many as 8 or 10 when the material is very technical. Indeed, while on the one hand we love the richness of detail that comes from doing an interview, the prospect of **transcribing** all of that can be daunting. A doctoral student that Ted supervises, for example, had interviewed 87 former gang members who were soon to be released from custody. It was a great sample to have access to, the student is an excellent interviewer, and the information the participants shared about their former lives and aspirations for the future was rich in detail. The main problem was that it was an embarrassment of riches. Much of the material was so sensitive and potentially of such interest to third parties that Ted and the student decided that they did not want to "farm out" any of the transcribing, feeling that they should keep the transcribing and anonymizing of the information to themselves, but a year later, the student was still transcribing. Ted encouraged her to break it down into smaller manageable parts because there was so much there to write about.

In part to try and address these sorts of challenges, the two of us started experimenting in our own work with automated transcription processes using voice recognition software. The program we use is called Dragon Naturally Speaking

(DNS), which is generally recognized as one of the top voice recognition programs available at this time. Once installed, DNS requires a brief training process in which the user reads standard passages for approximately 15 minutes. This trains both the researcher and the program—the researcher to speak in a manner that is most recognizable to the program, and the program to recognize the researcher's unique speech—and is remarkably accurate once trained. This can be supplemented with other user-generated material such as documents, which allows you to introduce vocabulary that is unique to your interests and research. For example, Ted does face-to-face and legal research with Indigenous peoples whose traditional tribal, place, and personal names are far beyond the program's default capability, but can be produced unerringly by DNS with a few minutes of training. The same would be true of any technical vocabulary.

Our first experimentation using DNS for transcription involved simply inputting a taped interview to the program for transcription. This yielded a highly error-filled copy that required almost as much time to edit as a traditional transcription would have taken. Our next step was to exploit the fact that the program knew each of our voices by making us the medium through which the interview was taken from digitized audio file to transcript. This involved wearing headphones, slowing the recording down by 20–30 percent (using another program such as the freely available Express Scribe, the commercially available Adobe Soundbooth, or the playback provisions in NVivo), and then speaking out what we heard into DNS as the recording played. Because this process used our own voices, which had already been trained in the program, the error rate was quite small and easily edited with only a few interviews of practice, while the total time taken dropped from 4 to 6 hours of transcription time for 1 hour of interview to about 1.5–2 hours of transcription time, i.e., a substantial time saving. It seems others have discovered this process as well, and that it has the official label of **shadow speaking**.[2]

Another option would be to actually begin or end an interview by putting the respondent through the training process, the basic version of which only takes about 15 minutes. While such sessions would not be particularly useful or feasible for single interview studies even when each interview lasts for more than an hour, they may be highly useful for something like an oral history project where a given participant is sometimes interviewed for dozens of hours. That would allow any digital recordings simply to be input into DNS and auto-transcribed. Because some training of the program will have occurred already, accuracy will be high from the start. By

---

[2]For example, see http://www.accessibletech.org/access_articles/multimedia/captionsGeneratedAuto.php.

correcting errors from the first interview and thereby further training the program, subsequent accuracy will be even higher.

No matter how you slice it, transcription is still a painstaking process. The one redeeming characteristic we see to the process is that, by the time you get to the end of doing a transcription, you are *very* familiar with your data, and in all likelihood will have ideas about data analysis to bring forward from it. However, our bet is that the sort of transcription we are describing here soon will be a thing of the past. Voice recognition software is improving rapidly. One place you see this is in captioning, which is provided to people who are unable to hear, but which once involved a transcriber, and now involves software that turns speech into text. Google introduced a captioning service called "Live Transcribe" that works on its Android Q operating system in late 2019 as a first developmental step.[3] Eventually, the service is expected to work with any video that is run on Android, and news reports indicate that you will be able to do the same with any material—like the audio tape of an interview?— that you supply as well, and that the service will be available offline as well as on.

Our main concern with the service being operated by Google is that the company's predatory history with respect to other people's information (e.g., see Zuboff, 2019) means their service should not be used for confidential data without a solid assurance that they will not suddenly consider your data their own. Indeed, we would much prefer the development of dedicated software like Dragon NaturallySpeaking, which can be used offline without concern that confidential data will be taken.

FOCUS GROUP INTERVIEWS

The focus group interview involves the researcher bringing together groups of anywhere from five to a dozen people to be interviewed together. Although at one level it is no more than a group interview, in practice it is so much more than that. Researchers who bring together focus groups are typically interested in doing so to accomplish two main things: (1) using the group to brainstorm ideas, on the assumption that the collective whole will come up with more alternatives than will the same number of individuals one at a time and (2) creating an opportunity to observe the group dynamic as members of the focus group discuss the topics that are presented to them.

---

[3]For example, see https://techcrunch.com/2019/05/07/live-transcription-and-captioning-in-android-are-a-boon-to-the-hearing-impaired/?yptr=yahoo; see also https://play.google.com/store/apps/details?id=com.google.audio.hearing.visualization.accessibility.scribe&hl=en_US.

Some History

Focus groups entered the academic world in the 1930s (Krueger, 2015). It was a time when social researchers were moving heavily into the use of surveys and interviews to gage public opinion and advance social science knowledge, but neither practice was without its critics. A major concern with surveys was that respondents were given only a few categorical responses from which to choose, while with interviewers the worry was that it was far too easy for them to lead the interviewee in discussions. For example, in one early methods text, Stuart Rice (1931) lamented that,

A defect of the interview for the purposes of fact finding in scientific research, then, is that the questioner takes the lead. That is, the subject plays a more or less passive role. Information or points of view of the highest value may not be disclosed because the direction given the interview by the questioner leads away from them. In short, data obtained from an interview are as likely to embody the preconceived ideas of the interviewer as the attitudes of the subject interviewed. (p. 561, cited by Krueger, 2015, p. 2)

The search was on for techniques that would reduce researcher presence while providing more room for the participant to take the discussion down paths that were more meaningful to them. Although various researchers seem to have toyed with the idea of group interviews, the two researchers most often identified with what we now recognize as focus groups were Paul Lazarsfeld and Robert K. Merton of Columbia University. The seminal meeting that launched their collaboration occurred in November, 1941, a month before the bombing of Pearl Harbor that brought the United States into World War II.

As Merton (1987) would later recount, Lazarsfeld invited Merton to attend his lab in which he was testing different methods of assessing audience response to radio broadcasts. The basic technique involved playing radio broadcasts for groups of a dozen or more people who would sit in the lab and listen to a program and press a red button whenever they heard content that evoked any sort of negative response in them—anger, anxiety, boredom, disbelief—and a green button whenever they heard content that evoked a positive response. As this was going on, a primitive instrument known as the Lazarsfeld-Stanton Program Analyzer would compile all the negative and positive responses and provide an ongoing polygraph-type image of the waves of negative and positive emotion. Merton criticized the way the postprogram interview was done; he felt the interviewer was leading the group far too much and asking overly generic questions about likes and dislikes instead of focusing on specific reactions to specific segments of the program. The union of the two researchers was sealed when Lazarsfeld apparently noted that another group was just about to enter, and would Merton care to show them how it should be done? Merton did so, and the rest is history (Morgan, 2019).

Like many other academics at that time, Lazarfeld and Merton would join the war effort in a research capacity and used their focus group techniques to analyze training films and war propaganda designed to boost citizen and troop morale. An important lesson for the mixed methods theme that runs through this book is that the two also recognized the limitations of the focus group method and how its utility was strengthened in combination with other techniques. For example, Merton (1987) recalled the parallel work using experimental methods that Carl Hovland was doing in another portion of the research group. While Hovland's experiments could show whether a particular film or broadcast could exert a significant effect on attitudes or behavior, it was the focus group interviews that could shed light on why and how those changes occurred:

> [B]oth kinds of data were required for sound conclusions: the rigor of the controlled experiment had its costs since it meant giving up access to the phenomenological aspects of the real-life experience and invited mistaken inferences about the sources of that experienced response; the qualitative detail provided by the focussed group interview in turn had its costs since it could lead only to new hypotheses about the sources and character of the response which in turn required further quantitative or, in this case, further experimental research to test the hypotheses. (p. 557)

Academics seem to have lost interest in focus groups after the war, but by the 1950s the method was commonly used by market researchers, who were charged by advertisers with the task of improving existing products, designing new ones, evaluating advertising campaigns, and simply better understanding customers and their wants. These days, focus group research is a major part of marketing and advertising industries. They have also been finding ever-increasing use by academics since the 1990s (see Figure 10.1).

When Are Focus Groups Useful?

Krueger (2015) describes three different "styles" of focus groups depending on the primary domain in which they are used: (1) in market research; (2) in academic research; and (3) in public/nonprofit agencies and settings.

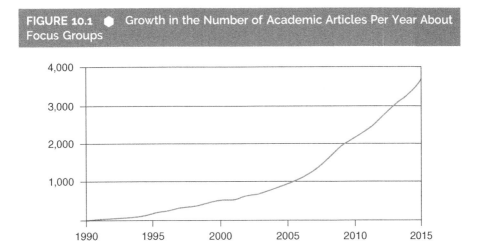

FIGURE 10.1 ● Growth in the Number of Academic Articles Per Year About Focus Groups

Source: Morgan (2019, p. 5).

The Marketing Context

In marketing, a group of typical consumers might be brought together to discuss their preferences, what they value in an existing product, or what they might like to see in a developing product. General Motors, for example, might be interested in designing a new truck and would hire a research agency to bring together a group of truck owners to discuss what features they believe should be included in the design of a pickup truck so that it would be most useful to carpenters or ranchers or whomever. Marketing researchers also use focus groups to assess other types of products and their packaging, such as politicians.

These groups are typically brought together in dedicated facilities with elaborate audio and video recording equipment and one-way mirrors to enable observation by senior members of the research team and/or sponsors. Participants are usually paid with money and/or catered food, with the amount of money offered rising depending on what amount of incentive is needed to bring in the group for a particular topic or product. Group sizes tend to be larger than for the other two styles—often around a dozen people at a time to ensure there will be a good cluster of talkers—and attention may or may not be paid to ensuring demographic diversity among attendees depending on the product and its intended customer profile. Discussion moderators often go through lengthy apprenticeships before they are able to run their own groups.

Corporate executives like focus groups because it allows them to see their products through the eyes of those who already or might in future consume their products, giving ideas of how to market their product and/or features to include in future product development. Turnaround time is often very important in the marketing context, especially in more volatile contexts such as political campaigns where candidates and their political messaging will often be reviewed and revised extensively over the course of a campaign, depending on the outcome of their own initiatives as well as that of their competitors.

The Academic Context

Academic approaches to focus groups differ in several noticeable ways from those used in marketing. One major difference is in secrecy. In the marketing context, focus group information has been paid for by a client who has a specific purpose in mind and any report that the work generates, and anything else about the groups that might be beneficial to the competition is considered proprietary. In contrast, academic researchers are required to be transparent about their research objectives, methods, recruitment strategies, and results as part of the analysis and dissemination of the research. In that context, rigor is expected and to be demonstrated. And while a marketer's report may almost be written by the end of a few focus groups—"Here are the six top strengths and weaknesses with your product or candidate that our participants identified"—academics are expected to use the same tools we see in relation to other methods (e.g., transcriptions, thematic, or content analysis). Krueger (2015) also notes that academic focus groups are less likely to meet in dedicated facilities with one-way mirrors that many noncorporate participants would find intimidating, and are more likely to do them in a home or other on-site settings. This may maximize comfort, but can make for greater challenges to the researchers to adequately record the proceedings for later analysis.

Focus groups may serve several purposes for researchers. Morgan (1988) explains that focus groups can be used productively when,

> orienting oneself to a new field; generating hypotheses based on informants' insights; evaluating different research sites or study populations; developing interview schedules and questionnaires; [and] getting participants' interpretations of results from earlier studies. (p. 11)

Focus groups also may provide provocative and/or insightful information to the researcher who is looking for unanticipated consequences to organizational interventions; is interested in determining issues of importance to those in the research setting or in acquiring new insights about the phenomenon from those who have experienced it; and/or is trying to develop research instruments (e.g., questionnaires, interview schedules, sampling, and solicitation strategies) that speak to the phenomenology of those under study. After a piece of research is completed and the researcher has done a preliminary analysis and interpretation of the data, these results might be imparted to additional focus groups for discussion. Such discussions may help the researcher gather alternative interpretations for further consideration and generate additional hypotheses and/or research questions on which to focus subsequent research.

The Public/Nonprofit Context

Krueger (2015) distinguishes this domain of focus group research from the other two in part because it shares some features of both marketing and academic research. Similar to the marketing context, Krueger notes that governmental and nonprofit agencies often share the marketing concern with trying to understand clients and their needs, finding out how their products and services are perceived and used, figuring out ways to attract or keep members, and evaluating impacts of the programs and services they provide. As in the marketing realm, the information need generally emphasizes the practical more than the theoretical.

Public health researchers were among the first to follow the lead of marketing researchers by incorporating focus group methods into their methodological repertoire:

> *Public health professionals were among the first to embrace focus group interviewing. Those working in prevention campaigns or in the emerging field of social marketing were quick to see the potential that focus groups offered. The social marketers borrowed many of the strategies from consumer marketing and adapted them to new products, services, and audiences. It was these public health professionals who were most aggressive in reaching new audiences. Academics had made some inroads, but it was the public health professionals who went into the neighborhoods, schools, Women, Infants, and Children (WIC) clinics, and migrant worker camps and listened. Low-income, disadvantaged, young, and other marginalized populations were included when new programs were designed. Public health professionals listen widely when they design programs to increase breastfeeding or vaccination rates or to prevent tobacco use, teen pregnancy, and violence. (Krueger, 2015, p. 179)*

Government agencies, religious groups, and service agencies followed their lead.

The public/nonprofit context shares more with the academic style of focus group research in the depth of analysis that is often involved in evaluating program successes, and in the range of methods that will be employed. Recall, for example, Merton's (1987) recognition of how mixed methods can provide a more comprehensive assessment in any program context than any one method alone: experimental and quasi-experimental methods can be used to evaluate program success; focus groups can help provide reasons how and why that success (or lack thereof) occurs; and methods such as surveys can establish how broadly those attitudes and opinions are distributed within and between user populations.

Focus groups in this style are also more likely to engage agencies and their clients in the community, and groups are likely to be smaller than in marketing research—more in the 5–8 range rather than 10–12. Also, moderators are more likely to be people familiar with the agency and the community it serves rather than a professional or academic with no prior connection to the community. Final reports are more likely to be broadly available even if not published, as opposed to the secrecy and proprietary approach take in the marketing realm, although confidentiality of individual participants normally would be provided and maintained.

Some Common Issues Across Focus Group Styles

A Decentered Process. Although focus groups have much in common with the traditional in-person interview, Morgan (1988, 2019) argues that their structure and inherent social dynamic gives them at least two unique advantages. Structurally, the decentered position of the interviewer or moderator means much greater emphasis will be placed on letting participants do the talking. Socially, the more decentered approach creates the opportunity for more interaction between participants, allowing them to place opinions "on the table" where similarities and differences between perspectives can be highlighted and discussed. This process allows participants to embellish on positions, discuss related dynamics, and articulate the rationale(s) underlying their perspective. Gray (2014) adds that the social dynamic in focus groups can provide a "cascade effect" where one person's statements trigger memories and other associations in others that otherwise may have been forgotten by the interviewee and never queried by the interviewer. He notes this can be particularly helpful when you have groups of people who share a common experience, even in very sensitive situations such as groups of people who have been victims of abuse, or who have lost a close friend or family member through tragedy.

Leveling the Playing Field. While some advantages accrue from the social composition of focus groups, the particular mix of participants can also pose problems. Some people will be less comfortable than others in expressing their opinions publicly; people with more extreme or unique views may be reluctant to expose them to possible ridicule; and people undoubtedly will be more concerned about maintaining their image in a public setting than in a one-to-one interview. Fontana and Frey (2003) suggest that three skills are particularly important in the group interviewer's repertoire:

> *First, the interviewer must keep one person or small coalition of persons from dominating the group; second, the interviewer must encourage recalcitrant respondents to participate; and third, the interviewer must obtain responses from the entire group to ensure the fullest possible coverage of the topic. (p. 73)*

The place to start is with the first question, which should be an easy one that you ask everyone in the group to respond to. The question should be relatively straightforward and answerable in a half minute or less. Doing so serves at least two purposes. First, it gets everyone talking right from the start; very often the hardest comment to make is the first one, and the longer it takes to get there, the greater the resistance to making it. Second, it is a final opportunity to ensure your recording equipment is working properly. One caution we suggest here is that you try and make your question as neutral as possible to minimize any status hierarchies that can get in the way of equal participation. For example, it would be better to ask a focus group of professors what department they work in or to give a short statement of their research interests rather than to ask them about their academic rank; if interviewing a focus group of entrepreneurs, asking them to describe the products or services they deliver would be preferable to asking them the size of the companies they operate. In each case the first question would be equally answerable by all, while the second is equally answerable, but also creates an immediate hierarchy.

Questions. A good second question will take people right into the topic that brought the group together. You might ask everyone to recall briefly their first or most recent or most memorable experience with the organization or product or service, or to ask them to reflect on what some concept—e.g., "a comprehensive education," or "good service," or "quality health care"—means to them. Such a question hopefully will start to shed light on different views that participants bring to the discussion and the interaction begins from there. You want to get away as soon as possible thereafter from the group interview approach of asking one question and getting an answer from each person, and into discussion, given that the opportunity to hear people with different perspectives encounter each other is one of the major reasons why you would want to do a focus group in the first place.

Group Size and Composition. One challenge with focus groups is to find a group size that ensures you have enough people to promote discussion and not be dominated by one or two more vocal people, but is not so big that you have a difficult time managing the group and you end up with the chaos of multiple conversations going on at the same time. Group sizes in the 5–8 range are typical of academic focus groups and 12–15 for marketing research groups. The more specialized the topic, however, and the more targeted the people you want to include, the more difficult you will find it to schedule a time and place that is equally convenient for all. Marketing researchers tend to have the easiest time of it for two main reasons: (1) they will pay whatever amount it takes to provide sufficient incentive to acquire participants and (2) there are usually minimal selection criteria for participation beyond a very general category (e.g., people who bought a Honda recently; homeowners; clients of a walk-in clinic).

Although one of the strengths of focus groups is that they create the possibility of interaction among people with differing perspectives on some issue, more homogenous groups tend to be preferred, particularly with respect to more sensitive issues. In order to share their views in a group setting, people need to feel comfortable and safe in expressing those views. Mixing white nationalists and Antifa in a group to talk about racial equality is more likely to end in disaster than to be an engaging conversation of diverse points of view. A better tack would be to do separate groups where each set felt comfortable comparing and contrasting their points of view with others who at least share some of the same assumptions; the moderator in this instance could introduce elements from one group into the other through a question that might be framed as something like, "So how do you respond to the criticism that …?" The same is also true of groups where there is something of a status hierarchy embedded in the roles people occupy. For example, if you were doing focus groups in a hospital setting over the question of how service delivery might be improved, you would probably want to create separate groups of doctors, nurses, and staff, given the likelihood of staff to defer to medical personnel, and for nurses to defer to doctors and/or for doctors to expect nurses to defer to them. The ideal would be to have some diversity within each group.

Finally, bringing strangers together is generally preferred to bringing in people who know each other. Friends or work colleagues will already have role relationships that will influence their participation in the group, and there is the added problem of potential consequences after the group is over for what they said during the session.

As Bernard (2015) explains, the best situation is one that mimics what happens when you sit beside someone on an airplane for a few hour flight; you hit it off, find issues of common interest, and have an engaging exchange of views only to get off at your destination, never to see each other again.

Confidentiality Issues. Notwithstanding your best intentions to protect research participant confidentiality in most of your research, focus groups represent a unique challenge insofar as the behavior of other people is not within your control. You can promise strict confidentiality on all the information you manage—the recordings and notes and transcriptions that will result—but cannot guarantee what others will do. We always draw this to participants' attention, while also saying how important it is to respect other people's confidentiality and hence to please leave whatever is said in the room in the room. Berg (2007) suggests getting people to sign promises of confidentiality. While not likely enforceable in any way, he sees the use of a form and signature as a way to drive home the importance of maintaining confidentiality and to at least get people to make a psychological commitment to maintaining it. Although noting that the confidentiality of what they share is dependent on the others in the group may lead some participants to hold some things back, we would rather err on the side of caution in such situations rather than fostering a false sense of security that might adversely affect a participant.

Challenges of Recording and Transcription. Focus groups are more limited in where they can occur relative to the one-on-one interview, given that the mobility that is possible when interviewing one person is difficult to replicate with a group. Controlling sound quality is the biggest challenge, even in a controlled and confined space; ensuring that everyone in the group is equally audible will require more audio expertise and equipment than is required for a one-on-one interview. Even assuming acceptable audio quality, transcription can become substantially more challenging when there are multiple voices, not all of which can be distinguished easily, and the possibility you sometimes will have more than one person speaking at the same time. For this reason, many focus group interviewers prefer to have a second person join them as note-taker; this frees the interviewer to focus on managing the group while the note-taker keeps track of who is saying what.

Chris made an interesting discovery about focus groups during the COVID-19 crisis that saw many of us working from home and not being able to hold meetings because of social distancing requirements. Prior to the declaration of a pandemic, Chris had been travelling to various towns and cities in the region to hold focus groups with people involved in the social–emotional development of children under 6 years of age. The study called for some overall discussion within a larger group as well as having participants break out into smaller groups from time to time. While the discussions went splendidly, setting up the situation so that both the aggregate group and the various breakout sessions could be recorded was a significant challenge. During the COVID outbreak, however, rather than suspend the research, Chris decided to use the *Zoom*™ videoconferencing app to do the focus groups. This solved the recording problem immediately in both the larger and smaller groups because both could be recorded, and the images and name identifiers associated with each participant made it easy to know who was speaking when. The experience showed considerable promise with multiple benefits definitely worth considering even after the pandemic is behind us.

In sum, focus group interviews are compatible with an array of research objectives and are useful for answering a variety of research questions, and while they possess their own limitations, they also can contribute unique and complementary information in a mixed-methods context. Although their use continues to grow, they remain an underutilized addition to the social and health science researcher's procedural repertoire.

ORAL HISTORIES

Broadly defined, "history" is everything that happened before you read this sentence. And now even that sentence has receded into history. We can never know *everything* about history, but that hasn't stopped historians and the rest of us who are interested in history from trying to understand it. In trying to do so, we realize one of the fundamental challenges of understanding history: it isn't here anymore. We thus cannot study history directly, but must do so by looking at those pieces and remnants of history that remain.

What's in the Box?

Now, let's imagine that the history we can study is all contained in a huge box. Of all that happened in that huge period of time we know as "history," the only things we can base our study of history on are the things inside that box because those are the only things that remain. And while many things get inside the box, many things do not. For example, Ted's children were always interested in sports, and Ted would always go to their games and ended up coaching all of them as they went through Little League baseball. The experience produced many wonderful father–child moments. But 100 years from now, when some historian sits down to write something about early 21st century humanity—even if they are writing about "father–child relationships in the early 21st century"—there isn't a chance in the world that this future historian will write about Ted and his sons and all those moments Ted appreciated so much that they shared at the baseball diamond. Why? Because that bit of human history, while as real as the fact that Lincoln is the capital of Nebraska, will never make it into the box of human events out of which future historians will manufacture history.

Or will it? Ironically, our describing that experience here makes it possible that some historian in 2120 actually *will* see some dilapidated old copy of this book and discover the fact about Ted and his sons and how they all loved playing baseball. Because we've put it in writing, a fact that would otherwise be recalled by no one besides Ted and his sons is now part of the contents of the box of study-able human history. It's actually a very interesting example of selective deposit, a phenomenon we'll discuss in more detail in Chapter 12. This term reflects the recognition that some things have a higher likelihood of being put into the box than others, and that some people and groups have better access to the box than others. It's interesting, for example, that, in Ted's role as dad, he has very little likelihood of accessing the box. No one outside his immediate family will probably ever have any sense of him as a parent. But in his roles as university professor and author, he has somewhat more access to the box, as evidenced by this book, which is now part of the historical record.

One of the tragedies of history is that so much that would be interesting to know will remain forever beyond our grasp because it was never placed inside the box. It's interesting to consider what sorts of biases have entered into that process. What people or groups have been systematically *less* likely to have had a chance to put something in the box? And what people or groups have had much *better* access to the box, allowing them to influence our sense of history by placing their experiences into the box?

Clearly, some people have had better access to the box than others. Governments, the wealthy, the powerful, the upper classes, and the educated all have had better access to the box than individual citizens, the poor, the vulnerable, the lower classes, and the illiterate. Similarly, it is also the case that men—because until relatively recent times, it was primarily they who formed the governments, controlled the property and wealth, and had better access to education—have had better access to the box than women. When historians open the box to try to understand history, the "facts" they look at are therefore not *all* the facts, or even a representative sample of facts, but only the facts placed there by those who had access to the box.

Rectifying the Imbalance of Written History

Oral history is partly a way of trying to deal with the problems of access just outlined. It recognizes and to some extent shares the general western European bias in favor of written documentation, and therefore tries to get material into the box that wouldn't otherwise be there. Oral history is consequently seen by many as "an interview technique with a mission." Fontana and Frey (2003), for example, note that "oral history differs from other unstructured interviews in purpose, but not methodologically" (p. 79), where the purpose is to take material that otherwise might have been forgotten and make it part of the written record. Reinharz (1992) adds that "oral history ... is useful for getting at *people* less likely to be engaged in creating written records and for creating historical accounts of *phenomena* less likely to have produced archival material" (p. 131; emphasis in original). By interviewing people about their past, we "recover" parts of history that otherwise might have been lost; by interviewing people about their present, we help ensure that their record is available for future generations.

Although examples of collected oral history narratives go back to antiquity, "its modern formal organization can be traced to 1948, when Allan Nevins began the Oral History Project at Columbia University" (Starr, 1984, p. 4, cited by Fontana & Frey, 2003, p. 79). That quotation, of course, has a certain delicious irony, since it's another example of how people with access to the box of history (like academics at prestigious universities) are the ones whose contributions we remember and can cite because they're part of the written record.

Because of the nature of the mission associated with oral history, you shouldn't be surprised to discover that the technique has been particularly popular among people who are on the margins of society—minorities, the poor, street people, laborers, and women, for example—and those who are interested in engaging in research with such people. Oral history narratives exist *en masse* for many of the "common people" of history whose experience otherwise would be ignored or forgotten. Examples include collections in which people talk about their working lives (e.g., Terkel, 1975), as well as more specific projects that focus on Pennsylvania steelworkers and their families, women working in Baltimore canneries (e.g., Olson & Shopes, 1991), the experience of Blacks in the Vietnam War (Terry, 1984), Palestinian women engaged in resistance activities (e.g., Gluck, 1991), IRA (Irish Republican Army) and UFV (Ulster Volunteer Force) combatants during "The Troubles" in Ireland and England in the latter half of the 20th century (Moloney, 2010), and a staggering array of other groups. No doubt many others haven't yet seen the light of day; as Fontana and Frey (2003) note, "often, oral history transcripts are not published but may be found in libraries, silent memoirs awaiting someone to rummage through them and bring their testimony to life" (p. 79).

Oral history methods found particular favor among many feminist researchers, who saw oral history methods as a way to rectify the gender imbalance in the largely male-dominated documentary archives of history. Gluck and Patai (1991) note that,

> The first major body of literature on women's oral history appeared in late 1977 in a special issue of Frontiers: A Journal of Women Studies. This ground-breaking issue served as the key reference on women's oral history for many years, and the suggested outlines for women's oral history interviews that appeared at the back of the journal were xeroxed, dittoed, and mimeographed by women in communities and classrooms around the country. (p. 4)

Emphasizing the gathering of women's oral histories is thus a way to include women's voices in history: "Refusing to be rendered historically voiceless any longer, women are creating a new history—using our own voices and experiences" (Gluck, 1984, p. 222). Reinharz (1992) suggests that women's oral history actually serves a threefold function: drawing women out of obscurity, repairing the historical record, and providing stories of people with whom women readers and authors can identify.

Archiving and Contextualizing the Past

While acquiring someone's life story or hearing about some part of it through an oral history can be an interesting endeavor in its own right, the next question is what you will do with it. Sometimes oral histories are intended for no other purpose than to archive them for future generations to look at as little time capsules from the past. For example, a number of years ago, the first Chair of Ted's department, Ezzat Fattah, the person whose vision had created that department in the first place, was retiring. Ted recognized that a decade later only the older veterans of the department would remember him, and that students probably would not even know his name or connection to the department. Although Ted had never done an oral history before, this seemed like an appropriate occasion to do one so that Dr. Fattah's recollections of the history of the department would be captured for posterity. They decided to conduct a series of interviews, with each one covering a period of his life (in chronological order). In the end, 12 hours of interview were recorded on video, and given to Dr. Fattah to be deposited in the university archives whenever he thinks it appropriate to do so, where it will remain until some historian of science decides to look at it and incorporate it into some broader analysis—another "silent memoir awaiting someone to rummage through it and bring it to life" (to paraphrase Fontana & Frey, 2003).

Past Meets Present

One thing you need to be careful of when doing oral histories is in looking at the past through contemporary lenses because we may end up imposing a framework that makes no sense to those who lived it. The question that arises is one of interpretation and the issue of "voice" and, especially, whose voice (if either) should dominate the final look of the text that's produced from the oral history. Katherine Borland's (1991) self-critical analysis of an oral history interview she did with her grandmother highlights the dilemma well.

The oral narrative that Borland analyzes concerns a day in the 1940s when her grandmother, who at that time was a recently divorced young woman in her twenties, was invited by her father to attend the harness races being held at the county fair. There are two things you need to know before we continue the narrative. First, unlike thoroughbred races where the horses run once in a day and then are likely to train for a week or two before their next race, in harness racing the horses will race multiple times in a day, such that a nine-race card might involve three groups of horses racing each other three times. Second, race tracks allow betting, and to encourage that practice produce a newsletter of sorts—a racing form—that shows each horse's performance in their previous races. This provides knowledgeable patrons the opportunity to place bets knowing something of the driver's and horse's performance history.

To make a long story short, the father considers himself something of an expert and, after consulting the racing form and viewing the horses, places his bets on Black Lash, "a horse with an established reputation for speed." Beatrice, Borland's grandmother, instead looks for what she thinks is the perfect combination of horse and rider, and decides to bet on Lyn Star. The father, upon hearing his daughter's choice, declares that her horse will never win and that betting on it would be a waste of money. Undaunted, Beatrice bets $2 on the horse to win, and it does so. Beatrice 1, Father 0. When the same group of horses gets ready to race again, the father declares Beatrice's horse's win to be a fluke, urges her to bet on his horse, which she ignores and bets $6 on Lyn Star again. And Lyn Star wins again. Beatrice 2, Father 0. As Beatrice tells it, the father is beside himself with frustration both at his own losses and Beatrice's wins, but ups the ante yet again with a loud denunciation of Beatrice's decision to bet $10 on Lyn Star to win in the third and last race between these horses. And of course it does, by a long shot. Beatrice 3, Dad 0. The know-it-all father is silenced while Beatrice and all those around her are drowned in gales of laughter at her good fortune.

That was the narrative. But what does it mean? Borland (1991) clearly recognizes that interpretation is a meaning-constructing activity:

> *Oral personal narratives occur naturally within a conversational context, in which various people take turns at talk, and thus are rooted most immediately in a web of expressive social activity. We identify chunks of artful talk within this flow of conversation, give them physical existence (most often through writing), and embed them in a new context of expressive or at least communicative activity (usually the scholarly article aimed toward an audience of professional peers). Thus, we construct a second-level narrative based upon, but at the same time reshaping, the first. (p. 63)*

So what did it mean to her?

> *What do I as a listener make of this story? A feminist, I am particularly sensitive to identifying gender dynamics in verbal art, and, therefore, what makes the story significant for me is the way in which this self-performance within the narrated event takes on the dimension of a female struggle for autonomy within a hostile male environment. (p. 67)*

Borland continues by noting that Beatrice was a female interloper in a male sphere. She notices that even before the first race, Beatrice's father did not want her to bet, something that Borland describes as a "risk-taking" activity, to which she adds, "Men take risks; women do not" (p. 68). She lauds Beatrice for holding her ground against her father's "denunciation," raising the stakes with increasingly large bets, and taking great pleasure by showing up her "know-it-all" father: "Thus, at the story's end, Beatrice has moved herself from a peripheral feminine position with respect to the larger male sphere of betting *and* talk, to a central position where her words and deeds proclaim her equal and indeed superior to her male antagonist" (p. 68).

There was only one problem with Borland's interpretations of "what was *really* going on" and "what was *really* being said," which was that her grandmother was buying none of it. Upon reading Borland's first draft, Beatrice wrote what Borland describes as a "fourteen-page letter" that rejected Borland's analysis. While appreciating Borland's recognition of the grandmother's personal strength that she demonstrated in so many ways—not only at the racetrack but in doing things that women just didn't do at the time, such as divorcing her first husband—the grandmother attributed the confidence underlying that strength to the many strong people in her life, including her father, who did nothing but encourage and take pride in her achievements. Rejection of the interpretation by her grandmother after reading the first draft led to further discussion, further revising, and some movement on the parts of both women as they tried to reach some jointly satisfactory resolution of the meaning of the original episode.

One of the central tenets of feminist research is that women must be able to say things in their own voice and that voice must be heard. Or do some women know better than others? Anderson and Jack (1991) appear to open the door to exactly that possibility. They begin by arguing that male-dominated science is an inappropriate model to the extent that it embodies hierarchical relations between the researcher and those researched, where an "expert" researcher "extracts" data from "subjects" and then reinterprets it according to a "culturally sanitized" (i.e., male-dominated) "spin."

> We need to hear what women implied, suggested, and started to say but didn't. We need to interpret their pauses and, when it happens, their unwillingness or inability to respond. We need to consider carefully whether our interviews create a context in which women feel comfortable exploring the subjective feelings that give meaning to actions, things, and events, whether they allow women to explore "unwomanly" feelings and behaviours, and whether they encourage women to explain what they mean in their own terms. (p. 17)

Anderson and Jack's (1991) assertions seem to question any face-value acceptance of what women say, seeing the task as one of reading between the lines and finding what the women being interviewed are "really" saying and what they "really" mean by it. But when does that reinterpretation become just another imposition?

Many feminist researchers (including Borland, 1991) and others have wrestled with these issues. Their analyses can make us all aware of how professional zeal and arrogance may lead us to usurp others' voices and take for granted some things that perhaps shouldn't be accepted. Black feminists, for example, argue that sisterhood has its limits if it means homogenizing women's experience in a way that doesn't do justice to the equally meaningful and simultaneously marginalizing experience of race (e.g., see Collins, 1991; Etter-Lewis, 1991; Fine, Weis, Weseen, & Wong, 2003;

Olesen, 1994), while others make the same point regarding Latina (e.g., Benmayor, 1991), Native (e.g., Greschner, 1992; Monture-Okanee, 1993; Petersen, 1994), and Third World women (e.g., Hale, 1991; Patai, 1991; Salazar, 1991). All call for research considerations that acknowledge and respect cultural differences. In Borland's case, the relationship she had with her grandmother allowed her to go back and negotiate a resolution that was satisfactory to both of them. Her experience suggests we should trod carefully when that self-correcting mechanism is not present, as when we look at historical archives of people no longer with us, or do our interviews and go back to our offices to analyze and write without reconnection with our participants.

When the Past Bites Back

Although oral history serves the various functions we have noted—allowing us to rectify the imbalance of history by giving otherwise marginalized sources an opportunity to tell their stories and include them in "the box" of analyzable history—another way we need to be careful is when the past we are capturing has relevance to those who are still around. A case in point is the Belfast Project, an oral history project organized by Boston College that began with the noblest of motives, but ended in disaster (e.g., Palys & Lowman, 2012).

To understand this story, you need to know a little bit about The Troubles, a 30-year war from 1969 to 1999 that was just the most recent eruption of conflict that goes back hundreds of years over Northern Ireland's relation with Great Britain. The conflict also had a religious dimension to it to the extent that the Unionist/loyalists who wanted to remain a part of Britain were mostly Protestants, while the Irish nationalist/republicans, who were mostly Catholics, viewed themselves as an oppressed minority and sought independence from Britain in a united Ireland. The Troubles erupted when protests that were being held in an effort to end discrimination against the Catholic minority were met with police brutality. The conflict escalated over years until there were veritable armies attacking each other and engaging in activities we now categorize as terrorism—disappearances of opposition members, bombs blowing up in public places and killing innocents—coupled with the involvement and intervention of British security and police forces whose tactics were often as despicable and deadly to innocent bystanders as those they sought to control.

The Troubles generally are considered to have ended with the signing of the Good Friday Peace Agreement in 1998, which took effect in 1999. It was not long thereafter, in 2001, when archivists at Boston College—a US institution with many historic ties to Ireland—sought to design an oral history study in which front-line combatants from all sides would have an opportunity to talk about their involvement in the conflict. Ed Moloney, an Irish journalist who had written extensively about The Troubles, was hired as project director. As Cote (2012) explained in a magazine article, Moloney was impressed with a similar oral history project that had been conducted after an earlier eruption of conflict in the 1920s, and was happy to see there was interest in something similar that could make a similarly positive contribution to understanding why and how ordinary people become involved in conflict.

> [The Irish oral history project] was a very, very valuable historical archive and it was conducted and paid for by the government," Moloney said in an interview. "I had always been an admirer of this. I had thought, 'Wouldn't it be great to do something like this in Northern Ireland and the Troubles?' for a very simple reason, and that is that history books and accounts of history are normally written by the leaders—by the people who are the generals and politicians, who emerge at the end of the day at the top of the heap. Very rarely do they reflect the views or the experiences and life stories of people who are at the ground level in these conflicts. (Cote, 2012)

Anthony McIntyre, a former IRA member who had spent 18 years in Northern Ireland prisons and went on to earn a PhD after his release, was hired to interview former IRA combatants, while Wilson McArthur, who was familiar with the unionist Ulster Volunteer Force (UVF), was hired to do interviews with loyalists. These were excellent choices, given the trust that members of each side would have had in the two interviewers, which was essential if participants were going to feel comfortable discussing how they came to fight in the conflict, as well as acts of violence in which they had been involved.

A second important component was of course a guarantee of confidentiality, which Boston College was prepared to extend. The donor agreement prepared by Boston College assured participants that the tapes and transcripts of interviews would be held in the secure "Treasure Room" of the Boston College library where they would remain under the complete control of the participant until their death, at which time control over the interview would be transferred to Boston College.[4]

It is hard to imagine a topic more central to contemporary events. With violence coming from extremist groups of all stripes, how worthwhile would it be to better

---

[4]In RE: Request from the UK re Dolours Price. M.B.D. No. 11-MC-91078. Agreement for Donation. Attachment to Moloney affidavit, p. 9. Retrieved from http://bostoncollegesubpoena.wordpress.com/exhibits/affidavit-of-ed-moloney/.

understand processes of "radicalization" as they occurred among members of the IRA and UVF? Clearly it was an important study. Boston College found funding for the project, and it went ahead. Interviews were completed in Ireland, transcribed, and transferred to the United States where they they were to sit in the Treasure Room until the respondent died. The first two to do so were Brendan Hughes of the IRA and David Ervine of the UVF, at which point their transcripts were released and Ed Moloney wrote a book about their involvement entitled *Voices From the Grave* (Moloney, 2010). Shortly thereafter, one of the interviewees who was still alive—Dolours Price—gave an interview in which she alluded to the existence of the study and the archive of information it had produced. At that point, the family of Jean McConnvile, who had been killed by the IRA 40 years earlier for allegedly informing on them to the British, and whose murderers had never been identified, wondered whether the interviews might contain material that would shed light on their mother's murder. They approached the Police Service of Northern Ireland, who in turn approached the British Government, who in turn asked the US government to send the interviews to them under the terms of an MLAT—Mutual Legal Assistance Treaty—that Britain had with the United States.

Suffice it to say at this point that everything that could go wrong did. Boston College at first were simply going to hand over the interviews, but were stopped in their tracks when Ed Moloney found out about the prospective betrayal and publicized the subpoenas in an effort to get Boston College to live up to their promises to maintain the confidentiality of the information. As legal proceedings continued and the number of transcripts subpoenaed started to grow, some of the participants still alive sought to get their files—which they had been told were theirs until they died—and those who did so successfully burned them. What a travesty. We will not go further in the sordid details of the case (but see Palys & Lowman, 2014 and the archive of documents at the Boston College Subpoenas website at https://bostoncollegesubpoena.wordpress.com/) other than to point out again that third-party threats to confidentiality may be rare, but when they occur their effects can be devastating both to the people involved and the data they have produced. The biggest mistake made by the researchers in this instance was to trust Boston College's assurances that the data would be safe and confidential as the participation agreement outlined, and to lose control over the data by archiving it in the Treasure Room of the Burns Library at Boston College (see Palys & Lowman, 2015). Although the researchers were ready to take the materials and bury them somewhere to ensure the project's pledge of confidentiality was upheld, Boston College would have none of it.

However rich and interesting they may be, most oral histories involve more innocuous stories of being a mine worker or being a teenager in the 1920s, i.e., nothing that is very likely to engender some third party to initiate a legal case to retrieve and interview. The Boston College case is an unusual one because it is the only time we are aware of that an international treaty has been used to obtain confidential documents from a research project. It is also the first oral history we know of that has ever had its archive subpoenaed. For Boston College, its main legacy is of how not to organize an oral history research project and how to fail abysmally at protecting research participant confidentiality.

SUMMING UP AND LOOKING AHEAD

This chapter reviews three types of interview techniques that involve direct interaction between researcher and participant: (1) one-on-one interviews; (2) focus group interviews; and (3) oral history interviews. The advantages and disadvantages of each are discussed, and some of their similarities and differences noted. Considerable time was also spent outlining the various ways that questions can be phrased, some of the strategies and techniques used in the overall organization and implementation of an interview, and some of the obligations and responsibilities entailed in dealing with a respondent on a human-to-human basis.

The broader theme of this chapter, then, isn't that you must declare allegiance to one method (and the associated cluster of researchers) or another. Instead, look at the different methods as different ways of compiling and understanding people's views that have unique strengths they can bring to any given project, but also have much to offer each other in the context of mixed-method inquiry. Different methods will be useful to you at different times, depending on your objectives in a given project, but using multiple methods that complement each other is a strong research strategy that can offer a more comprehensive understanding than any one method alone can reveal.

For example, in the evaluation of a police mobile data access system described in Chapter 8 on case study designs and Chapter 9 on surveys (Palys, Boyanowsky, & Dutton, 1984), the researchers used both interview and questionnaire techniques, knowing that they'd complement each other in supplying the information sought. Because the researchers came in after the system had already been in operation for more than a year, and the archival record on the system's development and implementation was at best sporadic, interviews helped fill in the gaps, giving a more human face to the multiplicity of meanings that people place on a new technology.

By doing target interviews with people throughout the organization, Ted and his colleagues were able to get a good handle on the perceived positives and negatives of the data system they were evaluating. But because of the limitations of target interviewing, they weren't sure whether the views they were picking up were held broadly or just by a few vocal people. Accordingly, they used the results of the interviews to design a questionnaire that was meaningful to the people involved, both in how it was worded and in the issues it addressed.

Similar issues will arise in subsequent chapters. Whether the topic is observational methods (Chapter 11), archival techniques (Chapters 12 and 13), or the variety of experimentalist approaches (Chapters 6–8), you'll see that different clusters of researchers have tended to construe each set of methods in different ways, using them to largely different ends and eschewing the way others have used them. Our approach throughout will be to articulate their diversity in a way that will help us understand how we can all benefit from them both individually and in combination.

Key Concepts

Background/demographic
  questions 400
Clarification probes 405
Echo probe 404
Experience/behavior questions
  400
Feeling questions 401
Interview schedule 402

Knowledge questions 400
Opinion/values questions 400
Probe for examples 404
Probes 403
Selective deposit 425
Semi-structured interviewing
  402
Sensory questions 401

Shadow speaking 413
Silent probe 404
Structured interviewing 402
Tell-me-more probe 404
Transcribing 412
Unstructured interviewing 401

STUDY QUESTIONS

1. Create a 3 × 2 table where the three columns are the three types of interviews discussed in this chapter, while the two rows represent strengths and weaknesses. Compare and contrast the different types of interviews by filling in the cells of the table.

2. What are some situations where it would be advisable to take a more unstructured approach to interviewing and when would a more structured approach be preferred?

3. Rosa is conducting interviews with women who work in "nontraditional" occupations, i.e., occupations that have traditionally been dominated by men. What are the relative advantages and disadvantages in this case of (1) taking general written notes during the interview and trying to write any "juicy" quotes down verbatim; (2) using a tape recorder to tape the interviews; (3) taping the interview and writing down key points as the interview proceeds?

4. Compare and contrast the feminist and dramaturgical views of the interview that were discussed in this chapter.

5. What unique advantages do focus group interviews have to offer? What limitations do you have to be aware of? What can you do to try to minimize those limitations?

6. What is "selective deposit," and how is it related to the study of history? In what sense do oral history methods address some of the problems of selective deposit?

7. Explain how Katherine Borland's oral history of her grandmother's day at the races illustrated both the difficulties and responsibilities of interpreting other people's lives. Was the resolution they came down to a fair one in your view?

OBSERVATION, ETHNOGRAPHY, AND PARTICIPATORY ACTION RESEARCH

CHAPTER OUTLINE

Because observation is something that all of us do all the time, we begin by dispelling the idea that observation as a research method involves no more than "just looking." Observation as a research strategy involves *looking in a planned and strategic way with a purpose*:

> *As members of society, we also make observations of the everyday world. These guide us in forging paths of action and interpreting the actions and reactions of others ... What differentiates the observations of social scientists from those of everyday-life actors is the former's systematic and purposive nature. Social science researchers study their surroundings regularly and repeatedly, with a curiosity spurred by theoretical questions about the nature of human action, interaction, and society. (Adler & Adler, 1994, p. 377)*

Indeed, you could easily argue that observation—watching what people do—is in many ways the most fundamental of methods. Talking to people is a great way to find out about people's attitudes and the values they hold, to be able to ask them about a broad range of activities and hear them tell us what they do and how they came to be doing it. But if behavior is what we are interested in understanding, then the most direct way to see what people actually do under whatever conditions interest us is to watch them do it.

There are of course limitations to observational strategies on their own. It leaves us to speculate about *why* the people we observe are doing what they are doing. Further, because there can be many reasons for any given behavior—is that wink happening because the person is being flirtatious? or are they signaling that they are just pulling our leg? or did a speck of dust fly into their eye?—it is very easy for us to be wrong. This once again encourages us to consider observation as particularly useful as an integral part of a mixed methods strategy where we can see the behavior and ask people about it and triangulate with other sources that will give us a comprehensive picture of when/why/how some phenomenon of interest occurs.

THE RELATIONSHIP BETWEEN OBSERVER AND OBSERVED

Weick (1968) and others (e.g., Angrosino & Mays de Perez, 2003; Bernard, 2013; Gray, 2014) suggest that a major element differentiating observational studies is the nature of the relationship between observer and observed. The traditional continuum of roles that many researchers envision (see Gold, 1958) can range from the complete participant to the complete observer, as depicted in Figure 11.1. Although the continuum is not as widely held as before for reasons that will become apparent below, it is a helpful place to start because it sensitizes us to the variety of relationships that might exist between observer and observed, each of which has its own advantages and limitations. We'll examine the two extremes of the continuum first and then try to make some sense of the middle ground.

The Complete Participant

With the "complete participant" role, the observer does not reveal to others that they are a researcher. From the perspective of those being observed, the researcher *is* a participant. Doing so gives you an excuse to be in the setting, while also helping avoid detection. One famous example of this type of research is Laud Humphreys's (1970) *Tearoom Trade* (described in Chapter 4), where Humphreys played the role of "watch queen"—acting as a lookout—in order to observe intimate sexual encounters between men in public washrooms.

Another example is a classic study entitled *When Prophecy Fails*, by Festinger, Riecken, and Schachter (1956). While most groups who foretell the end of the world are vague about when exactly Armageddon will arrive, this study began when Festinger heard about a doomsday group that had made a very specific prediction about when the world would end. What would happen when it didn't? From a strictly rational perspective you would think that people would say, "I guess we were wrong" when they predict the world will end at 10:56 PM on the 14th of January and it doesn't. Festinger became interested in the group because his theory of cognitive dissonance predicted the exact opposite, i.e., that when the world didn't end, those who were committed to it happening would believe even more strongly in the truth of their prediction and develop a new explanation to

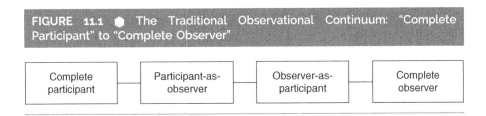

FIGURE 11.1 ● The Traditional Observational Continuum: "Complete Participant" to "Complete Observer"

Complete participant	Participant-as-observer	Observer-as-participant	Complete observer

explain the inconsistency. Two graduate students working with him decided to join the group in order to see what would happen within the group when the world did not end.

A third example is the pseudo-patient role that David Rosenhan (1973) and seven collaborators played at different mental hospitals in a famous study entitled "Being sane in insane places." Each person was to arrive at the admissions office and complain about "hearing voices" that said "empty," "hollow," and "thud." Beyond that, however, the pseudo-patients were instructed to act as they normally would—engaging in conversations, eating meals, writing notes—and to tell anyone who would listen that they now felt fine and were having no symptoms. They would only get out when they could convince the staff they were ready to be released. The objective was to better understand the processes by which labels of mental illness are conferred and maintained. The study was highly successful; once the "mentally ill" label was applied, it seemed everything people said or did was interpreted within the context of that label. One unexpected benefit of this was in the pseudo-patients' fieldnotes; while note-taking in most cases of surreptitious observation can be a challenge, in the psychiatric context, their note-taking was interpreted as just another illustration of their mental illness:

> *Nursing records for three patients indicate that the writing was seen as an aspect of their pathological behavior.... Given that the patient is in the hospital, he must be psychologically disturbed. And given that he is disturbed, continuous writing must be a behavioral manifestation of that disturbance, perhaps a subset of the compulsive behaviors that are sometimes correlated with schizophrenia. (p. 182)*

Ironically, the only people who recognized that the patients were actually pseudo-patients were other patients! The staff never recognized them as pseudo-patients, gave all but one a diagnosis of "schizophrenia" (the eighth was diagnosed as "manic depressive"), and, after stays ranging from 7 to 52 days, discharged them with a diagnosis of "schizophrenia in remission."

Of course, the lack of informed consent and the presence of deception in these examples should wave red flags for you in the realm of ethical concerns. For many people, the idea of going "undercover" and deceiving those in the site about your identity is anathema to the relationships that researchers should be striving for. Others are willing to consider the possibility if a number of criteria are met, including (1) if the study concerns an issue of importance that cannot be conducted in any other way; (2) whether the situation is "public" or not; (3) whether the data that are gathered involve identifiable persons; and (4) whether publication of your observations can be done without violating confidentiality to ensure that those who unknowingly participated in the research are nonetheless protected from harm. Those who have a stomach for it also argue that from a purely scientific perspective the "surreptitious observer" role cannot be dismissed, since it combines the dual advantages of being an observer (and hence being prepared, systematic, etc.) while also minimizing the reactivity of participants through the shared participant role.

When a decision is made to engage in **covert observation**, other issues arise. For example, assuming a strictly participatory identity in the setting, while still maintaining your observational motives, requires you to assume multiple roles, a situation that can create role conflict (e.g., see Cicourel, 1964; Marquart, 2001; Riecken, 1969). The problems are twofold. First, because (by definition) the "real" participants can't know that you're an observer, in most cases you can't take notes while observing. As a result, you must either make numerous trips to the bathroom in order to create voice memos, jot down notes or write down a choice quotation, or wait until the end of the day to write daily synopses. In the former case, if not perceived as having a bladder problem, you may be viewed suspiciously. In the latter case, the longer the delay between when you make your observations and when you actually write them down, the greater heed you must pay to distortions of recall or the bias of selective memory. Cicourel (1964) argues that such distortions represent one of the biggest problems in research involving the unknown, participating observer.

A second problem arises from the fact that, in order to continue the participant guise, you must *participate*. But by doing so, you potentially alter the very process you are trying to observe. When Festinger's graduate students joined the doomsday group in order to study them, did the mere act of their joining and participating in the group's activities help convince the original group members of the veracity of their vision? And once you've joined, what do you do when someone turns to you during discussion and asks, "So what do *you* think?" If you say something and people follow your suggestion, you may have influenced the group to go in a direction it might not otherwise have gone. If you say something and your suggestion is *not* followed, this sequence of events might be the beginning of disharmony or factionalism within the group. But if you *don't* say anything, you may engender suspicion about your presence or contribute to feelings of indecisiveness or ambiguity among members of the group. The challenge is to participate while still remaining a neutral influence; this is one instance where politicians, many of whom seem quite expert at sounding like they're responding to a question while really saying nothing, may provide a useful model.

Few people have any problem with the idea of doing observational research on the way that people use public spaces such as waiting rooms, elevators, shopping malls, and parking lots. Lyn Lofland (1973), for example, has spent a considerable amount of time sitting in bus depots and other public places observing the way strangers use space in public settings. And John Lowman (1989), as part of his study evaluating the effects of changes in the laws regarding street prostitution, followed a strategy of simply going out every few weeks and counting the numbers of sex workers who could be observed working the streets and mapping their location; this allowed him to assess the effects of changes in the law that sought to move street prostitution away from some neighborhoods and toward others.

You can easily imagine other examples: examining crowd behavior while attending a sporting event or music concert; spending time in the emergency room of a hospital watching interactions among paramedics, police, nurses, and doctors. In each case, the researcher sits down and is just another person in the room. Is observing such behavior a violation of privacy? Those who do this type of research argue you are examining only those actions people reveal in public. Bernard (2013) refers to it as "passive deception." Because this type of research rarely involves any attempt to acquire people's names, anonymity is preserved. The people are not identified and cannot be after the study is over. Institutional review boards by and large accept that view.

But what if you want to video record the way people spontaneously order themselves as they enter buses or get on escalators? For some researchers, public behavior is still "public" regardless of how it is recorded, and possible identifiability is not a concern. Others would be concerned about consent issues while still others would have no problem with it as long as individual identities are camouflaged or the only people who see the recordings are members of the research team so that confidentiality is preserved. All of these approaches are potentially valid; no doubt the particular behavior(s) being observed would play a role in determining which course would be most appropriate.

Also, we have glossed over any difficulties with separating "public" from "private" spaces, but there are times the line is not so easily drawn. What about meetings of Alcoholics Anonymous (AA), for example? They are open to anyone who wants to attend, and in that sense are "public." Or is the "open" invitation implicitly limited to those with a drinking problem who want to seek help? Can the "open" invitation also be exploited by researchers, journalists, and so on? Lofland and Lejeune (1960) did exactly that in their study of AA and were chastised by some and praised by others when they published their work.

Similar questions are asked about cyber opportunities such as discussion boards, some of which are completely open; others require "memberships" that are simply a matter of registering, while others are more surreptitious and closed (see Atchison, 1999 and Kitchin, 2002 for discussions about these issues as they pertain to cyber-research). Is it acceptable for researchers to "lurk" in such cyber-settings in order to observe the interaction and then to write about it without the consent of those involved? For example, Soothill and Sanders (2005) did a focused study of ten prolific clients of sex workers in Britain by analyzing the information they posted on a website for patrons of commercial sex. They justified their ethical choices thus:

> *What seems to be at the heart of this debate, and indeed our own data collection, is what material is considered public and what is considered private. … [T]his research has abided by the rules of the group that has been studied, and has not put individuals in a position that could cause them harm or disruption.*
>
> *Although Fox and Roberts (1999, p. 651) argue that researchers should be mindful of the difference between Internet information "that is publicly* accessible *and that which is publicly* disseminated*", the use of data without specific permission is defensible. First, the information is public and accessible to anyone. The open status of the website and all information that is posted is frequently acknowledged on the message board with the expectation that journalists, police authorities and Home Office researchers are frequent "lurkers". Second, there is no way of identifying the case studies in this paper as they all adopt pseudonyms. Also, remaining anonymous and taking steps to protect their own identity is a defining feature of the sex industry. Individuals have invariably given considerable thought to the issue of anonymity before contributing to a public forum about such a private act. (Soothill & Sanders, 2005, 6.3–6.4)*

Social and health scientists continue to be divided about the wisdom of doing surreptitious research. Some maintain that a lack of informed consent is never acceptable. Others argue that such an approach is reasonable as long as (1) the research question is of sufficient merit; (2) those being observed are not adversely affected or diverted by your presence; and (3) appropriate precautions are taken to ensure confidentiality. Still others suggest that even those restrictions are too cumbersome and that when observational research is designed to expose and analyze abuses of power and other corruptive practices, anything goes (e.g., see Punch, 1994 for a discussion of that perspective and Miller & Tewksbury, 2001 for a broader discussion about the utility and ethics of covert methods).

The Complete Observer

This position is epitomized by researchers who identify themselves as being engaged in observational research and who either set up a study in their own setting (such as a laboratory or clinic) or gain access to another setting (such as an organization or group) by seeking and obtaining permission. Once in the setting, the complete observer typically does their best to remain relatively inconspicuous, doing nothing other than observing with the full knowledge of all who are present that that's why the researcher is there. Although this type of observation is done in both the lab and the field, we'll begin by looking at the most contrived and obvious observing situation first, i.e., the observational setting where the researcher in white lab coat creates situations based on a particular hypothesis and observes what happens when a research participant is placed in it.

Observing on Home Turf

There's an extensive tradition of observational research in the laboratory, particularly among experimental social psychologists and those who study child development. Such studies typically involve setting up a particular situation, with the observer then retreating behind a one-way glass to make notes or systematically code the behaviors that emerge. There are two advantages to this approach. First, it's ethically non-problematic (assuming participants aren't misled about the purpose of the research), because participants know from the start that they are participating in a study where their behavior will be observed. Second, because it happens on the researcher's own turf in a predetermined manner, the researcher is ready to observe, using checklists or other coding schemes that have been prepared ahead of time.

Countering Reactivity

The biggest disadvantages associated with observational research with a known observer are the often artificial nature of the setting and the reactivity that can occur when research participants know they are being observed, i.e., when the researcher's presence and the mere act of observation somehow "change" the behavior of those being observed from what it would have been had the researcher not been present. The fact the researcher is not participating in any of the activities being observed only heightens the feeling of being observed. Who could feel comfortable seeing someone standing on the side with clipboard in hand, watching your every move? Experimental psychologists, the researchers who most commonly use this sort of method, have often resorted to deceiving participants about the "true" purpose of the study in order to counter reactivity effects. Recall, for example, the Donnerstein and Berkowitz study that we discussed in Chapter 6 on experiments. From the participants' perspective, they were helping the experimenter by delivering electric shocks to a female participant when she made mistakes in a learning task—a presumably helpful behavior they were required to perform. Meanwhile, from the researchers' perspective, the participants were exhibiting aggressive behavior to a woman that was hypothesized would vary depending on the type of film material they were being shown—a negative behavior they could deliver in doses at their discretion.

Outside the lab, active deception is much less likely in part because it is less needed. Other factors, some of which the researcher has some control over, can minimize reactivity in most observational field settings. An obvious one is the *conspicuousness of the observer*. All else being equal, a researcher who is in the middle of the action will be more conspicuous than one who stands discreetly at the edge. Related to this are the *characteristics of the observer*, particularly the *similarity* of characteristics between the observer and observed. In general, the greater the similarity between observer and observed (in age, dress, race, for example), the less conspicuous the observer will be and, hence, the less reactivity that will be generated.

The *characteristics of the participants* also affect reactivity. Children, for example, seem to forget about an observer's presence a lot more quickly than adults do, although the novelty of being observed wears off fairly quickly for both groups. Indeed, another important principle is that *the longer the observational period*, the more reactivity is reduced. This is so for several reasons: (1) novel stimuli in a person's environment (such as an observer) dominate the person's attention initially but soon fade into the background; (2) rapport is often established between the observer and those being observed, so that the observer becomes a less threatening presence; and (3) although it's easy to construct and maintain an image for a short time, most people find it very hard to keep up a false front over a longer period.

The *rationale for observing* given to participants also plays a role in the defensiveness they exhibit. For example, in the evaluation of a police department's radio data system that gave officers access to various data banks from a computer terminal located in patrol cars (MRDS) that we described previously, the research team went out of their way to assure officers that it was the *system* rather than *them* that was being evaluated (although it took some time before patrol officers actually became convinced that was the case). Also, the fact that several of the research assistants had prior policing interests and/or experience seems to have minimized reactivity (note that the factor used to their benefit was one of trying to maximize the similarity between observer and observed).

Ted and his colleagues also were fortunate in that study to have a way of assessing the extent to which the presence of observers generated reactivity, since they were able to scrutinize computerized archival records of system use that allowed them to compare how officers used the system when observers were present versus how they used it when observers were not. As this example suggests, *the nature of the phenomenon the researcher is observing* also will influence reactivity. The more deviant or stigmatized the activity being scrutinized, the more reactive the situation, and the longer it will take to build appropriate rapport.

Finally, another way that researchers attempt to deal with reactivity in the field is to participate on occasion, but to do so in as innocuous a way and as infrequently as possible. In this regard, there are a variety of things that researchers can do to be helpful, which also helps build rapport, without influencing the actual activity of the group. You can be the person who goes to get the coffee, or helps with the photocopying, or helps bring in the groceries, i.e., the role of "thoughtful guest," where you do small things that help the group function but do not alter its direction.

Structured Observation

Within the more lab-based observational tradition, the preference has been for more structured observation used in concert with a deductive approach that relegates the act of observation to the testing of hypotheses or the gathering of data that are defined by the researcher as important. The tradition is not limited to the lab, however. For example, when Ted and his colleagues did the evaluation of MRDS we refer to above (see also Chapter 8), the observation they did in patrol cars followed a highly structured protocol where each access of the system by a patrol officer was coded by the researcher riding with them in terms of what kind of information was accessed. When a highly structured coding scheme is used, a high priority for the researcher is to show that the scheme they are using can actually be used reliably—consistently—and that the researcher is indeed measuring what they think they are measuring—validity. Accordingly, we need to discuss how to develop, assess, and implement a reliable and valid coding scheme.

Checklists and Coding Schemes. As a first dimension to consider, coding schemes might be conceived of as either *static*, where particular attributes of the setting are noted (e.g., age and sex of participant, public or private setting), or *dynamic* (i.e., focusing on behavior and its unfolding). Dynamic coding schemes may include simple categorizations (e.g., whether someone gives change to a busker) or more complex ones (e.g., whether eye contact is made, how the initial verbal appeal is delivered, whether there is a movement to check for funds).

There are two main types of observational coding schemes: **sign systems** and **category systems**. With *sign* systems, the researcher essentially waits, noting each time a predetermined criterion behavior occurs. For example, a researcher investigating the incidence of prosocial behavior among children in a playschool setting might observe the children over the course of a day and (after having taken care to develop an operational definition of what kinds of acts will be considered "prosocial") note each time a prosocial act occurs. In contrast, *category* systems attempt to create a set of mutually exclusive and exhaustive categories into which any given behavior might be classified. Thus, rather than noting each prosocial act, the researcher might code on a minute-by-minute basis and, within each minute, code (at its simplest) whether the behaviors the children are exhibiting are prosocial or non-prosocial or (in a more complex coding scheme) whether the dominant behavior was prosocial, affectionate, communicative, aggressive, or whatever.

The sign system would give a better indication of *how many* prosocial acts were witnessed (since every act is counted), whereas a category system would give a better indication of the *temporal flow* of the prosocial acts during the day (e.g., Was the amount of prosocial behavior greater in the morning, when the children were fresh, or in the afternoon, when they were more tired? Was there more prosocial behavior before they watched a film in which the characters had to cooperate to achieve a collective objective or after?).

Assessing Reliability. Whichever alternative is chosen, researchers who develop structured coding systems are obliged to consider the reliability with which their coding scheme can be implemented. A "good" coding scheme is one where different individuals are able to code the same material or events independently and do so in the same way. Thus, if we're using a sign system to code incidents of violence in a mixed martial arts event, we're in big trouble if you count 30 incidents and another researcher counts 700 when we watch the same fight. Clearly, the researcher should assess the reliability with which a coding scheme can be applied *before* doing the actual study, since doing the study is a waste of time if you cannot have any confidence in the reliability of the numbers the observational scheme is generating.

In general, this is done by having different individuals code the same material independently. The reliability of the category coding scheme is the extent of inter-rater agreement. For example, in a 1-hour observational period where two raters were using a category system to code the "types of fight moves" in each 1-minute period, what percentage of the time did the two raters make the same categorizations, and what percentage of the time did they differ? If the inter-rater agreement is above 80 percent, and especially if it's above 90 percent, then you're doing pretty well and can feel comfortable going ahead and coding "for real." If it's lower than that, a better coding manual and/or more training might be required. In either case, the data should be examined carefully to determine exactly where the disagreements are occurring; this approach will help highlight what aspects of the coding scheme or training program need to be rectified.

A number of factors are known to influence the reliability of coding schemes, including the following:

- The more *clearly defined* and *nonoverlapping* the coding system, the higher the reliability.

- The shorter the period of time between the event and the coding of it, the greater the reliability of the recording; coding while observing is obviously optimal here.

- Reliability is lower when inference is required. For example, observers can agree more easily whether people are "walking" or "running" (two overt behaviors) than on whether people are "happy" or "sad" (two emotional states or feelings that involve more inference) about heading to their destination.

- Reliability is higher when the number of categories is small. A larger number of categories generally require finer, more difficult distinctions.

- Coder training will affect reliability. The researcher needs to determine just how much training is required in order to maximize the reliability of the observational scheme.

Reliability is particularly enhanced by carefully defining the construct(s) under consideration. For example, in one graduate-level methods class he taught, Ted told students that they were going to study coding schemes the next week. In preparation, they were each to watch the first period of a hockey game that was to be broadcast that weekend and were to come to class the next week ready to state how many violent acts occurred during that first period. When the students returned and gave their counts, the numbers ranged from 0 to 140!

Clearly, "violent" meant different things to different people, so Ted asked the students to explain what the term had meant to them. The person who counted "0" considered "violent" to be synonymous with "fights" and noted that there were none during the period that was observed. For the person who counted 140, "violent" meant any nonaccidental physical contact between players, and there were many incidents of bumping, boarding, and such during the period. Others argued for definitions that recognized professional hockey as a contact sport and hence focused on "gratuitous" contact as the defining aspect of "violence." Still others felt that, to meet their definition, the contact had to be gratuitous *and* outside the rules; these people focused on penalties emerging from contact (e.g., "tripping" would be a violent rule violation, but "delay of game" would not). They spent much of the class discussing which definition was "best" for their purposes. Once they agreed on what definition to employ, each of the students independently counted incidents of violence in a videotaped period of hockey. This time, there was very little variation in their counts. In other words, their coding was now *reliable*; independent observers could code the same material and come up with essentially the same results.

Validity. There are several other comments to make about this example. First, recall the distinction between reliability and validity. Although Ted's students had become *reliable* in their coding, the *validity* issue still remained. In one sense, all four of the definitions supplied were "valid." All you can do is choose definitions consistent with your research objectives and theoretical approach and then articulate these choices for scrutiny by other researchers. The "best" choice will vary depending on the theory and objectives that guide you, as well as the context. If one player intentionally bumps another during a football game, we may consider it "nonviolent" because it is "within the rules" and "part of the game." But the same behavior on an escalator at Nordstroms might be considered "violent" because it's gratuitous in that setting. The challenge is to derive a definition that is useful in your research context and to articulate your choices so that others can judge the utility of your definition to them.

However, sometimes doing so is not enough as real theoretical differences between researchers leave one group or another unwilling to budge. For example, in the area of prostitution research, some people argue that there are many reasons why women engage in sex work, which range from them being trafficked to engaging in it for "survival" reasons (e.g., drug addicted, poor, no other skills) to simply choosing it as a profession. While some theorists acknowledge this range and see the challenge of legislation being to ensure that women who engage in the profession are there by choice and can do so safely, others are adamant that all prostitution is sexual slavery and thus inherently violent. These differences also raise the issue of where the power to define should lie—with researchers who bring whatever their own theoretical perspective happens to be, or with the people who are the subject of their theorizing—as it did with Katherine Borland and her grandmother's day at the races that we discussed in Chapter 10. In anthropology, the choice is said to be between emic and etic understandings—emic refers to the understandings that exist within a social group, while etic refers to understandings from the outside, i.e., the observer's perspective.

The Complete Observer in the Field
Gaining Access

Field relationships are best developed over time, and one of the hallmarks of a lengthy career as a field researcher is that you are successful at building trusting relationships with particular communities. When you first meet members of a community, all you can offer them are promises: you will do this and that; you will give them this and that; you will protect them in this way and that. But over time it is your performance that does the talking. They see you deliver on your promises, or not. They see you sticking your neck out for them, or not. They see you being fair in your reporting, or not. They see you doing concrete things that will help the community, or not. You will have lots of decisions to make along the way about how close a relationship to have, whether you will compartmentalize your research life from the rest of your life, and what you will put in your published reports, but these relationships can be very enriching for your life, and it is a real honor to be trusted by a community and to live up to their trust—and they to yours—over time.

It's that first time that's the hardest, in part because the people or organization or group you want to approach know nothing about you, and depending on the sensitivity of their situation and the information you would be gathering, they need to make that leap of faith that says not that they will trust you—nobody does that right away—but that they will give you a chance. Understand that while we hope that your motives will be honorable and your intentions the best, you may also be competing for their attention with various hit-and-run researchers who just want to gather the data and get out of there, some of whom will have huge grants and try and simply buy access.

The basic issue you have to address when you first make contact with a person or group or organization of interest is why they should let you—a stranger—observe their behavior. Although we might like or hope for the prospective participants to trust us immediately after we parachute into a particular setting because we are affiliated with a university and/or have a project due next month and/or are basically honest and well-meaning, reality is rarely so benevolent. Instead, the complete observer often must be prepared to deal with a gatekeeper (Broadhead & Rist, 1976) and talk their way into the group. Lofland and Lofland (1984) suggest that you'll be most effective in doing so if you come armed with connections, accounts, knowledge, and courtesy.

With respect to *connections*, Lofland and Lofland (1984) suggest that, if you're not connected with the target group or organization already, you'd do well to cast about among your friends and acquaintances to find someone who is and who would be willing to provide an introduction. They recount the experiences of Joan Hoffman (1980), who was herself a member of an elite family and who had attempted to talk to community elites who were serving on hospital boards:

> *Introducing myself as a sociology graduate student, I had very limited success in getting by the gatekeepers of the executive world. Telephone follow-ups to letters sent requesting an interview repeatedly found Mr. X "tied up" or "in conference." When I did manage to get my foot in the door, interviews rarely exceeded a half hour, were continuously interrupted by phone calls ... and elicited only "front work" ... the public version of what hospital boards were all about ... By chance during [one] interview, my respondent discovered that he knew a member of my family. "Why didn't you say so?" The rest of the interview was dramatically different than all my previous data. (Hoffman, 1980, p. 46; cited in Lofland & Lofland, 1984, p. 25)*

Even when you know no one in the setting, connecting with one person who can act as an "in" and/or "key informant" can make all the difference between getting a project off the ground or not. For Whyte (1943), in his classic *Street Corner Society*, for example, the person who made all the difference was "Doc." For Duneier (1999) in his study of sidewalk entrepreneurs in *Sidewalk*, it was seller of "black books" Hakim Hasan, with whom he struck up a conversation when he noticed Hasan was selling a book Duneier had written previously. For Horowitz (1983), the beginning came with a mixture of persistence and luck:

> *I chose to sit on a park bench where many youths gathered from noon until midnight. On the third afternoon of sitting on the bench, as I dropped a softball that had rolled toward me, a young man came over and said "You can't catch" (which I acknowledged) and "You're not from the hood [neighborhood], are you?"*

This was a statement, not a question. He was Gilberto, the Lions' President. When I told him I wanted to write a book on Chicano youth, he said I should meet the other young men and took me over to shake hands with eight members of the Lions. (p. 7; cited in Berg, 2001, p. 146)

Once a preliminary connection is made, Lofland, Snow, Anderson, and Lofland (2006) argue that you also should be prepared with *accounts*, by which they mean "a careful explanation or account of the proposed research" (p. 43). Use words and concepts that are meaningful to the prospective sample, and while you should be prepared to offer an academic justification for your project, that's probably not what's being sought here. Instead, you should be ready to offer a simple, straightforward, and honest explanation that addresses the question "Why are you interested in us?"

In Chris's research on the sex industry, he frequently finds that he has to navigate his identity with participants when in the field. This is particularly the case since the people he observes and interacts with are frequently marginalized, stigmatized, and criminalized. He often finds that sex workers and their clients are very suspicious of him and his motives for wanting to observe in different physical and virtual settings. Some assume he is an undercover police officer, others believe that because he is an academic researcher he will judge them or their involvement in the sex industry. To calm their nerves and suspicions, Chris takes on the role of the naïve but informed newcomer who is interested in learning from them in order to address the stereotypes and preconceived notions that people might have about the sex industry and the people involved in it.

Chris is not alone in representing himself as a "learner," which indeed any researcher is (otherwise, there'd be no need to engage in the research). The advantages of taking that approach are twofold. First, it reduces the extent to which you might be perceived as threatening. Second, the process of "teaching" reveals much about a person's understandings.

However, difficulties can arise when adopting the role of "naive observer" that can end up interfering with the acquisition of rich data. In some situations being perceived as unknowledgeable may lead to you receiving little more than what Hoffman (1980) referred to above as "front work," that is, superficial information of the type that usually appears in brochures or on guided tours. Particularly when people are very busy and/or are more senior members of the organization, you must demonstrate that you're worth their time and that they, in particular, are the only appropriate sources for what you need to know. Showing that you've done your homework, that you don't ask the same basic questions that everyone else asks, that you can speak "the language" of that profession, and that you know something about the phenomenon you wish to observe (but do not have too many preconceived notions and are willing to watch and listen) is a good recipe for being treated seriously.

Finally, Lofland et al. (2006) emphasize that you must show *courtesy* and respect in negotiating for entry. This means emailing or phoning ahead to make appointments at a time convenient to your guide(s); taking the time to tell everyone who's interested a little bit about your research (using language that is accessible, relatable and understandable), even if a given person isn't directly involved; and ensuring that you also get permission from dependent or subordinate populations as well as from those who act as gatekeepers (e.g., asking the kids for their permission and not just their parents and the daycare person).

How and What Do You Observe?

Assuming that you *do* get access to the setting or group that you wish to observe, your next challenge is to make specific decisions about what, and then how, to observe. A detailed inventory of all the various techniques and alternatives is beyond the scope of this text, but various sources offer us a few basic points to consider.

Options Regarding Structure. We mentioned at the beginning of this chapter that we would be making distinctions between different approaches for pedagogical reasons that might be difficult to sustain, and the one we made between structured and "unstructured" approaches to observation is one of them. This is so for two main reasons. The first is that it is becoming more and more commonplace to combine observational techniques and indeed to combine observation itself with other methods to gain the benefits that arise from mixed methods inquiry.

The second is that, particularly with field-based research, very often the general strategy is not to have a singular plan and follow it rigidly, but to start off with broader observational coverage and gradually develop a focus after spending some time in the field. Ted recalls his time during a previous sabbatical when he had the opportunity to spend time with Howard Becker when he was at the University of Washington and join him in a graduate class on field research that Becker offered each week. Students were continually frustrated when they would ask him what sorts of things they should write down in their fieldnotes and he would always respond by saying "everything." His admonition was another way of saying that you should write down as much as possible because you never know what will turn out to be important later and become your eventual focus of study.

During the preliminary phases, you are trying to contextualize the phenomenon of interest, gather basic descriptive information that will inform subsequent analysis (e.g., How frequently does the phenomenon occur? Who's involved in the process? What other aspects of the process warrant scrutiny?). This is also a time to sharpen research questions, to consult with people who are knowledgeable in the field along with those who are most likely to be affected, and to decide what particular types of data will be used as indicators for the key concepts of interest.

A primary hazard to avoid here is in *not* making the transition to more focused observation. Certainly a more focused research question facilitates this transition, as does the imposition or generation of theory. The danger, as Cicourel (1964) notes, is that without theory or a clearly focused research question, you have no guide for your activity—it is the research question that determines what is "relevant" or not to pursue—in which case the method may amount to little more than a never-ending "pilot study" that accomplishes little.

Some Places to Start

Characteristics, Causes, Consequences. What you look for will depend on your particular research question(s) and objectives and understanding of the phenomenon of interest. Nonetheless, an inventory of some "basic" attributes may be considered. Most generally, John Lofland (1971) argues that, when you boil it all down, everything we call "social science" can be said to address one or more of the following three questions:

> *What are the* characteristics *of a social phenomenon, the forms it assumes, the variations it displays?*
>
> *What are the* causes *of a social phenomenon, the forms it assumes, the variations it displays?*
>
> *What are the* consequences *of a social phenomenon, the forms it assumes, the variations it displays? (p. 13)*

As you might expect when all of social science is summarized in three sentences, Lofland's synopsis subsumes considerable complexity. Consider how time is represented in these questions. Questions about *causes* direct our attention to the *past*. What are the antecedents of the phenomenon? Which of these are noteworthy in the generation or emergence or shaping of the phenomenon? Questions about *consequences* direct us to the *future*. In what sense is the phenomenon itself an initiator or cause of subsequent events? How does variation in the phenomenon relate to subsequent variation in other phenomena of interest? Finally, in pointing to *characteristics* or attributes of the phenomenon under study, Lofland is talking about *now*, the present. Implicit is a detailed description of the phenomenon as it is. But what characteristics are of interest to us?

Participants. Since the social and health sciences most often focus on human behavior, it seems reasonable to focus on the humans who inhabit our chosen milieu. Thus, as a minimum, you should describe participants in terms of demographics (e.g., age, sex), as well as other variables of interest that you note when observing, that appear in the literature as identified correlates, or that your particular theoretical dispositions dictate. *Who are these people?*

Acts and Activities. What people *do* is clearly of interest to social and health scientists; their behavior in the setting of interest will be one component of any complete observational account. Such behavior may include anything from relatively brief, situationally-constrained acts to elaborate activities that occur over more extended periods of time. What is happening? Involving whom? What aspects of the behavior are of particular interest to you (e.g., the way strangers are socialized into the setting; the way friendships form; the informal social rules that guide action)? Observation that extends over time helps researchers identify regularities and idiosyncrasies in behavior patterns that will in turn help focus subsequent research.

Words and Meanings. Related to but not necessarily synonymous with what people do is what they *say*. This element of the observational process can obviously include a lot: for example, the attitudes and beliefs that are espoused during ongoing activity, the explanations and accounts that people offer for what they do and how they do it, and the personal and social meaning that people see in and derive from what they do.

There are many decisions to be made about how to capture speech. One choice will pertain to how passive or provocative the researcher chooses to be in relation to the participants. Will you listen to ongoing and spontaneous conversation, or will you actively question and unearth information of interest to you? These two stances should not be seen as mutually exclusive. You might, for example, wish to be more passive during the initial, exploratory phases of the research, in order to acquire information about spontaneous activities and utterings, but later take a more provocative role in asking questions or seeking explanations/accounts. Often these will occur "offstage" in debriefing sessions with a key contact with whom you have rapport and to whom you can say, "What just happened there?"

Relationships/Networks. The elements listed above focus on individuals, but people exist—both implicitly and explicitly—in relations with other people in the production of phenomena of interest. Many aspects of relationships might therefore be of interest to us in an observational setting. You'll want to know, for example, who's a "regular" in the setting and who's more transient or tangential. You also may wish to ascertain the formal and informal roles different people occupy in the setting, and what these roles mean to them. And of course, all sorts of doors open up to you when you begin focusing on relationships: Who talks to whom? How and with whom is information shared? How are individuals recruited or screened for participation in the setting? Who is left out? What power relations exist? How do friendships and animosities evolve? How is status reaffirmed? What brings these people together?

The Setting or Environment. Action must happen somewhere, and the "somewhere" will tell you something about the individuals or group in question and potentially influence the action. What is the setting, and how is it perceived by both participants and the broader society? How do participants personalize and utilize the setting? To whom is the setting open, and to whom is it closed? How is accessibility conveyed? What objects are present, and what do their nature and position convey about the group or individuals being observed?

History. Social scientists rarely study situations that just appear. Our presence on site often in itself signifies that the group or setting we're observing has been around at least long enough to have caught our attention. Many observers in the social and health sciences view knowledge of the history of any setting or group as an integral part of understanding its current complexities.

Any study of history will be partly *descriptive* (e.g., certain persons or groups participated; certain events occurred on particular dates) and partly *interpretive* (e.g., we make inferences about why certain people were involved and the role they played, or we articulate what we feel is the broader significance of the processes we observed). Thus, historical accounts are themselves worthy of study *as* accounts, since they reflect the perspective of the person or group offering the account. Who the heroes and heroines are, what events are identified as "important," and the nature of myths and legends all tell something about the individual, group, or setting under study.

At the same time, you always should be aware of history as a social construction and its openness to revision. We have always been struck by the profundity of the statement "History is a justification of the present." History is, virtually by definition, always written from the writer's vantage point. And since those in power are the ones who write mainstream histories, their samplings of past events comprise all those things that were "important" (from that perspective) in getting to where we are today. To the extent that certain events are impossible to ignore (such as world wars or changes of government), the "spin" placed on them typically makes "our" people the heroes and heroines, while others are ignored or their contributions minimized, and the vanquished are deemed unworthy of mention. Current events and characteristics are assumed to be "natural" or "inevitable," and history is the name given to accounts of the glories and errors we encountered en route to the enlightened present. Still, as Yogi Berra is reputed to have said, "It ain't over 'til it's over"—that is, no history can ever hope to be "complete" until there's nobody left on earth to write it. In the interim, social scientists should be as interested in and as cautious about historical accounts—which tell you something about both history and the historian—as they are concerning other data sources.

Combining Elements. The components listed above shouldn't be seen as an inventory of things to include or as a rigid outline for your ultimate report. To quote Lofland (1971), "what have been outlined … [are nothing more than] … *elements* with which to sort and classify observations and to build some *other kind* of analytic scheme for one's observational materials" (p. 54; italics in original). Your challenge as a researcher is to ascertain what is important and what isn't, and then to build or test a theory or account of how the relevant elements interact over time to produce the phenomenon of interest.

Fieldnotes. As we suggested at the beginning of this chapter, many novice researchers fail to distinguish "observation" from "just looking." "Just looking" is something we all do whenever we enter a setting. "Observation" is an empirical technique that involves looking for a purpose—you have an analytical interest and are prepared to gather "relevant" data, however those terms are defined.

In more formal/structured settings, your role is clear: you will arrive with clipboard or a tablet or smartphone and coding scheme in hand, and there will be predetermined rules you will have established (when you decided how to operationalize your variables of interest) that specify whom to observe and at what times. But even when all your formal data coding is done on prescribed sheets or digital forms, we strongly advise that you either include a space for "comments" at the bottom of your coding scheme or have a digital recorder or small pad of paper at the ready. In some settings, a video recording may be made of the activity for future analysis. And in even less structured situations, the researcher who doesn't have easy access to paper and pen or some kind of digital recorder is being very shortsighted.

Even for structured observation methods, but especially for less structured ones like participant observation and ethnography, fieldnotes are integral to observation. No observational session is complete until those notes have been done. The notes should specify the time and place of observation, the people present and their spatial distribution and interaction, and any other details you as observer deem of interest.

Fieldnotes are normally very personal documents, and they have a crucial role, particularly in less structured observational research, because they're the raw data on which your analysis will be based. They are rarely shown to anyone but members of your research group and would virtually never be published as is (see Malinowski, 1967 for an exception). Accordingly, you should feel free to insert comments, make queries to yourself, and speculate about what might be occurring.

Richardson (1994), for example, distinguishes between several different types of fieldnotes via a shorthand she has developed for herself:

- **Observation notes** (ON): These are as concrete and detailed as I am able to make them. I want to think of them as fairly accurate renditions of what I see, hear, feel, taste, and so on.

- **Methodological notes** (MN): These are messages to myself regarding how to collect "data"—who to talk to, what to wear, when to phone, and so on. I write a lot of these because I like methods, and I like to keep a process diary of my work.

- **Theoretical notes** (TN): These are hunches, hypotheses, poststructuralist connections, critiques of what I am doing/thinking/seeing. I like writing these because they open up my text—my fieldnote text—to alternative interpretations and a critical epistemological stance. It is a way of keeping me from being hooked on my "take" on reality.

- **Personal notes** (PN): These are feelings statements about the research, the people I am talking to, myself doing the process, my doubts, my anxieties, my pleasures. I do no censoring here at all. I want all my feelings out on paper because I like them and because I know they are there anyway, affecting what/how I lay claim to knowing. Writing personal notes is a way for me to know myself better, a way of using writing as a method of inquiry into the self (p. 526).

Our systems aren't so differentiated, although we try to include the same variety of notes that Richardson (1994) reports. Ted simply distinguishes between things he's describing (on the basis of observing, hearing, etc.) and remarks he makes to himself that bear on personal feelings, tentative interpretations, questions to consider, future information to acquire, and so on. He just writes the former directly, enclosing the latter in square brackets to set them off as notes to himself.

Since most of the research that Chris does these days is with larger, interdisciplinary, teams of people that frequently reside and conduct their portion of the research in different geographic locations, the process and form that fieldnotes take for him is slightly different. Chris and his team use private access wikis or blogs to chronicle their individual fieldnotes detailing their observations and experiences of the various physical and virtual spaces in which they have immersed themselves. While each member of the team has considerable latitude when it comes to how they format their fieldnotes (e.g., as a stream of consciousness or in a more orderly fashion using headings and sub-headings), all members use an agreed upon set of colors to highlight text or other materials that correspond with different types of information. For example, fieldnotes regarding themes of people or things they are engaging with or observing are coded in yellow, the locations where the engagement or observation takes place (which can be real or virtual spaces) in blue, and any personal reflections, observations, and/or insights about the research process more generally in green. Each member of the team sets aside time each week to read and, where appropriate, comment upon the entries of other team members; in this way the team is recording and coding fieldnotes as the research progresses. The communication keeps them working as a team instead of spiraling off in multiple directions (although that is not an alternative, we would dismiss out of hand either).

Regardless of the particular style you develop, such notes are important. Because they create an ongoing record or personal/team archive over the course of your study, they act as a diary of the process you've gone through. You can look back over them to see how your knowledge and understandings of the situation have changed over time, to check whether all your ongoing speculations have been tested, or to discover any discrepancies or inconsistencies that might have become evident over time.

Of course, it may not always be comfortable or feasible to actually take notes in the setting itself, although it's always advisable to at least jot down very brief notes or key-words that will help you remember the chronology of the session. Whatever the case, always leave time at the end of each observational session to retire to a private location as soon as possible, *before* engaging in any other activities, to flesh out and organize the notes you've taken, which often are written all over the paper, in the margins, and with circles and arrows and perhaps little maps all around. And don't underestimate the length of time it'll take you to do so; many experienced observers suggest that you can expect to spend 4 hours formalizing your notes for every hour of observation (e.g., see Adler & Adler, 1994; Berg, 2007; Lofland et al., 2006). The longer you wait, the more other events will intervene to interfere with your recall and the poorer the record.

If you make note-taking a habit, your skills will improve substantially with experience. For example, Ted now finds that as long as he's able to jot down a few notes and keywords that reflect the overall chronology of a session, he can use them to generate detailed descriptions of events that have left people wondering whether the session was actually digitally recorded. A good place to practice such note-taking is in your classes. You probably take notes on lectures. If you do not already do so, try sitting down as soon as possible after each class and rewriting your notes, embellishing important points. With practice, you should soon be able to recreate the narrative of the whole lecture, and you'll find your later notes far better organized and thoughtful than the ones made during class, where the lecture's pace can cause you to leave points out. The worst thing you can do (besides taking no lecture notes at all) is take your lecture notes and then not look at them again until it's time to study for your exams. By that time, the train of thought will have been lost, the cryptic abbreviations that seemed so meaningful at the time will appear completely unfathomable, and you may have trouble following your notes, although they seemed perfectly logical when you first wrote them.

And finally, note that this practice of generating "notes to self" that begins in fieldnotes does not end when the data gathering is finished. Qualitative data analysis programs such as NVivo, for example, which we will describe in greater detail in Chapter 13, allow you to create memos to yourself or your research team members as you go through the process of listening to interviews, watching video, or reading transcripts or other text and begin the process of coding your data and develop that more in-depth understanding that will end up in written reports and accounts.

Mixing Participation and Observation

The two middle roles in the observational continuum are labeled *participant-as-observer* and *observer-as-participant*. As their titles suggest, both involve a mixing of the participatory and observational roles, with the difference based on which of the two predominates. This in itself may not be particularly clear-cut, and participant observers often float back and forth between the two, depending on the particular situation.

One perfect example of a mixture of roles was chosen by Muzafer Sherif in his famous "Robber's Cave" studies (see Sherif, Harvey, White, Hood, & Sherif, 1961). Sherif was interested in studying group dynamics, particularly with respect to group formation, cohesiveness, and conflict, and used a boys' summer camp as the context in which to perform his research. As far as the boys were concerned, it was summer camp and nothing more. But for Sherif, it was also an opportunity to manipulate different aspects of the situation (e.g., setting up teams, facilitating the development of rivalries, setting up a situation where an obstacle could be overcome only through cooperation) to systematically investigate their effects. Everything that happened involved typical summer camp experiences; Sherif's interest was in making things happen at particular times rather than leaving them to chance.

The ideal from Sherif's perspective was to be a participant—to avoid reactivity effects and to be close to the center of the action—while at the same time remaining detached from the action so that he didn't inadvertently influence it. If you were Muzafer Sherif, what role would *you* occupy in order to ensure that you didn't interfere unintentionally in the course of events? He obviously couldn't pretend to be one of the boys. He might have chosen to be a camp counselor, but then might have become a special focus of attention for the kids. The brilliance of Muzafer Sherif is revealed in that, even if you were at the camp, you probably wouldn't have given him a second glance. He was the janitor and part-time maintenance person, one of those invisible service people who are always there but in some way socially nonexistent or outside the action, perhaps raking leaves, picking up litter, or fixing a faucet. His presence likely would go unnoticed.

Of course, the Sherif example comes close to being surreptitious observation insofar as the children who attended the camp knew little or nothing about the field experiments and observational research they were a part of. Most participant observation and ethnographic research is more transparent than that to those involved and involves a more cooperative relationship between researcher and participants. In such cases, participant observers look for ways to be helpful while at the same time doing their best to avoid directing the action. Although being helpful and "going with the flow" are great for building rapport, one challenge you will face is when you are asked to do something that begs the question of where you will draw the line. For example, William Foote Whyte, in the years he spent in "Cornerville," at one point helped out his group by voting four times in a municipal election—once in his own name and three other times under an assumed name. Years later he expressed regret for this action:

> *I had to learn that, in order to be accepted by the people in a district, you do not have to do everything just as they do it. In fact, in a district where there are different groupings with different standards of behavior, it may be a matter of very serious consequence to conform to the standards of one particular group.*

> *I also had to learn that the field worker cannot afford to think only of learning to live with others in the field. He has to continue living with himself. If the participant observer finds himself engaging in behavior that he has learned to think of as immoral, then he is likely to begin to wonder what sort of a person he is after all. (Whyte, 1993, p. 317)*

In many ways, mixing participant and observer roles overcomes the problems of each role in isolation. To the extent that your status as an observer is honestly presented, ethical concerns about deception or lack of informed consent are minimized. And to the extent that you act as a participant in the setting, reactivity is often reduced because, as a participant, you more quickly fade into the group.

The Participant–Observer Continuum Reconsidered

We mentioned earlier that not all researchers subscribe to the "traditional" continuum of roles from "complete participant" to "complete observer" that we have outlined in this section. Many ethnographic researchers, in particular, began to express reservations with the role continuum to the extent it implies that you *can* be a "complete observer" devoid of any preconceived notions of what you are observing. But as Atkinson and Hammersley (1994) point out,

> [A]lthough it is important to recognize the variation to be found in the roles adopted by observers, this simple dichotomy is not very useful, not least because it seems to imply that the nonparticipant observer plays no recognized role at all … In a sense all *social research is a form of participant observation, because we cannot study the social world without being part of it.* (pp. 248–249)

This statement reflected the growing recognition that we cannot study the world without acknowledging the "we" that is doing the studying. As Denzin and Lincoln (1994) remind us, "any gaze is always filtered through the lenses of language, gender, social class, race, and ethnicity. There are no objective observations, only observations socially situated in the worlds of the observer and the observed" (p. 12). Our collective and individual biographies—whether because of the experience or the *lack* of experience (and hence perspective) they entail—cannot help but enter into and influence our work. Left at that, the challenge becomes one of trying to understand the role that our biography might play in our work and either make an effort to counteract it or simply be forthright about its existence and let the reader decide what to make of it.

The problem becomes magnified when we consider the power relations that have traditionally existed whenever we carry out a piece of research. We may try to be thoughtful about how we consider the research participant(s) we're observing and may do our best to listen to them carefully as they tell us about their world; at the end of the day, though, it's typically we alone who take the data home and "make sense" of it. The power of the text is ours:

> Many voices clamor for expression. Poly-vocality was orchestrated and restrained in traditional ethnographies by giving to one voice [that of the researcher] a pervasive

authorial function and to others the role of sources, "informants" to be quoted or paraphrased. (Clifford, 1986, p. 15)

This issue is not unique to observational or ethnographic research—recall the oral history study where Katherine Borland and her grandmother could not agree on what the grandmother's day at the races signified. But the debate has been particularly resonant in the ethnographic literature to this relationship between "self" (the observer) and "other" (the observed). bell hooks (1989) captures the attitude well:

Often this speech about the "Other" annihilates, erases: "no need to hear your voice when I can talk about you better than you can speak about yourself. No need to hear your voice. Only tell me … your story. And then I will tell it back to you in a new way. Tell it back to you in such a way that it has become mine, my own. Re-writing you, I write myself anew. I am still the colonizer, the speak subject, and you are now at the center of my talk." Stop. (p. 70)

The concept around which much of the debate has centered is that of "privilege," a term that refers in this context to the control that being the researcher gives over the content and form of the final text (for example, the book or article that emerges from a piece of research). The very nature of the research and publication process gives us the last word. Recognizing that fact reminds us of the weighty responsibility and ethical obligations that being a researcher entails. People entrust their views to us, and part of our moral obligation is to ensure that we treat them with respect, fairness, and a sense of justice. Indeed, many would argue that part of the academic mission is to facilitate our own obsolescence by helping create the social conditions in which people generally, and the disadvantaged in particular, can speak for themselves.

Whatever role the researcher takes in relation to their participants, a question to consider is always how the character of that relationship influences for better or worse, or neither or both, what the researcher is allowed to discover.

ETHNOGRAPHY/PARTICIPANT OBSERVATION/FIELD RESEARCH

One very interesting thing about being a known observer in some interesting cultural context is how difficult it is to remain "just" an observer. People talk to you, and you want to talk to them. As you get to know each other, other sources start to catch your attention. You are given access to archival files that tell you more about the history of the group and show you the transitions they have gone through over the years. Perhaps you discover there are other data sets from previous surveys by the organization or government that shed further light on their situation. You hear war stories about previous events and encounters and people start pulling out pictures to show how things were back then. When "observation" starts to push into "mixed method," we start to get into an area known variously as "**participant observation**" (in sociology), "**ethnography**" (in anthropology), or simply as "**field research**" (in various other disciplines).

In many ways these methods share some of the same challenges that we have already discussed with respect to observation more generally—gaining access, dealing with reactivity, recording fieldnotes, figuring out what and who to observe. However, the techniques we want to describe now go beyond these others in several respects. One is the commitment of time. Instead of an hour in a lab, or a couple of weeks in an organization, the classic ethnographic study involved anthropologists going and spending months or even years in a community, learning the language, taking part in cultural practices, and literally living in the community for extended periods. Second is the breadth of the analytical field. Instead of a focused research question or specific hypothesis being tested, ethnography is much more broadly concerned with "culture" as a whole, trying to understand a community as a broad organism in terms of how it defines itself, how it produces or acquires members, how they are socialized into the group, what the rules of membership are, the diversity of beliefs that are held, and so on. By way of background, Vidich and Lyman (1994) explain that

> ethnos, *a Greek term, denotes a people, a race or cultural group. When* ethnos *as a prefix is combined with* graphic *to form the term* ethnographic, *the reference is to the subdiscipline known as descriptive anthropology—in its broadest sense, the science devoted to describing ways of life of humankind.* Ethnography, *then, refers to a social scientific description of a people and the cultural basis of their peoplehood.* (p. 25; italics in original)

Historically, these methods have been the favored ones for trying to gain understanding into the phenomenological world of the "other," that is, coming to know people who are different from you.

Understanding the Culture of the "Other"

The history of ethnography conveys much about the history of social science and its attempts to grapple with the understanding of an "other," that is, someone other than ourselves. Vidich and Lyman (1994, 2003) suggest that ethnography grew out of Europeans' interest in understanding the cultures they encountered when Columbus stumbled across what to him was a "New World." Trying to understand someone so completely different poses a very big problem. As Vidich and Lyman (1994) phrased it,

> [I]n practice, it becomes this question: By which values are observations to be guided? The choices seem to be either the values of the ethnographer or the values of the observed—that is, in modern parlance, either the etic or the emic. Herein lies a deeper and more fundamental problem: How is it possible to understand the other when the other's values are not one's own? (p. 26)

The Early Ethnographer

Good question! Early cultural ethnographies (in the 15th and 16th centuries) by Europeans were done from a clearly European perspective and evaluated Indigenous practices and beliefs using a European yardstick. Most of these written accounts were produced by explorers, missionaries, and colonial administrators. Not surprisingly, when the implicit question was "how European" Indigenous cultures were, the answer was "not very."

The beginnings of "modern" ethnography are typically said to have emerged in the late 19th and early 20th centuries, when anthropologists like Bronislaw Malinowski (1922) and Margaret Mead (1928/1960) actually left their homes and went traveling to see firsthand how these "others" lived.

> The field-worker, during this period, was lionized, made into a larger-than-life figure who went into and then returned from the field with stories about strange people. Rosaldo (1989, p. 30) describes this as the period of the Lone Ethnographer, the story of the man-scientist who went off in search of his native in a distant land … Returning home with his data, the Lone Ethnographer wrote up an objective account of the culture he studied. (Denzin & Lincoln, 2003, p. 20)

Once again, the criteria for analysis were clear. The application of Darwinian evolutionary theory to social matters—an approach that placed humans at the top of the natural order and was conveniently adapted by Social Darwinists to place Caucasians at the top of the human order—allowed any concerns about social relativism to be placed aside easily. If "we" were the top of the human heap, then surely "ours" were the most appropriate criteria to be used in understanding and evaluating other cultures. Thus, "objectivity" meant employing European standards and imposing a

European point of view. The scholar's challenge was to translate Indigenous beliefs and practices into terms that Europeans could understand. But when taken out of context that way, practices that might have played an important social role in Indigenous cultures for thousands of years could appear quaint, trivial, and trite, if not completely beyond "rational" belief. The result made some people wonder how contemporary North Americans might appear if they were studied and written about in the same manner (e.g., see Miner, 1956).

Discovering the "Other" Among Us

The next "moment" of ethnographic history (to use Denzin & Lincoln's (1994) term) featured a number of American sociologists who began to practice a similar method to understand the "other" that existed at home. Although there were other isolated examples of this "urban ethnography," it was at the University of Chicago's sociology department in the 1920s through the 1940s (the "Chicago School") where this approach was practiced with zeal. The names Robert Park, Ernest Burgess, W. I. Thomas, and Louis Wirth are prominent in such accounts. Central to their approach was the idea that American cities are brimming with heterogeneous people of differing lifestyles and worldviews and that an understanding of American culture requires some understanding of that diversity. Park was the one to conceive of the "natural area" as the appropriate unit to be studied:

> *Every American city has its slums; its ghettos; its immigrant colonies, regions which maintain more or less alien and exotic cultures. Nearly every city has its bohemias and hobohemias, where life is freer, more adventurous and lonely than it is elsewhere. These are called natural areas of the city. (Park, 1952, p. 196; cited in Vidich & Lyman, 1994, p. 33)*

Park encouraged sociologists to undertake case studies of these natural areas. And he, along with his colleagues and students, did so *en masse* for more than three decades. Studies were undertaken of "the Jewish ghetto, Polonia, Little Italy, Little Germany, Chinatown, Bronzeville and Harlem, the gold coast and the slum, hobo jungles, single-room occupants of furnished rooms, enclaves of cultural and social dissidents, the urban ecology of gangdom, and the urban areas that housed the suicidal, the drug addicted and the mentally disabled, and on the social and economic dynamics of real estate transactions," to name only a few areas (Vidich & Lyman, 1994, p. 33). It was in keeping with this tradition that William Foote Whyte actually moved into an Italian American neighborhood to engage in research he called "participant observation" and that resulted in his famed monograph, *Streetcorner Society* (see 1943/1993).

Despite the differences between these two earlier moments of ethnographic history, they also shared a certain similarity. Underlying both was a sense of social scientific mission born from a kind of Euro-American imperialism that romanticized the "others" they scrutinized, while at the same time seeing their eventual passing as tragic, but inevitable, in the march of "progress" and assimilation. For anthropologists like Malinowski, the study of Indigenous peoples was important primarily because it was a way to have a last brief glimpse of prehistory before it became ensnared by the inevitable onslaught of "progress" and "civilization" and faded into oblivion. For sociologists like Park, however much hobos or immigrants were lauded and romanticized, one senses the belief that the urban ethnographers' texts would ultimately stand as museum pieces once all lost their uniqueness in the "melting pot" that was America.

But assimilation, it turned out, was not at all inevitable. Although challenges to theories that touted its inevitability were first raised in the 1930s (even by Park himself), a third moment of ethnographic history laid these views to rest. Vidich and Lyman (1994) describe the process: "During the two decades after 1970, ethnological studies of African American, Amerindian, Mexican American, and Asian peoples also cast considerable doubt on whether, when, and to whose benefit the much-vaunted process of ethnocultural meltdown in America would occur" (p. 37).

Multiple Forms of Contemporary Ethnography
New Ethnographers

Contemporary ethnographic approaches have undergone yet another shift in recent decades, a shift we attribute in large part to the gradual diversification of the academy that began in the latter part of the 20th century. The most common image of "the researcher" in the first half of the twentieth century would have been a white male who would go into the netherworld of another culture and come back with stories of "the other" that would be translated into the hegemonic understanding that was held out as the standard of "objectivity." Researchers were the ones who posed the important questions; research participants were expected to go ahead with their lives and let us observe and then write about them.

But the world and ethical sensibilities have changed. First, the formal laws and informal rules that kept women and minorities out of educational institutions or particular programs were challenged. Although Black students were occasionally admitted into US universities in the 1800s, more than a century later the admission of Black students into universities, particularly in the south, was still causing riots. Figure 11.2 shows the scene when James Meredith first attended the University of Mississippi in 1962. His admission required troops to be present to ensure his safety. Most students boycotted his first class, and neither any of those who did attend nor the instructor stayed to have their picture taken with him. Years later, the various "liberation" and "power" movements of the 1960s pushed for universities to offer courses that focused on the experience of African Americans, Indigenous peoples, women, and citizens of the "undeveloped" world, where they heard the often strange things that were being taught about them, and began to understand how white/male/straight experience defined "normal" and the standard of "objectivity" that went along with that. Those same students were soon going to graduate school, getting their PhDs, teaching those classes, and doing that research themselves. Among Indigenous peoples, for example, the favorite of anthropologists, we see more and more works by Indigenous authors extolling both the desirability and necessity of

FIGURE 11.2 ● These Pictures Show the Day in 1962 When James Meredith Attended His First Day at the University of Mississippi

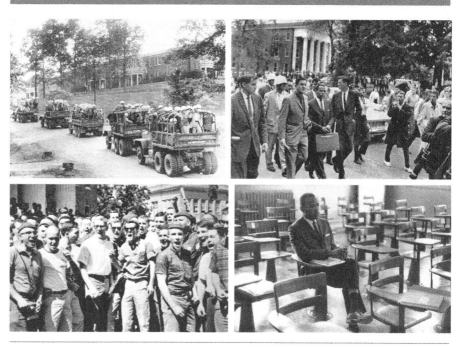

research with Indigenous peoples being done by Indigenous researchers incorporating Indigenous methods and epistemologies (e.g., Deloria, 1991; Duran & Duran, 2000; Hoare, Levy, & Robinson, 1993; Smith, 2001; Wilson, 2008). As Wolf (1992) reminds us,

> We can no longer assume that an isolated village will not within an amazingly short period of time move into the circuit of rapid social and economic change. A barefoot village kid who used to trail along after you will one day show up on your doorstep with an Oxford degree and your book in hand. (p. 137)

With the diversification of the academy came a broadening of interests in methods like ethnography. Instead of the typically white male researcher telling stories about the "other," the new ethnographers started detailing the ways that individuals and groups "fashion culturally meaningful expressions and fields of experience in which meaning is routinely contested, and where culture is perennially under construction" (Denzin & Lincoln, 2003, p. 398). Instead of researchers from "outside" coming to research an "other," many contemporary ethnographers do research from inside the culture of which they are a part, providing insights into the social-relational dynamics and lived experiences of power.

New Ethnographies

Autoethnography. With a more diverse core of academics dissatisfied with many existing methodological models that did not speak to their experience, perhaps it is not surprising that researchers would experiment with other ways to gather and interpret data. One such development is **autoethnography**, which combines the self-reflection of autobiography with the cultural analysis that is integral to ethnography. As Ellis, Adams, and Bochner (2011) describe it, autoethnography "is an approach to research and writing that seeks to describe and systematically analyze (graphy) personal experience (auto) in order to understand cultural experience (ethno)" (1). Perhaps not surprisingly, many of those who engage in autoethnography are members of groups that have felt excluded from and oppressed by traditional methods that saw them as an "other" and did not try and understand them on their own terms.

Ellis et al. (2011) suggest the primary objective of an autoethnography is for the writer to recount critical life experiences—epiphanies—that arise from being part of a particular culture in a way that can educate people both within and outside the culture as to the nature of that cultural experience. This often will take the form of storytelling, but it is at the same time more than that because of the analysis that should accompany the story. As Allen (2006) explains in this account from Ellis (2011), an autoethnographer must

... look at experience analytically. Otherwise [you're] telling [your] story—and that's nice—but people do that on Oprah every day. Why is your story more valid than anyone else's? What makes your story more valid is that you are a researcher. You have a set of theoretical and methodological tools and a research literature to use. That's your advantage. If you can't frame it around these tools and literature and just frame it as "my story," then why or how should I privilege your story over anyone else's I see 25 times a day on TV? (cited by Ellis et al., 2011, p. 3)

Grounding itself in the central principle of postmodernism that there are no "foundational" epistemologies and specifically dismissing traditional western science's claims to that crown, autoethnographers have sought to articulate their own procedures and criteria. Questions about reliability are reframed in terms of the narrator's credibility, i.e., whether the author has created a believable story consistent with factual evidence. Closely related to this are questions of validity, which are reframed in terms of whether the author has succeeded in bringing the reader into the author's life world and produced greater understanding. Issues of generalizability can be assessed either by contextualizing the story in existing literature or by comparing the author's account to other autoethnographies. Impact and utility are major criteria—does it help understanding? Does it resonate with others within or outside the culture? Does it foster better communication? Does it offer readers a way to improve their lives?

Although these goals are admirable, we doubt it will surprise you to hear that autoethnography has not been without its critics. The list of criticisms is a long one—too emotional, involving too little fieldwork, not rigorous enough, not analytical enough, too much navel gazing—that in large part can be summarized by saying that it is not traditional social or health science, which is of course exactly what it tries not to be. As Ellis et al. (2011) explain,

[A]utoethnographers find it futile to debate whether autoethnography is a valid research process or product. Unless we agree on a goal, we cannot agree on the terms by which we can judge how to achieve it. Simply put, autoethnographers take a different point of view toward the subject matter of social science. In Rorty's words, these different views are "not issue(s) to be resolved, only" instead they are "difference(s) to be lived with" (1982, p. 197). Autoethnographers view research and writing as socially-just acts; rather than a preoccupation with accuracy, the goal is to produce analytical, accessible texts that change us and the world we live in for the better. (p. 8)

For our part, we go back to Donald T. Campbell's reminder that "there are no royal roads to truth" and thus "should let a thousand methodological flowers bloom." With neither of us yet having done an autoethnography—the only method in this book that we have not yet undertaken at one time or another—any judgment about the method's ability to achieve its objectives would be premature. Our main concern is with the conflict of interest that seems inherent to the method; there are few people we know who are so open about their lives and so little concerned about what others might think of them that an authentic account devoid of self-censorship and image management would result.

Critical Ethnography. Another contemporary variation on ethnography, **critical ethnography**, has been defined as "conventional ethnography with a political purpose" (Thomas, 1993). Its roots lie in many ways with dissatisfaction where traditional ethnographers drew their analytical boundaries. On the one hand, there was recognition of the virtue of understanding "the marginalized other" up close and on their own terms. On the other hand, however, was a noticeable absence of structural analysis that questioned where that marginalization came from in the first place, and how existing social structures imbued with classism, racism, and patriarchy contributed to ensuring the group stayed there (Cook, 2008). Anthropologists would go into the field and understand the newest exotic tribe in some distant part of the world, but where was the analysis that drew attention to and questioned the colonial structures that usurped their resources, denied their self-determination, and kept them impoverished in the very territories that had sustained them since time immemorial?

Starting from the premise that the structure of contemporary society is fundamentally unequal (e.g., women, racial and ethnic minorities, and others are disadvantaged relative to the rest of society), the goal of critical ethnographers is to understand the relationship between societal structures and ideological patterns of thought that limit our ability to confront and change unjust social systems (Harvey, 2019). As Madison (2005) explains,

> *Critical ethnography begins with an ethical responsibility to address processes of unfairness or injustice within a particular lived domain. By "ethical responsibility," I mean a compelling sense of duty and commitment based on moral principles of human freedom and well -being, and hence a compassion for the suffering of living beings. The conditions for existence within a particular context are not as they could be for specific subjects; as a result, the researcher feels a moral obligation to make a contribution toward changing those conditions toward greater freedom and equity. The critical ethnographer also takes us beneath surface appearances, disrupts the status quo, and unsettles both neutrality and taken-for-granted assumptions by*

> *bringing to light underlying and obscure operations of power and control. Therefore, the critical ethnographer resists domestication and moves from "what is" to "what could be." (p. 5)*

When Madison (2005) talks about researchers resisting "domestication," she reminds us that the way we do research—the way we design our studies, the relations we have with research participants, the data we choose to gather, and the way we interpret it—will have implications for real people insofar as everything we do can either reaffirm or question the status quo (Madison, 2005). There are far too many pressures that encourage us to think of the status quo as inevitable, thereby constraining our imagination about what can be. As Thomas (1993) describes it, effective critical analysis requires an attitude of "intellectual rebellion":

> *The roots of critical thought spread from a long tradition of intellectual rebellion in which rigorous examination of ideas and discourse constituted political challenge. Social critique, by definition, is radical. It implies an evaluative judgment of meaning and method in research, policy, and human activity. Critical thinking implies freedom by recognizing that social existence, including our knowledge of it, is not simply composed of givens imposed on us by powerful and mysterious forces. This recognition leads to the possibility of transcending existing forces. The act of critique implies that by thinking about and acting upon the world, we are able to change both our subjective interpretations and objective conditions. (p. 18)*

In sum, the most emancipatory acts we can promote involve exercising the freedom to *think* differently about what the world might look like, because thinking about the world differently is a necessary precursor to achieving a different world. Critical ethnography is thus the methodological manifestation of critical theory that shows the linkages between the theoretical constructs that critical theories invoke and the social structures that construct and maintain them.

Doing critical ethnography thus means beginning with critical theory and choosing research sites that allow for a theoretically guided deconstruction of some phenomenon in terms of the power structures that underlie and reaffirm it. The idea here is that knowledge is power to the extent that recognizing how existing power structures thwart equality and reaffirm injustice is a first step to alleviating it by encouraging us to go beyond what is to what can be. Toward that end, Carspecken (1996) outlines a five-step process to guide critical ethnographic research, though he sees it as a general methodological approach with applicability beyond ethnography per se. These include "building and analyzing a record of observations, fieldnotes, and natural interactions between participants in the social site; using interviews and videotaped observations or interactions with participants; and examining broader social structures and systems that interact with and influence the site" (cited by Cook, 2008, p. 149). Although Carspecken for the most part encouraged looking at interactional spaces where marginalized individuals bumped into corridors of power, he also encouraged going beyond such sites to analyze policies, documents, books, television shows, and music—cultural artifacts that in many cases would also embody, or question, broader cultural understandings.

As you might expect, the overt desire to change the world for the better and to do so in a way that does not recreate the hierarchy of knowledge that proclaimed academics as the knowers and analyzers while the people they ostensibly cared about were relegated to the status of "data sources" had other implications as well. The push was on for more collaborative forms of research interaction wrapped around a desire for change:

> [A]lthough researchers have suggested that the methodology of critical ethnography could be used by practice-focused disciplines, such as health promotion and social work, to instigate action around research findings, writers on the development of critical ethnography have criticized the lack of action resulting from such studies. To this end, it has been suggested that the focus in critical ethnographic projects be placed on developing the skills of participants to enable them to continue researching their own lives and settings long after the researchers have departed. Some have also recommended moving critical ethnography farther into the realm of action research where the power differentials that exist between the researcher and the researched dissolve. (Cook, 2008, p. 150)

Those aspirations would be reflected in the development of participatory action research (PAR)—known affectionately (and abbreviated) as PAR—a collaborative model of research with the express purpose of "giving voice" and triggering social change.

PARTICIPATORY ACTION RESEARCH

Some History

The literature on **participatory action research (PAR)** indicates that the concept grew and took root in at least three different places in a history that Jordan (2003) describes as "complex and elusive" and thus "difficult to map with any precision."

One strand is European/American. The notion of "Action research" is typically attributed to Kurt Lewin, a researcher who arrived in the United States from Germany as a refugee in the 1930s and went on to be considered the father of contemporary social psychology by the time of his death in 1947. Lewin believed that the scientific method could and should be used in applied settings to improve social conditions. He was particularly interested in raising the self-esteem and social involvement of minorities and helping them get beyond conditions of exploitation and colonization that were so common and unquestioned at the time. He was also a believer in democratic processes and showed in some of his earlier work in the field of organizational behavior that more democratic groups in which employees were involved in the identification of problems and decision-making regarding possible solutions performed consistently better and had higher morale than groups run autocratically. Although he did not call it *participatory* action research, the participation of those who were involved in whatever site was the focus of study was integral to his process (Adelman, 1993).

It is interesting, however, that Lewin's approach to research and his promotion of action research was no runaway success. Perhaps it was because the academy became entrenched at that time with those who believed in a separation of knowledge and action, theory, and practice, in much the same manner you often see in the natural sciences—the physicists do the theorizing while the engineers build the bridges. Perhaps it was because Lewin died too soon from a heart attack without ever fully articulating methods that could be used in applied contexts where classical experimental methods were difficult to implement. That did not happen until the late 1950s and early 60s when Donald T. Campbell came along and not only talked about "the experimenting society" but also outlined a vocabulary by which we could evaluate interventions and an array of experimental and quasi-experimental designs through which that could be accomplished (e.g., Campbell, 1969b, 1991; Campbell & Stanley, 1963; see also Chapters 6 and 7).

A second strand of origin for PAR comes from the Third World, and especially Indigenous experience in the Third World, particularly Africa and South America, where Indigenous peoples engaged in anticolonial struggle were tired of people doing research *on* them and instead sought people who wanted to do research *with* them (e.g., Jordan, 2003; Smith, 2001). Kemmis and McTaggart (2007) point to the influence of liberation theology and neo-Marxist approaches to community development in South America and rights-based activism in Asia, both of which pushed for professionals engaging in collaborative relationships with communities working to achieve real change. Those approaches often met with resistance, but were also the source of important social change, which contrasted with the academy's worst excesses, such as the "hit-and-run research" that saw researchers place their own interests ahead of the community being studied (Hagey, 1997). This is also known as parachute research, an exploitative research activity where researchers who have no previous connection to, or involvement with the community come to the community, extract data and knowledge without due acknowledgment of local partners and collaborators and then disappear.

As MacDonald (2012) explains, a third strand of origin lay in the dots being connected between a variety of other groups and movements that each sought a more diverse world free of domination:

> *Participatory action research has also emerged from movements that shared a vision of society free of domination. These movements occurred within the fields of international development, the social sciences communities, and adult education. Participatory action research was linked to the following trends: (1) the radical and reformist approaches to international economic development assistance; (2) the view of adult education as an empowering alternative to traditional approaches to education; and (3) the ongoing debate within the social sciences over the dominant social science paradigm. For this reason, other groups of researchers, such as feminists, extended participatory research by analyzing power differences on the basis of gender, and supported the importance of collaboration between the researcher and participant. (p. 37)*

General Principles

PAR thus was developed with the intention of departing completely from hierarchical and exploitative models of research that placed the interests of academics ahead of the interests and plight of the community. There would be an "action" orientation—the whole idea of engaging with groups in the community would be about improving their situation and developing practical plans for that to happen. "No action without research; no research without action," Lewin would say (Adelman, 1993). As Kidd and Kral (2005) frame it,

> *[T]he focus is less on a research question or questions (and the attendant emphasis on knowledge gathering) and more on a problem to be solved. Knowledge is thus derivative. Rather than driving the project, areas of inquiry will be explored and the process examined to determine whether that inquiry effectively informs action, with some questions seeming and being crucial in the beginning of the project proving*

fruitless, replaced by others that emerge later. The first question may be, What are the questions? becoming more specific as group members work together (e.g., How do we deal with discrimination in the workplace? How does employment contribute to wellness? How can we have a stronger voice at the next policy meeting?). The exploration of these questions is the research component of PAR.

People in the community would not just participate and then wave goodbye while the researcher looked at them in the rear view mirror; they would be involved as genuine collaborators from the inception of the research project to the end.

At some level, this shift of focus suggested a major paradigm shift away from the models of research that dominated, and continue to dominate, the academy. In addition to rejecting the idea of knowledge for its own sake in favor of knowledge in the service of social justice (e.g., Kelly, 2005), early advocates of PAR questioned many of the academy's sacred cows in much the same way that critical ethnographers questioned the colonial base of classic ethnography. Primary among these was the notion of the "lore of objectivity" that mainstream social science had ascribed to itself. Advocates of PAR talked about how research too often embodied "relations of ruling" in which university "experts" would tell communities what their problems were and rarely questioned the social structures that created and maintained those problems in the first place (e.g., Jordan, 2003). In its place, PAR researchers and communities demanded analyses that put their problems in a broader context without losing touch with the need to address their day-to-day manifestations.

Although many lengthy articles and books have been written about PAR and its many variations, as McTaggart (1991) explains, at some level the principles that drive PAR are pretty simple and straightforward:

> *At one level of analysis, the idea of participatory action research is straightforward enough. The inventor of the term "action research," social psychologist Kurt Lewin, described action research as proceeding in a spiral of steps, each of which is composed of planning, acting, observing, and evaluating the result of the action. In practice, the process begins with a general idea that some kind of improvement or change is desirable. In deciding just where to begin in making improvements, a group identifies an area where members perceive a cluster of problems of mutual concern and consequence. The group decides to work together on a "thematic concern."*

As you might expect with a technique known as *participatory* action research, a major emphasis is on the notion of participation, which is far more than mere "involvement" (McTaggart, 1991; Santos, 2013). Participation in the sense of PAR is said to require a nonhierarchical mutually respectful relationship in which each party is recognized to bring a certain expertise to the task. Researchers bring some expertise about methods and data analysis, but members of the community are the ones who bring local knowledge, a better idea of what "the problems" are that need to be addressed, and are in the best position to decide on the feasibility and desirability of proposed solutions:

> *[U]nlike conventional forms of research methodology where authority is vested in the researcher-academic, PAR aims to shift responsibility for the research process on to individuals and groups who are directly affected by these inequalities. Insofar as professional researchers have a role within PAR, it is to set their expertise alongside the lay knowledge, skills and experiences of those people who constitute the object of their investigations. In this way the research process is conceptualised as an encounter, where equal partners meet, enter into dialogue and share different kinds of knowledge and expertise on how to address issues of exploitation and oppression. In this respect PAR is unashamedly committed to a politics of equity and social transformation that many other research traditions would dismiss as ideological. (Jordan, 2003, p. 190)*

Indeed, "collaborative" might be a better word than "participatory" in that it speaks more directly to the shoulder-to-shoulder and egalitarian relationship that is envisioned.

The Power of Participatory Action Research

Notwithstanding all the complexities that arise when the decision is made to begin a process of PAR, it is clear employing PAR can advance knowledge in a variety of different disciplines and community contexts in ways that would be unlikely to emerge from more orthodox research. The technique can create spaces for dialogue and foster more integrated horizontal and vertical processes of inclusion around the principles of social justice and cultural citizenship that include rights, recognition, respect, and redistribution. It allows for all stakeholders who can make a difference to problems identified by communities, including communities themselves, to be engaged in the process, and part of the research, debates, and dialogue. PAR also encourages us to access a richer understanding of the complexities of an issue or phenomenon and to develop our knowledge and analysis in ways that might foster a more radically democratic outcome. Finally, it also allows the community to be seen in a different way both by others and by the group or community itself, reflecting people with diverse histories engaging each other in a creative process of exploring what might work better.

Challenges and Concerns

Before we all head outside ready to join hands and sing *Kumbaya*, some of the many challenges and concerns that have been raised with respect to PAR also need to be considered.

Square Pegs and Round Holes

High on the list of challenges for PAR are concerns about researchers, the organization and reward structures of universities, and what Kidd and Kral (2005) recognized as deeply embedded beliefs about the value and power that comes through our expertise:

> *Given the centrality of power in PAR, at all levels from conscientization[1] to the gathering of knowledge and action, researchers must be prepared to engage in what can be a very personal struggle with their own deeply embedded beliefs. The researcher can, in very subtle ways, silence voices and undermine the entire process. Indeed, the potential frustrations, anxiety, and ambiguity of many PAR contexts are breeding grounds for researcher insecurity and the temptation to fall back on the comfort of one's power and social position. (p. 190)*

There are also pressures on many academics—those who work in universities and departments where only certain prestigious journals "count" when applying for tenure or promotion and/or when the volume of peer-reviewed publications expected is high—that can make participation in PAR projects a career-limiting or even career-ending move (e.g., see the case studies in Foley & Valenzuela, 2005). PAR projects do not happen overnight. It takes time to build a relationship with a community, and for the project itself to move through enough stages to be producing publishable material. If you are being truly collaborative, then it is not possible to say at the beginning of a project what will come out the other end, and the concerns that arise

---

[1]Kidd and Kral (2005) explain that, "Paulo Friere (1982) used 'conscientization' to describe the developing awareness that occurs among people engaged in self-inquiry" (p. 188).

in some projects may involve unique and local issues that are never publishable simply because no issues arose that might engage a broader audience (Gray, 2014).

"Cultural Critique" vs "Activist Research"

Within the academic community there also has been considerable debate about the "proper" relationship between researcher and community with respect to the extent of our political engagement. Hale (2006) identifies the opposing points of view as "cultural critique" versus "activist research." For him, **"cultural critique"** refers to researchers who retain their primary allegiance to the academy and whose political implications are "…manifested through the content of the knowledge produced, not through the relationship established with an organized group of people in struggle" (p. 98). There is a shared interest with activists in championing the causes of the oppressed and in deconstructing power, but beyond that a certain independence that harkens back to academic notions of objectivity and impartiality in the actual research and its write-up. He contrasts this with **"activist research,"** by which he means "… a method through which we affirm a political alignment with an organized group of people in struggle and allow dialogue with them to shape each phase of the process, from conception of the research topic to data collection to verification and dissemination of the results" (p. 97), i.e., more clearly serving the interests of the particular group with whom you are allied, and acting as their advocate when the opportunity arises. Although Hale puts himself more squarely in the "activist" camp, we appreciate his observation that the two need not be in opposition, may actually complement one another, and that both can benefit from the dialogue.

The story that provides the fuel for his analysis is his participation in a land rights trial in which the Awas Tingni, an Indigenous people, sued the government of Nicaragua in the Inter-American Human Rights Court for violation of their property rights, which they construed as a collective right belonging to them as a people. There is a tantalizing vagueness about his account, however. He describes the contributions of three core expert witnesses in the case—two eminent scholars of international law, Rodolfo Stavenhagen and James Anaya, and him. The former two both have served as Special Rapporteur on Indigenous Issues with the UN Human Rights Council. While Hale praises the other two, and rightfully so, and gives a summary of his own role in the case, he gives no analysis of the court decision, which in the end was successful, with respect to the evidence that the courts found most persuasive. The impression you are left with is that his activism helped sway the day, which it may well have, but we would not be so quick to draw that inference given our knowledge of Stavenhagen and Anaya and the weight their expertise and experience would command.

Our caution also arises from having seen similar issues play out in Canada in a trial in which several sex workers argued that Canadian law with respect to sex work made it impossible to do their work safely and thus was a violation of their rights to security of the person embodied in the Canadian *Charter of Rights and Freedoms* [*Canada (Attorney General)* v *Bedford* (2013) 3 SCR 1101]. In that case, there were several groups of researchers who presented evidence as recognized "experts" on the basis of their research with various actors involved in the sex industry and legal community that engages it. In the end, the court made a clear distinction between those researchers whose understanding of the industry and opinions about how to go forward grew from the research they had done over time and those who came into the debate with certain opinions and whose research seemed more directed at showing the validity of their views than in actually putting them to any sort of test by actively engaging other points of view and considering rival plausible explanations. Stated in the categories used by Hale (2006), the "activists" were seen as less credible true believers whose research was designed to find a certain conclusion, while those who engaged in "cultural critique" were seen as credible voices whose findings and conclusions were the ones the court found more persuasive (Lowman, 2014).

Community Diversity

Kidd and Kral (2005) also encourage us to avoid overly romanticizing the process or underestimating the pain it can take to achieve the benefits that PAR promises. The solutions that community members come up with may be at odds with those we think reasonable, and "the community" itself is rarely a homogeneous entity. Different factions may highlight different problems and embrace different solutions that can be completely at odds with one another. And while the researchers may come in with an egalitarian attitude, any given community will have its bullies and know-it-alls or no-it-alls who dominate discussions and can hijack a project with their insensitivities. Along those lines, Kidd and Kral (2005) mention the problem of "**consensus tyranny**," where the diversity of perspectives within the community is lost because of pressures that some members of the community exert for unanimity.

Empowerment for What?

Finally, while the name of the game in PAR is presumably one of the "empowerment" of communities, Jordan (2003) encourages us to take a step back and ask, "Empowerment for what? And for whose benefit?" In his view, the growing pervasiveness and acceptance of PAR in the academic mainstream has created a certain degree of "domestication" (Madison, 2005) or co-optation of PAR principles for limited ends and within a limited frame of reference. Jordan (2003) notes, for example, that many corporations are using the PAR model to engage employees in discussions about decision-making within the corporate context. Why? To maximize productivity and corporate competitiveness, which sounds to us like more of a corporate definition of success than an employee-generated one. Similarly, he notes the use of PAR by institutions such as the World Bank who use the feel-good, participatory language of PAR to show they care about those in less developed countries, while stating on its website that doing so will create the sort of "social learning" that will help them become better "'clients' who are capable of demanding and paying for goods and services from government and private sector agencies" (p. 194). The critique of PAR ventured here parallels the discussion we noted earlier about ethnography that resulted in the development of critical ethnography. How is the participation framed? And how broadly can the discussion be expanded?

Two Examples

An excellent example of the more collaborative approach envisioned in PAR is a piece of video ethnography conducted by Margolis (1994) in coal mining communities in Colorado that had seen better days. The process began with Margolis contacting the communities and beginning to identify purposive samples of individuals who could be interviewed on video about different periods in the communities' history. By involving the community in telling their own story, the study soon became a victim of its own success. Participants started lining up to be interviewed and began bringing out supplementary materials—old newspapers, photographs, family albums, documents—that gave an even more comprehensive community record. The product that Margolis was seeking to produce was a documentary film, and the collaborative nature of his process continued into the analysis and editing stage. A first "draft" of the film was shown to those in the community who were given an opportunity to comment on its strengths and weaknesses before Margolis went back and re-edited a final product. Margolis (1994) recounts the process:

> I intended to use the editing process to produce "documents" rather than documentaries. My role as editor was not that of providing the sociologist's standard of objective truth, but rather to arrange an order that reflected the living relation between biography and history. I wanted to capture the emphasis of knowledge held in common by communicating people's analysis in their own words. As much as possible I wanted to avoid relying on a narrator or expert commentator to impose an overview or legislate meaning. The process was designed to avoid forcing a preconceived analysis on the material. Ethnographic editing techniques allowed the raw materials to inspire both form and content. Certain topics brought up in almost every interview suggested scenes: immigration, ethnic

relations, changing techniques and technology of mining, exploitation in the company town, the struggle to organize, the Ludlow strike, the IWW Strike, disasters, etc. Each individual biography lent unique content even as people recounted history that they made in common. Historical categories were not imposed by the editor but were nominated by coal people out of their own experience.

A study that Ted was recently involved in that we described in Chapter 8 on case studies can be looked at through a PAR lens as well. The study (by Palys, Schaefer, & Nuszdorfer, 2014) involved looking at the relations between an Indigenous justice program (VATJS) and a subsequently created Downtown Community Court (DCC) and the negative effect that the latter had on referrals that were supposed to be heading to the former. It was an explicitly problem-solving piece of research that engaged personnel at both venues in a collaborative project to determine their respective views of what "the problem" was and how it might be addressed. Because it addressed both the history of the development of VATJS and the aspirations that members of both the DCC and VATJS expressed for their future relationship, the final report (Palys et al., 2014) provided a foundation for the development of an updated protocol agreement between VATJS and the Regional Crown. It was the beginning of a new relationship that seems to have flourished in the years since.

SUMMING UP AND LOOKING AHEAD

This chapter gives preliminary consideration to the extensive range of activities subsumed under the notion of observational research. We've seen that observational strategies are very flexible techniques that can be used in a broad variety of research settings. Indeed, "observation" is a highly generic term that can describe activities ranging from casual to formal and from structured to "unstructured" activities that may or may not involve interaction between researcher and participants and that may or may not be mixed with other methods as part of a multimethod strategy. The chapter emphasizes some of the many issues that weigh on the researcher up to and including the process of gathering data. Little is said, however, about how to make sense of those data, which is addressed in subsequent chapters.

An observational approach offers several advantages, not the least of which is that it often (although not necessarily) involves behavior in its real-world context. But observation is rarely used alone. Instead, it is either a precursor to more intimate research, where the researcher starts by checking out the scene, or an important element in a comprehensive participant-observation or ethnographic situational analysis in which observation of behavior in situ is combined with supplementary strategies (e.g., interviews, questionnaires, archival analysis).

The importance of supplementing observation with other techniques (especially self-report) cannot be overemphasized. Most obviously, it allows you to compare what people say with what they do. Sensitive observational study may greatly assist in the generation of new interpretive information that may inform the overall analysis, which in turn may suggest further elements of the setting to observe in greater detail.

Both more and less structured approaches to observation are discussed. Besides differing in degree of structure, the two approaches also are shown to differ significantly in the way they conceive of the observational setting itself. Researchers engaged in quantitative research, particularly those rooted in positivist traditions, are more likely to engage in structured observational strategies and to see themselves as separable from the act of observation, i.e., that it is possible to be an aloof, detached, and totally objective observer. In contrast, researchers conducting more qualitative and ethnographic or field-based research are more likely to see such divisions as artificial and question whether the act of observation can ever be separated from the issue of who does the observing. Related to this are questions concerning the standards or criteria used to make judgments based on observational data. Recent trends challenge us to consider the implications of trying to understand the "other" without autocratically presuming that our particular way of knowing is necessarily "privileged" or "authoritative." Even more common these days is a form of ethnography and observation that goes under the name of PAR where researcher and participants engage each other collaboratively to produce something that enhances the researcher's understanding of the group or site under study while simultaneously helping to advance participants' interests.

Instead of observing *people*, the next chapter moves into the observation of *things people create and leave behind* as a function of their activity—archives, files, videos, memoirs, official statistics.

Key Concepts

Activist research 479
Autoethnography 469
Category system 447
Coding scheme 446
Complete observer 439
Complete participant 439
Consensus tyranny 480

Covert observation 441
Critical ethnography 471
Cultural critique 479
Emic 450
Ethnography 464
Etic 450
Field research 464

Hit-and-run research 475
Parachute research 475
Participant observation 464
Participatory action research
  (PAR) 473
Reactivity 444
Sign systems 447

STUDY QUESTIONS

1. Louise wants to do an observational study of cocaine use among Atlanta's upper class. But she's unsure about what role to adopt on the continuum from "complete participant" to "complete observer." (1) Discuss each of the possible roles in terms of the ethical issues and reactivity involved. (2) What other advantages and disadvantages do you see to the various roles in this situation? (3) Indicate how you might approach this situation, and what you might look for at your first cocktail party.

2. Anne-Marie is designing a study of how Baltimore's major newspapers go about investigating, defining, and portraying "crime news." The study will involve an observational component, and Anne-Marie recognizes that her study may induce some degree of reactivity among the sample group. She comes to you for advice. Explain what reactivity is and give two suggestions about what Anne-Marie might do to minimize reactivity in her study. In each case, explain why you believe the suggestion you make will lead to a decrease in reactivity.

3. What is the difference between a *sign system* and a *category system* in observational research? Show that you understand the difference by indicating how each would be used in coding a children's cartoon show for its violent content.

4. Zelda is a professor teaching research methods who asks her students to do an observational study where they code what people do when they encounter a person begging in the street in response to different begging strategies. What are some of the things that she and her students can do to maximize the reliability of their coding scheme?

5. Several years ago, a study was conducted regarding the social content of video pornography. The study incorporated scene-by-scene coding of video content in terms of sex, aggression, and sexual aggression. Each scene was viewed and coded as to whether it included sex and/or aggression and/or sexual aggression, or none of these. (1) Did the video study utilize a *sign* system or a *category* system when coding scene content? Show that you understand the difference between these two by explaining your choice. (2) Describe one way you could assess the reliability of the coding scheme.

6. Is it ethically acceptable to you to observe people without them knowing they are being observed? In what sorts of situations would you think it appropriate and inappropriate?

7. Pick a social setting of interest to you (e.g., your classroom, a video arcade, a bowling alley, a bus, an elevator), and approach it as an observer engaged in preliminary exploratory analysis. Keep fieldnotes, and speculate on the "rules" that govern behavior in that setting. Also consider the ethical issues involved in observing in such a manner.

8. Differentiating possible observer roles on a continuum ranging from *complete participant* to *complete observer* was standard for many years. Why is that continuum now seen by many researchers as problematic?

9. What is *reactivity* and why is it a concern for observational researchers? What factors affect reactivity? What constructive suggestions would you offer to another researcher who asks what she/he can do to help reduce reactivity when she/he goes out to do field research? If your answer is "it depends," what would it depend on?

10. Jamal wants to do research on how people adapt to catastrophic news in relation to their health and finds that there are several discussion forums on the internet where people recently diagnosed with cancer exchange information about how this diagnosis is affecting the lives of them and their families. These discussion forums are not completely open—you have to be a member to participate and see what others are saying—but anyone can join. Jamal himself is not in that position now, although something like that happened to him years ago when his mother was diagnosed with cancer and passed away shortly thereafter. Discuss whether you agree with Jamal's decision to join the group and "lurk" there as a passive observer of the group's discussions.

11. When engaged in participant observation/ethnographic research, researchers often try and be helpful as part of a respectful exchange—they help you by allowing you access; you help them in whatever small way makes you useful to them—but the issue often arises as to where you will draw the line. For example, if you are studying people who engage in illicit drug use, should you feel obliged to participate if they offer you some? Or let's say you are doing research in a hospital and a nurse asks you to hold a patient down for the nurse to administer a drug that the patient clearly does not consent to. Would you do it? Discuss some scenarios that might arise in research areas that you are interested in to see what range of opinion exists among you and your peers on where that line should be drawn.

12. *Can* men do research about women? *Should* men do research about women? Discuss this issue in a study group or in an essay.

13. Why is it important to allow time immediately after any observational session to sit down alone and flesh out your fieldnotes?

14. In what way does participatory action research overcome some of the problems associated with earlier approaches to ethnography?

15. How does critical ethnography differ from traditional ethnography?

16. Is there something particular about being a marginalized population that makes the balance of power between researcher and participant "inherent"?

17. In participatory action research, the researcher is aligned with marginalized individuals and communities for the express purpose of improving their well-being and social conditions. What does this mean for researchers when it comes to walking the line between researcher and activist?

18. How realistic or practical is participatory action research? What are the main challenges that you need to be sensitive about when you engage the community?

19. What are some ways we could address the ethical issues in participatory action research?

ARCHIVAL SOURCES

We began the chapters on methods for gathering data by focusing first of all on interactive methods (surveys, interviews, and oral histories) and followed that with observational techniques and the mixed method approaches that go beyond straight observation (different forms of ethnography and participatory action research).

In this chapter we look at other material out there in the world—artifacts of human existence—that can be made into data by being content analyzed or thematized to capture how it reflects on the human condition. The sorts of materials we have in mind include contemporary products (e.g., newspapers, television, magazines, Webpages, Twitter feeds, YouTube videos) and a wide variety of historical material (e.g., old newspaper reports, books, historical documents). The chapter concludes by looking at data that come prepackaged as it were—data produced by government statistics bureaus and secondary data from other studies—which are more and more frequently being made available online for analysis on their own or as part of a broader multimethod inquiry.

CONTENT ANALYTIC APPROACHES

When we give surveys to people, interview them, observe them, or do experiments, we invite people to give us material we can work with to better understand the human condition. In doing so, we often impose a structure on what people say or do, even if that structure is no more than asking an open-ended question that is designed to tell us about some particular aspect of our participants' lives, or their point of view on some issue. Doing so makes it easier for us to analyze, but we do so at the cost of constraining what people would say or do if left to their own devices. Indeed, the more we structure, the more we make it easier on ourselves, but the more we take away the voice or spontaneity of their behavior.

But if the challenge of the social and health sciences is to understand humans and what we do, then scrutinizing the artifacts of our existence—things we leave behind—offers yet another way we can shed light on that understanding. The techniques we discuss in this chapter offer a counterpoint to interactive methods such as experiments and surveys by taking the world as it comes and recognizing that patterned behavior leaves trails that reflect on us both individually (e.g., the way the searches we make via Google or DuckDuckGo reflect our ongoing thoughts and curiosities) and collectively (e.g., the way the wear on floor tiles reflects the relative popularity of museum exhibits, or how the art on pottery reflects the practices and beliefs of bygone cultures). A primary advantage is that we are allowing the world to behave as it does without any intervention on our part, and hence without reactivity.

The commensurate challenge is that we need to translate all that information that can come in literally any size, shape, or form into a format we can work with, using analytical tools that are up to the task. For the most part, those tools are the methods of **content analysis** and thematic analysis.

Some History

Although Bernard (2013) and Krippendorf (2019) give examples of content analyses from the 17th century, our contemporary version of content analysis arose in the early 20th century. There were two primary foci to that early work. The first involved the analysis of newspaper content. One seminal article by Woodward (1934) outlined a method by which it presumably could be done. Recall that the 1930s was a golden time for survey research and attitude measurement, what with researchers such as George Gallup trying to understand "the will of the people" through the survey techniques he was developing and Rensis Likert (1932) showing that attitudes could be measured. Woodward was interested in an ongoing debate at the time over whether newspapers *influenced* public opinion (i.e., the media shape public attitudes) or *reflected* public opinion (i.e., the media give people what they want). He suggested that the question could be answered by measuring both public attitudes and newspaper content at regular intervals over time and observing which changes first. He did not actually do the study, because neither the tools nor the infrastructure to do the research were available at the time, but outlined the desirability of being able to do so and argued for the creation of a "Research Bureau for Newspaper Analysis" to do that work on an ongoing basis.

The second focus of study that put content analysis on the contemporary methodological map occurred during World War II and involved the analysis of propaganda. It was in that context that content analysis was first accepted as a reasonable basis of proof in court in the trial of William Dudley Pelley for sedition (*State v Pelley* 20 S.E.2d 850, 221 N.C. 487). Bernard (2013) describes how Pelley was accused of sedition by the Department of Justice for publishing pro-Nazi propaganda that was critical of US involvement in the war in Europe. Harold Lasswell, "a political scientist and expert in propaganda analysis," analyzed 1,240 statements from Pelley's publications by comparing them to 14 common Nazi propaganda themes and found that 1,195 of Pelley's statements (96.4%) were consistent with the Nazi themes. Pelley was convicted and the admissibility in court of evidence based on content analysis was established (Bernard, 2013).

Content analysis of Nazi propaganda also played a big part in the US and British war effort. Military authorities wondered whether content analysis of propaganda could give them insights into the German "war mood" and if it would be possible to better predict and thereby be better prepared for German attacks. Part of the difficulty in engaging in this sort of analysis is that it is difficult to validate whether you are correct in the inferences you are drawing because you have no access to what is "really" happening on the other side. However, there were some small but important validations during the war. For example, analysts developed the notion of "preparatory propaganda." They started by noting in retrospect—after a German military initiative had occurred—that, "In order to ensure popular support for planned military actions, the Axis leaders had to inform, emotionally arouse, and otherwise prepare their countrymen and -women to accept those actions; the FCC analysts discovered that they could learn a great deal about the enemy's intended actions by recognizing such preparatory efforts in the domestic press and broadcasts" (Krippendorf, 2019, p. 16). Once the form of the preparatory propaganda was understood, the analysts became sensitized to recognizing it as it was happening and *before* the military campaign actually began. This allowed them to prepare for the projected initiatives, as well as to better understand factors they could use to undermine the confidence and morale of the German military leadership.

At the end of the war, personnel in the Foreign Broadcast Intelligence Service of the Federal Communications Commission had an opportunity to assess just how accurate all the inferences they had drawn during the war had been. Alexander George, a former employee of the unit, compared a sample of inferences drawn by the propaganda analysts with information in Nazi archives that were surrendered after the war and found that 81 percent of their inferences were accurate, much higher than you would expect on the basis of chance alone. His resulting book (George, 1959) went into considerable detail on the analyses that were done and some of the reasons behind their hits and misses, and made a major contribution to the development of content analysis as a technique (Doob, 1959).

Content analysis became much more popular after World War II as it was picked up by disciplines beyond journalism. Sociologists and political scientists became interested in content analysis to assess and track shifts in public attitudes on myriad social issues. Psychologists began to use content analysis as an indirect way to assess motivation and personality characteristics, as well as to identify themes and patterns in interview transcripts. Anthropologists started to use the technique in their analyses of folklore and cultural stories and even began to think of their field notes in content analytic terms. Historians had of course always been interested in analyzing documentary evidence, and were ready to embrace the more systematic techniques of content analysis in their work. As Krippendorff (2019) describes, "Everything seemed to be content analyzable, and every analysis of symbolic phenomena became a content analysis" (p. 10).

Krippendorff (2019) concludes his historical analysis by noting how content analysis has taken off exponentially since the 1970s, something he attributes in part to the bourgeoning use of computer-assisted content analyses. He notes that a Google search for the phrase "content analysis" turned up 1,650,000 hits in 2011, compared to 275,000 hits for "survey research" and 894,000 for "psychological testing." When we repeated those searches as we were writing this in 2020, we found 11.6 million hits for "content analysis" and 5.0 and 3.6 million hits for "survey research" and "psychological testing," respectively.

A Broad Range of Materials

Brancati (2018) talks about the wonderful diversity of material that is amenable to content analysis, reaffirming Krippendorff's (2019) comment that you can content analyze just about anything. Brancati (2018) offers three primary categories:

1. *Written materials*: The most common here are newspapers, which, as we described above, have a long history as a source of data for analysis. Other examples of this category include books, documents, policies, laws, Twitter feeds, blog posts, comments left on various websites, and reviews.

2. *Verbal materials*: Although there is nothing in this category as common as "newspapers" have been to the content analysis of written material, "verbal material" is nonetheless a broad category that includes such raw material as film dialogue, music lyrics, television talk shows, podcasts, radio documentaries, and speeches.

3. *Visual materials*: This is another huge category that includes materials such as television programs, YouTube videos, music videos, comic books, video games, and photo collections.

We would add one more to her list:

4. *Official Statistics and Secondary Data*: Statistics produced on an ongoing basis by government—as "official" records produced by government—fuel a tremendous amount of research every year and thus deserve scrutiny as yet another archival source. The existence and utility of secondary data sources was discussed in Chapter 9, but we analyze an example here to show how such sources can help understand the strengths and limitations of official statistics.

We'll begin by using Brancati's categories, which offer a very workable and helpful set of categories to get us brainstorming about possibilities. That said, trying to draw any rigid lines between them would be fruitless. Take films. Although we included "film dialogue" among the verbal materials, we could just as easily have focused on the film script that gave rise to the film and call it "written material." Similarly, we could just as easily have focused on film scenes and called it "visual material." In many ways it is all just a question of emphasis. Nonetheless, Brancati's three general categories are helpful in organizing our presentation of the rich array of material that has been and can be content analyzed.

Working With Written Materials

Content analysis requires you to have some clear idea of what you are after. However the focus is derived—from your personal interests, from theory, or from exploratory study—you need to begin with a clear specification of your research question(s) and objectives. With written materials, we begin with a study that was done by Simon Davis, whose content analysis of personals ads offers us an extended example of how nonnumeric data can be analyzed in this deductive manner.

Examining Mate Selection Through Personals Ads

Defining the Focus. For Simon Davis (1990), the interest was in looking at mate selection. Previous research had indicated that the selection of opposite-sex partners often follows traditional sex-stereotyped roles. In Davis's terms, stereotypical media portrayals have a long history of emphasizing women as "sex objects" (preferably attractive, alluring, seductive), while for men, the emphasis has been on portraying them as "success objects" (preferably intelligent, wealthy, professional). In keeping with this pattern, the evidence on mate-selection practices had found that men emphasized physical appearance more than women as a factor in mate selection, while women emphasized personality, commitment, and financial security. However, much of the research that showed those tendencies was dated, which left Davis (1990) wondering whether it was still the case in the more progressive 1990s: "Were traditional stereotypes still in operation, that is, [were] women being viewed as sex objects and men as success objects?" (p. 45). Although his study is an older one, we like it as an example because Davis was so clear about the methodological choices he made, and because the issue has not gone away (e.g., see a similar study reported in Krippendorff, 2019).

The Research Site. Davis's research question could have been addressed in many ways. He could have created a survey or interview study in which he asked people to indicate the characteristics they were looking for in the "ideal mate," or he could have approached married or cohabiting couples and asked them to explain what it was about the other person they had found so appealing. But if men are most interested in ensuring that they couple with a woman who looks good on their arm, will they admit it? And if women most value someone who is smart and successful, thereby providing social status and financial security, would they confide that to him? Davis was worried about the "social desirability" bias that might permeate these methods. Accordingly, he looked for a research venue where social desirability influences would be minimized.

The location he decided on was the newspaper, specifically, the "personals" columns, which was the main place people would advertise for a prospective partner or mate in those days before the Internet. It seemed to meet the criteria: here, men and women seek mates; in the process, they must decide which aspects of themselves they think are most "relevant" to specify, as well as which aspects of the prospective mate they feel are most important. Even better, they're doing so because they really do want to find a partner, and reactivity would be negligible because they are unlikely to be thinking about the possibility that some social or health scientist might ever read their ad as part of an analysis of factors involved in mate selection.

Of course, many different kinds of newspapers, magazines, and online sites included such "personals" in their classified advertising. Many catered to specific audiences, such as lesbians, gays, executives, or people who sought sexual kinkiness. Although the mate-selection practices shown by such groups may be of interest, Davis chose to start with more "mainstream" ads, particularly those that involved prospective heterosexual relationships. Accordingly, the newspaper he scrutinized was his city's main daily newspaper, which in Davis's words is perceived as a "conservative, respectable journal" (1990, p. 45), rather like the *San Francisco Chronicle, Detroit Free Press, Miami Herald*, or *Denver Post*.

Many libraries would keep old copies of the local newspaper as part of their document archive, and it was to the city library that Davis went to check for old editions of his local paper. A preliminary examination of these papers revealed that, although you could place a personals ad on any day of the week, Saturday was clearly the "big" day for such ads: 40–60 ads appeared every Saturday, as opposed to between 2 and 4 ads per day during the week. He thus decided to focus only on Saturday editions. Of the 52 Saturday editions in the year before he started the study, Davis chose to randomly sample six from throughout the year, subjecting *every* ad in each of those editions to analysis. The random sampling would ensure that the editions he analyzed could be considered theoretically representative of the issues published during that year; at 40–60 ads per weekend edition, he could expect to end up with several hundred ads, which seemed a reasonable number to analyze. But how to analyze them?

Operationalizing the Variables of Interest. Davis had stated that he was interested in this notion of women (in men's eyes) as "sex objects" and men (in women's eyes) as "success objects." But how do you analyze the typical personals ad for those elements? That is, how do you determine whether any given ad is or is not an example of those phenomena?

Davis approached this question by looking for particular words that could be taken as indicative of the concepts of interest to him. First, he decided to analyze only that part of the ad in which the ad's writer specified the attributes they sought in a prospective mate. Within that portion, he decided (after reading many ads to see what kinds of words and phrases were typically used) on the codes shown in Table 12.1.

Three other attributes the ads were coded for included the sex of the ad's author; the age of the ad's author, but only if a *specific* age was indicated; and the ad's length (expressed as the number of lines).

Note, by the way, that the first nine codes fall neatly into the general categories Davis had been talking about with respect to his primary study objectives. The notion of the "sex object" is reflected by the first four categories—words or phrases that mention "physical attractiveness," "physique," or "sex" or that request a "picture." The notion of the "success object" is addressed by the "employment" cluster contained in the next three categories—"profession," "employed," and "financial"—as well as the "intellectual" cluster represented by the categories "education" and "intelligence." The remaining four categories—"honest," "humor," "commitment," and "emotion"—all related to a "personality" cluster that had been found in the literature to be more commonly concerns of women; hence, although they were of interest to gather data about, they didn't explicitly relate to the focal concepts of "sex object" and/or "success object."

Davis's elaboration of categories took what had been a very ephemeral idea—the notions of "sex object" and "success object"—and began translating them into fairly concrete, operational terms. Certainly one positive outcome of doing so would be that the coding could probably be done with a high degree of reliability, since such categories reduce the amount of inference required of the coder. Note also how his study design involved a step-by-step approach, in which each step builds on the one preceding; as a result, the data address his objectives adequately and clearly.

TABLE 12.1 ● Coding Scheme Employed by Davis (1990) for an Analysis of Mate-Selection Patterns Evident in Personal Newspaper Advertisements

#	Code	Explanation
1	Attractiveness	Coded when the author of the ad indicates that he or she seeks someone who is *pretty, attractive, handsome*, or *good-looking*.
2	Physique	Similar to category 1, but focused more on the body than on the face; relevant key words here would include *muscular, fit, and trim, good figure*, or *well-built*.
3	Sex	Used when reference is made in the ad to desirability of *high sex drive, sensuous, erotic*; or where there is a clear message that author wants to find someone interested in engaging in sexual activity (i.e., *lunchtime liaisons-discretion required*).
4	Picture	Some ads request that respondents send along a photo of themselves, while others do not. Davis (1990) assumed that if a picture was requested, appearance was important.
5	Profession	Used when the author indicates that prospective partner should be a *professional* person.
6	Employed	Coded when the ad specifies that the person should have a steady *job or steady income*.
7	Financial	Used whenever the ad indicates that the person sought should be *wealthy, financially stable*, or *financially secure*.
8	Education	Coded whenever an indication is given that the prospective mate should be *well-read, college-educated*, or *simply well-educated*.
9	Intelligence	Key words for this category include a request for someone who is *intelligent, bright*, or *intellectual*.
10	Honest	Coded when the ad requests someone honest or states that respondent should have *integrity*.
11	Humor	Coded when reference is made to the desire for the prospective mate to have a sense of *humor*, to be *cheerful*, or to enjoy a good laugh.
12	Commitment	Used when the author explicitly indicates that he or she seeks a liaison that would be *long-term, might lead to marriage*, or similar phrasing.
13	Emotion	Used when there are indications of the desirability of emotional expressiveness, such as *romantic, expressive, sensitive*, or *responsive*.

You should see, for example, that if we were now to go ahead and code the various ads to ascertain how often ad authors of each sex used terms like "attractive," "professional," and "well educated," we should have a fairly clear answer as to whether men are indeed more interested in meeting "sex objects" as defined in this study and whether women are more interested in meeting "success objects" as defined in this study. And that's exactly what Davis went on to do.

While Davis might have been able to get away without undertaking a reliability assessment because his coding essentially involved little more than looking for specific key words and thus would be expected to be quite reliable, normally content analysis would require you to demonstrate that the coding scheme that has been developed can be implemented reliably. This is most commonly done by having two or more coders sit down and independently code a sample of the same material (i.e., you don't have to use every single item in the sample). Several different statistics can be used to compute **inter-rater reliability**, depending on the type of data you have (see Krippendorff, 2019). The simplest is simply to look at the percentage of codes on which the pair of raters agree. Eighty percent or more would be considered acceptable.

Aggregating and Coding the Data. With his 13 coding categories in hand, Davis could use them to code the various ads. One problem he anticipated was that a few particularly zealous "sex object" seekers or "success object" seekers could really throw off the data if they said the same thing a dozen different ways; that is, if each of the 13 phrases were counted as an instance of the phenomenon of interest, the total number would inflate the average for their group (i.e., for men or for women). Accordingly, Davis decided to code each of the categories as either "present" or "absent." Operationally, this meant that he would sit down with each ad, ask whether each of the 13 categories was evident, and then code it on a purely yes-or-no basis.

Thus, if an ad said that its author was looking for someone "with a great body," that ad would be coded as a "yes" for the "physique" category. If another ad expressed its author's interest in someone who was "muscular, fit, with great body tone, and curves and bulges in all the right places," that ad, too, would be coded as a "yes" for the "physique" category, even though its author repeated essentially the same thing four times in succession.

Davis then went through each of the randomly sampled Saturday editions, finding a total of 329 ads. He decided to omit one of them from the analysis (appropriately noting the decision in his article) because it involved a gay relationship rather than the heterosexual relationships on which he had decided to focus. Of the 328 remaining ads, 215 (or 65.5 percent) were placed by men, while 113 (or 34.5 percent) were submitted by women.

Because he had coded for the age of the person in each ad, he also was able to tell us a bit about who these people were: the average age of those who reported it was 40.4 years, with very similar average ages for the men (40.7 years) and the women (39.4 years) who had included that information. The biggest problem here was that a full half of the women (50.4 percent) and almost a third of the men (32.6 percent) did not report their *exact* age.

Once all the ads were coded, Davis had only to begin making the appropriate comparisons. His first analysis scrutinized the differences between men and women in each of the 13 categories. These data are reported in Table 12.2: where Davis found significant differences, we've shaded the side with the significantly higher percentage. All the differences, significant or not, were in the anticipated direction, and most (10 out of 13) of the individual comparisons were statistically significant (i.e., the differences were found to be larger than would be expected on the basis of chance variation alone; see Chapters 6 and 14 for discussions of statistical significance). Thus, for the "sex object" cluster, men were more likely than women to specify that they were seeking someone who was attractive, had a

TABLE 12.2 ● Gender Comparison for Attributes Desired in Partner

Variable	Desired by Men (n =215)	Desired by Women (n = 113)	Chi-Square
Attractiveness	76 (35.3%)	20 (17.7%)	11.13(*)
Physique	81 (37.7%)	27 (23.9%)	6.37(*)
Sex	25 (11.6%)	4 (3.5%)	6.03(*)
Picture	74 (34.4%)	24 (21.2%)	6.18(*)
Profession	6 (2.8%)	19 (16.8%)	20.74(*)
Employed	8 (3.7%)	12 (10.6%)	6.12(*)
Financial	7 (3.2%)	22 (19.5%)	24.26(*)
Education	8 (3.7%)	8 (7.1%)	1.79(ns)
Intelligence	22 (10.2%)	24 (21.2%)	7.46(*)
Honest	20 (9.3%)	17 (15.0%)	2.44(ns)
Humor	36 (16.7%)	26 (23.0%)	1.89(ns)
Commitment	38 (17.6%)	31 (27.4%)	4.25(*)
Emotion	44 (20.5%)	35 (31.0%)	4.36(*)

Note: (*) means that the difference between the male- and female-authored ads was statistically significant at the $p < .05$ level; (ns) means that the comparison was nonsignificant, that is, the difference observed was no greater than what you would expect on the basis of chance variation alone.

Source: Davis (1990). Reprinted with permission from Springer Science and Business Media.

nice physique, and/or was interested in sex, and were more likely to request a picture of the respondent.

For the "success object" cluster, women were more likely than men to express a preference for someone who was a professional, employed, and/or financially secure. The data on the "intellectual" cluster were a little less clear: there were no statistically significant differences between the sexes in the extent to which they mentioned the desirability of "education" (although women had the higher percentage again), yet the category "intelligent" was noted significantly more often by women than men.

As for the "personality" cluster, women were more likely than men to specify attributes that fell into all four of these categories. But the size of the difference was statistically significant only for "commitment" and "emotion," and not for "honesty" and "humor."

Another way to look at these data is to group them into the overall categories of interest, for example, to aggregate all the "sex object" categories—appearance, physique, sex, picture—to create one overall index. This is shown in Table 12.3, which reaffirms the overall differences between male-authored and female-authored ads that were already evident when we scrutinized the individual categories. Men were shown to be more likely than women to state in an ad that they were seeking someone who was physically attractive; women were more likely than men to say that they were seeking someone who was financially stable and well educated.

Alas, despite all the gains that have been made in the realm of sexual equality, Davis's (1990) data would seem to show that many men and women—at least in the early 1990s—still followed very traditional patterns when seeking a mate.

TABLE 12.3 ● Gender Comparison for Physical, Employment, and Intellectual Attributes Desired in a Prospective Partner

Variable	Gender		Chi-Square
	Desired by Men (n = 215)	Desired by Women (n = 113)	
Physical (aggregating variables 1–4)	143 (66.5%)	60 (44.2%)	15.13(*)
Employment (aggregating variables 5–7)	17 (7.9%)	47 (41.6%)	51.36(*)
Intellectual (aggregating variables 8–9)	29 (13.5%)	31 (27.4%)	9.65(*)

Note: (*) means that the difference between the male- and female-authored ads was statistically significant at the $p < .05$ level.

Source: Davis (1990). Reprinted with permission of Kluwer Academic/Plenum Publishing Corporation.

Caveat and Critique. Or did they? Probably the most positive element of Davis's analysis is the use it makes of an unobtrusive and nonreactive archival measure to scrutinize "real" processes involved in searching for a mate (i.e., the people who placed the newspaper ads were in fact searching for partners). But we still should be careful about how much confidence we place in the conclusions.

Davis expresses caution related to the apparent age of his sample. Having determined that the average age of those ad authors who cited their exact age was around 40, he is cautious about the generalizability of his results (their external validity), suggesting that the results may merely reflect the particular age cohort represented in the ads. Just because the 40-ish people who placed these ads seem to follow very traditional patterns of mate selection does not mean that people in other age cohorts—those in their teens and 20s, for example—also do so.

We also have to question the selection bias associated with those who use ads as a way of selecting mates, rather than what at that time were more conventional means such as introductions through friends, meeting at social events such as parties, and/or meeting at venues of common interest such as the gym, library, or opera. Indeed, the fact that those who placed ads were in their 40s and were still (or newly) unattached may suggest that ads in the 1990s were a venue for mate selection largely for those who were unable or unwilling to meet people through conventional means and/or for those who may still be unattached precisely *because* they had a rigidly sex-typed and traditional conception of roles and desirable attributes. People who were more socially egalitarian may have met someone already, and hence did not need to place an ad.

As this implies, those who chose mates *not* because they sought someone with a great body or a large bank account, but because they sought a well-rounded person who combined many positive attributes, may well be sitting out there happily ensconced in and enjoying their relationships, and may never even have considered placing a personals ad. Thus, although Davis's findings are indeed consistent with his hypothesis regarding differential bases for mate selection, they may well have emerged precisely because people who sought mates for the attributes he hypothesized were the people who ended up placing personals ads in those days, and not because they reflect the way men and women in general seek and select mates.

That said, we do wonder if the generalizability of results has run its course. While placing a personals ad was an unusual thing to do and held some small degree of stigma in the 1990s, these days matchmaking sites like Tinder and Harmony seem pretty much par for the course, just another way that people get to bring new people into their lives for possible romantic ends. We've included a study question at the end of this chapter encouraging you to consider how you might replicate Davis's study today with the dating sites now available.

Working With Verbal Sources

The domain of "verbal materials" includes all sorts of audio sources such as dialogues, speeches, music lyrics, and podcasts. Interviews could appear in this category as well, but we prefer to leave that discussion to the chapters dealing with interviews as well as the next chapter on analyzing nonnumeric data because one of the attributes of content analysis that is not typically met with the classic interview is the absence of reactivity.

Examining Populism Through Political Speeches

One example of just such a content analysis appeared in *The Guardian* magazine concerning what appears to be a growing trend toward "populism" in politics around the world. A report from Britain's Tony Blair Institute for Global Change (Kyle & Gultchin, 2018) states that between 1990 and 2018 the number of populist leaders in power increased fivefold, from 4 to 20. While it was formerly the case that populist leaders were more likely to appear in fledgling democracies, much of the recent growth in populist leadership has come in formerly strong democracies like the United States, Italy, and India. *The Guardian* sought to further understand this growth by collaborating with "Team Populism," a network of academics who have published extensively on the topic over the last decade, on a study of contemporary leaders.

What Is Populism?. We were fascinated with this study for several reasons. The topic itself is a fascinating one because "populism" is not associated with any particular kind of democratic government—there are populists on both the "right" and the "left," as well as others who fit neither category particularly well. Instead, it refers to a particular style of government that begins with two basic tenets: (1) the idea that the country's "true people" are at war with "others"—both "outsiders" who threaten the "true people's" interests, as well as insider politicians who are dismissed as "establishment elites" and (2) nothing should constrain the will of the people (e.g., Kyle & Gultchin, 2018; Mudde, 2004). Team Populist and *The Guardian* add a third element implied by the first two, which is that, (3) at stake is nothing less than a battle between good ("us") and evil ("them").

At some level, the idea that governments should be influenced by "the will of the people" seems uncontentious; after all, isn't the "will of the people" what democracy is all about? However, for many years "populism" was seen as a bad thing, a perversion or pathology of democracy that seemed governed by paranoia, the threat of the other, resulting in oppressive and inherently undemocratic measures—undermining freedom of the press, denying rights, removing checks on government abuse of power, mobilizing against groups that are scapegoats for society's problems—that are justified as "necessary" for "national security" to avert "a crisis," to preserve life as "we" know it. As Mudde (2015) explains, however, there is often at least a grain of truth in the critique that populists bring; the "good" side of populism is that it comes with an insistence that governments should open a dialogue on issues that have been ignored that are nonetheless meaningful to "the people," and where those in power have effectively closed off the opportunity for meaningful debate. The bad side is what happens when populists get in power, when who "we" are is defined in homogeneous terms, outsiders are demonized, and the legitimacy of political opponents is questioned. As Mudde (2015) explains,

> In short, populism is an illiberal democratic response to undemocratic liberalism. It criticises the exclusion of important issues from the political agenda by the elites and calls for their repoliticisation. However, this comes at a price. Populism's black and white views and uncompromising stand leads to a polarised society—for which, of course, both sides share responsibility—and its majoritarian extremism denies legitimacy to opponents' views and weakens the rights of minorities. While leftwing populism is often less exclusionary than rightwing populism, the main difference between them is not whether they exclude, but whom they exclude, which is largely determined by their accompanying ideology (e.g., nationalism or socialism). (p. 2)

Operationalizing Populism. If our objective is to understand populism and assess the roots of its emergence, then the first thing we need to do is to find a research site that will provide the raw material for that assessment. In the case of *The Guardian/* Team Populism analysis, that began by choosing which countries to look at. *The Guardian* settled on a list of 40 countries, including the eight countries in the Americas with the largest populations (the United States, Brazil, Mexico, Columbia, Canada, Argentina, Peru, and Venezuela) as well as the seven largest in Europe (Russia, Germany, Turkey, the United Kingdom, France, Italy, and Spain). A second choice was what to look at in order to assess populism, and the choice made there was to look at leaders' speeches. A third choice involved how to operationally define "populism" so that you could reliably categorize any given politician as populist or not.

There are numerous methodological challenges that arise when attempting to do an international study like this. One is the challenge of language, given that you want to have speeches in the politician's native language. *The Guardian* addressed this by hiring research assistants who were fluent in whatever language was involved. The downside of doing it that way is twofold: (1) with multiple content analyzers working on different material, you need to worry about inter-rater reliability in the way they are coding and (2) it would be very difficult to ensure the person doing the coding is "blind" to whichever politician's speech is being coded, which creates a situation where any preconceptions the coder has about the politician may interfere with them paying attention only to the content of the speech they are analyzing.

A second challenge is to ensure that there is some comparability of the types of speeches that each leader is being assessed on because you want to ensure that any differences you find between politicians is due to actual differences between them and not because one politician's campaign speeches are being compared to another politician's postelection speeches, for example. In that regard, *The Guardian* decided to sample four speeches from each politician, with the same four types of speeches being chosen for each one: (1) a campaign speech; (2) a "ribbon cutting" speech given to a local audience; (3) a "famous" speech that had been widely circulated and showed off each leader at their eloquent best; and (4) an international speech given to an audience outside the country.

With some degree of standardization brought in to ensure as much comparability as possible, the next step was to decide on the procedures that would be used to determine each politician's degree of populism. For *The Guardian*/Team Populist project we describe here, the decision had been made to use four speeches per politician, but what would the basic unit of analysis be? They could go line by line, or paragraph by paragraph, or section by section, any of which might be defensible. In this case, however, the Team decided to ask coders to do "holistic coding," i.e., each coder was to read the speech as a whole independently and assign a rating as to "how populist" the speech as a whole was judged to be. In most cases, two coders coded each speech; when coders disagreed, the score assigned was the average of the two. The scale ran from 0 (no indication of populism) to 1 (clear populism, but used inconsistently or with mild tone) to 2 (clear populism used consistently and with a strong tone). A given leader's score was their average score across all four speeches (Lewis, Clarke, & Barr, 2019; see also; Team Populism & *The Guardian*, 2019).

Newspapers and magazines rarely make detailed methodological notes available when they report research results, but that was not the case here. *The Guardian* referenced various publications at the Team Populism site that explained conceptual and methodological choices, and the news magazine itself reported on the way that coders were trained to ensure they were doing so consistently, and also reported on reliability and validity. With respect to reliability, the statistic computed was Krippendorff's alpha, which can run from 0.0 to 1.0, where 1 is perfect agreement between the two. After training, Krippendorff's alpha for the populism data was 0.82, which is both quite high and quite acceptable (see Krippendorff, 2019).

Validity was assessed in several ways. One was simply to look at **face validity** of the coding scheme (see Team Populism & *The Guardian*, 2019)—whether, on the face of it, the measure seems to capture what it is supposed to measure—which does indeed seem to get at populism in the way it has been defined. A second is to see whether differences you know should be there do indeed occur. For example, of the four different kinds of speeches, you would expect campaign and "famous" speeches (delivered in contexts such as inaugurations or state-of-the-union addresses) to score higher on populism than "ribbon cutting" and international speeches. "Ribbon-cutting" speeches are local with a smaller audience, while international speeches normally would be less "political" because diplomacy often prevails given the diplomatic tradition that leaders should not meddle in the affairs of other countries. And that did indeed prove to be the case, with average scores of 0.60 and 0.42 for campaign and "famous" speeches, and 0.23 and 0.20 for ribbon-cutting and international speeches.

There were, however, a few surprises. One was that former US President Donald Trump, who was typically seen as more populist and certainly pressed all the buttons associated with populism, only scored as "somewhat populist" on the basis of his speeches that were analyzed. In his case, an interesting finding was that there were significant differences between prepared speeches he read versus those where he improvised. His prepared speeches were found to be more populist than when he improvised. Although at some level counterintuitive, *The Guardian* explained this was because, when he improvises, he tends to talk about himself rather than to focus exclusively on the "others" who are blamed for the world's problems (Lewis et al., 2019).

Findings. There were two general foci to the analysis. One was how the leaders compared with each other. Table 12.4 shows a subset of leaders from *The Guardian/*Team Populism analysis and their scores in descending populist order. The second analysis looked at changes over time, given that the leader data for the 40 countries on which they had complete data extended over the period from 1990 to 2019. In that regard, Lewis et al. (2019) note that the average scored has doubled across all 40 countries from the early 2000s to today, and that the number of countries with

TABLE 12.4 ● Comparative Populism Scores for 11 Political Leaders		
Politician	Country	Populism score[a]
Hugo Chávez	Venezuela (1999–2013)	1.9
Nicolás Maduro	Venezuela (2013–2019)	1.6
Evo Morales	Bolivia	1.5
Recep Tayyip Erdoğan	Turkey	1.5
Viktor Orbán	Hungary	0.9
Silvio Berlusconi	Italy	0.8
Donald Trump	United States	0.8
Narendra Modi	India	0.6
Jair Bolsonaro	Brazil	0.5
Tony Blair	United Kingdom	0.1
Angela Merkel	Germany	0.0

[a]Scores could range from "0" (not at all populist) to "2" (very populist).

Source: Derived from information presented in Lewis et al. (2019).

leaders who are at least "somewhat" populist (i.e., defined as scores of 0.5 or above) has also doubled, from 7 to 14.

Another interesting finding was that Latin American populists tended to be on the political left, while those in Europe tended to be from the political right. In that regard, they seem to confirm the distinction that Kyle and Gultchin (2018) make between "cultural populism" and "socioeconomic populism":

Cultural populism claims that the true people are the native members of the nation-state, and outsiders can include immigrants, criminals, ethnic and religious minorities, and cosmopolitan elites. Cultural populism tends to emphasize religious traditionalism, law and order, sovereignty, and painting migrants as enemies.

Socioeconomic populism claims that the true people are honest, hardworking members of the working class, and outsiders can include big business, capital owners, and actors perceived as propping up an international capitalist system.

The distinction is a useful one, for example in distinguishing in the United States between politicians Donald Trump and Bernie Sanders, both of whom have been referred to as "populist" in the media. The evils Donald Trump wanted to save us from include immigrants, ethnic and religious minorities and liberals, and his calls to "drain the swamp" seems to have been to drain it of politicians and replace them with captains of industry. Bernie Sanders, in contrast, sought to save us from greedy capitalists who get rich while failing to pay honest working people a decent living wage, and avoid paying taxes that could sustain a universal health-care system and broader access to education.

Limitations and Further Research. It is also unusual for a newsmagazine to include a discussion of the limitations of a research project, but *The Guardian* does exactly that. Lewis et al. (2018) write that,

> *This research is not intended as a definitive or final determination of how populist any given leader is. Textual analysis is just one approach for gauging the populism exhibited by a politician. No methodological approach is foolproof. Speeches are just one of many ways politicians communicate their ideas, particularly in a social media age; some politicians may tend to be more or less populist depending on the mode of communication.*
>
> *The average score given to any political leader's term in office is also dependent upon which speeches were selected. Analysing more speeches per leader may have yielded a more reliable average score.*

A by-product of the collaboration between *The Guardian* and Team Populist is that all the data on which these analyses are based are available for downloading at the Team Populism site, which we encourage you to check out for your own curiosity or for a project.[1]

Working With Visual Sources

Archival visual data are everywhere: images in print media such as magazines, pamphlets, or posters; television programs, films, cinema verité, and documentaries; video sharing websites such as YouTube; photographic or digital images that appear in family albums, social networking sites such as Facebook, Pinterest, and Snapchat as well as in public and private archives; the art that adorns the walls and halls of

---

[1]See the "data" link at the Team Populism web site at https://populism.byu.edu/.

museums such as the Louvre; and the graffiti you see on subway and bathroom walls. While students of cultural and media studies, communications, and visual anthropology will know the utility of using visual media as a rich source of data for answering a range of research questions, these sources also can be very useful for people working in a range of other social and health science disciplines for obtaining critical insights into social life.

It is often said that a picture is worth a thousand words. It is certainly true that images and video are capable of providing rich data to answer research questions that conventional observations and data collection techniques simply would not be able to accurately and comprehensively record. Visual data offer social and health researchers a way of actually *seeing* aspects of phenomena that we otherwise would only be able to hear or read about through secondhand accounts obtained through the range of more obtrusive methods we have discussed in previous chapters. Photo and video allow us to access basic information such as the number of people attending a particular event or complex social interactions and narratives such as the movements, activities, and conflicts of those individuals who participated in the riot in Boston in 2004 after the Red Sox won their first World Series in 86 years.

Pictures and videos are historical documents. As representations of often complex historical activity, visual data are incredibly useful for documenting historical change in a way that is generally possible only through expensive and time-consuming longitudinal studies. For example, Kimberly Neuendorf and her colleagues (Neuendorf, Gore, Dalessandro, Janstova, & Snyder-Suhy, 2010) were interested in determining whether prevailing societal norms about women and female sexuality have changed over time. While there are many ways that Neuendorf et al. could have addressed this question, they did so by studying the idealized portrayals of female beauty that are perpetuated through films. Out of countless television programs and movies they could have selected, they decided that the long-running and popular James Bond movie franchise with its infamous "Bond girls" was particularly well suited for achieving their research objective. The researchers carefully coded and analyzed 20 Bond films beginning with 1962s *Dr. No* and ending with 2002s *Die Another Day*.

The Bond films are an excellent vehicle for looking at portrayals of women because you have the same central character and even the same production company over time, and a changing historical backdrop against which the films are being produced. The results from Neuendorf et al.'s (2010) analysis indicated that "despite social progression of feminist ideology, the women of Bond continue to be portrayed in rather limited sex-stereotypical manner" (p. 758). While the number of female characters represented increased over time and the roles of women in the franchise expanded with women becoming more autonomous, the characters have become more sexually attractive and are more likely to be the recipients of physical harm.

Just as the information contained in pictures and videos offers researchers rich opportunities for finding answers to a diverse array of research questions we also should acknowledge that the people, places, or events that *do not* appear in visual images sometimes can offer important information for answering a range of research questions. For example, while Chris was studying at the University of Toronto he would routinely walk the halls of buildings where the pictures of graduating classes from as far back as 1870 were displayed. While the images of these early alumni revealed much about the dress and decorum of the time with each photo displaying mostly wealthy Caucasian men wearing double breasted waistcoats with pocket watches, Chris was more fascinated by what was *not* present in picture after picture, year after year. Very few of the pictures were of women and racial minorities, a condition that did not appear to change dramatically until the 1950s. Are there similar photographic images of graduating classes at your university or college that would allow you to pose questions about changes in gender, race, and class of students over time?

Notwithstanding the many research possibilities that exist with visual data, they are also not without challenges. Perhaps the most significant challenge facing researchers wishing to use visual data relates to the fact that it is sometimes difficult to ascertain the authenticity and credibility of images or video since such medium can easily be forged or manipulated. For example, it is quite common to hear people say "before I put that picture up on Facebook I'll have to 'Photoshop it'." All computers come prepackaged with basic image and video editing software and social media applications such as Snapchat provide users with access to a wide array of filters and lenses, allowing anyone to edit the "reality" that is present in the video and digital images that they preserve. Individuals and groups with access to greater resources will find it even easier to edit visual materials. This manipulation can be as simple as removing the red eye from a picture or as complex as removing full segments of time from a video.

Just as elements of the "reality" captured in an image or video can easily be removed they also can be added. Such additions or removals can be almost impossible for the untrained eye to detect. So while image and video offer researchers the opportunity to observe aspects of a phenomenon, in a digital age we need to be increasingly aware of the possibility that the "reality" that we think is being represented in a picture or video is nothing more than a clever recrafting of a particular event.

Even when an image or video remains unaltered, we need to keep in mind that visual representations are merely snapshots or clips of selected aspects of social reality and these clips reflect the gender, class, and racial position of the person who took the photo or created the video (see also our discussion of Becker, 1979 in Chapter 8). Historically, cameras and video-capture devices were available only to those who could afford such technologies, as a result much of the visual data that are preserved in physical and virtual archives represent another example of selective deposit that will overrepresent particular class interests and perspectives. With the increasing pervasiveness of smartphones with built-in high-resolution cameras, this situation may be changing.

It is also important to keep in mind that pictures and videos frequently contain a performative element. When individuals or groups are the subject of a picture or video they frequently "perform" or pose for the camera consciously representing themselves in a particular light. Somewhat related to the performative aspect of visual media is the fact that the content that people choose to capture in pictures and video frequently is that which has particular significance or tells a particular story as they see it. It is exceedingly rare to see people taking pictures or video of mundane events. More frequently photos and video either depict the best or worst of the human condition or the specific story that the person creating the visual wants to relay. As a result, visual records may not tell us much about the typical conditions underlying a phenomenon of interest.

Visual records also more commonly deal with *anticipated* events owing to the more cumbersome weight that bringing along a video camera involves. This is rapidly changing with the newest generations of smartphones; now huge numbers of people are carrying image- and video-capable phones in their pockets, creating situations where there can be high-quality videos by the hundreds in significant events such as the "Occupy" events around the world and during protests and state repression in what came to be called the "Arab Spring"; YouTube, Facebook, Snapchat, and Twitter ensured that messages, images, and video about these events were being beamed to the world within moments of their occurrence.

The quality of the images and video can greatly impact the "reality" that is captured and a researcher's ability to extract the information from the visual data. While it is increasingly common for images and video to be captured with high-resolution digital cameras or high-definition digital recorders, much of the visual data contained in public and private archives that are available to social and health researchers are stored on microfilm, microfiche, 16 mm or 8 mm film reels, beta or VHS tapes, computer disks, or in the pages of dusty old books or photo albums. The detail that is captured by these media varies dramatically. Microfilm and microfiche often store only low-resolution black-and-white images of original photographs that may themselves have been in a heightened state of erosion at the time they were archived. While 16 mm and 8 mm film formats store both video and audio tracks, the resolution of the film and the accuracy of the color are inferior to that of even the most basic modern-day smartphones. The relative disparities in the quality of the visual content of differing media dramatically impact the depth and breadth of data that researchers can extract, which in turn impacts the reliability and validity of their results and conclusions.

In addition to dramatic differences in the quality of the original recording media, the temperature and relative humidity as well as the lighting and air conditions of the public and private archives where visual media are stored dramatically impacts the quality of the archived material over time. It is not uncommon for photographs or video to become faded or yellowed over time or for microfiche and 8 mm film to dry and crack. As a result of the ravages of time librarians, archivists, and private collectors are often faced with difficult decisions about what data they are able to continue to preserve and what format they should preserve it in. There is currently much debate among archivists about whether it would be more effective to preserve text and images contained in old books on microfiche or as digital PDF files. While only time will tell what preservation format will be selected, with new technologies emerging at such a rapid rate it is only a matter of time before these preferred archival formats once again become obsolete and another collection of valuable visual archive material is lost.

As was the case with content analyses based on written and verbal materials, content analyses of visual materials can range from highly structured analyses that involve coding material into a series of mutually exclusive and exhaustive categories, to more thematic or discursive analyses that attempt to identify visual metaphor and the underlying message to a given production. An example of a more structured analysis is the Neuendorf et al. (2010) content analysis of the James Bond films that we noted above. An integral part of their process involved creating a content coding manual, testing inter-rater reliability across the eight coders who were involved, and further developing the coding manual until an acceptable standard of reliability was met. On the other hand, we could equally easily imagine a more semiotic analysis of the Bond films that was more focused on the roles and image that the women in the films were expected to portray. Indeed, as an example for this section of the Chapter, we thought it best to balance our discussion of Simon Davis's (1990) analysis of mate selection and Neuendorf et al.'s (2010) analysis of the Bond films with a more thematically driven analysis that Ted did involving the portrayal of Indigenous people/s in film.

Images of Indigenous People in Film

Ted is interested in both film and Indigenous issues, and so it should perhaps be no surprise that he would be drawn to examining how Indigenous people have been portrayed in film. There had been previous studies that looked at how Native peoples had been portrayed in books, films, and other media, but Ted's interest was in looking not only at what those portrayals were and how they had changed over time, but particularly in linking those portrayals to other types of "portrayals" that appeared in other venues of life, particularly in science and policy. This essentially involved taking several different sets of analyses and weaving them together to see how each of those domains—film, science, and policy—both reflected broader attitudes and helped reaffirm them over time.

Given that Indigenous-settler relations have been ongoing in North America for more than 500 years, one limitation you have to keep in mind immediately is that film only came into existence in 1895 with Louis Lumière's introduction of the *cinématographe*. Accordingly, Ted found it helpful to connect with an analysis of portrayals of Indigenous people that had been done by Trigger (1988) that showed how Indigenous people were portrayed in written histories that had been prepared by missionaries and amateur historians from the 1700s onward. To summarize briefly, what he found was that when Europeans needed Indigenous people as guides for exploration, or as military allies, or as partners in the fur trade, Indigenous people were portrayed very positively. However, when most of the continent had been explored, the US revolutionary war and skirmish with Canada in the War of 1812 had ended so that military alliances with Indigenous peoples were no longer useful, and interest in the fur trade was replaced by an interest in establishing agricultural economies where the Indigenous penchant for hunting and fishing got in the way, portrayals became very negative. It was that finding that inspired Ted's title of "Histories of convenience"—affirming the adage that history can sometimes be no more than a justification of the present—given that it appeared that the way Native people were portrayed said a lot more about the aspirations of the settlers at any given time than it did about Native people themselves.

Given that the Trigger (1988) study was cast largely in the 1700s and 1800s and ended with histories produced in the late 1800s and early 1900s, film provided a way to extend that coverage to see whether the same sorts of dynamics operated into the twentieth century. Ted's analysis then proceeded by dividing the years from the beginning of film in 1895 to the present into recognizably different policy periods to see how the science and policy of each time was related to the sort of film content that was being produced both by Hollywood and various documentarians. Readers who are interested in more of the detail are welcome to check out Palys (2003), as we will only give a general summary here.

The first period Ted identified where film was available, which he characterized as "A tragic but inevitable oblivion," extended roughly from 1895 to 1925. In science, Darwin's theory of evolution had been taken up by social Darwinists who transformed his notion of "survival of the fit" to "survival of the fitt*est*" to explain why European culture was the inevitable future while Indigenous people were destined either to be trampled in the process or absorbed into the North American gene pool. In policy the emphasis was on preparing Native people for this future by placing them in residential schools and taking as much of their land as possible given the pervasive belief they would not be needing it anyway. Film of the time reaffirmed that view, as the emphasis was on filming native people in their traditional dress (even when they no longer wore it on a daily basis) and engaged in traditional practices. You may have seen some of the beautiful photos and films done by Edward Curtis for the Smithsonian Institute. The "inevitable" demise of Indigenous cultures that was promoted at that time was used to justify the pillaging of Indigenous art and cultural artifacts; the assumption at that time was that the only place Native culture would exist in the future would be in museum exhibits. Exemplary documentary films of the time include Curtis's *In the Land of the Head Hunters* (1914), later retitled as *In the Land of the War Canoes*, and Flaherty's (1922) *Nanook of the North*. A representative Hollywood film would be Zane Grey's (1925) *The Vanishing Race* (also known as *The Vanishing American*).

The second policy period Ted identified went from about 1920 to the end of World War II in 1945, which he characterized as "Justifications for genocide and control." While a demographic graph of the population of Native people in North America would be a downward line from first contact onward, thanks to diseases the Europeans brought as well as various wars in the United States, in the 1930s the line started to shown an upward turn as birth rates started to exceed death rates and it became more and more clear Native peoples were not going to simply fade away. The impression you get from reading policy documents of the time was that if Native people weren't going to simply disappear, then the government would help them do so, as federal policies in various settled countries in the English-speaking world—the United States, Canada, Australia, New Zealand—started enacting extremely restrictive policies designed to impose a forced assimilation. Films of the time responded by supplying your parents and grandparents with many of the stereotypical myths many still believe today—(1) the homogeneity, savagery, and inferiority of "Indians" and Indian culture; (2) the universal bravery and honor of settler populations; and (3) the myth that all North American Indians were "conquered peoples" (p. 25)—that showed that treatment was well deserved. Two well-known Hollywood films in that genre were John Ford's (1939) *Stagecoach* (whose riders were warned "You're all going to be scalped and massacred by that old butcher, Geronimo") and *They Died with Their Boots On* (one of many one-sided versions of General Custer's battle and defeat at the Little Big Horn).

The postwar period was a turning point in Native/settler relations both in North America as well as internationally. It seems fighting wars against two nations (Japan and Germany) who both believed they were destined to rule the world as the superior race was enough to encourage broader reflection on relations within our own backyard. The civil rights movement began to pick up steam in that period, as did Indigenous-settler relations, although the prevailing model was still an assimilative one. While Indigenous people were still seen in an inferior position, there was some recognition that at least part of the reason that had occurred was because of inefficient and insensitive policies on the part of the Bureau of Indian Affairs in the United States and the Department of Indian Affairs in Canada, not to mention endless broken promises in treaties. Exemplary Hollywood films of the time included *Broken Arrow* (1950) and *Cheyenne Autumn* (1964), both of which laid fault at the feet of a few "bad apples" whose prejudicial attitudes had caused problems that could be reversed by honest dealers like Richard Widmark and Edward G. Robinson. *Cheyenne Autumn* ends with the two Indian leaders, played by non-Indigenous actors Ricardo Montalban and Sal Mineo, lamenting they have no more tobacco for their peace pipe, at which point Edward G. Robinson suggests they embrace a new tradition, whereupon he passes out cigars. The message is that their salvation will come from embracing the new American way.

A final period, which extends from the 1960s to the present, was given the label, "Aboriginal Perspectives and Voices." It is a time when various liberation movements—for women, Indigenous peoples, African-Americans—were finding their contemporary voices and pushing for equal places in American society. Internationally, institutions such as the United Nations called for decolonization and courts started to recognize Indigenous territorial and cultural rights. One of the benefits of participation is that we now have a generation of Indigenous filmmakers adding their own voice in addition to non-Indigenous filmmakers engaging in more realistic and less stereotypical portrayals. Some in more documentary style revisit incidents in the past to reveal their inherent injustice—films such as *Incident at Oglala* (1992) in the documentary realm and *Thunderheart* (1992), its fictional companion. More recently we have Indigenous storytelling in such films as *Dance Me Outside* (1994), *Atanarjuat: The Fast Runner* (2001), *Rumble* (2017) and recent Academy Award winner *Roma* (2018), all of which show Indigenous people as more than characters from the past who wear headdresses and ride pinto ponies, but also have contemporary lives and continue to be proud of their heritage despite the impacts of colonization.

As you can see, Ted's (2003) "Histories of Convenience" was a far cry from the structured and standardized approach that Simon Davis (1990) took in his study of priorities in mate selection, which shows you something of the range of techniques that come under the title "content analysis," while also exhibiting the diversity of approaches you can consider when looking at your next content analytic project.

OFFICIAL STATISTICS AND SECONDARY DATA

Official Statistics

Archival measures comprise any information that is contained in "hard copy" or digital records or documents. You could argue that official statistics are nothing more than another type of archive, but they are sufficiently different and voluminous to be treated as entities worthy of consideration on their own.

Numerous advantages accrue from studying official statistics, not the least of which is that many statistical series, and particularly those produced by governments, allow time series analysis, as we saw in Chapter 7 regarding quasi-experimental design. More importantly, because they already exist and may cover an extensive time span, they allow that analysis to be done *now*; i.e., you needn't wait for 20, 40, or 100 years for the process to unfold. However, even government-produced data should be considered in light of notions like selective deposit and selective survival. What governments *don't* collect data on can be as interesting a statement as what they *do* collect data on. For example, with all the attention paid in the United States, particularly over the last few years, regarding the killing of unarmed Black men by police, it is fascinating that there are no government-produced statistics available that can inform research into these deaths, where they happen, when they occur, and whether they are increasing or decreasing in frequency.

Your challenge is always to consider the impact what is available to you for analysis—out of all the things that *could* be available—will have on your conclusions. Cook and Campbell (1979), for example, point out the bias toward "outcome" rather than "process" data in many series put together for monitoring purposes.

The existence of such tendencies in historical sources reaffirms the value of having your research question *guide* the research, lest you be seduced into believing that the *available* data are necessarily the most *important* or *relevant* data. We must be sensitive to the ways in which data availability constrains our conclusions and the range of theory that can be developed, while also recognizing the value in the treasures we have found.

Finally, researchers who delve into the archives should be on the lookout for possible shifts in how particular data series are defined and in the procedures for recording or saving material—what Campbell would call "instrumentation" threats. If the series is local enough to have been prepared by a single person, then you have to consider that any changes following that person's retirement might reflect little more than the presence of a different recorder, rather than changes in the phenomenon of interest. Similarly, policy shifts in recording practices, or digitization of a previously manual system, may produce differences in what otherwise look like continuous and comparable time-series data.

In sum, government-produced data are treasure troves of information that tell about society. They are necessarily secondary data that are unlikely to have been prepared for research purposes. This is both their limitation and strength; the information was prepared by someone else, and for some other purpose than for supplying evidence that might be useful to a researcher. The influence of the data's *context of production* must be considered (although this is no less true of any other data-gathering technique). The intermediary process between event and datum, or between having the thought and putting it to paper or on the screen, must be considered and articulated. We will do so in the next section by looking at one example of a government-produced statistical series that you've probably seen on the TV news or read about in newspapers or magazines. This topic has also received attention in one way or another from researchers in sociology, criminology, psychology, anthropology, economics, and education, to name but a few of the fields. The data series we refer to are crime statistics. We focus on them for no better reason than that we are most familiar with them and much has been written about them, but we hope that you see our analysis here in more generic terms, as the same could apply to almost any type of statistical series that comes out of agencies such as the US Census Bureau, Statistics Canada, or Britain's Home Office.

How Much Crime Is There?

Although several varieties of crime statistics are produced by criminal justice agencies, "crimes known to the police" typically receive the greatest attention from academics, the media, and the general public. Every month, in every jurisdiction in America (and in most of the industrialized world), the police compile and send off their statistics to their respective federal governments, who dutifully publish these figures, along with computed crime rates. Periodically, articles appear in the media along with various pet theories to account for any change. Many sociologists, criminologists, and others analyze these statistics to try to find out whether crime is up or down, and why; comparisons are made between various cities and countries. Crime statistics undoubtedly rank with the consumer price index and unemployment rates as one of the primary indicators of our quality of life. But what do they mean? And how are they compiled?

Perhaps the best way to begin answering these questions is to introduce the notion from test theory that every observed score (O) is a function of a "true" score (T) plus or minus some degree of error (e), that is,

$$O = T \pm e$$

Ideally, we seek to reduce error to zero so that $O = T$. That is, we want our observed scores (i.e., the crime rates published by FBI and the Bureau of Justice Statistics) to reflect nothing but the "true" situation (i.e., the actual amount of crime that exists in society). The problem, of course, is that we can never know reality directly; if we could, we wouldn't need crime statistics. Still, that should not stop us from considering the possible strengths and weaknesses of the measures we *do* choose. Thus, in assessing any measure, from crime statistics to survey results, we need to consider how systematic error might have been introduced in our measurements.

One way to do so is to look at how a given statistic is constructed. A simplified model of how crime statistics are constructed is shown in Figure 12.1 (adapted from Skogan, 1975). The process begins with the generation of a "true score," that is, the occurrence of a "criminal event," a behavior contrary to the laws of the United States.

Even in making that opening statement we're already in hot water, since the more we emphasize a country's laws as the defining measure of "real" crime, the more guilty we are of subscribing to status quo definitions of good and evil. An extensive discussion of such issues is beyond the scope of this book (but see Morden & Palys, 2019 if you are interested). What's important for now is that you appreciate how crime data are constructed *given* current laws.

FIGURE 12.1 ●   The Process by Which a Crime Statistic Is "Constructed"

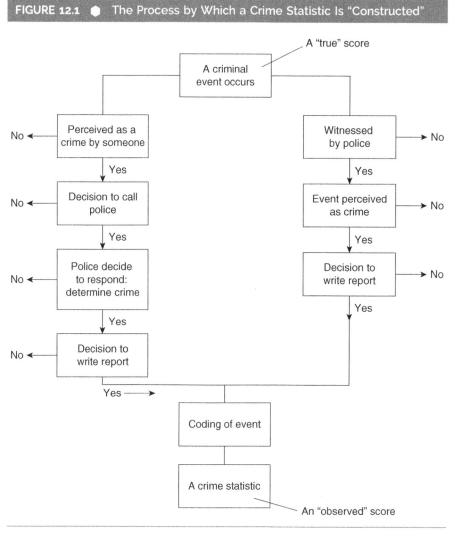

Source: Adapted from Skogan (1975).

We Start With a "True" Score

For exposition's sake then, we choose to accept "contemporary United States law" as our referent for "reality." We begin with an act, a "true" score, to see what filters it must pass through before it becomes a "statistic" (i.e., an "observed" score). The process begins in one of two ways. Either the "crime" is perceived as such by a private citizen or it is noted in some other way by the police. Let's deal with those two separately.

Chapter 12   ■   Archival Sources   517

Was the Event Perceived as a Crime?

Going down the left-hand side of Figure 12.1, we see that the first step in the process lies with the community: someone must first perceive the event as a crime. If no crime is perceived, nothing is likely to be done. Some reasons that the citizen might not perceive an act to be "criminal" could be that they may not have been aware that the act occurred or they might not know the act was illegal.

People's tendencies to perceive a given event as a crime also may vary depending on cultural factors (e.g., among different ethnic groups), as well as spatially and over time. For example, one study that looked at policing in different size communities ranging from extremely remote to highly urban (Dutton, Boyanowsky, Palys, & Heywood, 1982) found that the concept of "assault" clearly varied considerably by place; a certain amount of "roughness" that might be tolerated in a mining town likely would have been seen as "assaultive" in an urban suburb. The upshot is that comparing data regarding criminal and/or deviant behavior across time, space, and cultures can be extremely problematic.

Were the Police Contacted?

If an act *is* perceived as criminal, the next step in its becoming a statistic is that the police must be contacted. It's obviously difficult to ascertain from police records why people *don't* phone the police. But some hints have been forthcoming from victim surveys, where individuals who report having been victimized to the interviewer are then asked whether they contacted the police—and if not, why not.

Table 12.5 shows the results that were obtained in one US study. These data suggest that citizens who feel victimized will impose their own set of filters in determining whether the matter warrants attention, and if so whether it's specifically police attention (as opposed to medical attention, for example) that's warranted.

In sum, not all crimes are enumerated in crime statistics reports because, for varying reasons, the crime may not have been reported in the first place. It's usually these unreported crimes that are referred to as the "dark figure" of crime (e.g., see Skogan, 1975).

Did the Police Respond?. When a crime *is* reported, the ball is in the police's court. The first decision they make is whether to respond to your call. They must decide whether they agree that the matter is one for the police, and then whether it's possible or worthwhile to send someone out to the scene. In many instances, the police won't respond at all.

TABLE 12.5 ● Reasons Cited for Not Reporting Victimizations to the Police		
Reason	**Personal Crime (%)**	**Household Crime (%)**
Nothing could be done, lack of proof	30.8	36.1
Not important enough	25.6	30.1
Police would not want to be bothered	6.2	8.9
Too inconvenient or time-consuming	3.1	2.4
Private or personal matter	5.6	5.4
Fear of reprisal	0.8	0.4
Reported to someone else	15.9	3.2
Other, or not given	12.0	13.4

Source: National Association of Criminal Justice Planners/National Criminal Justice Information and Statistics Service. (1979). *Criminal victimization in the United States, 1977* (p. 70). Washington, DC: National Association of Criminal Justice Planners/National Criminal justice Information and Statistics Service. Reprinted with permission.

Was a Report Written?. If police *do* respond, one of the things they determine is whether or not a crime has been committed. But even if they agree that one has, officers have considerable discretion in deciding whether to write a report and whether to recommend the laying of charges.

Research by Black (1970) and by Black and Reiss (1970) showed that a variety of extralegal factors influence officers' decisions about whether to write a report. The officers in those studies were *less* likely to do a report when the relationship between perpetrator and victim was close, since they believed that such cases would less frequently make it to court (see also Rigakos, 1995). Officers were more likely to write a report when the victim was deferential or of high status.

Policy and Crime Data. Crime reporting and hence crime rates are sensitive to policy shifts, some of which can be self-serving. Seidman and Couzens (1974) examined reports for the Washington, D.C. police, concluding that a decrease in crime rate that city had appeared to enjoy was primarily a product of the police chief's orders to get the crime rate down, a task that was most easily accomplished by underreporting and downgrading crimes. Skogan (1975) notes that these tactics are particularly prevalent in those urban centers where police chiefs are evaluated by their ability to reduce the crime rate.

Crime statistics also change when recordkeeping practices change. In London, England, for example, "robbery" statistics formerly included only those cases where the robbery was certain or probable; "suspected" robberies were written in a separate book. But then a policy change called for *all* robberies, whether suspected or certain, to be recorded; a 220 percent increase in the "crime rate" was subsequently observed (Skogan, 1975). A similar shift in recording practices in New York City helped the robbery rate the next year go up 400 percent, while assaults with a weapon rose 200 percent, larcenies went up 700 percent, and burglaries rose by 1,300 percent.

And of course, a big policy change occurs when the law changes. Resulting shifts in the crime rate may thus not reflect any change in behavior; rather, they may merely reflect a change in the breadth or existence of a criminal designation or in the evidentiary rules that make cases more or less likely to be investigated and prosecuted.

Although this discussion has focused so far primarily on the left-hand side of Figure 12.1, many of the same arguments hold with respect to the right side of the figure, which refers to proactive efforts by the police to control crime. Suffice it to say that there will be much crime that the police will not witness and that much of the crime that *is* witnessed will be either ignored or not formally reported.

How Do We Count?

Whether the reporting source is a police officer or a citizen, some events will pass through the various filters noted above and be considered worth recording as an official crime statistic. Here we come to a bit of a problem: coding the event. Remember that we want to enumerate the amount of crime that exists in our society. To do so, we must agree on how to count, and such agreement is a lot harder to reach than you might expect. Brantingham and Brantingham (1984) offer the following example to illustrate the complexities involved:

> *Two men go on a crime spree. They enter a convenience store, rob the proprietor and three customers, shoot a police officer who attempts to apprehend them, knock cans and bottles off the shelves, and set the store on fire as they leave. (p. 51)*

How many crimes are involved here? An ambitious district attorney (DA) might find 16: (1 murder + 4 robberies + 1 vandalism + 1 arson + 1 weapons charge) × 2 defendants = 16 crimes. At the other extreme, you could argue that because there was only a single event, there must be a single crime—or perhaps two crimes, because there were two perpetrators. But if we decide to call it only one crime, what do we call it? The first one (i.e., robbery)? The last one (i.e., arson)? The most frequent one (i.e., robbery)? The most serious one (i.e., murder)? Another possibility is that we could count the number of victims (one proprietor, three customers, one police officer), and hence count five. So which is it? One? Two? Five? Sixteen? Something else?

In the United States and much of the rest of the industrialized world, Uniform Crime Reporting (UCR) procedures are employed in an effort to standardize (i.e., make more reliable) reporting across jurisdictions and police forces. The general rules are (1) for crimes of violence, you count the number of victims; (2) for crimes of property, you count the number of events; and (3) for multiple offences, only the most serious offence is recorded. In our example, therefore, the local police would tell Federal Bureau of Investigation or the Bureau of Justice Statistics that one murder had been committed.

The use of this scoring system has several implications. First, UCR procedures were not widely adopted until 1962, so you're courting difficulty if you are doing a more historical analysis that involves a comparison of pre-1962 and post-1962 crime figures or treats it as one consistent time series. It also suggests that crime rates overstate the relative frequency of violent crimes relative to property crimes, and that crime rates are an understatement of the number of offences reported to the police.

Final Comments on Crime Statistics

Crime statistics released by a government agency look terrifically official and precise. They're frequently perceived as "objective" indicators of crime. By now you should realize that this is *not* exactly the case: crime statistics (like any other statistics) are the result of a human process. As Skogan (1975) states,

> Every statistic ... is shaped by the process which operationally defines it, the procedures which capture it, and the organization which interprets it. (p. 18)

In other words, every statistic, regardless of whether it is the crime index published by the Federal Bureau of Investigation and the Bureau of Justice Statistics or a self-report to a survey, is in some sense a *social construction* that comes into being as a function of various psychological, sociological, and organizational processes. One of the big difficulties with archival statistics is that because of their assumed/perceived "objectivity," their reliability and validity often have been subjected to less scrutiny than is the case with perceptually oriented survey measures. To the extent that they have been assessed in this way, their validity and reliability appear questionable. More to the point, we must consider what they mean, as we must do for any data.

Those who frequently use crime statistics argue that even though crime statistics are invalid, they're nonetheless useful. Brantingham and Brantingham (1984), for example, compare them to a bathroom weigh scale that's miscalibrated and always reads 10 pounds too light. The weight readings are incorrect (i.e., invalid), they say, but could still be used to measure *changes* in weight or to compare different people, since the error is constant. However, the errors in crime statistics do *not* appear to be constant. The various "scales" in America are miscalibrated to varying unknown degrees; even given scales in given locations change their degree of miscalibration over time. Comparisons are still possible, but they must be done with some sensitivity to the changing context(s) in which crime statistics have been produced and with some understanding of how far any comparisons can be stretched (e.g., see Brantingham, 1991).

But if crime statistics don't show the amount of crime in an area, what *do* they show? Some authors (e.g., Ditton, 1979) argue that crime statistics are an indicator of police priorities and activity more than of crime per se. Certainly this argument is easy to support when considering victimless crimes, and there's evidence that the same is true to varying degrees with respect to certain crimes involving victims (e.g., assaults, spousal assaults). But such an argument becomes more difficult to make with other crime categories, such as murder, where the proportion of "social control" versus "real crime" probably tips in favor of the latter.

Crime statistics also reflect public confidence in and expectations about police performance. Some events are so trivial they'd probably *never* be reported, while some events are so serious that they'd virtually *always* be reported. But there's a big grey area between those two extremes, where "confidence in the police" can play a significant role in whether the police are informed. This is not to say that all official crime statistics produced to date should be scrapped or that people who produce them should be looking for other jobs. Instead, crime statistics should be treated the way we treat all other data we gather, i.e., as a social product that is related to, but is only an imperfectly mirrored reflection of, the phenomenon it aims to describe. Indeed, the trick is to understand the crime statistic (or whatever other data you gather or produce) as a part of the phenomenon you're scrutinizing.

SECONDARY DATA SOURCES

Alternative Views of Crime: Victimization Surveys

A discussion of victimization surveys might seem an odd inclusion in this chapter, since surveys were dealt with in Chapter 9 as part of our consideration of more interactive techniques. But including them here allows us to make several important points. First, we wish to reaffirm that *every statistic is a social construction*. Although we personally have less of a problem with self-report information (e.g., interviews, attitude scales) than with archival statistics produced by the Census Bureau or Statistics Canada or the Home Office, perhaps because we "produce" the former ourselves, we always should keep in mind the strengths and limitations of our data and consider the various sources of bias or error that might exist.

Second, "used" survey data have themselves become an important source of archival data for social scientists. When major studies are done, the raw data are frequently stored and made available to qualified researchers in anonymized form for secondary analysis. Other investigators can then peruse these data for far less than it cost to generate them.

Limited to Crimes With Victims

Victimization surveys have their own limitations, which are a product of the way the information is gathered. Figure 12.2 will help focus our discussion. Once again, our diagram begins with a "true" score (i.e., a "crime" that occurs). The first filter through which the event must pass is that the crime must involve a victim, since a victimless crime is unlikely to be reported in the survey.

Finding the Respondents

Next, the victim must be interviewed. Victimization surveys typically seek representative samples of target populations, usually the residents of a given urban centre. Of course not everyone will be interviewed. But as long as all people and all victimizations have an equal probability of being selected, a representative picture of victimizations can emerge. Unrepresentativeness occurs when all victimizations do not have an equal probability of being selected. So we must consider these systematic sources of bias.

One type of person (and hence crimes against such people) that will not appear in victimization surveys is the nonresident victim (i.e., commuters, transients, tourists). We interview people from a particular area, but not everyone who was victimized there is from that area. Skogan (1975) notes that an average of 13 percent of the daytime population in US cities are commuters, in addition to varying numbers of tourists and transients. People in these categories can be victimized and can even report their victimizations to the police, but won't be around to be interviewed later.

FIGURE 12.2 ● The Construction of Crime Statistics via Victimization Surveys

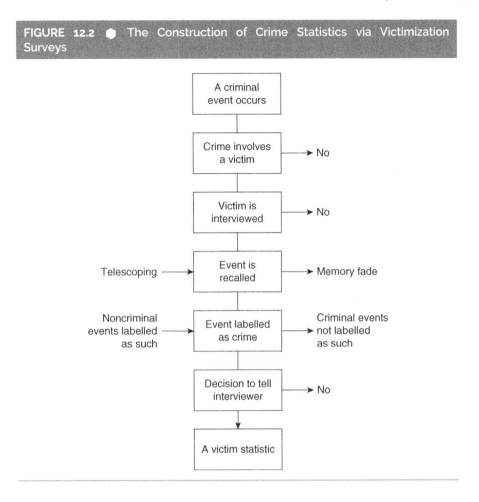

Recall: Memory Fade and Telescoping

Given that the victim *is* interviewed, the event must first be recalled. You need to guard against two problems here. One is **memory fade**, the tendency for events to be forgotten. Memory fade has been investigated in two ways. In one strategy, *known victims* (as revealed by police records) are interviewed to see if their victimizations are reported to the interviewer; overall, such studies suggest, about 75 percent of known incidents are recalled. Given that *known victimizations* are generally of higher saliency (they were considered important enough to have been reported to police), the implication is that memory fade for less serious incidents is probably greater. In the second strategy, investigators ask a sample of respondents about victimizations and plot these against time. Monthly crime rates decrease visibly as you go back in time, especially after 3–6 months, which suggests that memory fade has occurred.

While memory fade refers to the tendency of events during the sample period to drop out, **telescoping** refers to the propensity of respondents to bring events that were *outside* the sample period into it. In answer to a query about victimizations within the last year, for example, respondents may include events that actually happened more than a year ago. Part of the reason may be that people are responding to implicit or explicit demands to report victimizations if you've contacted them about, and they've consented to, a victimization survey. Another reason may be the generally fuzzy definition of "a year ago" as a boundary for thought; an event may be described as "about a year ago" regardless of whether it was really 10, 12, 14, or even 16 months ago. This problem of telescoping is reduced by **bounding** (e.g., instead of saying "in the last 6 months," you might cite a more memorable event, such as "since Christmas") or by successive administrations of the survey (where the sample period is bounded by the prior visit). Victims require signposts to guide their recall. (The degree of error in unbounded situations is 17–21 percent.)

Labeling the Event as a Crime

As Figure 12.2 shows, the next step involves labeling the event as a crime. The victim must categorize the event both as a crime and as belonging to a particular crime category. But this may or may not be the "right" crime category, and the event might or might not "really" be a crime. The evidence suggests, though, that this isn't an especially big problem. In a pilot study in San Jose, California, legal authorities and respondents classified an event in the same category 88 percent of the time (Skogan, 1975).

But Will You Tell the Interviewer?

Even if the event *is* accurately recalled and labeled, the respondent must decide next whether to tell you about the event. In validational studies where known victims (i.e., people identified through prior reports filed with the police) are interviewed, decisions about whether to tell the interviewer seem to be affected by some of the same variables that influence decisions about whether to report the incident to police. One of these is the relational distance between victim and perpetrator. "Known victim" respondents recalled and reported victimizations by strangers 75 percent of the time, those by acquaintances 58 percent of the time, and those by relatives only 22 percent of the time. Rapes were reported very cautiously; in one pilot survey in San Jose, California, *all* rapes were described as "attempted" (Skogan, 1975).

Just Another "Take" on Crime

Recall Skogan's (1975) statement, cited earlier with respect to crime statistics of the UCR variety: "Every statistic … is shaped by the process which operationally defines it, the procedures which capture it, and the organization which interprets it" (p. 18). We hope you see now that this warning applies equally to victimization surveys. Neither type of data gives the truth about crime, although each contributes a truth. In G. Morgan's (1983) terms, each engages crime, giving its own particular "take" on the phenomenon. However, when taken together, we hope you will also see the merits again of multimethod approaches to understanding a phenomenon where different methods have strengths that make up for the weaknesses of others and complement one another to give a more complete picture overall.

BIG DATA

We close this chapter by making what for now must be a brief note about an emerging archival source that leaves its advocates beside themselves in zeal and its critics enveloped in concern—"big data."

Imagine a database that includes everything about you there is to be known, including your genetic information and health history (from government health records), to your institutional past (from government records regarding justice, education, and labor at every level), to your behavior (e.g., financial records recording every transaction; every movement through Google locations), to your social networks (through Facebook and Twitter and your smartphone), to your habits (through the internet of things), to your physical state (via your Fitbit device), to your thoughts (through your use of search engines). Burrows & Savage have referred to big data as the "digital by-product of routine transactions between citizens, consumers, business and government" (2014, p. 2). Like dust, our **behavioral exhaust** (Zuboff, 2019)—the information we leave behind with every click, query, and transaction—is everywhere. Government agencies, public institutions, private corporations, and various trackers are all too willing to pick up each and every particle with or without our knowledge, with or without our informed consent, toward ends that may or may not be transparent.

Such an archive would create unprecedented opportunities for health and social scientists, which leaves many of them salivating at the prospect. When we evaluate such a database on three standard dimensions, the 3 Vs—volume (the amount of information available), variety (the range and form of information available), and velocity (the speed with which it is created)—we begin to understand just how unique, powerful, and unprecedented such a database could be. The sheer volume and variety of data and our ability to link together different archives would allow social and health researchers to ask and answer research questions that have been unanswerable using traditional methods. The continuous ongoing creation of these data—their velocity—provides us with an opportunity to study human relations not just over time but relationally in real time. Even very specific, small, and hard to study populations can be scrutinized in an empirically rigorous manner when the number of data points is so huge. It surpasses anything that has existed in human history (Golder & Macy, 2014).

But bigger doesn't always mean better. Collecting huge volumes of data in a wide array of forms and formats in real time can compromise data quality. Data are often fragmented, incomplete, or formatted in a way that render them difficult or impossible to use. We may be seduced into thinking that big data involves "everything" about us, but as our discussion of crime statistics illustrated, every datum bears the stamp of the institutional process that gathers it, and thereby reflects that subset of our activity that is of interest to those who collect the data. Selective deposit is as relevant here as any other database, and health or social science researchers are rarely the ones deciding what information will be gathered and kept, which means the archives often do not contain the type of information that we might be interested in, and even if so, are rarely in the form we would like to facilitate the type of analyses we might want to do. Linking disparate databases creates an even more complex challenge. Even when successful, sometimes there is simply too much data and we do not have the capacity to make sense of it, i.e., **information overload**. Other times the analysis may require immense computing power that we cannot access. Furthermore, extant social and health science analytical approaches are not well suited for the analysis of this type of data (Tinati, Halford, Carr, & Pope, 2014).

Working with big data also raises a host of ethical concerns. Who owns and controls the data contained in these data archives? Government? The public or private organization that collected it? The individual citizens who provide it? Is it ethical to use data for purposes other than for which it was originally collected? While you might have consented to Google or Amazon to use your online browsing or purchasing information to "enhance your shopping experience," did you understand that the information also could be used to determine your eligibility for health or life insurance?

Lastly, big data has the clear potential to place individual privacy and security at risk. Big data are able to be rapidly processed and analyzed, allowing for the identification of correlations and patterns in human action and relations that would not be visible with smaller datasets. Merging or joining small pieces of data from seemingly innocuous and disparate datasets—even datasets that have been anonymized—has the potential to lead to the identification of individuals which could result in harm to persons (McFarland, Lewis, & Goldberg, 2016). This is particularly the case when these individuals are from marginalized, stigmatized, or isolated communities.

Over the past 20 years, with the digitization of society, and the evolution of **surveillance capitalism** as the primary economic model (Zuboff, 2019), we have seen a shift in data collection from collecting information *from* people and events to collecting information *about* people and events. This information has been stored en masse in big data archives. One thing is certain, while big data is an emergent area for social and health researchers it is one that we simply cannot ignore. As we have seen throughout the book thus far, choices with respect to how we go about conducting research are rarely black and white. This is certainly the case when it comes to working with big data, which combines incredible potential for research with equally incredible prospect for the trampling of privacy and other rights.

SUMMING UP AND LOOKING AHEAD

This chapter focuses on data sources that are growing in importance to many social and health scientists as they broaden their investigative strategies beyond interviewing or direct observation to include a historical dimension in their research and/or to take advantage of existing archival sources. The first portion of the chapter considers some of the variety of archival sources of data—textual, verbal and visual—and considered several examples in detail that show how content analytic approaches can range from highly structured analyses of keywords to more thematically and theoretically driven approaches.

We then go on to consider some of the data available to researchers who seek to take advantage of existing statistical data archives that are produced by government agencies and private researchers as a way of finding answers to their research questions.

The first type of data considered in detail are "official crime statistics," which are analytically deconstructed in an effort to show how a statistic of this sort is produced and to show the many qualitative elements contained in its construction. The reason for doing so is not to cast any sort of pejorative light on crime statistics per se, but rather to make the point that the same range of considerations should be implemented when one considers any set of archival statistics, no matter what government, agency, organization, or institution produced them. At the root of this view is the idea that we must always be prepared to ask questions about what the numbers mean, an approach that requires understanding something about the procedures and perspectives that combined to produce them.

Our discussion of victimization surveys revealed again the strengths and weaknesses that come along with using that particular type of data, but also revealed how mixed methods approaches—in this case a combination of official statistics and victimization surveys—when taken together can give a more comprehensive understanding of a phenomenon than either method can alone. It also allowed us the opportunity to introduce you to the availability of secondary data archives that are available online. Check with your university or college library to see what other archives may be available at your institution. Many of these archives took tens if not hundreds of thousands of dollars to produce; it makes good sense to make the fullest use of them rather than attempting to recreate the wheel on your own.

Just as we saw in earlier chapters that questioning (in Chapters 9 and 10) and observation (in Chapter 11) give one a "take" on reality (rather than "truth" itself), archival measures must also be considered in the light of the methodological and organizational procedures and assumptions by which they were produced. Each technique and each data source offers only a slice of truth—using a certain implement to reveal a certain perspective. Ultimately, the researcher's task is not only to uncover these truths but also to articulate the perspectives that gave rise to them.

A final section of the chapter notes the increasing attention being paid these days to what has come to be known as "big data," i.e., huge troves of data that are compiled from the myriad activities we do in the digital world that are so easily collected and await analysis. The section suggests we are only beginning to understand the strengths and weaknesses of such data; like all data they are artifacts of human processes and their existence and decision to store them say as much about those who gather it as they do of those whose activity is being recorded. There are also unique challenges that arise about how to analyze such data, particularly more qualitative data that defy easy aggregation and summary.

In the next chapter we continue our consideration of archival measures that were not originally intended for research consumption and thus also avoid reactivity, including textual, audio, and video sources that reflect human existence, where the method of choice is content analysis or one of its variants.

Key Concepts

Bounding 524
Content analysis 489
Face validity 503
Information overload 526

Inter-rater reliability 496
Memory fade 523
Surveillance capitalism 527
Telescoping 524

Variety 525
Velocity 525
Volume 525

STUDY QUESTIONS

1. Find out which newspapers your college, university, or municipal (public) library keeps and how many years' worth of issues they've retained. Design a quantitative and/or qualitative study that compares the way newspaper reports from different time periods treat an issue of interest to you. For example, you might look at (1) how women are portrayed in articles from the 1960s, 1970s, 1980s, 1990s, 2000s, and 2010s; (2) how environmental issues and/or environmental activists are portrayed in the 1960s and in the 2000s; or (3) whether the composition of the newspaper's front page is different now than it was at the turn of the 20th century.

2. In the study of populism, why was it important for the same types of speeches to be used for each of the politicians included in the analysis?

3. Choose your five favorite songs, obtain the lyrics from the Internet, and develop a coding scheme that you could use to identify and code words or actions that reflect themes of gender, race, or class.

4. Crime statistics suggest that about 90 percent of the crimes that are committed in the United States each year are nonviolent, while about 10 percent are violent. Does the coverage of crime news in your local newspaper reflect that state of affairs? Using Davis's (1990) study, reported in this chapter, as a guide, design a content-analytic study to answer that question.

5. What advantages accrued to Davis by using newspaper personals ads as opposed to surveys or interviews to study mate selection?

6. The content analysis of political leaders in *The Guardian*'s study of populism was done using "holistic coding," while Davis in his study of mate selection used more of a key word search. Would it have been possible to do these the other way around, i.e., by a key word analysis of speeches and a holistic analysis of personals ads? Consider what advantages and disadvantages might have occurred if you did so.

7. Davis's study of mate selection came at a time when relatively few people placed personals ads, which appeared in newspapers in the days before the Internet. Design a replication of Davis's study based on the kinds of information people include in an online matchmaking/dating site.

8. Pick some textual source of data that exists at your college or university and design a study to systematically compile and content code that data. The examples we have in mind would include projects such as (1) analyzing washroom graffiti to see whether there are any differences between the arts and sciences or between men and women in what is written; (2) analyzing the messages and images on people's T-shirts; or (3) analyzing the messages on bumper stickers displayed in your university or college's parking lots.

9. Skogan (1975) states that *"every statistic … is shaped by the process which operationally defines it, the procedures which capture it, and the organization which interprets it"*(p. 17; italics in original). In what sense is this claim true of the crime rate estimates produced by the police for the Federal Bureau of Investigation and the Bureau of Justice Statistics? In what sense is it true of the crime rate estimates that are produced by victimization surveys? Is it also applicable to the compilation of "big data"?

10. Some criminologists (e.g., Ditton, 1979) argue that crime rates based on police data have nothing to do with crime and everything to do with police involvement in social control activities. To what extent do you agree or disagree with that perspective?

11. In what ways do crime statistics exemplify the advantages and limitations of archival data cited in this chapter?

12. Three people go on a crime spree. They break into a sporting-goods store and steal several shotguns, shoot and kill the store's owner, steal a nearby car, drive the wrong way down a one-way street to make their getaway, and then speed off down the highway. How would these activities be coded using the UCR system of crime-counting?

13. A researcher wants to evaluate the impact of a 1962 Massachusetts law that changed the rules of evidence regarding crimes involving gun violence, and decides to use a time-series design. What difficulties do you see immediately with a study of that type?

14. This chapter has subjected crime statistics to considerable scrutiny aimed at demonstrating the relationship between particular events and our archival record of them. Try to apply the same type of scrutiny to any other archival statistic(s) of interest to you (e.g., suicide rates, unemployment rates, hospitalization rates, abortion rates, or rates of adolescent drug use).

15. What are some of the prospects and challenges that exist in the world of big data?

ANALYZING NONNUMERICAL DATA

When a researcher sits down and is confronted with hundreds of pages of transcribed interview text, thousands of image files, or hours of video footage, it is not uncommon for them to feel overwhelmed at the task of trying to make sense of this wealth of rich data. The situation is worsened by the fact that many researchers have never been exposed to formal techniques for making sense of data that emerge from interviews, focus groups, newspapers, magazines, institutional/agency files, textbooks, speeches, photographs or digital images, films or videos, television programs, diaries, and letters. Making sense of nonnumeric data is often presented as the product of some form of mystical revelation rather than implementing a particular set of analytical techniques. Published qualitative analyses are often criticized for lacking transparency with authors rarely making the data analysis process explicit or systematic (Miles & Huberman, 1994; Ragin, 1987). Perhaps the most negative effect of the mystic quality of the analysis of talk, text, images, and video is that it can serve to delegitimate these types of data and the resulting analyses in the minds of individuals who hold more naive realist positions on social and health research.

The previous chapter described some of the content analytic techniques that can be used with nonnumeric sources. In this chapter, we go a step further to demystify the processes involved in analyzing and interpreting nonnumeric data. We begin with an overview of inductive and deductive strategies, followed by consideration of some of the advantages, disadvantages, and applications of computer-assisted qualitative data analysis software (CAQDA).

CODING AND MEMOING

The "unstructured" nature of nonnumeric data presents a challenge when it comes to detailing techniques of analysis. Unlike its numeric counterpart, there are few well-established and accepted rules for analyzing text, images, audio, and video. The way that data are understood varies depending on the disciplinary interests and theoretical perspective of the researcher. While a discussion of these varying approaches is beyond the scope of this chapter, we mention this variation here simply to point out the connection that often exists between theory and method. The approach we take will have implications for what sorts of data we might look at and the range of meanings we draw from them. Regardless of the particular technique you choose, almost all analytical techniques that focus on nonnumeric data involve coding and memoing.

Coding

Coding helps achieve the goal of data management and data reduction; that is, when a researcher codes the volumes of data they have collected, they are in essence organizing and reducing the data into smaller more manageable segments that can be retrieved easily and compared with other coded segments of data. A coded segment might represent or illustrate a specific theoretical or analytic concept, or it can simply reflect elements of the data that we want to highlight or think about further, just as we might use a yellow highlighter to draw our attention back to a specific quote or idea that we see in a book. Applying a coding scheme might be as simple as deciding whether, in a given passage, a certain word or type of behavior or theme is present or absent or may involve more complex judgments about the thematic content of a paragraph or scene or segment of the source material.

Deductive Approaches

Codes may be generated and assigned to research data in deductive or inductive fashion, or some combination of the two. **Deductive coding** sees the researcher coming to the data with a well-specified or predefined set of interests. For example, when Ted was doing research on the social content of video pornography for the Fraser Committee on Pornography and Prostitution, there was a clear interest from the outset to focus specifically on sexual, violent, and sexually violent content (Palys, 1986). Similarly, when Neuendorf, Gore, Dalessandro, Janstova, and Snyder-Suhy (2010) set out to content code all of the James Bond films, their interest from the outset was to focus on relations between men and women in the films—and especially those between Bond and the "Bond girls"—and how those had changed, if at all, over time.

Inductive Approaches

In contrast, **inductive coding** generally begins with the identification of general themes and ideas that emerge from a very literal reading of the data (often referred to as **open coding**) and can proceed in either direction, i.e., sometimes elaborating a category by making finer and finer distinctions, and sometimes beginning with very specific descriptive coding categories that are subsequently combined to create more general categories that bring disparate events or descriptions under the same conceptual umbrella. Generally speaking, the preferred order is to go from more specific codes to more general categories rather than the other way around; while it is very easy to combine smaller codes together to make bigger ones, it is more work to disaggregate larger categories into smaller ones.

For example, Chris began his analysis of in-depth interviews of sex buyers by reading through each transcribed interview and highlighting passages that appeared to stand out, such as where his participants talked about why visiting sex workers appealed to them, how prices for services were determined and paid for, and how they described their interactions with sex workers. This initial stage of reading and coding allowed him to begin to identify some of the themes that emerged from within interviews and then to create some broader categories by combining more specific categories (e.g., aspects of the solicitation, negotiation over price, and the service sought and delivered were all seen as part of "relationship with sex seller") as well as finding it useful to distinguish within categories (e.g., distinguishing between different participants—such as heterosexuals, bisexuals, and homosexuals—who seemed to approach the exchange in different ways for different reasons).

Ted was in a similar situation when he was serving on a federal committee mandated to look at the impact that the federal government's ethics policy was having on research in the social sciences and humanities. A first task of the committee was to find out just what social science and humanities researchers felt the problems with the initial policy statement were. An open solicitation brought scores of replies from researchers and research groups across the country, and the first analytic task involved going through the responses, coding each one in terms of the ethics and research issues that were being identified, using the results to help establish priorities, and reporting back to the research community what had been found and the plan of action the committee envisioned to address those difficulties (see SSHWC, 2004).

Memoing

While the processes of open and focused coding involve attaching theoretically relevant labels to segments of our nonnumeric data, **memoing** allows us to record and reflect upon the observations and insights accrued through the research and coding process. A memo is in essence a note that we write to ourselves where we elaborate upon the categories of meaning that are beginning to emerge from the research or coding process, just as we might write margin notes in a book we are reading, or include thoughts and other "notes to self" in our field notes as we think of them.

The two are not independent processes; we constantly move back and forth between coding and memoing. The memoing process allows us to clearly and concisely explain—to ourselves and any others involved in the project—the meanings we have attributed to particular codes that we have assigned to elements of our data. Over time, our series of memos will show the development and elaboration of our coding scheme. Memos also allow us to reference or link to other data or observations that help us demonstrate the validity and reliability of our coding. We often memo by placing **annotations**, in the form of margin or sticky notes, on or near coded content where we will comment on our general feelings about what the content means (i.e., conceptual definitions), possible links to literature, or other locations in his data where similar or different themes are present (e.g., other interviews, images, or news media reports). We use these annotations during subsequent analysis to help us start to make sense of the relationships among and between our data and to help us craft the resulting story that emerges from it.

Typologies

In many cases, coding involves either highlighting and labeling segments of interest and/or the straightforward application of coding rules to talk, text, images, and/or video. The coding itself may be more fluid and evolving or more highly structured and rigidly imposed. Coding may also be a stepping stone toward examining more complex concepts and relations within the data. **Typological analysis**, for example, sometimes referred to as cluster analysis, is a method of organizing coded material that involves placing similarly thematically coded information (e.g., people, places, events, or social artifacts that share common characteristics) into relational categories that allow the researcher to make distinctions among groupings or clusters of people, places, and so on that are meaningful to the researcher and/or participants. This process is similar to the creation of a contingency table in quantitative analysis, with the entries in the table this time being actual content—quotes from an interview; segments of a video; quotes from a newspaper article or from a Twitter comment—rather than numerical frequencies.

For example, a researcher interested in understanding the potential links between sexual safety behavior and drug use among teens might begin by classifying coded passages from interviews with teenagers that pertain to sexual safety behavior (e.g., condom use during differing types of sexual activities) and types of drug use (e.g., consumption of various types of legal and illegal drugs). Once the researcher decides what it is that they want to classify, the next step in typological analysis is to map the relationships among and between similarly coded content. The researcher might then start building a typology of drug users, organizing participants' accounts about their drug use according to the class and "severity" of the drugs they use (e.g., differentiating between (1) opiates such as heroin, crack or powder cocaine, (2) methamphetamines such as ecstasy, molly, gamma-hydroxybutyrate (GHB); (3) hallucinogens such as lysergic acid diethylamide (LSD); and (4) anesthetics such as ketamine, anabolic steroids, hashish, cannabis, tobacco, and alcohol). Organizing coded material according to such groupings would allow the researcher to start to look at differences and similarities among participants' accounts of sexual safety behavior on the basis of the type or severity of the drugs they indicated using.

Typologies are very useful ways of classifying and organizing similarly coded material and, as is the case with coding more generally, can be done deductively or inductively. More deductive approaches will see researchers arrive with particular categories of theoretical interest in mind; more inductively minded researchers will want to ensure that the typologies they create reflect groupings that are meaningful for those they are investigating instead of merely reflecting their own preconceived notions of what is important. In our example of teenage drug use, for example, a more medically minded researcher might be tempted to identify drug clusters based on their pharmacological similarity, while a criminologist might be tempted to identify drug clusters based on the way the various drugs are treated (or not) within the law. The teenagers involved, on the other hand, might be more likely to cluster the drugs on the basis of the social context in which they are consumed, such that ecstasy, ketamine, methamphetamine, LSD, and GHB might be strongly associated with raves; alcohol, hashish, and cannabis with recreation; and steroids and some forms of methamphetamine such as diet pills with "health," "fitness," or "body image."

In order to guard against developing typologies that do not reflect "real" aspects of the phenomenon under investigation, it is important that the researcher establish a clear and concise reasoning for the typologies they develop. In order to do this, they should consider the nature of the categorical membership by asking the following types of questions:

- Is the coded content a type of a larger class of things? (e.g., is the drug part of a larger class of drugs? Adderall, Dexedrine, and Benzedrine, for example, are all part of a larger class of drugs called amphetamines.)

- Is the coded content part of some other phenomenon? (e.g., is drug use part of some other phenomenon such as crime, social activity, health, and fitness regimes?)

- What conditions precede the occurrence of the coded content? (e.g., what activities or mental states do participants identify as occurring before they use drugs?)

- What conditions follow the occurrence of the coded content? (e.g., what happens to participants after they use drugs?)

- What factors are responsible for the coded content occurring? (e.g., what reasons do participants provide for using drugs? What is the particular drug generally used for?)

- Where does the coded content occur? (e.g., are there any particular locations or situations where/in which people use different types of drugs?)

Asking questions such as these that are relevant to the phenomenon under investigation and the unit of analysis selected helps the researcher avoid developing meaningless typologies that hinder their ability to reveal valid and reliable patterns underlying coded content.

Once the researcher has coded content into meaningful and relevant categories, the next step is to begin the process of identifying the spaces where overlap exists between the categories in relation to the phenomenon under investigation. In our example of sexual safety behavior and drug use, once we developed categories of drug use based on social behaviors such as going to raves, general recreational activities, and "health, fitness, and body image," we would next want to determine if teens who engage in risky sexual activities (e.g., intercourse without a condom) do so across social contexts or vary their behavior depending on context (e.g., do teens who use drugs at raves report similar or different sexual safety routines than those who use drugs as part of a "health" and "fitness" regime or those who use them purely for recreational purposes?).

This process of comparison continues until we have exhausted all of the coded categories of drug users and sexual safety behavior and we are able to then create meaningful labels for the various unique categories of the phenomenon under investigation (e.g., "high-risk drug users," "medium-risk drug users," and "low-risk drug users"). We might visually display our typology in a Venn diagram, network map, or flowchart as appears in Figure 13.1.

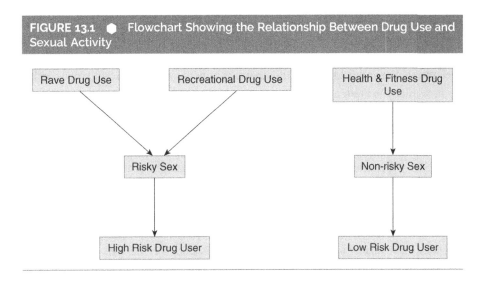

FIGURE 13.1 ● Flowchart Showing the Relationship Between Drug Use and Sexual Activity

COMPUTER-ASSISTED QUALITATIVE DATA ANALYSIS SOFTWARE

While studies by Davis (1990) on mate selection and by Trigger (1988) on images of Indigenous people that we described in Chapter 12 exemplify the sorts of procedures that are involved in more thematic/qualitative and more structured/quantitative analysis of media, both studies were done at a time when there was no such thing as software for the analysis of nonnumeric data. It was a time when researchers began the process by typing up their handwritten field notes or tape-recorded interviews, photocopied their visual data, and plopped themselves down on a wide open floor. Once situated in their space they would organize the mountain of paper into smaller hills and begin the time-honored tradition of slowly and methodically perusing the data, highlighting transcripts and photos with markers, scribbling annotations in the margins, and recording memos on sticky notes and index cards. This inevitably would lead to countless attempts at restacking and reorganizing the data into progressively smaller piles that at times might resemble typologies, taxonomies, or mental maps. This painstaking ritual would proceed until the researcher emerged from the ruins with their finely crafted typed analysis.

While this image of the procedure for analyzing nonnumeric data might conjure up feelings of nostalgia for people born long before the advent of the personal computer in the early 1980s, many social and health researchers who work with nonnumeric data now use technology to assist in various aspects of the research and analyses process. We now digitally record interviews, field notes, and memos and use word processing software to transcribe them; use electronic file and referencing software to organize and link our literature and research data files; use electronic search tools to locate details or perform word counts; and use audio, image, and video editing programs to edit our rich media data and field notes. Still other programs allow us to develop visual displays or models of our thinking about the relationships in our data. In the remainder of this chapter, we discuss how to use some of these technologies in order to analyze nonnumeric data, note what new possibilities arise because of the efficiencies that these developments—and particularly the development of qualitative data analysis (QDA) software—represent, and consider some of the implications of doing so.

Technological Options

While the contribution that developments in digital and computer hardware and software have made toward improving the efficiency of the data collection and analysis process is undeniable, it can be rather daunting for any one researcher or research team to have to acquire (sometimes at considerable cost) and master such a wide variety of software. This can leave those of us who are faced with having to make sense of mountains of nonnumeric data with the sinking feeling that we have to "go old school" whether we like it or not.

Fortunately, an increasing number of specialized software applications for making sense of both numeric and nonnumeric data have emerged in the mainstream market place over the past 30 years. While we will discuss applications created for numeric data in the next chapter, the most popular applications for working with nonnumeric data include QSR NVivo, Atlas.ti, MAXqda, HyperRESEARCH, QDA Miner, and Ethnograph.

Despite the growing availability of specialized software packages designed to improve the speed and efficiency of coding and analyzing the diverse forms of nonnumeric data that social and health researchers are likely to collect, there are still some people who object to using computers to code and analyze rich textual, audio, and visual data. Many social and health researchers who were born before the Internet or who were taught how to analyze this type of data by someone who refused to accept and/ or learn new technologies and techniques still prefer going "old school" to analyze talk, text, image, and video using highlighters, sticky notes or index cards, and scribbling in the margins of printed paper. Some argue that using a computer removes the researcher from the analytical process and from the research data itself, blunting our senses and removing us from the data in ways that dramatically and negatively impact the depth and breadth of the resulting analyses. Still others accuse these programs of being nothing more than an attempt to "quantify" qualitative data, a process that could very well result in increasing demands that the data meet solely quantitative criteria for rigor, thereby undermining the way data integrity is defined in the more qualitative context.

The two of us see QDA software as simply another tool in our research tool belt. Software programs help us make sense of our data; they cannot do our analyses for us. No matter how sophisticated the software becomes, strong analyses will always require us to painstakingly and meticulously code the material, thinking through the meanings and various possible interpretations and returning to the data to test our assumptions in an effort to develop both nuanced and comprehensive explanations and theory.

Selecting a Software Package

Although no single program is superior in all respects to all others at present, each of the packages listed above provides an excellent range of features for the analysis of nonnumeric data. When selecting a QDA package, there are several things you should keep in mind. First is the amount and type of data you are going to be working with, as each of the programs has particular strengths and weaknesses. Some deal with text files only while others allow you to work with images, video, audio, hypertext, posts on social networking sites (e.g., Twitter feeds), GeoData (e.g., Google Maps), or structured questionnaires. Further, some programs are limited in the amount of data they can handle; some place a physical cap on the number of objects (i.e., interview transcripts or images) you can analyze while others simply become unstable and crash when you attempt to bring in too many files.

What you wish to describe, understand, or explain through your analysis and your approach to analysis are also important considerations when selecting a program. While all the software applications we have named will provide you with the tools to conduct a basic search, code and retrieve style of analysis, if you want to conduct a more sophisticated analysis involving linking data elements, complex visual displays or models, or integrative analyses of mixed data, you need to take a careful look at what different software can do before you invest the time and money to adopt one.

While open source and freeware QDA programs are available (e.g., Weft QDA, RQDA), they tend to offer a very limited range of features and little to no user support. The more sophisticated programs such as NVivo, Atlas.ti, and MaxQDA offer educational and student pricing. However, even these are not cheap, with educational licenses ranging from $500 to $700 and student licenses ranging from $99 to $199. Ted's university now offers NVivo leases for free to graduate students and faculty and has installed it in every computing lab on campus, but it took several years to convince the university of the program's utility, and we expect his university is still among the minority. If your institution does not have any of the QDA programs available and you are curious about these programs, we encourage you to take a firsthand look by downloading the fully functioning free 30-day trial versions of the software that are available online through each company's website. All are relatively easy to learn as they are all built upon the menu-tool bar–based user interface that is standard in the word processing software we all use on a daily basis. That said, as with any program, there is a learning curve that will be steeper for inexperienced users than for technophiles. Fortunately, the popular commercial applications offer very good learning resources in the form of instruction manuals and online tutorials and community forums.

As we have mentioned throughout the book, both of us do research in a wide variety of academic, government, nonprofit, and commercial settings where we sometimes work alone and sometimes work with teams of researchers from different disciplinary backgrounds. The projects we are involved in can range in size from a few focus groups or in-person interviews to large-scale mixed methods investigations that involve hundreds of in-depth interviews, dozens of focus groups, community and research meetings, and seemingly limitless numbers of PDF documents, image, and video files. Because we are involved in such a wide range of projects with a diverse array of researchers our research questions fall all along the inductive-deductive/constructionist-realist continuum, so the types of analyses we are called upon to perform can range from discourse analysis to classical content analysis and beyond. When we were trying to decide on what QDA program to use, we needed to find one that was adaptable to the widest range of conditions possible. While programs such as Atlas.ti and MaxQDA both offer an excellent range of features and are certainly ones you should consider when making your own choice, we ultimately decided that QSR's NVivo was best suited for our needs.

USING NVIVO FOR SOCIAL AND HEALTH RESEARCH

The utility of NVivo begins with the manner in which it duplicates digitally what researchers and students who are working qualitatively have been doing manually for years. Instead of using your yellow highlighter to emphasize a certain passage, NVivo does so digitally. Instead of writing little notes to yourself in page margins or on yellow stickies, NVivo allows you to create digital memos or annotations that accomplish the same thing. Even on these simple tasks, however, there are benefits to working with software like NVivo instead of manually. An analogy would be to say that word processing is to writing on a piece of paper what NVivo is to the manual coding of nonnumeric data. In each case you are doing the same activity—writing with ink on a pad of paper or writing with keystrokes on a computer using word processing software are two means to accomplish "writing" and neither medium guarantees or precludes you winning the Nobel Prize for Literature—but the flexibility and possibilities that the word processor brings to the activity of writing are far richer than the possibilities that come with ink on paper.

NVivo does all of the things that you might do with a yellow highlighter and a pencil, but does so digitally in a way that maximizes the amount of information that you can deal with and the number of different ways you can conceptualize and reconceptualize your "data," whatever those data happen to be. We put "data" in quotes here because we are using the term in its broadest sense to refer not only to formal data that are gathered in a research context but also include any other information—journal articles, books, field notes, pictures—that you want to retain and manage. It is as if you have an infinite number of highlighters in every conceivable color for each one of the categories of information you want to highlight and can call up any single color or set of colors you want at any time. There also is no more worry about "now where did I see that quote?" because any quotes we've coded are immediately retrievable, and even if we didn't code it, the program's search capabilities mean that we should be able to locate the quote with a few well-chosen search terms.

We also appreciate the range of material NVivo allows us to work with. While our yellow highlighter works well with text, it comes up short when we want to include a video or picture or radio interview or piece of music in our project. NVivo allows all those types of sources to be coded using what is essentially a digital highlighter, which makes them all retrievable as well. Because we also have been known to change our minds from time to time as our familiarity with and understanding of our data develops, we also like the flexibility that NVivo offers us to change our coding labels, disaggregate or aggregate coding categories, or do the work for us in finding all references to a certain kind of content that we have an interest in.

Just these basic features make us wonder why anyone out there still uses yellow highlighters and stickies in any research project, but there is far more that the program can do. While providing step-by-step "how to use NVivo" is beyond the scope of this book, there are several very good introductory instruction manuals available that we would recommend, such as Kristi Jackson and Patricia Bazeley's (2019) *Qualitative Data Analysis with NVivo* and Lyn Richards's (1999) *Using NVivo in Qualitative Research*.

Project Planning and Organization

Part of the appeal of NVivo for us is that we see it as more than just a QDA application. As illustrated in Figure 13.2 below, the program can deal with virtually any kind of content—text, images, video, audio files—and, as such, does double duty as a central file management facility where we can store (1) digital copies of relevant literature as well as bibliographic reference information imported directly from Zotero, Refworks, Mendeley, or Endnote; (2) project organizational materials such as meeting notes, email, research instruments, and spreadsheets; and (3) research data and observations such as field notes, memos and annotations, digital recordings and transcripts of interviews, images and video files (see Palys & Atchison, 2012), and social media posts from Twitter, Facebook, and YouTube. Having all the material relating to a particular research project in one central location, called a project file in

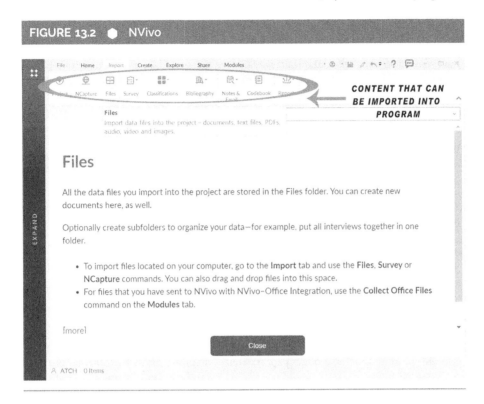

FIGURE 13.2 ● NVivo

NVivo, allows us to work more efficiently and effectively both alone and in team environments. One of the first things we do when we are starting a new project is create an NVivo project file so that we can import or link to all relevant materials that we produce as the research takes place, in this sense the project file is an organic entity that grows with the project.

Working With Data

NVivo allows us to import a wide range of data and file formats directly into our project file. The data and file formats supported by the program include text files (doc, docx, rtf, txt), image files (bmp, jpg, tif, gif), mixed text and image portable document format (PDF) files, audio files (mp3, wma, wav), and video files (mpg, wma, avi, mov, qt, mp4). In addition to allowing us to work with a wide range of text, image, audio, and video data directly within the program, we can work with websites and peripheral digital files either by way of external links that open Web browsers or other programs or by directly importing the content of the sites using a feature of the program called NCapture. This feature is particularly useful when conducting research with online communities or social network sites (e.g., YouTube, Facebook, or Twitter) or when working on mixed or multimethod projects where we have collected numeric data that we analyze in spreadsheet or quantitative data analysis programs such as Microsoft Excel or SPSS.

In addition to being able to import a wide variety of digital material directly into NVivo as well as being able to link up to external material, the program also allows us to create and edit text-based documents with its built-in word processor. The embedded word processor and audio player allow us to transcribe digitally recorded data and observations such as interviews and field notes right in the program. We also use it to create memos to assist us in our research and analysis as it progresses. The memos become "data" as well and can be compiled and coded the same as any other sources.

Since an increasing number of books and articles are available digitally as PDF files, we get digital copies of textual materials whenever possible and treat these sources as "data" that we read and code as part of the research process. In fact, since a large part of our research begins with our reading of the available literature relating to the topic we are investigating, we generally begin most of our projects by importing all of the relevant journal articles, policy papers, book chapters, and print media into our project file where we can easily read and code it for use during the design, collection, and analysis stages of our research (see Palys & Atchison, 2012). For example, we did exactly that when we started working on this book, with source material for each chapter comprising a subset of the larger project. A great advantage of having all these materials under an NVivo project umbrella is that all of the text contents are searchable—rather like having your own personal search engine that is specific to your project.

Labeling Nonnumeric Data Through Codes

NVivo offers a variety of ways to label any piece of information that you feel is relevant to your project including literature, memos, interview audio files or transcripts, social media, open-ended survey responses, or image and video from the field or the archives. The basic labeling unit that the program uses is referred to as a code (or "node" in older versions of the program). A code is quite simply a short label representing an idea, theme, persona, place, interest, or concept. In NVivo codes, as seen in Figure 13.3, are used to store all of the references from the data (e.g., segments of text, image, video, or audio material) that correspond to a particular theme, topic, idea, or concept we identify. Codes can be created in several different ways within the program including (1) *a priori* based on our identification of factual,

FIGURE 13.3 ● NVivo Coding

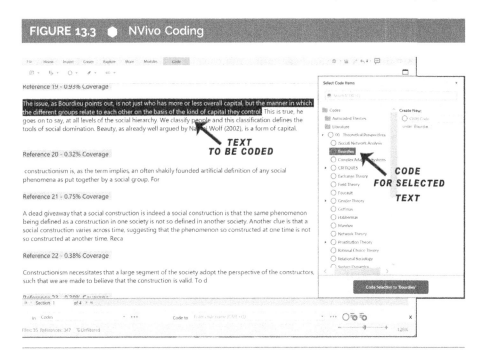

thematic, or theoretically relevant ideas; (2) *in process* on the basis of our reading of the data; (3) *in vivo* using the exact phrasing of our participants; or (4) *automatically* on the basis of the formatting of our data or using a text or word search to identify the most commonly occurring words or phrases in your data. As this makes clear, use of the program is equally compatible with inductive, deductive, and mixed approaches.

One advantage of the digital highlighting NVivo allows is that any given segment of data can be assigned a unique label or be assigned to any number of different codes, unlike your yellow highlighter, which gets confusing if you try to code any given section using more than one color of highlighter. Furthermore, as the coding progresses and we begin to develop more specific ideas about the data and the relationships among and between coded content, codes can be grouped together by merging them or dragging and dropping them into folders, sets, or models where they can be organized into hierarchies (e.g., taxonomies) or visual displays (e.g., typologies or mental maps).

For example, if we are reading through the medical records of people diagnosed and treated for attention deficit hyperactivity disorder (ADHD) in order to answer research questions about the different treatment options that have been utilized by doctors and psychologists, we might create a code labeled "treatment options." Once created, any time we come across information in the patient files that refers to ways that ADHD is treated, we can simply highlight the material and assign it to the "treatment options" code. As we read through more and more of the medical records files, we could continue to identify examples of treatment that we can add to the "treatment options" code. At any time, the program can be asked to produce a report that compiles and shows all of the sections that have been highlighted with a given code.

Codes can be disaggregated as well. For example, the "treatment options" code might be further subdivided into therapeutic, education or training, and pharmaceutical by creating three new "child" or branch codes under our main "treatment options" code and then rereading the content we have coded at "treatment options" and reassigning or recoding each entry into the new treatment categories. Passages where multiple treatment options are used can be coded in multiple overlapping code categories.

It is incredibly helpful to be able to rapidly compile a particular concept every time it appears or every time a quote includes reference to or illustrates a particular position or point of view. Analytically, it allows us to see all instances of a particular concept, which allows us to reflect on the concept itself and perhaps also to ask what elements are missing that have not yet been sampled. It also provides a basis for more systematic comparative analysis by allowing the researcher to, for example, subdivide the quotes you have for different subgroups. At the writing stage, it becomes easy to compile all quotes about a particular topic in one place, thereby facilitating your choice of what quotes to include to ensure that the range of ways the topic is discussed is illustrated.

Coding Static Attributes Through Classifications

While the majority of the coding of nonnumeric data is accomplished through the use of codes, we are also frequently interested in coding more static elements such as the demographic characteristics of a particular participant, the publication and content information of a book chapter or journal article, or the geographic coordinates where a digital image or video was created. This type of information might be referred to as the "quantitative" content in qualitative data.

The classification facility of NVivo, illustrated in Figure 13.4, is an ideal place to catalog the static attributes of nonnumeric data. There are two main types of classifications—*file* and *case*—with each serving different purposes. We use file classifications to record information about the static and comparable details of the literature

FIGURE 13.4 ● NVivo Classification

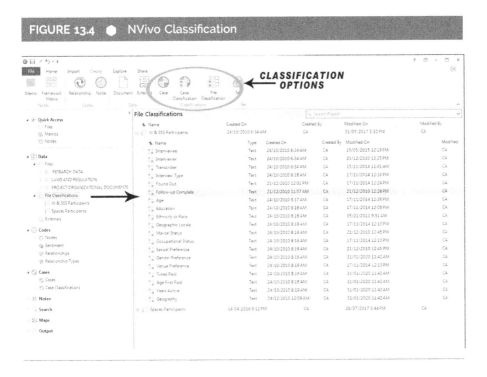

we include in our project file. For example, when Ted was working on an article related to the confidentiality case that arose out of Boston College (see Palys & Lowman, 2012; see also Chapter 10), he had more than 400 source files from the year the case had been before the courts—including newspaper articles, legal submissions, affidavits, radio interviews, videos, blogs, letters, and so forth—and one issue of interest to Ted was in how the different source files compared in their coverage. NVivo allows each file to be coded as to the type of source, which would allow him to generate a report that includes all of the entries that address a particular issue, or to subdivide them by type of file, which would allow him to inspect whether the type of file is associated with different views about the case. Alternatively, case classifications can be used to code demographic information about our units of analysis (individuals, locations, pictures, or videos). In Ted's case, for example, he could code whether particular comments about the case are uttered by a researcher, university administrator, journalist, or politician, which again allows him to either look at comments about a particular issue (i.e., code) as a whole or to subdivide the report so that the different commentators are separated, thereby making it easier to inspect the entries to compare the views of these different groups.

Readers of this book who are familiar with programs such as Microsoft Excel, Open Office Calc, or SPSS will already be familiar with ways of storing information in tabular form. For those who are not, spreadsheets, data files, and classification sheets all store and display information in columns and rows. Generally, each column represents the attribute or variable (e.g., sex, age, data collection technique, publication type, year of publication, file type) you are classifying and each row represents the individual case or unit of analysis (interview participant, audio recording, image, or video file). Each case or unit can be classified in terms of the value they possess for a particular attribute. For example, if we decide to code participants on the attributes of age, sex, sexual preference, and racial background, we can then create categories within that attribute that will allow us to code our next respondent as male, 18 years old, bisexual, and Caucasian, while the one after that might be female, 26 years old, heterosexual, and Asian. Classification sheets, like spreadsheets and data files, allow us to record, code, and analyze the static attributes of our research data. When retrieved, attributes are displayed in the form of a spreadsheet that can be used to perform advanced queries and analyses within NVivo—for example, we might want to compare how men and women talked about the risks and benefits associated with condom use—or can be exported to quantitative data analysis programs such as SPSS for quantitative analysis.

Recording Observations Using Memos and Annotations

The most basic way we can record our more lengthy ideas, insights, interpretations, and understandings of our research throughout the process is through the use of **memos**. In addition to acting as catalogs of our thinking process, in NVivo memos are also pieces of data that we can code and link to other elements of our research data such as research participants, segments of image or rich media, or attributes in a classification. While memos are standalone documents that we create inside the program, we can also create shorter annotations—virtual sticky notes—that we attach to a particular element (section of text or area of image, video, or audio) of any project document. Unlike memos, annotations are limited to 1,024 characters and their content cannot be retrieved using the program's various search functions. Figure 13.5 provides an illustration of both a memo (the main text content) and an annotation (the note at the bottom that refers to the section of main text highlighted in blue).

Memos and annotations serve a variety of functions during the project design and data collection stages. We use theoretical memos and annotations as a way of cataloging the theoretical insights that we have as the research and analysis progresses. For example, in the early stages of research design, we might come across a particular

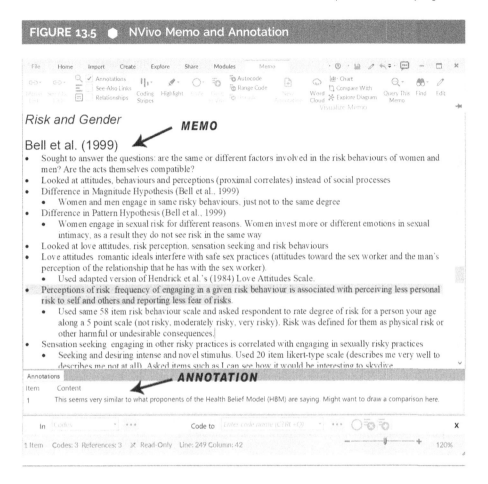

FIGURE 13.5 ● NVivo Memo and Annotation

Risk and Gender

Bell et al. (1999)

- Sought to answer the questions: are the same or different factors involved in the risk behaviours of women and men? Are the acts themselves compatible?
- Looked at attitudes, behaviours and perceptions (proximal correlates) instead of social processes
- Difference in Magnitude Hypothesis (Bell et al., 1999)
  - Women and men engage in same risky behaviours, just not to the same degree
- Difference in Pattern Hypothesis (Bell et al., 1999)
  - Women engage in sexual risk for different reasons. Women invest more or different emotions in sexual intimacy, as a result they do not see risk in the same way
- Looked at love attitudes, risk perception, sensation seeking and risk behaviours
- Love attitudes romantic ideals interfere with safe sex practices (attitudes toward the sex worker and the man's perception of the relationship that he has with the sex worker).
  - Used adapted version of Hendrick et al.'s (1984) Love Attitudes Scale.
- Perceptions of risk frequency of engaging in a given risk behaviour is associated with perceiving less personal risk to self and others and reporting less fear of risks.
  - Used same 58 item risk behaviour scale and asked respondent to rate degree of risk for a person your age along a 5 point scale (not risky, moderately risky, very risky). Risk was defined for them as physical risk or other harmful or undesirable consequences.
- Sensation seeking engaging in other risky practices is correlated with engaging in sexually risky practices
  - Seeking and desiring intense and novel stimulus. Used 20 item likert-type scale (describes me very well to describes me not at all). Asked items such as I can see how it would be interesting to skydive

Annotations

Item	Content
1	This seems very similar to what proponents of the Health Belief Model (HBM) are saying. Might want to draw a comparison here.

1 Item   Codes: 3 References: 3   ✗ Read-Only   Line: 249 Column: 42   120%

passage in an article or book we are reading discussing a certain theory that we think might be useful at some point in the research. We might create a memo we call "theoretical note" that briefly details the theory and provides a couple of key references to the people responsible for creating the theory or we might create an annotation that records our immediate thoughts or insights about the specific passage where the theory is mentioned.

Methodological memos we create in our project are often based on our thoughts and reflections on particular aspects of our research such as the sampling or solicitation approaches we are using or ideas on how to better record interviews or notes when we are in the field. Project memos are similar to methodological memos, but we use these to record our thoughts and observations on key details, goals, assumptions, and decisions we make during the research that may impact the information we gather and our subsequent analyses. Similarly, we use case or field memos to record our observations about a particular interview participant, research setting, or other unit of analysis. These memos are great for summarizing our thoughts about an interview or our impressions of a particular participant. They are also very useful for highlighting some of our initial ideas about what is going on in our research that frequently find their way into our coding of the research data.

In addition to offering ways of recording insights regarding theory and methodology as well as ongoing observations about your research, memos and annotations are helpful for tracking our developing analysis and help ensure that we are being as transparent as possible in making sense of the data.

Analyzing Data

While we see NVivo as an excellent tool for file and data management and project organization that provides a great space for recording and cataloging our thoughts and observations and coding our research data and field notes, one of the program's greatest strengths lies in the range of options it provides for the analysis of coded material. Analysis in NVivo can take a wide variety of forms, allowing researchers to employ any or all of the analytic techniques we highlighted earlier in this chapter and in Chapter 12. The technical procedures for analyzing data within the program include simple point and click retrieval of coded content, retrieval and display through framework matrices and advanced queries (searches), and retrieval and display through advanced visualizations and modeling.

Retrieving Coding Using Point and Click

One of the most useful and basic ways to quickly retrieve and display all the materials that we have identified under a specific code within NVivo is simply to ask the program to retrieve and display the contents of whichever code we are interested in. This allows us to see all the locations in the data where a particular theme or concept is present as well as allows us to look more closely at the coded content to make sure that it has been consistently and accurately coded.

When we conduct simple thematic analyses, we often code our data over successive readings and then retrieve the content of each individual code when we are ready to sit down and begin writing. Quite frequently we organize our different codes thematically as typologies, taxonomies, or mental maps using features of the program that allow us to group content into sets (folders for elements with equal or shared features), code hierarchies, or models (a chart-creating feature that allows us to visualize the relationships among and between codes or cases). We often find that this code and retrieve style of analysis is more than suitable for the identification of the key themes that we piece together as we write since specific references can be quoted, summarized, synthesized, compared, and contrasted further during the writing process. This approach to analysis is particularly well suited for the thematic analyses that students writing extensive literature reviews, substantive papers, or comprehensive exams are often required to do, demonstrating once again that NVivo has uses far beyond formal research environments.

Queries and Word Frequency Analysis

While the simple code and retrieval functions of NVivo are far more efficient than conventional non–computer-assisted approaches for analyzing data, the techniques we've described are just the tip of the iceberg in terms of what NVivo offers when it comes to analyzing coded data. The program also offers a range of sophisticated query (e.g., search, organize, and retrieve) options that support a wide variety of analytical approaches. The analytical tools available include simple and advanced text and word frequency searches, coding queries, compound queries that combine searches for text and coding, and framework matrix and coding analyses that allow you to see patterns in coding, just to name a few! We'll describe just two of those in the introductory treatment we intend here.

The **text search** facilities that are built into the program allow you to quickly find and retrieve all the places in your data (including our memos and annotations) where particular words, phrases, concepts, ideas, or themes are present or intersect with one another. It can be used to perform a range of analytic searches from basic identification of every instance where an exact word appears in the research data to complex queries involving wildcards, conditional statements, and proximity specifications such as those we would use for **KWIC (key-word-in-context) analyses**. An added feature of these searches is that they can be done with all or any identifiable subset of sources, which allows you to do both focused and broad searches.

Moving from a text search to a KWIC analysis is quite simple since results of text searches are presented in a way that we can ascertain the number of times a particular word appears in each piece of our data (e.g., in each interview), can see the exact points in the text where the word appears, or can view the word context visually in the form of a customizable word tree that allows us to see a branching display of a specified number of words appearing before and after our keyword across all or part of our data. A simple text search can be extended using the compound query option to combine two separate text search terms, which allows us to locate spaces in our data where they occur together in the same sentence or passage.

The program also has a sophisticated **word frequency query**, illustrated in Figure 13.6, which allows us to determine which words or concepts appear most often in any textual data we have in our project. In addition to being able to specify the minimum size of the words we wish to include in our search, the program also allows us to specify how close of a match we seek (e.g., the exact word, or synonyms as well, or, even more broadly, words sharing generally the same meaning). The program displays the results in the form of numeric summaries showing the frequency and percentage of the appearance of words in the data or visually in the form of a word cloud, tree map, or cluster analysis. While we rarely use word frequency alone to analyze our data, we find that it is an excellent tool for quickly identifying potential themes or frequently occurring concepts in our data or to get a deeper understanding of the language that participants use to describe certain concepts or phenomena.

FIGURE 13.6 ● NVivo Word Frequency Query

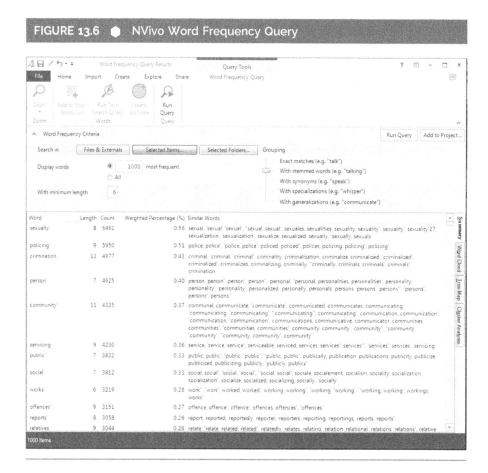

Analysis Through Visualizations

For many, visually displaying relationships between people, places, things, themes, codes, and concepts is the most efficient way to make sense of nonnumeric data. Accordingly, the final set of NVivo facilities for analyzing coded unstructured content that we will highlight are those relating to visualization and modeling of coded data.

Charts in NVivo are particularly useful for identifying how frequently a particular theme is coded across cases or for determining if a particular code is more or less likely to be associated with specific case attributes. For example, if we are interested in visually displaying which interview participants discuss "recurrent thoughts of death or suicide" and how frequently each participant mentions this in their interviews, we could generate a chart that summarizes our coding for "recurrent thoughts of death or suicide" for all of our participants. The result would be a chart that would not only show us differences in frequencies of experiences but also one in which each of the bars representing these frequencies could be clicked on to retrieve the actual text where we have coded participants "recurrent thoughts of death or suicide."

A more intricate way of visualizing the patterns in our coding of people, places, things, or themes in our data is through cluster analysis. This technique allows us to visually display the grouping (clustering) of sources or codes that share similar wording, attribute values, or coding. Cluster analyses are incredibly useful for identifying patterns in data since they graphically display relationships between elements of our data; the closer clusters of elements are to each other in the visual display the more similar they are to each other. So if we were interested in seeing how similar the wording that various women who have experienced postpartum depression use to describe their experiences is, we could accomplish this through a cluster analysis.

Tree maps are another useful way to visualize patterns in our data. A tree map is a diagram that displays the hierarchical relationships among coded content. Tree maps display coding frequency in the form of a series of nested rectangles presented horizontally from left to right with the largest rectangle on the left-hand side of the display representing the code with the greatest amount of content and nested rectangles becoming increasingly smaller in size as one looks to the right-hand side of the display.

A Final Note on User Friendliness

Although our lengthy inventory of NVivo features—which is still not exhaustive—may leave readers feeling a bit overwhelmed by the apparent complexity of and range of possible strategies within the program, we close by noting two things about NVivo that contributed to our decision to adopt that program.

First is that it is a program that does *not* require you to know too much to begin, but allows you to wade in slowly. Using the program's excellent online help section and accompanying user tutorials, you can learn the basics of the software in an hour—how to create a project; how to do searches; how to create codes; and how to retrieve the coded material—which is sufficient to begin using the program for whatever literature or other data you want to code. Those basic skills alone make the program usable for a wide range of projects, while other skills can be added on as needed whenever you get to one of those "I wonder if I can do 'x' with this program?" moments.

A second element that adds to NVivo's user friendliness is the wealth of tutorial material available at the QSR site as well as on its YouTube channel. While the hour-long webinars are helpful to see the various ways one can deal with a data set, we especially appreciate the large number of skill-specific videos that last from one to no more than 3 minutes to give a quick overview when you need a reminder or brief introduction to how to accomplish a specific task.

ANALYSIS OF DATA FROM MIXED METHODS RESEARCH

One of the greatest benefits of mixed methods designs comes at the data analysis stage when the different types of data can be brought together and used to shed light on each other. Data from mixed methods investigations are capable of providing you with a much greater diversity of views (Teddlie & Tashakkori, 2003), and it is divergent views that give you the opportunity to falsify aspects of your theory or to question the assumptions upon which your understanding of a phenomenon are based. Mixed methods analysis allows you to have greater confidence in your research by the opportunity it provides to interrogate more thoroughly the plausibility of your conclusions.

Bazeley (2012) notes that in mixed methods studies, integration occurs when diverse analytic strategies and techniques are applied to the diverse sets of numeric and nonnumeric data in such a way that the results of the analyses can be used inter-dependently to answer a range of research questions that traverse the boundaries between qualitative and quantitative. Bringing together different forms of data at the analysis stage to achieve the ideal that Bazeley details has been notably difficult

(Bryman, 2007). The major issue confronting most researchers is whether to transform one type of data so that it is directly comparable and compatible with the other or to maintain the integrity of each form of data and develop analytical and interpretive techniques that effectively integrate both forms. Since quantitative data are already structured and cannot easily be transformed to become less structured, one of the toughest decisions you have to make during analysis is how you are going to handle your qualitative data. Transforming qualitative data and observations into a more quantitative form by assigning elements of talk, text, or image into static and structured categories can defeat the purpose of collecting the rich qualitative data in the first place. Alternatively, ensuring different types of data "speak" to one another can be very challenging.

To this end, Jackson and Bazeley (2019) propose three frameworks for the analysis of mixed data:

- A **concurrent** or **complementary approach** where we use one data source to complement and expand on the analysis of another. An example of this would be when we use interview or focus group data to provide details on the context or processes underlying the patterns revealed through quantitative analyses of structured survey data.

- A **sequential approach** where we use the results of our analysis of one type of data to inform or shape how we go about analyzing the second form of data. An example of this would be when our inductive analysis of qualitative data produces a theory that we then use to generate hypotheses that we test through the analysis of quantitative data.

- A **convergent approach** where we merge the two forms of data into a single data set in order to compare and contrast the results. An example of this would be when we combine qualitative data with quantitative data to produce a social network analysis. In this approach we might take data gathered from interviews with participants where we asked them to describe their working relationships with people in their office and combine it with data from a survey where we asked these participants to identify all of the people they collaborate with in the office on a daily or weekly basis. We would then take both sources of data and use them to develop an adjacency matrix (a numerical table depicting the ties between actors), which we would use to produce a variety of statistical analyses of the composition of the network as well as a visual display of the relations among and between individuals (called a network graph or sociogram).

Despite the development of these frameworks, at this point there are no analytical techniques we are aware of that have been developed specifically for the concurrent analysis of qualitative and quantitative data. While quantitative data analysis programs like SPSS have the capacity to display and re-order qualitative data in the form of open-ended or "string" responses from self-administered or researcher-administered questionnaires, none of these programs include features that allow for more advanced analysis of nonnumeric data. If we want to further analyze this type of data, we are forced to either collapse it into structured categories so that we can analyze it quantitatively or export it so we can analyze it more completely using software such as NVivo.

While the developers of statistical software packages such as SPSS have done little in the way of including features and tools for the analysis of nonnumeric data in their programs, the same cannot be said for those developing QDA software. Over the past decade, many of the most popular applications that have been developed for working with nonnumeric data have begun to provide tools for the analysis of mixed data. NVivo began to provide features and tools for mixed data analysis in 2013 with its release of version 10 (SP3), although there is as yet no provision for even the most rudimentary of statistical analyses.

Mixed data analysis in NVivo begins when we import a structured data set into the program—usually a data matrix in tabular form with variables across the columns and cases down the rows—from a questionnaire or structured interview. This raw survey data can be in the form of an Excel spreadsheet, plain text (comma or tab delimited) file, or data provided from an online survey conducted through Survey Monkey or Qualtrics. Once the data is imported into the program, we have several options. In some cases we might want to begin by comparing responses to structured survey questions with those provided in open-ended questions. Converting the different closed ended questions into attributes in a classification sheet allows us to use the query functions of the program to select out subgroups of participants based on their attribute values (e.g., selecting out participants according to their political affiliation as republican, democrat, or independent). Once selected out we can begin the process of comparing and contrasting responses to the open-ended survey questions for each of these groups, along the way we would code the different patterns or themes that we identify to codes. After we finish our initial coding of the open-ended survey responses, we can dig deeper to look for additional patterns or themes by using the survey responses to generate a matrix coding query. This type of query produces a table that displays differently coded information (the columns of the table) according to categories of responses to specific survey questions. So we can produce a matrix to see how similar or different material at a specified code or across several different codes was for male, female, and trans* participants.

After we have completed our mixed analysis of the closed and open-ended data from the survey, we can link the data from individual survey respondents to other data we have collected from them. For example, say we have survey data for 500 participants and we have interview transcripts, videos, and still images that we have gathered from these participants during our research in the field. We can use NVivo to directly link the individual survey responses to the corresponding nonnumeric data in our project file. Once the different forms of data are linked, we can begin to use the survey data to help us dig into our other data in much the same way we did with the open-ended survey data.

QDA software like NVivo has taken the greatest strides toward providing a platform where social and health researchers can leverage the insights provided by more structured quantitative data to help us dig further into the richness and complexity of information contained within various types of qualitative data we might collect. Despite these advances, we are still a long way from being able to conduct truly integrative or convergent analyses that allow us to mine the potential of multiple forms of data in a way that allows us to determine and illustrate how such data "speaks to each other." At this point there is no single data analysis program that provides a set of analytical tools that can be used to conduct a fully integrated analysis of nonnumeric and numeric data. Perhaps with an increasing emphasis on "convergence" in the technological world, we will see programs like NVivo and SPSS merge into a single platform. For now, more sophisticated analyses of mixed data still require us to use at least two different programs and then integrate our analysis during the interpretive phase.

SUMMING UP AND LOOKING AHEAD

One of the great benefits of more qualitative approaches—their ability to produce reams of rich data—is also in some ways their greatest liability. What is a researcher to do when they sit down at the end of the day with hundreds of pages of interview transcripts, thousands of words of information in their field notes, and/or computer directories full of audio and video files? Unlike more quantitative research, where the researcher can take stacks of numbers and incorporate them into well-defined sta- tistical techniques to summarize and focus the analysis in the form of a few tables, charts, and graphs, the procedures involved in managing more qualitative data are rarely discussed. And yet never has the need for such a discussion been greater given the virtual explosion of text, image, audio, and video data that we can create and/or download, thanks to the digital revolution. Indeed, one of the biggest challenges facing researchers of any stripe these days is the simple question of how to manage all the data that is out there. The current chapter attempts to redress that inattention by outlining some of the issues and strategies involved in the collection and analysis of nonnumeric data.

The two main processes involved in analyzing text, images, audio, and/or video data are coding and memoing. In both cases the objective is to take the piles of data we have accumulated and find ways to present them in a manner that reduces the volume of information we are working with, transparently summarizes the patterns that exist in the data, and helps us to achieve our empirical objectives without doing any injustice to the data.

Coding can be deductive or inductive. Deductive coding occurs when your research focus and interest are well defined from the start so that decisions about what to code are made independent of the data in front of you. Common practices with the more deductive coding techniques include word counts and KWIC analysis, as well as classic content analysis. Notwithstanding a clear focus from the outset, deductive coding still often involves initial categories being fine-tuned and elaborated in contact with the data. More inductive approaches to coding are more squarely rooted in the data themselves, often beginning with a process known as open coding, where researchers begin simply by noting thematic elements of the data that are of interest. Subsequent coding then often involves aggregating specific segments together as common processes and related events are brought together and identified as theoretically interesting.

Memoing not only refers to the common practice in more qualitative research to write analytical notes to oneself in field notes as the data are being gathered but also extends to the coding process as categories are gradually defined and embellished and your memos to self become an archive of the in-project development of your understanding and the coding categories that go with it. Coding and memoing are not independent processes; researchers typically go back and forth between the two as they expose themselves to and begin to try to understand their data.

The chapter concludes with a discussion of QDA software. We describe the variety of these that are available, indicate some of the considerations to keep in mind when deciding which QDA software is right for you, and follow this with a discussion of some of the possibilities that arise in NVivo, which we rely on because it offers the most flexibility for the kind of work we do. The discussion makes clear that QDA tools such as NVivo are useful for more than simply data analysis and that it also serves as a general information management tool in the context of a project that allows you to input text, audio, video, images, code them, write memos, and where all the text is searchable. For example, this makes it an ideal program for managing all of the literature that you compile in digital files (which are increasingly becoming the way we store all sorts of data). The program also allows both thematic and attribute coding, with the latter allowing for separate retrieval for different groups, thereby enabling comparative analysis (see also Palys and Atchison (2012) on these points).

Notwithstanding our own interest in and affection for the data management and analytic power that QDA software like NVivo allows, we also note the resistance in some quarters to the use of computers for QDA and some of the reasons we have heard that lay behind that resistance (see also Palys & Atchison, 2012). In our view, QDA software is simply another analytical tool that is rooted in qualitative analytical practices of yesteryear—coding, memoing, highlighting, reflecting, searching—and that creates certain efficiencies, but does not do the work for you and still requires an engaged researcher to use effectively.

We argued that QDA programs such as NVivo make it easier for us to create, store, organize, edit, correct, and locate an increasingly diverse and expansive array of research data. They also provide us with a range of efficient ways to code multiple forms of data and to record, access, and link our thoughts (e.g., our memos and annotations) about our project and data to other aspects of our emergent analysis. We can also quickly search volumes of coded and uncoded material to extract relevant bits as we pursue ideas, clarify concepts, and develop models and theories. The programs also allow us to quickly and easily apply a variety of content analytic strategies ranging from simple word counts to KWIC to more complex matrix-based analyses. They further enable us to retrieve and display thematically coded material in a variety of visual formats including typologies, taxonomies, mental maps, flowcharts, and matrices. Finally, they also have begun to provide us with the capability to analyze mixed data and facilitate both individual and collaborative writing of the analyses that form the basis of our research reports, articles, and books.

Our biggest disappointment at the moment is that we know of few universities and colleges to date who have embraced and made available QDA software such as NVivo to the same extent that quantitative statistical packages such as SPSS or SAS are routinely available on campuses, even though one does not have to be a qualitative researcher to benefit from NVivo's information/data management capabilities. Although we hope the situation will have changed when and if a second edition of this book comes into existence a few years down the road, we have kept our discussion of the software more conceptual and introductory here in order simply to whet your appetite, knowing that opportunities to use the program at your university or college for free may be limited in the near future.

However, we strongly encourage more adventurous faculty members and students who pride themselves in being "first adopters" to go to the QSR website and download a free 30-day trial version of the program. The downloadable tutorials that have been prepared will get even the most timid user up and running very quickly; QSR also often holds Webinars to explain the program and answer questions from newbie and veteran users alike.

Having focused in this chapter on analytic techniques that can be employed in the analysis of more qualitative, nonnumeric data, in the next chapter we examine the other end of the continuum, i.e., some foundational techniques for summarizing, representing, and analyzing more structured, quantitative data.

Key Concepts

Annotations 534
Cluster analysis 535
Code 544
Coding 532
Concurrent mixed data analysis 555
Convergent mixed data analysis 555

Deductive coding 533
Inductive coding 533
KWIC (key-word-in-context) analyses 551
Memo 534
NVivo 541
Open coding 533
Project file 542

Qualitative Data Analysis (QDA) software 538
Sequential mixed data analysis 555
Text search 551
Tree maps 553
Typologies 535
Word frequency query 552

STUDY QUESTIONS

1. Discuss the main differences between numeric and nonnumeric data and briefly describe the major challenges that are associated with analyzing nonnumeric data. What similarities do the coding of numeric and nonnumeric data share?

2. Distinguish between deductive and inductive coding. Do you have to choose between one and the other in any given project?

3. Explain what memoing involves and indicate some of the ways that memoing is useful in the process of coding nonnumeric data.

4. What drawbacks do some people see to doing computer-based analyses of nonnumerical data using QDA software? What advantages are there to using them?

5. The section of this chapter entitled "Typological and Other More Complex Analyses" offers three different ways of creating a drug typology—by pharmacological similarity; by their categorization within the Criminal Code; and user-generated typologies based on where and how the various drugs are consumed. Imagine now that you are conducting a study on how drug use finds its way into a particular school subculture. What do you think would be the advantages and disadvantages of incorporating each of the three types of typologies into your analysis?

6. Why do simple word counts make sense to include as part of your analysis of nonnumeric data? What do they offer you? What extra information does KWIC (key-word-in-context) analysis give you?

7. Find out which newspapers your college, university, or municipal (public) library keeps and how many years' worth of issues they've retained. Design a quantitative and/or qualitative study that compares the way newspaper reports from different time periods treat an issue of interest to you. For example, you might look at (1) how women are portrayed in articles from the 1960s, 1980s, and 2000s; (2) how environmental issues and/or environmental activists are portrayed in the 1960s and in the 2000s; or (3) whether the composition of the newspaper's front page is different now than it was at the turn of the 20th century.

8. Choose your five favorite songs, obtain the lyrics from the internet, and develop a coding scheme that you could use to identify and code words or actions that reflect themes of gender, race, or class.

9. Pick some textual source of data that exists at your college or university and design a study to systematically compile and content code that data. The examples we have in mind would include projects such as (1) analyzing washroom graffiti to see whether there are any differences between the arts and sciences or between men and women in what is written; (2) analyzing the messages and images on people's T-shirts; or (3) analyzing the messages on bumper stickers displayed in your university or college's parking lots.

10. Develop a taxonomy of the course offerings of one of the departments in your college/university.

11. What are some of the advantages and disadvantages of using qualitative data analysis software such as NVivo to analyze text, images, audio, and/or video nonnumeric data?

ANALYZING NUMERICAL DATA

Numbers are a fact of life. They are also a tool of social and health science in the same way that they are a tool of everyday life: they help us describe, make comparisons, and express relationships. Of course, they can also be used to distort, mislead, and stonewall. Indeed, one of the implications of entering the information age seems to be that *everybody* can now point to *some* data *somewhere* that "prove" the correctness of their view of the world. It makes sense to try to understand data and how they're used.

Data needn't be intimidating, although many people seem to find them so. Indeed, some people assert—sometimes even with a sense of self-righteous pride—that they aren't "numbers" people. Don't get us wrong. You can do perfectly good, interesting, and valuable research *without* getting into razzle-dazzle multivariate statistics, as we hope the earlier chapters in this book have shown. But any researcher who skips through the data section of an article or a report and takes the writer's conclusions at face value, and any citizen who uncritically accepts the reportage offered in contemporary news media, is doing themselves a disservice. Any competent researcher and citizen needs to understand some statistical basics, and that's what this chapter will offer.

This chapter will address the sort of data that are most amenable to quantitative analysis, that is, structured, systematically derived data amenable to aggregation and statistical analysis. We'll consider two ways to represent and examine those data: through **descriptive statistics,** which present the data in summary form, and through **inferential statistics,** which analyze sample data to reveal relationships among variables and to make inferences about populations. You'll see that the latter may be used inductively, to suggest possible relationships, or deductively, to test hypotheses. This chapter will emphasize the conceptual underpinnings of numbers and some of the statistical procedures to which they might be subjected. The aim is not to turn you into a statistician, but to discuss some statistical fundamentals in a way that will help you understand the statistics you will likely be getting either in lab periods or some other course, as well as the sorts of data you will see reported in mainstream media.

VARIABLES AND CONSTANTS

In order to discern what it is about numbers that might interest us, we must take a step back and talk about the concept of variables. Stated simply, a **variable** is anything that varies. The opposite is a **constant,** which is something that *does not* vary. In your research methods class, for example, most likely all of you sitting in the chairs are students; that is, the social status of "student" is a constant in your class. Presumably all class members are also human beings, so we might say that "species" is also a constant in your class. But there are many *variables* in your class as well.

The declared major of your colleagues is probably a variable, for example, unless the class is a required one in which only majors can enroll, in which case "major" would be a constant. Other variables might include whether you are enrolled part-time or full-time, your ages, ethnicities, vocational aspirations, attitudes on social issues, and so forth. The whole task of the social and health sciences is to *explain* variation (e.g., why are the proportions of males and females so different in computing science compared to sociology?) in relation to other variations (e.g., variation in life history, competencies, aptitudes, interests).

As soon as you begin attaching numbers to things, several other processes are automatically activated. Numbers imply classification, for example, since the simple counting of objects implies that the objects are part of the category whose frequency you are counting. This is sometimes a relatively simple process, for example, if you count your fingers and toes or the number of people in your class. But on other occasions, the boundaries that define a category may be rather more blurred, as when deciding, for example, whether a death was an "accident" or a "suicide" or whether the punishment a parent delivers is "a spanking" or "physical abuse."

This chapter won't discuss the constructionist aspects of how social categories are derived, why some areas of life are more or less fully enumerated than others, or the social and political dynamics by which particular categories are negotiated (but see, for example, Lakoff, 1987, or anything by Michel Foucault). But don't forget that such issues permeate this chapter. Numbers always have an aura of precision about them, but behind every number is the product of a social process that has caused that number to exist (e.g., see Chapter 12's section on crime statistics and the discussion in Chapter 2 regarding operationalization). Maintain the same healthy skepticism about numbers that you do about any other information you might be presented with.

LEVELS OF MEASUREMENT

The types of descriptive and inferential statistics to use in any situation depend to some degree on the types of variables with which you are dealing, which in turn depends on how you've gone about measuring them. Remember that social and health science research involves a continuing interplay between theory and data. The variables that interest us are theoretical constructions—abstractions we draw from our experience—that we feel are useful in describing and interpreting human activity. But empirical research cannot be done in the abstract. We must give our variables empirical meaning by operationalizing them for a given research context. The correspondence rules by which those operationalizations are imposed (i.e., the way we take observations and change them into variables for analysis) define the type of measurement taken.

Nominal or Categorical Measures

The simplest way to measure an object is simply to categorize it, that is, say what it is and what it is not. Examples of **categorical variables** include whether a person owns or rents their abode, a student's choice of academic major, and whether a person is in a treatment group or a control group. In each case, any assigning of numbers to those categories would be completely arbitrary. We can code oranges as "1" and apples as "2," but that makes no more or less sense than coding apples as "1" and oranges as "2." The different values the variable can take on (e.g., apples or oranges, for the variable "fruits found in lunchboxes") are merely different from one another; one value doesn't embody or possess *more* or *less* of the variable under consideration. Apples and oranges, for example, are just different fruits, with neither being any more or less of a fruit than the other.

Ordinal Measures

A second level of measurement is called **ordinal measurement** because the numbers ascribed to our classification possess order. That is, not only are the values *different* from one another (as was the case with categorical variables), they also embody differences of *magnitude* with respect to the variable under consideration. For example, full-time research faculty members in North American universities are classified into three categories: (1) assistant professor, (2) associate professor, and (3) full professor. There's an underlying sense of *order* to these categories; each successive category is "higher" in the academic hierarchy than the previous one. Numbers imposed in order to code and analyze the distribution of "academic rank" are somewhat arbitrary—we could equally legitimately call the categories 1, 2, and 3; or 5, 10, and 15—but they aren't *totally* arbitrary, since using 1, 3, and 2 would destroy the underlying order we see.

At the same time, the limits of ordinal measures also are evident. In the real number system, the distance or interval between 1 and 2 is equal to the distance between 2 and 3, but that property does not hold for an ordinal variable like academic rank. The numbers are merely rankings; the order is important, but the distance between ranks is not consistent. Another example might be "order of finish" at a track meet. Runners come in first, second, third, and so on; the order is important, but the distance between the first and second runners may not be the same as the distance between the second and third.

Interval-Level Measurement

When the property of equal distance *is* met, **interval-level measurement** is said to exist. In the monograph that originally differentiated these measurement types, Stevens (1951) gave thermometer readings as an example. Note that a temperature of 30° is *different* from a temperature of 20° (i.e., it meets the requirement of categorical measurement). It's also *higher* than 20° (i.e., there are magnitude relations, as in ordinal measurement). But a new criterion applies: it is also possible to say that the *interval* between 20° and 30° is equal to the interval between 10° and 20°, or that 1° is of equal magnitude at any point in the scale. On the other hand, certain limits are imposed because the scale does not have a "true" zero point.

In the social world, suppose we ask faculty members at a university to indicate which they value more highly: the research or the teaching component of their jobs. To express their answers, we give them a five-point scale with the following verbal designations: (1) research is much more valued than teaching, (2) research is somewhat more valued than teaching, (3) research and teaching are about equally valued, (4) teaching is somewhat more valued than research, and (5) teaching is much more valued than research. Psychometric research (e.g., see Altemeyer, 1970; Dawes, 1972) has shown that people can use such scales quite easily and that unless the verbal designations are very poorly chosen, adults use such scales in a manner consistent with at least interval-level properties.

Ratio Measurement

The final level of measurement noted by Stevens (1951) is called **ratio-level measurement**, and the prototypical example is that of a ruler measuring distance or length. Ratio measurement embodies all three previous levels of measurement. A distance of 3 inches is *different* from a distance of 2 inches. We can also say that it's *longer* than 2 inches. Further, the differences between the points are meaningful: the interval between 1 inch and 2 inches is the same as the interval between 8 inches and 9 inches.

A notable new property of ratio-level measurement is that the scale has a true zero point; in other words, the number zero *means* something: namely, that there's none of the quality being measured. This property allows us to say, for example, that 2 inches is twice as long as 1 inch, or that the ratio of 2 inches to 1 inch is the same as the ratio of 8 inches to 4 inches (i.e., both are 2:1). Note that this situation differs from that in the thermometer example. The zero point on most thermometers is arbitrary: zero degrees, whether on the Celsius scale or the Fahrenheit scale, doesn't mean a total absence of heat or molecular activity. So you cannot say, for example, that 80° Fahrenheit is twice as hot as 40°, or that the ratio of 80°:40° is the same as the ratio of 30°:15°. Other examples of ratio scales include measures of time, mass, and volume.

Levels of Measurement and Statistical Analysis

Stevens (1951) argued that it's important to differentiate between these levels of measurement because the range of mathematical operations you can legitimately perform on your data is limited by the level of measurement. With nominal/categorical data, for example, it's reasonable to create frequency distributions and to indicate the most frequently occurring (or modal) categories, but it makes no sense to compute an "average" when the numerical coding of categories is completely arbitrary to start with (e.g., an "average" sex of 1.2). At the other extreme, with ratio-level data, you *can* meaningfully employ a wide range of mathematical operations.

There was a time when social and health science researchers bowed to Stevens's (1951) typology with the reverence otherwise reserved for works of scripture. But much has changed in the decades since that article was written. The onslaught began with a humorous article by Lord (1953) that focused on the relative merit of performing various statistical analyses with the numbers on football jerseys.

The numbers on football jerseys are obviously categorical: the fact that a quarterback wears number 12 while a halfback might wear 33 conveys no information at all about who is the better player. Computing average jersey numbers or comparing the average jersey number of one team to that of another would be a mathematical absurdity, according to Stevens (1951). But the central character of Lord's (1953) fictitious story—a certain mathematics professor at an unnamed university—does exactly that (in secret, of course) when the players on the university team complain that the other teams laugh at them because their numbers are "too low."

To address this question, Lord's hypothetical professor does what to Stevens (1951) would have been unpardonable: he compares the mean (average) football jersey number on his team to those of other teams and finds that his team's numbers are indeed significantly lower than those of their opponents. But given the particular question being posed, comparing the "average" jersey numbers actually made reasonable sense. The moral of Lord's (1953) story? You can do anything you want with numbers, since the numbers themselves haven't a clue what's "being done" to them, but it's up to you the researcher to make decisions about the range of operations that are meaningful to perform on given data in a given context. If the question (to continue Lord's example) is whether one team's numbers are significantly lower or higher than another team's numbers, computing the mean (average) numbers and comparing them is a meaningful and reasonable thing to do. But if the question were something like "Which team is 'better'?" then comparing the average number on football jerseys would be meaningless and absurd, since football numbers bear no relation at all to the variable "athletic skill."

We can indeed fault Stevens's (1951) scheme for the qualities ascribed to various measures, since the level of measurement is *not* inherent in the data itself; rather, you must always consider the use to which the data are being put. For example, Stevens argues that the ruler is a perfect example of a measurement scale (for distance or length) with ratio properties. In social and health science, though, our interests are *not* with the empirical variables per se, but with the underlying *theoretical* variables they're thought to represent.

As long as distance per se is all that interests us, in other words, the measures do have ratio-level properties. But rarely are we interested in distance per se in social and health research; instead, we're interested in distance as an operationalization or indicator of some theoretical variable of interest (e.g., social distance or interpersonal closeness). And it's the range of operations we feel comfortable using *when the measure is used as an indicator for the underlying theoretical variable of interest* that will influence the range of mathematical operations we can legitimately perform on the data. Thus, using a ruler to measure height is one thing, but using the same ruler to measure the distance between two people as an indicator of how much they like each other is something else. The first has ratio properties; the second may or may not. As this example reaffirms, the property lies not in the measure, but in how the measure is used.

This isn't the place to get into a lengthy review of statistical debates on the range of statistics that might legitimately be employed with any given type of data. Suffice it to say that numerous **"Monte Carlo" computer simulations** have shown that many statistical techniques, and certainly the ones in this chapter, can be quite robust to violations of the theoretical assumptions underlying them. You needn't, therefore, be as rigid as Stevens proposes, although you also shouldn't jump to the opposite conclusion, that "anything goes." Your research questions should guide your data analysis, with the caveat that it is up to you to consider how meaningful the analysis is, given the type of data and the theoretical use to which they are being put. The question for us, then, is what those uses might be.

DESCRIPTIVE STATISTICS

A very basic use of statistics is to summarize your data. Instead of saying that we have this marble, and this marble, and this marble, and so on, we can much more succinctly say that we have 10 red marbles and 12 blue ones. Such brevity is admired in the social and health sciences, where the nature of the scientific task requires us to *describe,* in conceptual terms, the nature of our social universe. Descriptive techniques fall into three general categories: depictions of the *distributions* of each variable, statistics that convey the *central tendency* of each distribution, and statistics that convey the *variability* or *dispersion* that exists in each distribution. Within each of these three categories various techniques may be most useful, depending on such considerations as level of measurement.

Depicting Distributions

The first and most straightforward step we can take toward summarizing our data is to create frequency distributions to summarize the number and percentage of persons occupying each of our analytical categories. Indeed, whenever you finish gathering and coding your data, the first thing you should do is prepare frequency tables for each of your variables, to better visualize how they are distributed. To illustrate the various types of descriptive techniques available to you, we'll continue the example of the faculty members at a fictitious university, which we will call State University (or StateU). Tables 14.1–14.4 show frequency distributions summarizing the number of male and female faculty members (Table 14.1), the number of faculty members at each rank (Table 14.2), responses to a question about the relative value faculty members ascribe to the teaching and research components of their job (Table 14.3), and the numbers of years faculty members have been employed (Table 14.4).

These four tables collectively demonstrate a number of different aspects of frequency distributions. Note that frequency distributions are appropriate for data at all levels of measurement: sex (Table 14.1) is a categorical variable, academic rank (Table 14.2) is an ordinal variable, responses to the query about research and teaching priorities (Table 14.3) may be treated as an interval-level variable, and number of years of employment (Table 14.4) represents a ratio-level variable. Because each of the tables shows the distribution for one variable at a time, they're called *univariate frequency distributions (uni* = one; *variate* = variable).

A second thing to consider about Tables 14.1–14.4 is how they are presented. Each table has a number to identify it and a title that describes its contents. Each table also has clearly labeled columns, the first naming the category being described (under Sex, Rank, Response, and Years Employed). Also included in each of the tables is a column titled *Frequency* that indicates the number of observations that fall into each

TABLE 14.1 ● Distribution of University Faculty by Sex

Sex	Frequency	%
Male	240	60
Female	160	40
All faculty	400	100

TABLE 14.2 ● Distribution of University Faculty by Rank

Rank	Frequency	%
Assistant professor	170	42.5
Associate professor	130	32.5
Full professor	100	25.0
All faculty	400	100.0

TABLE 14.3 ● Distribution of Responses to Question Regarding Relative Priority of Teaching as Compared to Research

Response	Frequency	%
Research valued much more highly	50	12.5
Research valued somewhat more highly	75	18.8
Research and teaching equally valued	150	37.5
Teaching valued somewhat more highly	75	18.8
Teaching valued much more highly	50	12.5
All responses	400	100.1

Note: Total percentage deviates from 100.0 as a result of rounding.

of the categories listed, and another indicating the percentage (%) of the total sample that is described by those categories. The bottom row of each table shows totals for each of the columns.

TABLE 14.4 ● Distribution of Number of Years Employed at State University				
Years Employed	Frequency	Cumulative Frequency	%	Cumulative %
1	13	13	3.25	3.25
2	12	25	3.00	6.25
3	12	37	3.00	9.25
4	11	48	2.75	12.00
5	11	59	2.75	14.75
6	9	68	2.25	17.00
7	9	77	2.25	19.25
8	8	85	2.00	21.25
9	12	97	3.00	24.25
10	13	110	3.25	27.50
11	16	126	4.00	31.50
12	17	143	4.25	35.75
13	19	162	4.75	40.50
14	20	182	5.00	45.50
15	21	203	5.25	50.75
16	23	226	5.75	56.50
17	23	249	5.75	62.25
18	25	274	6.25	68.50
19	25	299	6.25	74.75
20	23	322	5.75	80.50
21	19	341	4.75	85.25
22	18	359	4.50	89.75
23	16	375	4.00	93.75
24	13	388	3.25	97.00
25	12	400	3.00	100.00
All faculty	400		100.00	

TABLE 14.5 ● Distribution of Years Employed at State University, Using 5-Year Intervals				
Years Employed	F	Cumulative Frequency	%	Cumulative %
1–5 years	59	59	14.75	14.75
6–10 years	51	110	12.75	27.50
11–15 years	93	203	23.25	50.75
16–20 years	119	322	29.75	80.50
21–25 years	78	400	19.50	100.00
All faculty	400		100.00	

You can see from the bottom line on Tables 14.1–14.4 that 400 faculty members were involved in this fictitious sample and that complete information was obtained on all four variables for all 400 faculty. If data are missing for any of the variables, you'd normally include a category called "Missing" to show the completeness of your information. If total percentages deviate from 100, as occurs in Table 14.3, you'd also note the reason why. In this case it's because of rounding errors (as we've noted at the bottom of the table); this also would be the case if this was a "check all that apply" question where respondents are allowed to check more than one category.

The differences between the tables are also noteworthy. Table 14.4 is the only table to give *cumulative frequency* and *cumulative percentage (cumulative %)* across categories. These are included for Table 14.4 because it summarizes a sufficiently large number of categories and because there's a clear ordering on the "years employed" variable, from lowest to highest. Thus, it can be seen that approximately one-eighth (12.0 percent; $N = 48$) of the faculty have been employed at the university for 4 years or less; or it can be computed that approximately half the faculty (49.25 percent; $N = 197$) have been employed at the university for 15 years or more.

But using year-by-year categories in Table 14.4 leaves us with 25 different categories! Such a detailed inventory may be of interest in some situations, but hardly serves the purpose of data summary. Thus, you'd normally collapse so many categories into perhaps five to eight *aggregated categories* or *class intervals,* as has been done in Table 14.5. Category ranges should be of equal size (all those in Table 14.5 involve a 5-year range), should be based on an easily comprehended unit (e.g., 5 categories of 5 years each, rather than 7 categories of 3.57 years each), and should represent the full range of data. But note that such aggregation is achieved only at a cost; we've lost information on exact years of employment.

A second way to depict a frequency distribution is to graph it. Figure 14.1, which shows the distribution of the sex of the faculty members, is a simple *pie chart.* Such charts are best suited to situations in which a small number of categories are distributed reasonably equally (to avoid having many "slivers" of pie that are too small to be easily labeled) or for displaying how some entire entity (100 percent) is divided by category frequency.

Figure 14.2 uses a *bar graph* to show the distribution of academic ranks among the faculty in State University (or StateU), whereas Figure 14.3 shows a *histogram* of responses to the query regarding the relative value attached to teaching or research. Note that all three figures are numbered, and each has a title that identifies the variable being shown. Each segment of the pie, and each bar of the bar graph and the histogram, is also clearly labeled.

A fourth form of graph, known as a *frequency polygon* or *line graph,* is particularly useful when there's a relatively large number of categories. Figure 14.4 shows the distribution of the numbers of years of employment among university faculty members (using the data supplied in Table 14.4), while Figure 14.5 depicts a bar graph of the categorized years-of-employment variable (using the data supplied in Table 14.5). Once again, note that all figures are clearly numbered, titled, and labeled.

FIGURE 14.1 ● Faculty Membership by Sex

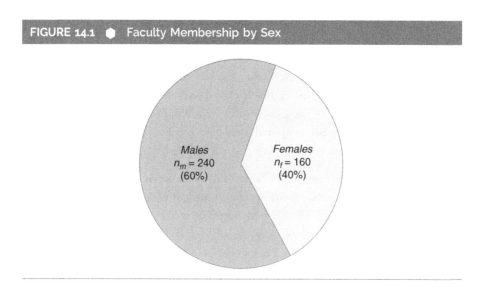

Males
$n_m = 240$
(60%)

Females
$n_f = 160$
(40%)

FIGURE 14.2 ⬣ Faculty Membership by Academic Rank

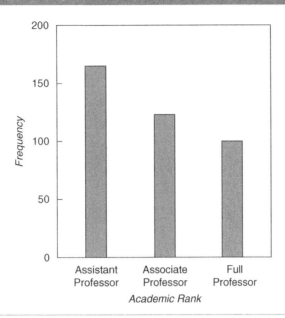

FIGURE 14.3 ⬣ Response to Query Regarding Priority Attached to Teaching as Compared to Research

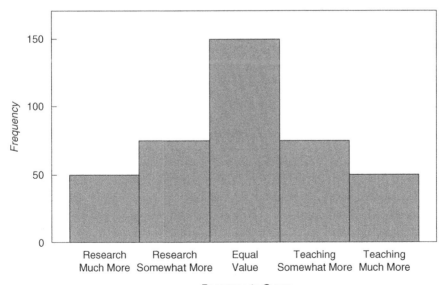

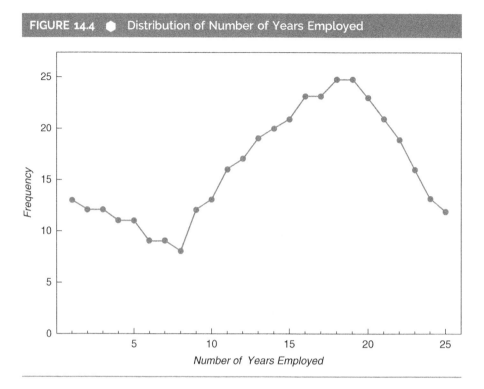

FIGURE 14.4 ● Distribution of Number of Years Employed

Measures of Central Tendency

After depicting the distribution of each variable, whether through frequency tables such as Tables 14.1–14.5 or graphically as in Figures 14.1–14.5, you are ready to begin describing the distributions statistically. First to be considered are measures of *central tendency,* or the "typical" datum for each variable. The three available to you are the mode, the median, and the mean.

The Mode

The mode identifies the score or scores that are "typical" in the sense that they represent "the most frequently occurring category." Thus, at StateU, the modal faculty member with respect to the sex variable is a male, and the modal academic rank is that of assistant professor. As for the query about the relative value attached to research and teaching, the modal response was that the two are valued equally. And finally, more of the current faculty were hired 18 or 19 years ago than at any other time. As these examples suggest, the mode can be used to describe data at any level of measurement.

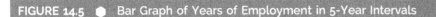

FIGURE 14.5 ● Bar Graph of Years of Employment in 5-Year Intervals

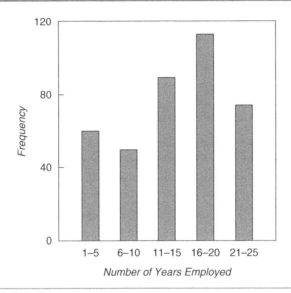

The Median

The second statistic for revealing central tendency is the **median**. This statistic identifies the "typical" datum as the one that splits the distribution in half: 50 percent of the sample data lie above it, and 50 percent lie below it. The median is thus the middle score, rather like the median on a highway that separates the two halves of the road. But note that the median is not always a meaningful statistic; the idea of a "median" sex, for example, seems absurd, since the "typical" case cannot even exist. Indeed, the median is useless with nominal-level variables because the order that is required to have a midpoint is absent. Medians can thus be used only with ordinal-, interval-, or ratio-level data. Returning to the data presented in Tables 14.2–14.4, you should see that the median academic rank at StateU is a relatively junior associate professor (since the middle case is only 7.5 percent beyond the assistant professor category), the median opinion on the attitude item is one of valuing research and teaching about equally, and the median number of years employed at StateU is 15.

The Mean

The final measure of central tendency to consider is the **mean**, or what you may know as the arithmetic average. It is computed by simply taking the sum of the values and dividing by the total number of scores. Thus, for example, if your midterm marks in the five courses you're taking were 76, 79, 82, 93, and 81, the mean would be the sum of those marks (76 + 79 + 82 + 93 + 81 = 411) divided by the number of courses (N = 5), or 411/5 = 82.2.

Since a mean is computed by adding and then dividing numbers, it has little meaning if the numbers are assigned arbitrarily. Thus, the mean has even more limited utility than the median when it comes to the kinds of variables for which it may be meaningful. Certainly it would be meaningless for nominal variables (e.g., a mean sex?), and it should be used cautiously or not at all with ordinal data (depending on the degree of arbitrariness of the coding scheme). One place you do see it used with ordinal data is with ranked data, where it is not unusual for people to compute an average rank. Problems are fewer with interval data and nonexistent with ratio-level data. Thus, if the five responses to the attitude item (Table 14.3) were coded 1 through 5, we could say with little discomfort that the mean response is 3.0 (research and teaching equally valued). And you should be able to calculate (from Table 14.4) that the mean length of employment at StateU is 14.3 years.

In sum, the mode, the median, and the mean are three descriptive statistics; each gives a picture of the "central tendency" of the distribution of scores you've obtained. Each expresses an "average" or "typical" score in its own way: for the mode, central tendency is identified as the most frequently occurring score; for the median, the typical score is the one that lies on the 50th percentile, splitting the distribution in half; for the mean, central tendency is defined as the arithmetic average. Let's review the results we obtained with the variables we observed at StateU.

Sex is a *categorical* variable, so the only measure of central tendency that seems appropriate to use is the mode. The modal faculty member at StateU is a male.

Our attention then turns to academic rank. Using the mode, we find that the most frequently occurring academic rank is that of assistant professor. The *ordinal* nature of the academic-rank data also leads us to use the median. But the median gives us a different indication of central tendency—that of junior associate professor—than does the mode.

Since responses to the query concerning the relative value associated with research and teaching represent an *interval*-level variable, mode, median, and mean are all appropriate statistics. Here, all three statistics point in the same direction: "equal value associated with research and teaching."

The last variable on which we have information is "years of employment at StateU." Because this is a *ratio*-level variable, mode, median, and mean are all appropriate statistics. But here they give three different answers regarding the "typical" faculty member. The *modal* faculty member was hired 18 or 19 years ago (see Table 12.4); the *median* faculty member was hired 15 years ago; and the *mean* faculty member was hired 14.3 years ago. Why do the mode, the median, and the mean point sometimes in the same and sometimes in different directions?

Symmetry and Skew

In order to answer that question, we have to consider one more characteristic of distributions: *symmetry* versus skew. A symmetrical distribution is any distribution in which the two sides are essentially mirror images. Thus, the three distributions shown in Figure 14.6(a)–(c) are all symmetrical, even though their shapes are otherwise very different. Whenever we have a symmetrical distribution (as was the case in Table 14.3 and its counterpart, Figure 14.3, with respect to the attitude variable), the mode, the median, and the mean will all lie in exactly the same place. When our distributions are *asymmetrical*, or "skewed," the situation changes.

Look at the three graphs included in Figure 14.7. You should recognize immediately that Figure 14.7(b) shows a symmetrical distribution, while Figure 14.7(a) and (c) show skewed distributions. In order to distinguish between the two kinds of asymmetrical distributions, mathematicians use the convention of describing the direction of the skew based on where the distribution's thinner end, or "tail," is. Thus, Figure 14.7(a) is referred to as a "positively skewed" distribution, since its tail is at the positive end of the number line; Figure 14.7(c) is referred to as a "negatively skewed" distribution, since its tail is at the negative end of the number line.

As noted above, when distributions are symmetrical, the mode, median, and mean all will lie in the same place; Figure 14.7(b) illustrates this situation. But when distributions are asymmetrical, or skewed, the situation changes. Since the mode is by definition the most frequently occurring score, it remains at the highest "bump" in the distribution. The mean and the median, though, will be differentially affected by the extreme scores that lie at the distribution's "skew" or "tail" end. The mean, which is particularly affected by that tendency, will be "pulled" farthest away from the modal value. The median also will be affected but less so; it normally will lie between the mean and the mode.

How to Lie With Statistics

While the statistics we have been dealing with thus far have been extremely "simple," they're also extremely important. *Any* data analysis should begin with an inspection of

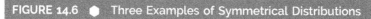

FIGURE 14.6 ● Three Examples of Symmetrical Distributions

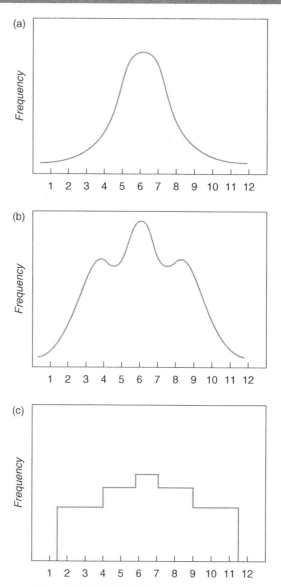

raw univariate distributions so that you can see how the variables are distributed and choose accordingly the type of statistics you report. In general, the more the better. Modes can be reported for any type of data. Medians are appropriate when the data

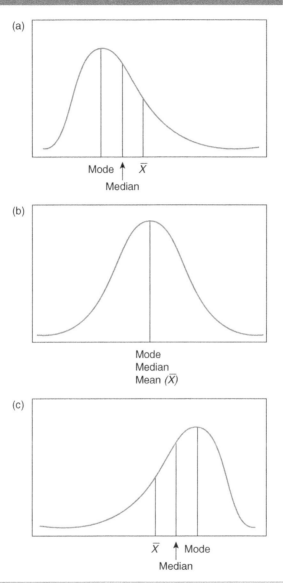

FIGURE 14.7 ● Examples of (a) a Positively Skewed Distribution, (b) a Normal Distribution, and (c) a Negatively Skewed Distribution

(a)

Mode ↑ $\overline{X}$
Median

(b)

Mode
Median
Mean $(\overline{X})$

(c)

$\overline{X}$ ↑ Mode
Median

have at least ordinal qualities; they are also the "better" statistic with interval- and ratio-level data when the distribution is skewed, especially when there are a few extreme scores (also known as **outliers**). Means always should be cited for interval-

and ratio-level data, but should be used more cautiously with ordinal-level data and with highly skewed distributions.

Not showing univariate frequency distributions and being selective in the statistic to report are favorite techniques of those propagandists who use statistics to provide distorted images. The whole idea of using statistics is to concisely summarize a set of data; implicit are the ideas that such summarization is a relatively neutral process and that summary statistics give a representative picture of the data as a whole. People's general faith in those suppositions allows the unscrupulous to manipulate statistics to their own ends. For example, tourist or investment brochures may extol how splendid an area Upper Oceana is, noting that tourism and property costs are very reasonable despite the fact that most Upper Oceanans live in comparative opulence—the average annual income is in fact a fairly comfortable $95,455 per year! Sounds great, don't you think? If only the rest of us were so well off! The impression we get is that the average Upper Oceanan is doing very well financially; perhaps some are doing better or worse, but the average standard of living, at least as measured in economic terms, seems quite high.

But examining the entire distribution of incomes leaves us with a rather different impression. It seems that for every Upper Oceanan who has an annual income of $1,000,000, there are 10 others who earn a measly $5,000 a year. Thus, it turns out that the "average" (i.e., the mean) masks a situation where a few individuals live in wealth, while the majority live in poverty. Generally speaking, the median should be reported along with the mean, since the median is less distorted by deviations from symmetry. Examining the univariate distributions is always a wise move, as is presenting them in a research report.

Examples of individuals and groups using statistics to mislead and distort are so numerous that they could easily fill a book. Indeed, readers interested in an enjoyable and thoughtful book on that topic should have a look at Darrell Huff's *How to lie with statistics* (1954; reissued in 1982 and 1993) or Daniel Levitin's (2017) *Weaponized lies: How to think critically in the post-truth era*. Both books do an excellent job of explaining basic descriptive statistics and showing how they're often misused to distort and mislead. An awareness of such tricks should be part of everyone's education as a citizen and consumer. As a social and health scientist, your job is to appreciate such techniques as things to *avoid*; as a prospective member of the social and health science community, your task is to be open and complete in your descriptions and analysis of data.

Measures of Variability

Measures of central tendency convey one aspect of the nature of the distribution: the "typical" or "average" score. But distributions also can differ in their *variability*.

While measures of central tendency attempt to describe a distribution in terms of *similarities* (by focusing on a "most common" or "typical" score), measures of variability focus on *differences* among the scores (by attempting to generate measures of *dispersion*). So variability represents a key stepping stone in our analytic venture, since it's the basic "stuff" that social and health science is trying to explain.

The Range

The most basic expression of the degree of dispersion that exists is given by the range. When dealing with categorical or ordinal variables, where any numerical coding that's involved is relatively arbitrary, providing the range involves giving a full enumeration of all the categories in which observations were obtained. This allows critical readers to inspect your categories to see what range of categories has been included. You also can articulate the range of frequencies that exist in your categories: this will tell your reader whether there is an approximately equal distribution of people across categories or whether they are more prevalent in one than another. Of course, such information also can be made available in tables or graphs of univariate frequency distributions.

With interval-level data, where the numbers begin to have some intrinsic meaning, the range is expressed as the difference between the maximum and minimum values. Thus, the range of responses on the "years employed" variable (see Table 14.4) was 24 years—from the most recent hiring, 1 year ago, to the earliest, 25 years ago (i.e., $25 - 1 = 24$).

Although the range is an important statistic to report, it's not sufficiently definitive. The difficulty is revealed by inspection of Figure 14.8, which shows two different distributions superimposed on each other. The distributions are symmetrical; have the same mode, median, and mean; and have exactly the same range, but only a cursory visual inspection is needed to see that they're still very different. One of the distributions is very dispersed, with scores spread across the whole range. The other is much more compressed, with a huge majority of scores squished in very close to the distribution's mean, a pattern that reflects very little variation.

Another problem with the range as a descriptive statistic is that it only takes one weird/extreme outlier to change it dramatically and thereby give an unrepresentative

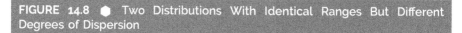

FIGURE 14.8 ● Two Distributions With Identical Ranges But Different Degrees of Dispersion

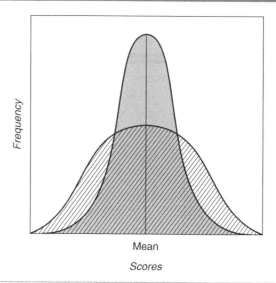

Frequency

Mean

Scores

impression of the degree of variation that exists. For this reason, many researchers prefer to use a measure known as the **interquartile range (IQR)**.

The "quartile" part comes from the fact you begin by dividing the distribution into quarters. If we look at the distribution of scores in Table 14.4 regarding "years of employment," for example, we can see that the 25 percent point (marking the "1st quartile") comes in the category of people who have been at StateU for "10 years"; the 50 percent point (marking the "2nd quartile" or median) comes in the category "14 years"; and that the 75 percent point (marking the "3rd quartile") comes in the category "20 years."

The "inter" part of the term comes from our desire to look at the distance between the first and third quartile points, that is, we want to lop off the extreme scorers in the top 25 percent and bottom 25 percent of the distribution and then look at the range that describes that middle 50 percent.

The IQR for the data in Table 14.4, therefore, is $20-10 = 10$ years. In and of itself, this statistic is not particularly meaningful, but it would be, for example, if we wanted to compare the distribution of years of employment at StateU to that at other universities. This brings us to yet another limitation of both the range and the

IQR as descriptive statistics: although they are useful for comparing relatively similar types of distributions using similar units and similar categories, they are relatively meaningless in and of themselves and cannot be used to compare different distributions.

Standard Deviations and Variances

The challenge, therefore, is to develop a statistic that not only can convey differences in variability between similar-based distributions such as the two superimposed in Figure 14.8 but also has broader utility across a wider range of distributions.

The place mathematicians began to look for this statistic was at the concept of deviations from the mean, which seems reasonable enough, given that the variability we are trying to get a handle on involves variability around that central point. We can follow through the logic of it by starting with a distribution of scores, computing its mean, checking out how much each score we have deviates from the mean, and then maybe finding an "average" deviation around the mean. The technique we will use here is to take a situation where we "know" what the answer "should" be—because we start with a situation that has been constructed to deal with a certain type of problem—in order to try out different possibilities to see what will give us an acceptable answer. In this case, we created the example in Table 14.6 to show how misleading the range can be and to pose the problem of how we can differentiate between two distributions that have identical characteristics in many respects (e.g., same range; same mean, median, and mode; same number of observations), but that are so clearly different in their dispersion.

Table 14.6 shows two distributions of scores, under the left-hand columns "Thin" and "Dispersed." Both columns have the same range (i.e., in each the lowest score is 1, and the highest score is 9), and the mode for each distribution is 5. We'll leave it to you to do the computations that show that they also have the same median and mode (5.0 in each case). The table's third and fourth columns show how much each of the scores deviates from the mean of its group; at the bottom of each of those columns you can see the sum of the deviations about the mean. Funny thing—the total works out to zero in both cases!

Indeed, it turns out that this will always be the case, since the mean is in fact the numerical value for which the sum of deviations is zero: all the pluses and minuses will inevitably cancel one another out, and they'll always add up to zero. Just adding up deviations from the mean would thus seem to be a dead end; they don't do the job we require of them.

TABLE 14.6 ⬡ Describing Thin and Dispersed Distributions					
Scores		**Deviation From Mean**		**Squared Deviations**	
Thin	**Dispersed**	**Thin**	**Dispersed**	**Thin**	**Dispersed**
1	1	−4	−4	16	16
2	2	−3	−3	9	9
3	2	−2	−3	4	9
3	3	−2	−2	4	4
4	3	−1	−2	1	4
4	3	−1	−2	1	4
4	4	−1	−1	1	1
4	4	−1	−1	1	1
5	4	0	−1	0	1
5	4	0	−1	0	1
5	5	0	0	0	0
5	5	0	0	0	0
5	5	0	0	0	0
5	5	0	0	0	0
5	6	0	+1	0	1
5	6	0	+1	0	1
6	6	+1	+1	1	1
6	6	+1	+1	1	1
6	7	+1	+2	1	4
6	7	+1	+2	1	4
7	7	+2	+2	4	4
7	8	+2	+3	4	9
8	8	+3	+3	9	9
9	9	+5	+4	16	16
Sum = 120	Sum = 120	Sum = 0	Sum = 0	Sum = 74	Sum = 100
N = 24	N = 24			Mean = 3.08	Mean = 4.17
Mean = 5.0	Mean = 5.0			$\sqrt{3.08} = 1.75$	$\sqrt{4.17} = 2.04$
				S.D. = 1.75	S.D. = 2.04

Not being the sort of folk who give up quickly, however, and always ready with a handy technique to take care of inconvenient things like pluses and minuses that cancel one another out, mathematicians next looked at the possibility of taking the absolute magnitudes of the deviations (i.e., ignoring the sign of the difference), but that didn't work out very well in more complex algebraic calculations. Then they came up with the possibility of *squaring* all the deviations about the mean. The nice thing about squaring each deviation is that it makes every number a positive number (e.g., −5 squared and +5 squared both equal 25); it also gives greater weight to deviations the farther they are away from the mean (e.g., a 1-unit distance, whether plus or minus, when squared, gives 1; 5 points of distance, whether plus or minus, when squared, gives 25). Columns 5 and 6 of Table 14.6 show what happens when we begin looking at the squared deviations; the sum of the squared deviations is given at the bottom of each column for the respective distributions. Do we have success?

The sum of the squared deviations about the mean is indeed greater for the dispersed distribution than it is for the thinner one. But our success is more apparent than real. Although the sum of the squared deviations about the mean is indeed successful at differentiating between the two distributions shown in Table 14.6, it turns out that other examples can easily be invented that make our success short-lived. More specifically, note that the dispersed distribution and the thin distribution in Table 14.6 have exactly the same number of people in them. What would happen if we took the thin distribution and simply doubled the number of scores we have? The range would be the same; the mean, median, and mode would all be the same; and the form of the distribution would be the same, but suddenly our sum of the squared deviations would be twice as large, suggesting that the thin distribution is even *more* variable than the dispersed one! That's a problem.

Fortunately, the problem is short-lived as well. The hint for a solution comes from the fact that our problem seems to be related to the number of observations. The solution comes when, instead of merely summing all the squared deviations about the mean, we then proceed to divide that sum by the number of observations, thereby giving us the *average* squared deviation about the mean. Once we do that, everything in the hypothetical examples works out splendidly. We see that the average squared deviation about the mean is substantially larger for the dispersed distribution in Table 14.6 than it is for the thin one (4.17 versus 3.08, respectively)—just as, logically, we feel it should be. And if you take the thin distribution and double the number of observations we made, it turns out that, when we divide that doubly large sum of squared deviations by the doubled number of observations, we still end up with exactly the same average squared deviation. Once again, this is consistent with the logical notion that indicators of the form of a distribution, in terms of its variability, should not be influenced by other considerations such as sample size.

If you follow the reasoning above, you now understand the basis of two incredibly important statistics that form the basis of analysis for a wide array of statistical techniques. The summary statistic we ended up with above—the average of the squared deviations—is known in statistical parlance as the **variance** of a distribution.

As for the second statistic of importance, the one weakness of the variance as a measure of dispersion is that it's expressed in *squared* units rather than in our original scale of measurement. To make our statistic more meaningful in our original context, recall that we originally squared all the scores to get around the problem of having the pluses and minuses cancel each other out. Thus, to get back to our original units of measurement, all we need do is take the *square root* of the variance statistic. Given that we originally squared the deviations and, after finding their average deviation from the mean, are now taking the square root, our new statistic simply reflects the average deviation about the mean that is present in our distribution. That statistic is called the **standard deviation**. We will hear of it again.

INFERENTIAL STATISTICS

As the previous section stated, the notion of variability is a crucial one in social and health science. It's the variance in life that we spend the most time trying to explain: Why are things one way one time and a different way another time? To use the example of the faculty at State University once again, it's all well and good to say that the largest number of faculty members are assistant professors, but an *understanding* of university life requires that we explain why some people are assistant professors, others are associates, and still others are full professors. And while it's nice to know the distribution of length of employment, things become even more interesting when we start asking why members of some social groups seem more or less likely to get hired than others, why and how these propensities might change over time, why more or fewer people are hired in 1 year than in another.

The rest of this chapter discusses two general classes of statistics that examine such relationships: *measures of association* (i.e., where the question of interest is in how two or more variables "go together" or are associated with one another) and *measures of difference* (i.e., where the general question of interest is typically whether the means of two or more groups differ). This distinction is to some degree contrived, but as you'll discover near the end of the chapter, it's a useful pedagogical distinction to make at this time.

Examining Relationships Among Categorical Variables
Cross-tabulation and Contingency Tables

The researcher who's interested in examining the relationship between two nominal or categorical variables will normally begin by cross-tabulating them, that is, creating a celled matrix or contingency table where the joint (or bivariate, where *bi* = two and *variate* = variable) frequencies are shown. For example, the State University (StateU) scenario involves two categorical variables: sex (male or female) and academic rank (assistant, associate, or full professor). The *univariate* frequency distributions for those two variables were depicted in Tables 14.1 and 14.2; their *bivariate* frequency is illustrated in Table 14.7. Such bivariate tables are a purely descriptive technique but are an important prerequisite for *inferential* analysis.

Like other tables, this one has an identifying number, a title that denotes its contents, and clearly labeled variable names and attendant levels. Across the table are three columns, each signifying an academic rank. At the bottom of each column are the (univariate) column *marginals* (i.e., totals): 170, 130, and 100 for the three ranks, as in Table 14.2. The two rows, labeled on the left side of the table, show the sex variable. On the table's right-hand side are the (univariate) row marginals: 160 females and 240 males, as in Table 14.1. The total number of faculty members, 400, is shown at the bottom right-hand corner of Table 14.7; there, we cross-check to ensure that the total number of faculty members by rank (170 + 130 + 100 = 400) is the same as the total number by sex (160 + 240 = 400), and it is.

Within each cell of the table are the bivariate frequencies; that is, the number of people who manifest the joint characteristics of a given sex at a given rank. The

TABLE 14.7 ● The Cross-Tabulation of Sex by Academic Rank for State University Data

		Academic Rank			
		Assistant Professor	Associate Professor	Full Professor	Row Marginals
Sex	Female	90 Ex = 68	50 Ex = 52	20 Ex = 40	160
	Male	80 Ex = 102	80 Ex = 78	80 Ex = 60	240
	Column marginals	170	130	100	400

number 90 in the top left-hand corner, for example, shows that there were 90 female assistant professors on the faculty at StateU. (Don't worry about the "Ex" numbers below those for the moment; we'll get to those in the next section.) You can see that the number of female faculty members decreases as you go up the ranks (90 assistants, 50 associates, 20 full professors), while male faculty members are spread evenly across the ranks (80/80/80). It's also easy to compute that while roughly 53 percent of all assistant professors are female (i.e., 90/170 $\times$ 100), only 38 percent of associate professors and 20 percent of full professors are females; conversely, 47 percent of assistants, 62 percent of associates, and 80 percent of full professors are males.

Inclusion of a bivariate frequency distribution (also called a **contingency table**) is a very helpful way to summarize and represent your data. In this case, we immediately get the impression that sex and rank are associated at StateU: female faculty members seem especially underrepresented at the senior levels of the academic hierarchy. Another equally appropriate way to represent the data would be to use a grouped or clustered bar graph. Figure 14.9 shows such a graph for the "Rank by Sex" data of Table 14.7.

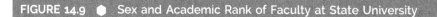

FIGURE 14.9 ● Sex and Academic Rank of Faculty at State University

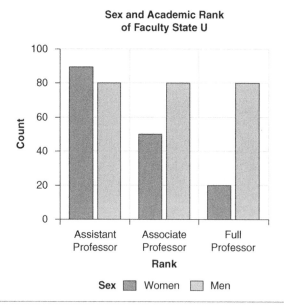

The Chi-Square Distribution

But a social or health scientist researching this situation would not stop there. They would first want to know whether the joint variation of sex and rank we observe is still within the realm of what we might expect from mere chance variation or whether it exceeds those bounds. This is a question of the *statistical significance* of the results. In order to determine it, we need some sort of measure by which we can decide how likely or unlikely we are to obtain the particular distribution we observe. This is given by a statistic known as **chi-square**, which allows us to assess whether two categorical variables are associated more strongly than would be expected on the basis of chance variation alone. Doing so requires us first of all to compute a chi-square statistic to describe the particular pattern of frequencies and then compare our chi-square statistic to the chi-square distributions to see how likely that particular chi-square value is to be observed.

The chi-square statistic is based on a comparison between what we'd *expect* on the basis of chance variation alone, i.e., if the two variables were indeed independent, and what we actually *observe*. To compute the expected values, we take the univariate marginals (i.e., row and column totals) as givens. An *expected frequency* is then computed for each of the cells, depending on the relevant column and row marginal for each cell. In essence, we thus say, "Given that there are more male (240) than female (160) faculty members, and given that there are more assistants (170) than associates (130), and more of both than full professors (100), how many female assistant professors would we expect there to be if there were no association between rank and sex?" We do that by taking the column marginal for assistant professors (170), multiplying that by the row marginal for females (160), and dividing by the total number of observations (400) to get the expected frequency of 68 that you see in Table 14.7 in the "female/assistant professor" cell (i.e., Ex = 68). Thus, if there were *no* association between sex and rank, we'd *expect* there to be 68 female assistant professors; in fact, we observe many more ($n = 90$).

The same procedure is followed for each and every cell. To obtain the number of expected female full professors, for example, you'd take the row marginal for females (160), multiply by the column marginal for full professors (100), divide by the total number of observations (400), and get Ex = 40, i.e., many more than the 20 female full professors we actually observe. We'll leave it to you to check our calculations on the other four cells; just follow the same rules noted above (i.e., relevant column marginal, multiplied by relevant row marginal, divided by total number of observations). You can check your calculations by summing your expected frequencies for each row and column; they should add up to the actual marginal totals (since the marginals are treated as givens). For example, note that the expected frequencies that we computed for males in each of the cells in that row (102, 78, 60) add up to 240, which is indeed the total number of males we have; similarly, the expected values for the associate professor column that we computed (52, 78) add up to 130, which is indeed the total number of associate professors among the faculty at StateU.

If the math of what we've just described seems a bit mystical, let's try and work it through a bit more conceptually. We start off with two basic facts, which is that there are more male faculty members than female ones (240 versus 160), and that the most common rank is assistant professor, next is associate, and finally full (170 versus 130 versus 100). Now, if we take as a given that, out of the 400 faculty members, 160/400 or 40 percent are female, then shouldn't we expect 40 percent of the professors at each rank to be female? But how many would that be? Well, we have 170 assistant professors, so 40 percent of that would be 68, which is in fact the expected value we computed. At the other end, there are 100 full professors at StateU, so if there was no association between sex and rank we would expect 40 percent of them to be women as well. The math there is easy—40 percent of 100 is 40, so logically we'd expect 40 of them to be full professors, which is indeed the expected value we computed.

Whichever way you get there, we now have *two* different bivariate frequency distributions: one of *observed* frequencies and another of *expected* frequencies. The chi-square statistic involves a comparison between the two. To compute it, we first take the *difference* between what we expected and what we observed for each cell. For example, in the "male/assistant professor" cell, we observed 80, but would have expected 102 if there were no relationship between sex and rank and if nothing other than chance had been operating—a deviation of $80 - 102 = -22$. But note that if we observed 22 *fewer* male/assistant professors than expected, then, given the marginal, we must have had 22 *more* female/assistant professors than expected; indeed, that is the case (i.e., $90 - 68 = 22$). We once again have the problem that a simple summation of all the deviations will add to zero; the mathematical solution, as with the variance statistic, is to square those deviations to get rid of the pluses and minuses. Thus, for the "male/assistant professor" cell, our squared deviation statistic is $(-22)^2$, or 484.

At the same time, we also must acknowledge that a deviation of 22 will be differentially "surprising," depending on the number we expected in the cell. If we had expected 500 people in the cell, for example, a deviation of 22 people might not seem especially large; if we had expected 50, on the other hand, a deviation of 22 would be quite substantial. To take into account the relative magnitude of the deviation, we take the squared deviation statistic we computed above (484) and divide it by the expected value for that cell (102), to come up with 4.7.

The final step is to *sum* these individual cell statistics across all six cells, in order to create our final chi-square statistic for our contingency table. You should compute these values and the total for yourself, but the values we obtained (running from left to right across successive rows of Table 14.7) are 7.1, 0.1, 10.0, 4.7, 0.1, and 6.7, which sum to 28.7.

But what exactly does 28.7 mean? Is that big? small? surprising? expected? We must take our sample statistic and compare it to the appropriate chi-square distribution in order to answer those questions. Appendix A shows a listing of critical values for different probability levels; pay particular attention to the .05 and .01 levels. These are values that our sample's chi-square statistic must *meet* or *exceed* before we're prepared to say, with 95 percent or 99 percent confidence, that the deviation between expected and observed values in our distribution was *statistically significant* (i.e., greater than we would expect on the basis of chance variation alone). But Appendix A gives a lengthy list of such criterion values. Which one is "ours"?

Degrees of Freedom. Note the column at the left of Appendix A, the one titled *df* (**degrees of freedom**). The reason we need that column recalls the problem we faced in calculating deviation statistics. The magnitude of a chi-square statistic will be sensitive to the number of cells included in the analysis. Our example table had two rows and three columns (or six cells), and we derived a chi-square value of 28.7. Would a table with three rows and four columns (i.e., 12 cells) have resulted in a higher chi-square value merely because of a greater number of cells? The answer, all else being equal, is yes. Thus, we must take the *size* of the contingency table into account, and we do so by considering the number of degrees of freedom it possesses.

Degrees of freedom *(df)* is a very hard concept to nail down, although you see it whenever an inferential statistic is being discussed. At its core is the notion that the theoretical distribution will vary in form depending on the number of parameters that are free to vary. That again sounds very mystical, but let us give you a trivial example. Have you ever watched *American Idol* or *America's Got Talent* or *So You Think You Can Dance*? They all follow the same general formula where thousands of people who want to try and win the competition start off by auditioning for a set of judges, and then, as the season progresses, there is round after round of eliminations until the huge mass of people who started the process are whittled down to three on the final night of the show. At the very end, the final three people stand on stage and the winner is to be announced. Let's call them Alejandro, Madison, and Laine. But of course, the show wants to build the suspense and maintain it as long as possible, so they go in reverse order. When the third place winner is about to be announced, how many people could be the third place winner? Well, at that point, it could be all three. Let's say that Laine is announced as number 3, and he goes off to the side. How many people are there who could be in second place? At that point, there is still lots of suspense because it could be either Alejandro or Madison. Let's say they announce that Madison has come in second. Is there any suspense at that point? No. Why? Because if Laine came in third, and Madison came in second, then it *has* to be Alejandro who won the competition. In statistical terms, we would say that there are two degrees of freedom in the announcements because for two announcements there is more than one possible outcome, but once we know who those two are, there is no more freedom to maneuver; it *must* be the one remaining who wins.

With contingency tables, where the distribution of data is framed in terms of certain numbers of *rows* and *columns,* the *df* we have in our example of Table 14.7 are constrained by the fact there are two rows and three columns in our table; the number of cell values free to vary, given the marginal values, is relatively small.

Let's try and follow the *American Idol* logic again by telling you how we went about creating that contingency table, in order to have an example that we could use as an illustration. Our earlier presentation of the univariate frequency distributions at StateU (Tables 14.1 and 14.2) had established our givens (i.e., the observed univariate marginals). Because we wanted to create a situation that in fact still exists at many universities, which is that sex *is* related to rank, we first decided that we'd put most of the "female" observations into the "female assistant professors" category. We could have chosen any number from 0 to 160 to put in that cell, but we chose 90.

Then we went to the next cell. What limitations did we have? We know (from the given marginals) that there are 160 females, and now we also "know" from our choice above that 90 of them are assistant professors; thus, when we went to create a number for the "female/*associate* professors" cell, we could choose any number from 0 to 70 (since $160 - 90 = 70$) as the number for the cell. Like the first (female/assistant) cell, it had constraints but was still *free to vary.* We chose to put the number 50 in that cell. The process continued: we went to the third cell—female full professors. But here our choices were no longer free to vary. Given that there were 160 female faculty members in total, and given our two choices in the female/assistant (90) and female/associate (50) cells, the number in the third cell *had to* be 20—the *only* number that could go there if the marginal was to remain as set.

The same was now true of all the other cells. There were 90 female assistant professors; if the column marginal for assistants ($n = 170$) is to remain, there *must* be 80 male assistant professors. Given there are 130 associate professors, and 50 of them are female, then there *had to* be 80 male associate professors. Similarly, the number of male full professors *must* be 80.

In sum, as we went through the process of creating the above example, there really were only two cell values where we could make choices when setting the observed cell values. Mathematically, you would say that in this 2 × 3 contingency table, despite the fact that there were six cells, we "really" had only two *degrees of freedom* that we could vary. After those two, *every* choice was "determined," *given* the marginals.

A formula has been derived that allows you to easily determine the degrees of freedom for a contingency table. Take the number of rows (2 in our case) and the number of columns (3 in our case), subtract 1 from each (i.e., $2-1 = 1$; $3-1 = 2$), and then multiply those two numbers together (i.e., $1 \times 2 = 2$). Mathematically, the formula is $df = (R-1)(C-1)$, where R is the number of rows, and C is the number of columns.

Thus, we now know that the particular values that are "ours" in Appendix A are the ones associated with $2df$; our chi-square value must meet or exceed 5.99 in order to be considered "statistically significant" at the 95 percent level of confidence (i.e., because the probability of observing our results on the basis of chance alone is less than 5 percent, or $p < .05$) and must exceed 9.21 in order to be considered statistically significant at the 99 percent level of confidence (i.e., $p < .01$). Both of these values are in fact handily exceeded by our chi-square statistic of 28.7. Thus, we can say with 99 percent confidence that the suggestion that rank and sex are *not* associated at StateU is probably false. The likelihood of our observing these results by chance variation alone is so improbable that we reject the "null" hypothesis—that rank and sex are *not* related—and infer that sex and rank probably *are* related.

Interpreting the Result. So what does our finding really mean? No matter how we slice it, males appear more likely to have been promoted up the ranks than females. Is this indicative of biased promotional practices at StateU? Is it yet another social example of how an "old boys' network" can make it hard for women to succeed? Certainly the data presented are consistent with that explanation; this is exactly the sort of bivariate distribution we would expect if discriminatory promotional policies were in place. But are there rival plausible explanations to consider?

One such explanation might assert that the significant association between sex and rank we observe is in fact not a result of discriminatory *promotional* policies, but rather the legacy of discriminatory *hiring* practices that acted to keep women out of university and graduate schools, and hence out of the academy, for many years. Thus, since women at StateU may not have been adequately represented on the faculty until recently, perhaps those who are at StateU are still at too junior a stage of their careers to have accumulated the sort of scholarly record that should lead to promotion.

If that were the case, then we'd expect to see it in our data. For example, we'd expect there to be a significant association between sex and length of employment, such as seems apparent in Table 14.8. We can see that the propensity to hire female faculty members has changed considerably over time. Of those still remaining from the hirings of 21–25 years ago, only 21.8 percent of the faculty hired were female,[1] while in succeeding 5-year categories, the hiring rate for females went up to 34.5 percent, then 47.3 percent, then 50.9 percent, and finally to 54.2 percent. We'll leave it to you to work out whether the chi-square value for that contingency table is indeed significant. If it is, any interpretation must still consider the impact of *mortality* on the results.

Even if we could take the bivariate frequencies of Table 14.8 at face value, the hypothesis that *promotional* practices are discriminatory has not necessarily been negated. We cannot simply ignore the earlier finding, which revealed proportionately fewer women appearing in the higher ranks. With this additional finding of differential likelihood of hiring females over time, several rival explanations remain plausible: (1) promotional practices favor males; (2) former discriminatory hiring practices mean that few women have been on faculty long enough to warrant promotion;

TABLE 14.8 ● Cross-tabulation of Sex by Length of Employment at State University

		Length of Employment					
		1–5 Years	6–10 Years	11–15 Years	16–20 Years	21–25 Years	Row Totals
Sex	Female	32 Ex = 23.6	26 Ex = 20.4	44 Ex = 37.2	41 Ex = 47.6	17 Ex = 31.2	160
	Male	27 Ex = 35.4	25 Ex = 30.6	49 Ex = 55.8	78 Ex = 71.4	61 Ex = 46.8	240
	Column totals	59	51	93	119	78	400

---

[1]The figure 21.8 percent is not in the table. We computed it by noting that in the column "21–25 Years," there were 78 people hired, 17 of whom were women. This works out to $(17/78) \times 100 = 21.8$ percent.

(3) both of the above statements are true to some extent; or (4) neither of the above statements is true, and some other variable(s) account for the result. For example, it may be that promotional and hiring policies have always been equitable, but the problem may lie elsewhere, for example, not enough women had access to university, entered graduate school, graduated with doctoral degrees, or whatever.

The next step in any comprehensive analysis would be to seek out data that bear on those various explanations. You might, for example, attempt to gather archival data on the comparative success ratios of male and female applicants for promotion, or the comparative research and teaching records of male and female faculty members at the time they were considered for promotion, to check for any evidence that more stringent criteria were imposed on female candidates than on males. Or you might want to consider whether the criteria themselves favor males over females, given existing social structures and vocational constraints. Alternatively, you might turn your attention to graduate-school admissions records or to proportions of male and female job applicants over time. Each set of data would shed further light on the dynamics of this microcosm of society and how it has changed (or not) over time. The only constraints will be the availability of data and the analytical intelligence of the researcher.

Examining Relationships Among Continuous Variables
The Limits of Contingency Tables

The chi-square statistic discussed above is a useful measure of association when dealing with two categorical variables where each has relatively few levels. Although it's possible to use this type of statistic with larger numbers of categories, you need reasonably large expected cell frequencies in order to do the analysis with some degree of mathematical integrity; thus, sample size requirements rapidly become prohibitive as the size of the contingency table increases. For example, the contingency table involving sex and rank was a 2 × 3 table with six cells; with a minimal requirement of 5–10 expected observations per cell (or 30–60 observations in total), the 400 observations we had were clearly adequate to perform the analysis.

But suppose we want to look at the relationship between the length of time faculty members have been employed at StateU and their opinions on the relative value of teaching and research. The length of time ranged from 1 to 25 years (i.e., 25 levels), and the scale they responded with had 5 levels. We *could* cross-tabulate those two variables, but the contingency table would be 5 rows deep by 25 columns wide—125 cells! With the requirement for minimal expected frequencies of 5–10 per cell, we'd need somewhere in the order of 600–1,200 observations before the statistical analysis even began to become meaningful. Suddenly, our 400 observations look very puny.

Of course, we could always collapse cells in order to help our data fit the statistical requirements. Instead of the 5 levels on the opinion item, we could collapse down to 3: (1) research valued more than teaching (i.e., categories 1 and 2), (2) research and teaching equally valued (category 3), and (3) teaching valued more than research (categories 3 and 5). Similarly, we could group "years of employment" data into 5 levels of 5 years each (as was done in Table 14.5). These two steps would reduce our 5 × 25 (or 125-cell) table down to a 3 × 5 (or 15-cell) table, which would clearly be more reasonable, given our total number of observations.

But while we *can* do that, most researchers would be reluctant to do so, other than for simplifying, illustrative purposes. We'd lose too much information. Another alternative would be preferred: the scatter-plot diagram. Then we could go further, assessing whether the relationship between variables is linear by using the Pearson product-moment correlation coefficient (otherwise known as **Pearson's** *r*).

Scatter-plot Diagrams

A scatter-plot diagram is a graph that depicts the status of each respondent on the two variables whose association we're interested in assessing. It offers the great advantage of allowing us to "see" the nature of the relationship that exists between the two variables. Scatter-plot diagrams are a useful way to see what *kinds* of relationships might exist between your variables. Figure 14.10(a)–(h) show some of the variation we might see; for discussion purposes, note that for each of the diagrams we've created a "best" regression line or have placed a "balloon" around the entire set of data points in order to visually illustrate the amount of variation in scores that exists around the regression line.

The first dimension to consider is whether the relationship appears to be *linear* or *curvilinear,* or whether there is no apparent association at all. Figure 14.10(h) shows a curvilinear, inverted-U-shaped relationship. As an example of this sort of relationship, consider the data from the StateU faculty members. It's conceivable that a curvilinear relationship exists between academic rank and the relative importance attached to the teaching and research aspects of the job. Assistant professors may value research more highly because they see it as an important element in tenure and promotion considerations. Associate professors may then pay greater heed to their teaching role, while full professors will undoubtedly include those whose research interest has won them international recognition for their work (since this is a criterion for promotion to full professor). We don't know how widely that pattern actually occurs, but it seems a plausible curvilinear relationship.

Other sorts of curvilinear relationships are also possible: U-shaped, circular, or any of myriad others. A consideration of those relationships is clearly important, since

FIGURE 14.10 ● Scatter-plot Diagrams of Eight Different Relationships Between Two Variables

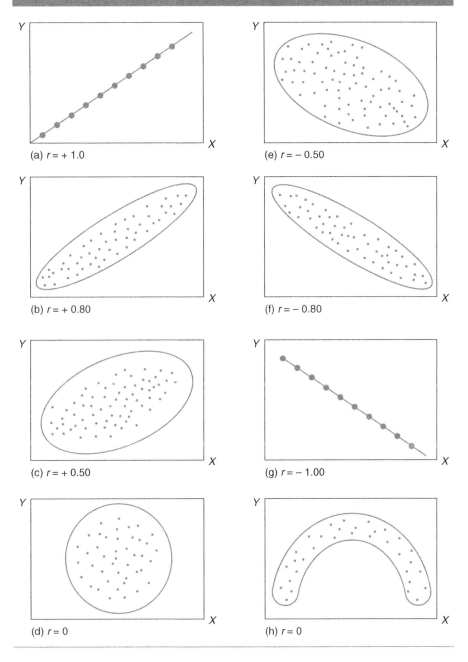

(a) $r = + 1.0$

(b) $r = + 0.80$

(c) $r = + 0.50$

(d) $r = 0$

(e) $r = - 0.50$

(f) $r = - 0.80$

(g) $r = - 1.00$

(h) $r = 0$

they're orderly and no less meaningful than linear relationships, although a detailed consideration of how to investigate them is beyond the scope of this chapter.

Figure 14.10(d) shows no relationship between the two variables at all. Points are strewn all over the scatter plot. These are of no great interest to us here, either.

The remaining scatter plots *do* concern us here. All depict *linear* relationships, albeit with varying strengths of association. In distinguishing among these remaining scatter plots, the first dimension to consider is that of the *direction* of the relationship: Are increases in one variable associated with increases or decreases in the second variable? The relationship is considered *positive* or *direct* if *in*creases in one variable are associated with *in*creases in the other; the relationship is considered *negative* or *inverse* when increases in one variable are associated with decreases in the other. Figure 14.10(a)–(c) represent positive or direct relationships, whereas Figure 14.10(e)–(g) represent negative or inverse relationships.

The second dimension of interest is the *magnitude* of the relationship. The highest-magnitude relationships are depicted in Figure 14.10(a) and (g), where all points fall along the same straight line (known as the *regression line*). Next are the relationships evident in Figure 14.10(b) and (f), where there's a little dispersion around the line, but where the "balloon" fits quite tightly. Figure 14.10(c) and (e) are still lower in magnitude; there's still a definite direction to the mass of points—positive in Figure 14.10(c); negative in Figure 14.10(e)—but there's also considerable dispersion around the regression line.

Quantifying the Relationship: Pearson's *r*

Not surprisingly, mathematicians have sought ways to quantify the direction and strength of the relationship between two quantitative variables. Karl Pearson's work around the turn of the 20th century resulted in the development of a statistic known as the Pearson product-moment correlation coefficient, or, more briefly, as Pearson's *r*. Note that Pearson's *r* describes only linear relationships.

There are two components to any correlation coefficient: a sign and a number. The *sign* indicates the *direction* of the relationship: a plus (+) sign indicates a **positive or direct relationship**, and a minus (−) sign indicates a **negative or inverse relationship**. For simplicity sake, the *number* component is defined so that its range is between zero and one. Zero is used when there is *no* linear relationship; 1.0 describes a *perfect* linear relationship, where every data point lies on the same straight line.

Figure 14.10(a)–(g) have been labeled with rough approximations of the Pearson correlation coefficients that might describe those data. You can see that Figure 14.10(a)–(c) differ from Figure 14.10(e)–(g) insofar as r values for the former all show a "+" while all the latter begin with a "−". Note also that the magnitude of the relationship decreases as you go from the perfect relationship in Figure 14.10(a) ($r = +1.0$) to that in Figure 14.10(b) ($r = +0.80$) to that in Figure 14.10(c) ($r = +0.50$), and similarly as you go from Figure 14.10(g) ($r = -1.0$) to Figure 14.10(f) ($r = -0.80$) to Figure 14.10(e) ($r = -0.50$).

The sign and numerical components together allow you to make immediate comparisons between relationships in terms of both their direction and their strength. For example, the relationships depicted in Figure 14.10(e)–(g) are all similar in direction but different in magnitude; those in Figure 14.10(b) and (f) are identical in the strength of the relationships but opposite in direction.

A Computational Example. It's fairly easy to compute a correlation coefficient for any given set of paired observations. We won't show the formula's derivation here, but conceptually, it can be understood as a weighted count of how often data points fall in quadrants "b" and "c" versus quadrants "a" and "d" of Figure 14.11.

Table 14.9 shows the computational sequence for a set of data involving the midterm and final exam grades for eight students taking a course in research methods. As you can see, the formula requires you to compute a number of different terms along the way. Generally speaking, the formula takes the scores on each variable, transforms them into "standardized" scores (so that the variables don't have to be on the same scale or expressed in the same units), and then compares how variation in one variable coincides (or does not) with variation on the other.

FIGURE 14.11 ● Four Quadrants of a Scatter-plot Diagram

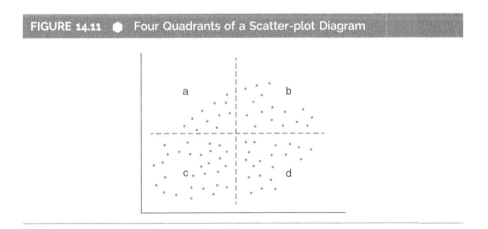

TABLE 14.9 ● Computing a Correlation Coefficient

Student	Midterm Score (X)	Final Exam Score (Y)	X^2	Y^2	XY
Wenona	18	18	324	324	324
Abby	19	23	361	529	437
Aaren	30	25	900	625	750
Tayler	33	28	1089	784	924
Jamal	27	34	729	1156	918
Marsha-Ann	32	38	1024	1444	1216
Michaela	41	37	1681	1369	1517
Kim	47	42	2209	1764	1974
$N = 8$	$\sum X = 247$	$\sum Y = 245$	$\sum X^2 = 8317$	$\sum Y^2 = 7995$	$\sum XY = 806C$

Computation

1. Take the sum $\langle \sum \rangle$ of the X scores: $\sum X = 247$
2. Square the sum of X : $(\sum X)^2 = (247)^2 = 61009$
3. Square each X score. Take the sum of those squared X scores: $\sum X^2 = 8317$
4. Take the sum of Y scores: $\sum Y = 245$
5. Square the sum of Y: $(\sum Y)^2 = (245)^2 = 60025$
6. Square each Y score Take the sum of those squared Y scores: $\sum Y^2 = 7995$
7. Compute cross-products by multiplying each X score by its associated Y score. Take the sum of those cross-products: $\sum XY = 8060$
8. Note the number of paired observations: $N = 8$
9. Insert the computed figures into the following formula to compute r, the correlation coefficient:

$$r = \frac{N\sum XY - (\sum X)(\sum Y)}{\sqrt{\left[N\sum X^2 - (\sum X)^2\right]\left[N\sum Y^2 - (\sum Y)^2\right]}}$$

$$= \frac{8(8060) - (247)(245)}{\sqrt{[8(8317) - 61009][8(7995) - 60025]}}$$

$$= \frac{64480 - 60515}{\sqrt{[66536 - 61009][63960 - 60025]}}$$

$$= \frac{3965}{\sqrt{(5527)(3935)}} \quad \frac{3965}{\sqrt{21748745}}$$

$$= \frac{3965}{4663.6} = +0.850$$

10. Compute the degrees of freedom, which is given by the number of paired observations minus two, that is, $df = N - 2 = 8 - 2 = 6$.
11. Determine whether the observed correlation is statistically significant by inspecting the critical values listed in Appendix B, for the appropriate degrees of freedom. You should see that for *6df*, the critical values that must be exceeded are $r = 0.7067$ and $r = 0.8343$ for $p < .05$ and $p < .01$, respectively, in our example, where $r = 0.850$, we would conclude that our correlation is indeed statistically significant at $p < .01$; that is, the correlation is greater than we would expect on the basis of chance alone, suggesting that the two variables are indeed associated.

The correlation coefficient of $r = +0.85$ derived in Table 14.9 indicates a strong relationship between performance on the midterm and performance on the final: those who do well on the midterm generally do well on the final, while those who perform poorly on the midterm tend also to do less well on the final. But the relationship isn't perfect, suggesting also that some changes take place: some students who do well on the midterm are perhaps overconfident, don't study as much for the final, and therefore blow it; others take their poor midterm performance to heart, work harder, and improve on the final; or illness that affects some students during one exam is not a factor during the other. Measurement error also occurs: tests are imperfect, thus allowing regression toward the mean to occur.

The next question is whether the correlation we observe is greater than what we would have expected on the basis of chance variation alone. Once again (as with chi-square), this is a question of the *statistical significance* of the results.

We use r distributions in the same way as chi-square distributions. Appendix B shows a listing of criterion values for r, the Pearson correlation coefficient. Once again, the criterion value depends on *degrees of freedom*. For correlations, the number of degrees of freedom is equal to the number of *paired observations* minus two. Thus, for our data, we have $8-2 = 6df$. Appendix B shows that for $6df$ we require a computed correlation of $r = 0.7067$ or higher in order for our relationship to be considered significant at the .05 level, or $r = 0.8343$ for the .01 probability level. (Criterion values are expressed only in terms of the *magnitude* of the relationship; the direction doesn't matter.) Our obtained correlation of $r = +0.85$ exceeds both those criterion values: we can therefore say with 99 percent confidence that the two sets of scores are related beyond the level you would expect on the basis of chance alone.

The Proportion of Variance Accounted for: r^2. While the correlation coefficient (r) conveys the magnitude and direction of a relationship between two variables, we'll also note here (but won't go into the proof) that the proportion of variance that's shared by two variables is equal to the square of their correlation coefficient. Thus, if we determine that the correlation between two variables is $r = .90$, then we also immediately know that $r^2 = (0.90)^2 = 0.81$ (i.e., that 81 percent of the variance in one variable is shared by the other).

Besides understanding the inherent relation that r and r^2 have with each other, a consideration of *how* they're related may give you a slightly different take on correlation coefficients. Figure 14.12 plots the relationship between r and r^2. You can see that correlations in the neighborhood of 0.10–0.30 look fairly puny in this light, since even a 0.30 correlation between two variables means that they share a mere 9 percent of their variances in common (since $0.30^2 = 0.09$). Even a correlation between X and Y of $r = 0.50$, which many researchers would normally get very

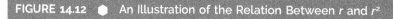

FIGURE 14.12 ● An Illustration of the Relation Between *r* and *r²*

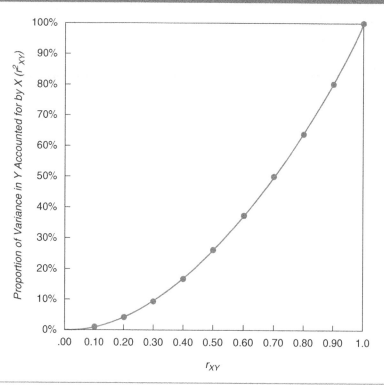

excited about, means that X accounts for no more than a quarter (25 percent) of the variance in Y; this still leaves another 75 percent of the variance in Y that is *not* yet accounted for. Not until correlations get into the 0.71 ballpark do you begin to account for even half of the variance in Y. Thus, while the un-squared correlation coefficient (r) may be useful in indicating direction, it may well give an impression of a stronger relationship than would be the case if you were to pay greater heed to r^2 and its proportion of variance interpretation.

What Correlation Coefficients Do Not Tell You. You've computed a correlation between two variables and found it to be significant. What does this mean? Literally, it means that the two sets of data you've correlated are associated more closely than you would expect on a purely chance basis. But before you jump to the conclusion that you've unearthed some immutable truth, look at some of the reasons you might have obtained the correlation coefficient you did. Consider the following:

1. *Whether the theoretical variables are related.* The discovery of a significant correlation is an *empirical* finding, which you may or may not be able to generalize to the theoretical domain. First, there's a question of the relationship between your theoretical variable and your operational one; that is, the epistemic relationship between the two. Second, as is true of any empirical finding, its *external validity* (or generalizability) must be considered; this is a separate issue.

2. *Whether the association is a causal one.* Every methods textbook will tell you that *correlation does not mean causation.* The fact that two variables happen to "go together" doesn't in any way mean that there's necessarily a causal connection between the two of them. It *may* be that the first variable causes the second; it *may* be that the second variable causes the first; or it *may* be that both variables are influenced by some third variable that you haven't yet recognized. Other variables may "share variance" with both sets of scores, such that the correlation you observe may not reflect a "real" association between the two variables you are investigating, but merely the variance they share with that third variable. For example, although we haven't done the calculation, we bet there is a correlation between the number of ice cream cones consumed in any given day and the number of drownings that occur. Does ice cream cause people to drown? Probably not. It's more likely that a third variable (the outside temperature) influences both.

A similar situation might be evident in the example of midterm and final exam scores. The correlation *may* reflect consistency in the evaluation of "competence in research methods" (as we hope), but it may also just reflect similarities in test-taking behavior (which is independent of research methods competence per se). Many social beliefs are clearly supported by people's erroneous belief that correlation implies causation. For example, the occasional covariation of visible-minority status and "low levels of social achievement," however selectively that observation is obtained in the first place, is often used to try to justify the racist belief that visible minorities in some way "cause" their "inferiority," when instead social structures, racism, and institutionalized poverty are often causes of both. The tendency to blame the victim is another manifestation of confusing correlation with cause. Victims might in some cases be the architects of their own misfortune, but just as clearly might not.

The example above urges you to be cautious about jumping to conclusions when you find a significant correlation. Similar caution is warranted when you *don't* find a significant correlation. Pearson's *r* is designed to test for a very particular type of relationship between variables—a linear one. Just because a correlation is not significant does not necessarily mean that a patterned, orderly relationship does not exist. When looking at correlations, you should always look at scatter plots to avoid indulging in interpretations that may turn out to be nonsensical.

Examining Differences Between Categories
A Slightly Different Way of Making Comparisons

Thus far in our look at inferential statistics, we've emphasized techniques for measuring association. Let us now introduce another set of techniques that tackle another very basic task one is often faced with in the social and health sciences, that is, making comparisons to look at difference.

To explain how that is done in different situations, consider a situation in which you, as a student, might often find yourself. Suppose you complete two midterm exams, later finding that you scored 22 out of 27 on the Anthropology 101 midterm and 41 out of 55 on your Philosophy 330 exam. Did you do better in anthropology or philosophy? To answer that question, you might look for some common ground on which to compare the two scores, perhaps by translating your scores into percentages. On doing so, you find that your anthropology grade was actually 81.5 percent, while your philosophy score was 74.5 percent. Comparing the two, you conclude that your performance was better in anthropology than in philosophy.

Social and health scientists who analyze such data would actually take the analysis a step or two further, as we'll soon see. But first we'd like to draw your attention to exactly what you did when you tried to compare your midterm exam grades in that way. You created an abstract, hypothetical situation in which a crucial element that made the two grades incomparable in the first place—the fact that one exam was marked out of 27 while the other was marked out of 55—was negated by looking at a theoretical distribution of numbers (who said you had no understanding of statistical concepts?) called percentages. Neither of the exams was actually marked out of 100. But you took the 22 out of 27 in anthropology and said, "Well, if this exam had been marked out of 100 points, and my performance and the marking remained constant, what would I have received as a grade?" And you came up with 81.5 percent. The same process with the philosophy grade led you to conclude you would have received a grade of 74.5 percent on that hypothetical exam. By establishing a common ground, you made the two grades comparable.

When we describe percentages as "theoretical," it isn't because percentages are unreal or completely abstract. Rather, the term implies that there's no particularly good reason, other than as a completely arbitrary standard of judgment on which people have agreed, to look at percentages or to have defined percentages as necessarily being a score out of 100. There's no law of mathematics stopping us all from deciding tomorrow that percentages will henceforth be computed with a base of 1,000 rather than 100 (although a desire for linguistic integrity might lead us to call them "per-millages" rather than "percentages"), if we so please. Percentages (or other such standardized ratios) may be arbitrarily defined, but given that we have defined them that way, the results we garner through them are anything but arbitrary.

Members of the social and health sciences go through a somewhat similar process, but they take a few more details into account. Since you've already learned the hard part—characteristics of distributions, and particularly the concepts of standard deviations and variance—the rest will be easy.

Z-Scores and the Normal Distribution

In the same way that percentages provide a common ground for comparing grades, social and health scientists have looked for a common ground on which to compare different distributions of scores. The creation they came up with is known as the **normal distribution**. It's "normal" in the sense that it's typical of many distributions we come across in everyday research; indeed, after more than a decade of gathering all sorts of data—from exam grades to attitude scores to aptitude measures to behavioral indices—we never cease to be amazed at how often we encounter distributions that are roughly normal in their form. There's a central tendency where scores cluster more closely together than anywhere else along the frequency distribution; as you move farther and farther away from that mean/median/modal point, you see fewer and fewer scores, until they disappear into infinity. Figure 14.13 depicts a standard normal distribution.

In the same way that "percentages" were arbitrarily defined as being out of 100, the standard normal distribution was also given some characteristics on a relatively arbitrary basis. The distribution's mean was set at zero, while the standard deviation was set at 1.0. Conveniently enough, this also implies that the variance is also 1.0, since the variance is the square of the standard deviation. Of course, no such choice is *completely* arbitrary. Making percentages out of 100 rather than out of 472 certainly

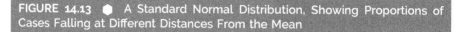

FIGURE 14.13 ● A Standard Normal Distribution, Showing Proportions of Cases Falling at Different Distances From the Mean

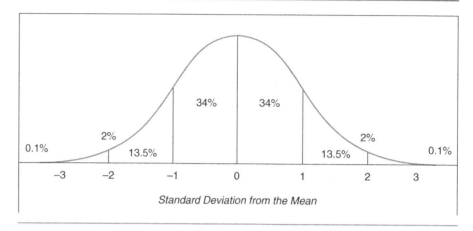

makes computation easier, as does setting the normal distribution with a central tendency (i.e., mean) of zero and with variability (i.e., standard deviation and variance) of 1.0.

Once the normal distribution is defined, it becomes possible to calculate, for a particular observation at a given distance from the mean, the probability of getting an observation at least that far from the mean. This requires first that we have some measure of deviation from the mean. Since we've already discussed the notion of a standard deviation, it should come as no surprise that social and health scientists seized on the "standard deviation unit" as the ruler to use for any given distribution of scores. They could have called these "standard deviation units" or "SDUs." Instead, mathematicians decided to call deviations computed in terms of standard deviation units "z-scores."

Let's return to the example of your midterm exam grades. A social or health scientist wouldn't be content with merely using percentages as a common ground of comparison. Treating those percentages as comparable assumes that both exams were equally difficult and that both professors (or their teaching assistants) marked with equal stringency. But as you may well have found in your own courses, that may be a tenuous assumption. So a social or health scientist would be interested in knowing whether the scores on that anthropology midterm are approximately normally distributed—and, if so, what the mean and standard deviation of the distribution are.

Suppose it was a particularly difficult exam, so hard that the mean score among your classmates was 15 out of 27, with a standard deviation of 10. That means that your score of 22 was actually 7 points above the mean, or $7/10 = 0.700$ standard deviation units above the mean. In other words, your z-score on that exam would have been $+0.7$ (the "+" signifies your score was above the mean; recall that the mean of the distribution is zero, and that deviations from it can be in a positive or negative direction).

Next we'd want to gain the same information for your philosophy midterm. Suppose that it, too, was a fairly difficult exam. Most of your classmates managed to pass, since the mean and median were both 30 out of 55, but very few of them did either very poorly or very well: the standard deviation was a mere 8.0. With a mean of 30 and a standard deviation of 8.0, your score of 41 was, in fact, $11/8 = 1.375$ standard deviation units above the mean; in other words, you achieved a z-score of $+1.375$. Thus, when we compare your performance to that of your classmates, we find that your score in philosophy (with a z-score of $+1.375$) was actually more exceptional than your score in anthropology (where your z-score was $+0.700$), even though your percentage grade in philosophy (74.5) was lower than the one you received in anthropology (81.5).

The process is similar in many ways to what you did in translating your two grades into percentages. In looking for a common ground, you chose percentages, which are arbitrarily established to be expressed out of 100. The logic was essentially to say, *"If both exams had actually been based out of 100, what would my two scores have been?"* The social or health scientist, however, says, *"If the scores on both these exams were drawn from normal distributions, then what is their comparative likelihood of being drawn?"* By referring your grades to the normal distribution, we could compute exact probabilities for obtaining at least any given score, or we could give percentile estimates of where you (or any other person) stack up in the distribution. But we'll leave that technique for your course professor to cover if they think it is useful. We now turn to a situation where we have two variables of interest—one categorical and one continuous—and we seek to determine whether the categories differ in their status on the continuous variable.

Comparing Group Means Through the t-Statistic. In looking at your score on the anthropology exam, we tried to understand it by placing it in its distributional context. But social and health scientists, and particularly quantitatively oriented ones, aren't often interested in single scores. Scores are interesting only in the context of distributions. Similarly, samples become more interesting when we link them to the populations from which they were drawn and/or start comparing different samples to each other.

In comparing distributions, we're usually interested in whether the means differ: the t-statistic is the measure that mathematicians have invented for us to use in this instance. People seem to rest so much easier when abstract concepts are reified—we relate so much better to Santa Claus than to the abstract ideals of harmony and sharing. Perhaps the *t*-test is little more than a tentative concrete response to the question "How big is big?"

One person who tried to answer that question was W. S. Gossett, who worked as a chemist at the Guinness Brewery in Dublin, Ireland, in the late 1800s. Apparently company policy forbade the publication of research, so Gossett published under the pseudonym "Student," which is why the *t*-distribution is known as Student's *t*-distribution and its descriptive statistic as Student's *t* (e.g., see McGhee, 1985). The story begins where the standard deviation left off.

When the question under consideration was the extremity of your anthropology exam score, we first found out where your score stood relative to the mean of the distribution of scores (i.e., we took the difference between score and mean). We then determined what the standard deviation of the distribution was, using that as a kind of ruler with which to measure your score in standard deviation (or *z*-score) units.

When a social or health scientist wants to know whether any two groups differ, the question is phrased in terms of whether there's a difference between the two group means. Not surprisingly, therefore, step 1 in computing a *t*-statistic involves finding the difference between the two means. But once we know the difference, how do we know whether it's a "big" difference or whether it might be expected to occur through chance variation alone?

Gossett grappled with that question by asking us to assume the null hypothesis, that is, that the two groups we're dealing with are actually just samples from the same population. Suppose we have an infinite number of observations of a variable that is normally distributed. We randomly sample one group of five observations and compute their mean score, sample another group of five observations and compute *their* group mean, and then compare the two means to see how close they are to each other. Then we take another two samples of five observations each, computing and comparing their group means, then another two samples, and another two, until we've made an infinite number of comparisons. If we looked at those comparisons, we'd see that purely on the basis of chance variation, group 1 sometimes scored higher than group 2—sometimes by a little, sometimes by a lot—while other times group 2 scored higher than group 1. We could begin creating a frequency distribution of all of those differences.

Because the two samples were always drawn from the same population with the same population mean, we'd expect that over the long run the most frequent difference we'd observe would be zero and that frequencies would diminish as we move away from that central tendency. Indeed, with extensive repeated sampling (as is done in Monte Carlo simulations), it can be demonstrated that a frequency distribution of differences between two sample means will be normally distributed, with a mean around zero, regardless of whether the population from which the observations are drawn is normal. If that's the case, it should be possible to determine the probability of *any* given difference, as long as we take into account the particular distributional characteristics we're working with. The *t*-statistic that Gossett developed was intended to provide us with exactly that information.

But how extreme is any given *t*-score? Not surprisingly (we hope), we determine that fact by checking our *t*-score against the Student's *t*-distributions, the critical values of which are reproduced in Appendix C. Just to put some flesh on this search, let's return to the example of the faculty members at StateU.

Suppose we're interested in comparing 10 male and 10 female faculty members in terms of the relative value they attach to the research and teaching aspects of their jobs. Table 14.10 shows these hypothetical data; the females have a mean of 2.3 on the 5-point scale, whereas the males have a mean of 3.4. As this suggests, the female faculty members have a mean opinion that's on the "teaching valued more highly" end of the scale, whereas the male faculty members have a mean that's closer to the "research valued more highly" end of the scale (recall Table 14.3). The difference between them is thus $3.4 - 2.3 = 1.1$ scale points. But is that difference "significant," or is it within the realm we might expect on the basis of chance variation alone? The computations necessary for deriving a *t*-statistic are shown in Table 14.10; we compare that *t*-value to the critical values summarized in Appendix C.

As with chi-square and *r*-values, critical *t*-values take into account degrees of freedom, which, in this case, are determined by sample size. This is because, all else being equal, two samples of 5 people each are much more likely to have divergent group means than are two samples of 100 people each. The various *t*-distributions reflect this, as do the critical values listed in Appendix C.

Thus, we first compute degrees of freedom, which, for the *t*-test, are given by the formula $df = N_x + N_y - 2$, where N_x is the total number of observations in one group, and N_y is the total number in the other. When the sample sizes of the two groups are equal, the formula is more simply stated as $df = N - 2$, where N is the total number of observations in the two groups taken together. Since we sampled 10

TABLE 14.10 ● Computing the *t*-Statistic

The distribution below shows responses for 10 male and 10 female faculty members to the query whether they value the research or teaching aspects of their role more highly; possible responses were (1) teaching much more highly valued; (2) teaching somewhat more highly valued; (3) teaching and research equally valued; (4) research somewhat more highly valued; (5) research much more highly valued.

Males (X)	Females (Y)	X^2	Y^2
2	1	4	1
2	1	4	1
3	1	9	1
3	2	9	4
3	2	9	4
4	2	16	4
4	3	16	9
4	3	16	9
4	4	16	16
5	4	25	16
$\sum X = 34$	$\sum Y = 23$	$\sum X^2 = 124$	$\sum Y^2 = 65$
$N = 10$	$N = 10$		
Mean $= 3.4$	Mean $= 2.3$		

Computation

1. Take the sum of the scores in group 1 (males): $\sum X = 34$
2. Square the sum of group 1 scores: $(\sum X)^2 = 1156$
3. Square *each score.* in group 1, and take the sum of those squared scores: $\sum X^2 = 124$
4. Note the number of scores in group 1: $N_X = 10$
5. Compute the mean score of group 1: $\bar{X}_w = 3.4$
6. Take the sum of the scores in group 2 (females): $\sum Y = 23$
7. Square the sum of group 2 scores: $(\sum Y)^2 = 529$
8. Square *each score* in group 2, and take the sum of those squared scores: $\sum Y^2 = 65$
9. Note the number of scores in group 2: $N_y = 10$
10. Compute the mean score for group 2: $\bar{Y}_w = 2.3$
11. Enter the appropriate figures into the following formula for the computation of t:

$$t = \sqrt{\left[\frac{\left(\sum X^2 - \frac{(\sum X^2)}{N_X}\right) + \left(\sum Y^2 - \frac{(\sum Y^2)}{N_Y}\right)}{N_X + N_Y - 2}\right] \times \left[\frac{1}{N_X} + \frac{1}{N_Y}\right]}$$

$$= \sqrt{\left[\frac{\left(124 - \frac{1156}{10}\right) + \left(65 - \frac{529}{10}\right)}{10 + 10 - 2}\right] \times \left[\frac{1}{10} + \frac{1}{10}\right]}$$

$$= \frac{1.1}{\sqrt{\left[\frac{(8.4) + (12.1)}{18}\right] \times \left[\frac{2}{10}\right]}}$$

$$= \frac{1.1}{\sqrt{(1.14)(0.2)}} = \frac{1.1}{\sqrt{0.228}} = \frac{1.1}{0.477} = 2.31$$

12. Compute the degrees of freedom by taking the number of observations in group 1, plus the number of observations in group 2, minus 2, i.e., $df = N_x + N_y - 2 = 10 + 10 - 2 = 18$.
13. Determine whether the observed correlation is statistically significant by inspecting the critical values listed in Appendix C, for the appropriate degrees of freedom. You should see that for 18df, the critical values that must be met or exceeded are $t = 2.101$ and $t = 2.878$ for $p < .05$ and $p < .01$, respectively. Thus, our observed difference in the current example would be considered statistically significant at $p < .05$, but not at $p < .01$.

female and 10 male faculty members, for a total $N = 20$, our $df = 20-2 = 18$. Accordingly, we must look at the line for 18 df in the list of critical values given in Appendix C; there, we see that the critical value for t to be significant at the .05 level is 2.101, while the critical value at the .01 level is 2.878. Thus, the difference between male and female faculty members on the attitude variable, which resulted in a t-score of 2.31, is statistically significant at the .05 level.

Limits of Two-Variable Analyses

Error Rates When Undertaking Multiple Analyses. Researchers rarely do studies that involve only two or three variables. It's far more common to have several independent variables, several dependent variables, or a dozen or more questionnaire or observational variables. As the size and complexity of your data collection increase, one possibility is to do more two-group comparisons via the t-test or more bivariate (i.e., two-variable) correlations to take the additional variables into account.

However, note that as the number of variables increases, the number of possible comparisons that can be computed increases dramatically. With two groups, for example, only *one* possible comparison (i.e., group 1 versus group 2) can be made. With three groups, there are *three* comparisons possible (1 versus 2; 1 versus 3; 2 versus 3). But with four groups, there are suddenly *six* comparisons possible (1 versus 2; 1 versus 3; 1 versus 4; 2 versus 3; 2 versus 4; 3 versus 4). And by the time we reach 10 groups, there are *45* different two-group comparisons that can be made! Substitute "variables" for "groups" and "correlations" for "comparisons" and you can see that the same is true for correlation coefficients.

You could always just go ahead and do each of those individual comparisons or correlations. But statistically that approach poses a problem. To understand why, recall that the notion of "statistical significance" suggests that we find a point on the distribution under consideration (i.e., chi-square, t, r) where we can feel confident that a difference is "real" or "reliable." We can never be certain that a difference is real; we can only be confident to varying degrees. Traditionally, the social and health sciences have adopted $p < .05$ as the default criterion, that is, the criterion to use unless there's some reason, articulated beforehand, to do otherwise. We choose that level because 95 percent confidence (i.e., in all likelihood being "right" 95 out of 100, or 19 out of 20, times) represents "good odds" that our decision to treat a difference (or correlation) as real is appropriate.

The other side of that figure, however, is that on approximately 5 out of 100 occasions, or in 1 out of 20 situations, we will be *wrong*—we'll proclaim a result to be reliable when in fact it is not. If we're making only one comparison or a few comparisons, we're prepared to live with that uncertainty. But if 20 or 50 or 100 comparisons are made, the odds are high that some of the comparisons we observe to be "statistically significant" will in fact be spurious. If only a few of those comparisons are significant, we probably shouldn't be terribly excited by them; they're probably mere ephemeral shadows that will disappear next time we look at them. If you compute 100 correlation coefficients, for example, the odds are that around 5 of them will emerge as statistically significant purely on the basis of chance variation alone. Accordingly, researchers must be particularly cautious when interpreting the results of numerous tests on the same set of data.

There are at least three ways around this problem, however. The **Bonferroni technique** involves splitting the adopted probability required for significance across the entire range of comparisons to be made (e.g., see Kirk, 1968; Pedhazur, 1982). For example, if you're adopting a significance level of $p < .05$ and plan to undertake 10 separate t-tests (or chi-squares or Pearson correlations), the Bonferroni procedure involves merely spreading the .05 (known as the *experiment-wise error rate*) across the 10 comparisons, with the result that a $.05/10 = .005$ significance level would have to be achieved on any given comparison before you'd be prepared to consider it "reliable." This approach makes for rather conservative testing (since a .005, or 5/1000, criterion is a very stringent one), but this is considered preferable to engaging in "much ado about nothing."

Alternatively, if you're in the luxurious situation of having a very large number of cases (e.g., 10 times as many cases as you have variables), your data are amenable to a procedure known as **jackknifing**. There are several ways to do this, but the simplest is to randomly split your sample of cases into *two* samples, do the analyses you want to do separately in the two samples, and then focus only on those results that emerge as statistically significant in *both* data sets.

The logic of this approach is that while some correlations or comparisons may well turn out to be statistically significant on the basis of chance error when you are doing a large number of these calculations in one sample, it's highly unlikely that specific chance occurrences will replicate on a second occasion. Only those with some substance to them will do so, and hence only those that can pass the significance hurdle *twice* are thought to warrant further consideration and discussion.

The third alternative is to learn some more techniques that have been developed precisely in order to overcome that error rate problem. The analysis of variance (ANOVA), for example, is conceptually akin to doing multiple *t*-tests on a given set of data, but controls for error rate in the process. Similarly, multiple regression analysis has been developed to deal with situations in which you are attempting to correlate many variables with some criterion (dependent) measure. But these techniques are beyond the scope of this book, so you'll have to await further courses in statistics to see how they work.

SUMMING UP AND LOOKING AHEAD

The chapter began with a discussion of variables and constants and then introduces the notion of levels of measurement, explaining the differences between nominal, ordinal, interval, and ratio scales. The level of measurement your variables possess will influence, to some degree, the range of statistics with which each variable may be analyzed. At the same time, it is not the empirical variable per se, but the underlying theoretical variable that's most important to consider when identifying our level of measurement—and hence which particular statistical operations are appropriate.

A number of descriptive techniques—frequency distributions, pie charts, bar charts, histograms, frequency polygons—are then discussed as ways of presenting distributions of obtained data. The task is to describe those distributions statistically. Indicators of central tendency include the mode, the median, and the mean; each is an appropriate summary statistic in some situations, but each can also be misused. Also included is a discussion of descriptors of distributional variability, including the range, the standard deviation, and the variance.

The focus then turns to inferential statistics that can be used to examine the relationships among variables. A distinction is made between those statistics that focus on the degree of association among variables (e.g., chi-square, correlation) and those that focus on examining the differences between groups (e.g., *z*-scores, *t*-tests). These tests are called inferential statistics because we're ultimately less interested in the sample per se than in using the sample as a vehicle through which to make inferences about populations.

The section on inferential statistics first examines relationships among categorical variables. The cross-tabulation or contingency table is a way to represent such bivariate relationships, while the chi-square statistic is the appropriate measure of the extent to which observed cell frequencies deviate from those expected on a purely chance basis. Comparing a computed chi-square statistic to its chi-square distribution gives the probability that the deviations we observe would occur on the basis of chance alone. Using the concept of degrees of freedom and Appendix A, you can determine the criterion value your chi-square statistic must meet or exceed in order to be proclaimed significant. A "statistically significant" result implies 95 percent or 99 percent confidence in stating that the distribution was unlikely to have been obtained by chance variation alone, suggesting that the two categorical variables are indeed associated with one another.

The chapter then focuses on relationships between two continuous variables. The scatter-plot diagram can be used to illustrate such bivariate distributions, and the Pearson product-moment correlation coefficient describes the direction and magnitude of a linear relationship. The critical values in Appendix B, along with the degrees of freedom, determine the particular criterion value that must be matched or exceeded in order for the correlation to be declared significantly greater than zero.

But a significant correlation coefficient does not tell us whether the underlying theoretical variables are, in fact, related or whether the association, however strong, is a causal one. A nonsignificant r-value doesn't necessarily mean that there's no relationship between the variables. Pearson's r tells you only about significant linear relationships; other curvilinear relationships may or may not exist and must be tested for separately.

Attention then turns to techniques that emphasize the assessment of difference; these normally involve looking at differences between groups (a categorical variable) on some continuous variable, that is, a comparison of group means. The t-statistic and t-distribution are useful in comparing two group means. But while a significant t-score leads us to conclude that the two groups do indeed differ, discerning the reasons why they differ remains an analytical (rather than purely statistical) task. Rival plausible explanations must be considered.

With the analysis of your data behind you, it's time to start writing it all up in a final research report. The next chapter looks at how to do that.

Key Concepts

Bonferroni technique 614
Categorical variables 566
Chi-square 591
Constant 564
Contingency table 590
Degrees of freedom 593
Descriptive statistics 564
Inferential statistics 564
Interquartile range (IQR) 584
Interval-level measurement 567
Jackknifing 614

Mean 577
Median 577
Mode 576
"Monte Carlo" computer
    simulations 569
Negative or inverse
    relationship 600
Normal distribution 607
Ordinal measurement 566
Outliers 581
Pearson's r 598

Positive or direct relationship 600
Range 583
Ratio-level measurement 567
Skew 579
Standard deviation 588
t-statistic 610
Variable 564
Variance 588
z-scores 608

STUDY QUESTIONS

1. Distinguish between *variables* and *constants*. Show that you understand the difference between them by identifying three variables and three constants that might be used to describe the people in your research methods class.

2. Give examples of one variable at each of the four levels of measurement, and explain in your own words why that is the correct label for each.

3. "Measures of length and distance are ratio-level variables no matter what theoretical variable they are being used as operationalizations for." Would you agree or disagree? Explain.

4. Prepare a brief questionnaire that includes variables at all four levels of measurement. Designate your variable names, and state explicitly what level of measurement you feel each is being measured at. Invent responses; then prepare frequency distributions and compute summary statistics for each.

5. Perform appropriate bivariate analyses on the data gathered for Study Question 4.

6. For what kinds of variables (or levels of measurement) are the mean, median, and mode considered appropriate descriptors of central tendency?

7. In a recent edition of your local newspaper, look for an article that offers statistical information. Would you consider the data well presented? Why or why not?

8. Why is the standard deviation a "better" indicator of dispersion than the range, for interval-, and ratio-level variables?

9. Acquire data from the relevant person at your educational institution (e.g., office of analytical studies, personnel office, faculty association, or union) regarding your university or college faculty (e.g., information concerning distributions of sex, visible-minority status, rank, salary levels, years employed, etc.) and undertake an analysis of those data. Are they consistent with the view that you're attending an egalitarian educational institution? Offer rival plausible explanations and indicate the sorts of data you might seek or generate to look into the matter further.

10. Encourage the professor in your research methods class (if they do not do so already) to tell you not only the class mean on your most recent or next quiz or exam but also the standard deviation. What was your grade on that exam? What z-score would that be?

11. Hollie gets 87 percent on her final exam in Syrian Epistemology, where the mean of the class was 80 percent with a standard deviation of 5 percent; she manages to get 93 percent in Neo-Gregorian Chants, where the mean of the class was also 80 percent with a standard deviation of 15 percent. In sum, she scored above the mean in both cases. Compared to her respective classmates, however, did she do better at Syrian Epistemology or at Neo-Gregorian Chants?

12. Why do we need to know the degrees of freedom in our data before checking whether the chi-square or r- or t-value we have is significant?

13. Why is a high, statistically significant r-value not necessarily indicative of a causal relationship between the two variables being correlated?

14. A researcher computes bivariate correlations between pairs of variables by hand and ends up with correlation coefficients of -0.46, $+0.52$, $+0.83$, -1.04, and -0.87.

    a. Which of those r-values *must* be incorrect? Why?

    b. Of the remaining values, which represents the strongest association between two variables?

    c. For the correlation coefficient you chose in 14(b), what proportion of variance do the two variables share?

15. A researcher asks a sample of 47 males and 52 females whether they support the idea of censorship for sexually violent films. Among the females, 37 say yes, 11 say no, and 4 are uncertain. In contrast, 22 of the males say yes, 19 say no, and 6 are uncertain. Create a contingency table to depict these data. Do the necessary computations to learn whether there's a significant association between sex and opinions regarding censorship in that sample.

16. A graduate student wants to test out the notion that there is an inverted-U-shaped relationship between anxiety and performance (i.e., whether performance is lowest with either very low or very high levels of anxiety, and highest with moderate levels of anxiety). Given that the relevant data are gathered, would the Pearson correlation coefficient offer a useful way of testing whether the hypothesized relationship is indeed found? Why or why not?

17. A student gathers data on 15 variables from a sample of 100 shoppers at a local mall and proceeds to intercorrelate all the variables, resulting in a total of 105 different correlation coefficients having been computed. Although disappointed at the fact that not many of the relationships prove to be statistically significant, he's pleased to see that seven of them are, and he writes up an analysis that focuses on those seven. Is that a reasonable thing for him to do? What if he increases his sample size to include 200 shoppers?

18. What is the *Bonferroni procedure,* and when and why might you use it?

DISSEMINATING YOUR RESEARCH

CHAPTER OUTLINE

You're in the home stretch now. Your research is done, you feel you have something to say, and now you're ready to disseminate it to the world. In other books we have written about research methods (e.g., Palys & Atchison, 2014), this chapter was called "Writing your research report," but as we enter the third decade of the 21st century, there are so many other ways to tell the world about your research that need to be considered.

There are two main reasons for this expansion of coverage. First is that in academe we see much greater emphasis on connecting to broader communities beyond just other academics. While peer-reviewed journals are still an important place to publish and a respected source of information because of the professional standards of rigor that peer review helps to maintain, the successful academic these days also will be writing op-eds for the newspaper, doing presentations in public forums, creating and updating a web page so that people interested in your work can find it, and maintaining a social media account that allows you to build and maintain a community of followers you can keep informed about your own and related work.

Second, not all of the people reading this book are going to end up in academe. Many, if not most, of you will probably end up in other venues of life where the skills you learn here will help you be critical consumers of the news and research reporting you see and hear there. Many of you also will end up in agencies or government departments or corporate settings where your job will involve some sort of research and/or presentation of information to an audience. In this chapter we'll start off by talking about writing, but will have some advice for some of those other venues as well.

THE WRITTEN REPORT

There are many splendid books and chapters within books that offer advice about how to write research reports. Howard Becker's *Writing for Sociologists* (2007) is a great one that continues to be used widely. Another is Harry Wolcott's (2009) *Writing Up Qualitative Research.* Psychologists can consult the *Publication Manual* published by the American Psychological Association (2010). *The Elements of Style* (1999) by William Strunk Jr. is another classic. In chapters, Lofland, Snow, Anderson, and Lofland (2006) offer useful advice on writing in *Analyzing Social Settings,* as does Berg (2007) in *Qualitative Research Methods for the Social Sciences.* And of course, more and more resources appear every year on the internet.

Although we will duplicate some of their coverage, our emphasis is on suggesting general organizational considerations that you should keep in mind when writing.

These considerations apply to your final research report, whether it's a term research project for a course, an article for publication, or a report you're writing as a consultant or agency researcher. We'll begin with some very general observations about the process of writing—and some of the problems people have with it—and conclude with more specific considerations that should be kept in mind for the various sections of your report and the linkages between them.

Some General Thoughts About Writing

Get Comfortable

One of the fascinating things we have found when we talk to our colleagues and students about writing is that everyone has certain habits—you might even call them rituals or compulsions—that go along with feeling comfortable and being able to write. These are highly personal practices that may make little or no rational sense and serve no apparent purpose other than allowing you to feel like you can sit down and write. Some people need to clean the house first. Some need to sharpen pencils. Some like to have music playing while others require complete silence. Some prefer to write on a computer; others would rather write on paper and transcribe to a computer later.

The two of us are no exception. Ted needs to play one game of Sudoku before he starts to write each day, prefers to be surrounded by silence and darkness, and is most happy writing on his home desktop computer with its three monitors that allow electronic documents and whatever else to be posted on the sides while focusing on the document he is writing in the middle. Chris has a multimonitor desktop setup similar to Ted's but prefers to work in the middle of what Ted would find multi-media chaos: lots of visual stimuli outside his third storey window; movies and/or TV programs and/or music (often more than one at a time) playing in the background.

Get to know what your rituals are and give in to them. While at one level they make "no rational sense," we view them like the sleeping rituals that people go through that are part of having a good night's sleep. In many cases they often are the transition time in which you get rid of other mental clutter and get your thinking focused on the task before you, and the monitor or paper in front of you, and what you want to say.

Spew It Out

If there is one thing common to professional life in all sorts of disciplinary domains, it is writing. We know that academics are supposed to write articles and books, but academics are not the only people who are expected to write on an ongoing basis. Most professions require you to have the skills to write reports, or memos, or letters, or report cards, or briefing notes, or press releases, or case summaries, or policy recommendations, and on and on. It is fascinating, therefore, that whenever the discussion in our classes turns to writing, one of the first things we find out is how many people actually do not enjoy writing. Most reactions seem to range from "can do it if I have to" to a kind of paralytic fear that leaves people staring at a blank page or computer monitor waiting for that magical opening sentence they hope will open the floodgates, and waiting, and waiting.

Becker (2020) suggests the biggest cause of this deer-in-the-headlights paralysis is the mistaken belief that one draft and perhaps at most a mini-edit are all it should take to produce a decent paper. This creates huge pressure, unrealistic expectations, and a sense of failure when students try and do their first college or university research paper in one late-night marathon and come up short. Step 1 is thus to get real and understand, first of all, that the typical university or college paper is more complex in terms of the ideas being knocked around than was the case in high school. Step 2 is to realize that there is a sampling problem here—all you ever see that anyone else has written is their final product; what you don't see is what it took to get there.

Writing is a bit like driving to a place you've never visited before in the days before GPS. Some general principles and a roadmap would help get you there, but it wasn't until you arrived and had a clear sense of your destination that you could begin to determine the "best" route and where you can flatly and easily reject some possibilities as "dead ends" or "the wrong direction." However, that is sometimes easier said than done when it comes to writing, where we often discover new things as we try explaining to someone else what we think we know. Gaps in our understanding begin to appear. We realize that the flow of logic we thought was so impervious to criticism is more porous than we imagined. Or we find the order in which we decided to tell the story turns out not to work that well after all. Discovering any of these is not a bad thing. These unanticipated problems are actually one reason we enjoy writing—not *really* knowing what we think about something until we have written it down and worked through all the details (e.g., see also Richardson, 2003).

Writing is more than a one-shot deal. To use the driving analogy again, think of your task as one of describing the best route to this new destination. The major accomplishment of your first draft is simply that it's done—and "getting there" is in itself no small feat—but that first draft still contains all the wrong turns, misreading of maps, traffic jams, dead ends, and so on. It's a route that got you there but is by no means the most efficient or direct route. Now, there *are* times when you might actually want to describe that *whole* journey, but in most cases the world just wants to know what your point is, how you came to that conclusion, and what it means for them. To do that, you need to take your first draft and start whittling it down to the essentials, the basic information your reader needs to know to understand and travel the route.

Good writing is a *process* that always takes more than one draft, and this is true regardless of how good and experienced a writer you are. It normally takes no fewer than 5, and often more than 10, drafts before we think of our work as done. First drafts stick out like a sore thumb: they wander all over the place; they sound like you are making it up as you go along; and they're generally pretty boring because it's never really that clear where you're taking the reader. How many drafts do you need to do? As many as it takes. There *does* come a point of diminishing returns, where you're better off getting the paper out there to have other people read it, or simply setting aside for a few days to look at it with fresh eyes, but a big part of good writing is being supercompulsive about wanting to get it right.

More and more we find we are asked to write to length—no more than 280 characters for a tweet, no more than 600 words for an op-ed, no more than 8,000 words for a journal article, no more than 15 minutes for a conference presentation or an hour for one to the community, no more than 100 pages for a master's thesis, no more than 250,000 words for a book. Ideally you will become practiced at being able to explain your research equally well in all those different forums. The idea is to say what you need with as much economy as possible, but doing so concisely—making every word count—is a very time-consuming process. It reminds us of a quotation attributed to Pascal, who is said to have written a long letter to his friend that concluded, "I have only made this [letter] longer because I did not have the leisure time to make it shorter."

Understanding that the first draft is no more than that—a *first* draft—should take the pressure off you to feel that the world will end if your first draft is not perfect. Like Becker (2020), if you are sitting there looking at an empty monitor, we encourage you to make your first draft nothing more than a "spew" draft where you simply spit out your story, saying everything you feel you might want to say as quickly as you can type or write it down, or dictate into a voice recognition program, without recourse to notes. Spewing it out gets it down so that you can work on it. By promising yourself that you will not look at any notes you give yourself permission to make mistakes because, after all, who can simply write a first draft off the top of their heads? After that comes reflection: Is the story complete? Or are there parts of the story that have not yet been told that need to be included? Are *all* the parts currently there necessary for the story? Are there "extra" parts that are not crucial to your story that can be discarded? Going through this exercise is helpful because it helps you identify all the essential pieces of the puzzle, helps you get rid of extra fluff, and shows you what work needs to be done in the second and subsequent drafts. In the end, the only draft that matters is the last one; no one will see the others, so say whatever you want in them because they are only a way of getting to the one that counts.

Speak to Your Audience

There is no One Right Way to do a paper. Any given story can be told equally well in several different ways, with the final look of it depending on what works for you in allowing you to tell the story you wish to tell, in the style that you are comfortable telling it, *and* that speaks to the audience to whom you are telling that story.

Knowing your audience helps you with two crucial elements—assumptions and vocabulary. "Assumptions" are important because what you can assume will vary from audience to audience. For example, if you are writing to a highly specialized audience who shares your exact research interests, you will already share understandings such as what the "classics" in the area are; what issues are current; and what methods are normally used to study your problem or question. In that case you can be very direct, use specialized vocabulary that you can assume people in the area will know, and will probably spend most of your time outlining your analysis, the elements that lead to your conclusions, and some of the implications of your work for other researchers in the area.

Knowing your audience also means that you take into account what their expectations will be, i.e., what elements must be there before they accept your story as both solid and complete. With a professional but more general interest audience, you will have to take the time to contextualize your problem or question a bit, but can probably still assume a fair amount in terms of shared understandings about methods and sampling, for example. Nonprofessional audiences will need more in the way of contextualization, and you will probably end up spending less time on the actual analysis other than to perhaps give an illustration or two and more time talking about the implications of your work for the community your audience represents. The papers you write for your professors represent a situation where it is probably best to assume a certain degree of ignorance because part of what you are trying to do is to show that you understand your course material well enough to apply it. Even though your research methods professor will no doubt know what "internal validity" is, for example, you will want to show how it applies to your research as a way of showing you understand. But no matter who your audience is, we have to disagree with the sentiment that Calvin and Hobbes express in Figure 15.1; there is no reason whatsoever for academic writing to be a boring, impenetrable fog.

FIGURE 15.1 ⬥ Academic Writing Doesn't Have to Be Esoteric and Boring

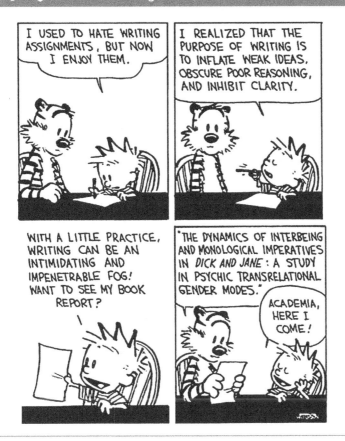

Pass It Around

Once you have a draft that you feel does the job, get someone else to read it. Faculty members who write alone are always looking for critical feedback and will often circulate papers among knowledgeable colleagues. Those who write collaboratively have each other to exchange views with as drafts go back and forth, but they, too, come to a point where another set of eyes is needed. This may come from simply passing the draft over to another colleague you know will be interested in the topic, by submitting the article to a journal so that it can undergo peer review, or, as is the case with this book, by involving a professional copy editor who goes through what we have written word-by-word and line-by-line to rein in our verbal excesses, ensure our language is consistent, and make suggestions about wording that makes our point more directly and efficiently.

Of course two things that faculty members often have are the luxuries of choice and time. We are the ones who decide that it is time for an article or book to be written, and although we often have deadlines to deal with, especially when we have agreed to write a chapter for a book or have signed a book contract, the choice of whether to commit to any of those projects in the first place is ours. In contrast, your deadlines are imposed by your professors and are typically within a single semester course, which means that being well-organized, getting an early start, and ensuring that you leave yourself enough time at the end for redrafting and perhaps exchanging drafts with a friend should be a high priority. As Howie Becker once told Ted, we learn far more from rewriting than from writing.

The main trick here is to understand that criticism is good—not something to shelter yourself from—because it can improve your final product and make you a better writer. Our writing took a giant leap forward when faculty members and friends we respected spent the hours it took to make line-by-line and word-by-word commentary on our work. Although a sea of red ink on a hard copy or dozens of "track changes" in a document file may be momentarily disappointing, the better way to see these responses is that they have been written by someone who cared enough about you and saw enough value in your work to take the time to give detailed commentary and encourage you along. Ted will always feel indebted to Bob Altemeyer and Lorna Sandler for the care they took in commenting on Ted's early papers as an undergraduate and graduate student, while Chris acknowledges the similar role played by John Lowman and Dalia Vukmirovich.

Telling Your Story

We title this section "Telling Your Story" because there are many parallels between writing a research report and writing a story or screenplay. Novelists, playwrights, and screenwriters will all tell you that every story has three parts to it: **a beginning, a middle, and an end**. Those same parts exist in every research report as well. Let's wander through each of those sections and discuss the kinds of considerations that are involved.

Beginning

The *Introduction* is where the characters are introduced and the stage is set; your "characters" in an academic article will be things like articles from the literature or perspectives on a problem (which typically are tied to sources in the literature) or positions in a theoretical or methodological debate. Which characters are appropriate for you to introduce will depend on the research questions that guided your research and what you want your report to focus on now that you're finished.

We make a distinction here between "your research" and "your report" because the two are not the same. During the research design and data gathering process, there's always a tendency to gather more data than you will actually use. The common view is "better too much data than too little," so we always stretch a little further than we originally intended to ensure we've covered all our bases and have some sense of the broader context in which our core research fits. Because of this, it is typical that you do *not* describe all of your research or detail all of your findings in a single report, in the same manner you will not cite everything you read or discuss everything you thought while you were reading the literature. The journey that research involves can be a lengthy one with assorted side trips and dead ends, but the objective of your final written report is to tell a focused, concise story. The only things that appear on paper are elements that help that story get told. Get to the point.

If you are writing a relatively short research report, like a journal article or term project (i.e., anything up to about 25 double-spaced pages), then your cast of characters will be lean; no one should be introduced who does not have an important role to play. Longer projects, such as honors or graduate theses, allow commensurately more room for character introduction. However, you still should be judicious about what is included, and everything that appears in your final draft should be there for a purpose. This requires having a preliminary sense of what your paper is about because that is a prerequisite to being able to decide what is "relevant" and "necessary" to include.

Making It "Interesting". Speaking to your audience means **making it "interesting"** for them, so one thing you want to do right at the start is to foster that interest by explaining why reading your paper is the most important thing a member of your intended audience can do. But what makes a paper "interesting"? Murray Davis (1971) asked a similar question when he decided to try and figure out what makes different *theories* "interesting." To address the topic he first determined which theories were most frequently represented in sociology textbooks—and took these as his sample of theories that were considered "interesting" enough to write about—and then considered whether there were any discernible differences between the theories that appeared frequently in texts and others that covered similar ground but did not garner the same attention.

Davis opened his article by suggesting we need to reconsider theoretical/ methodological lore, which tells us the theories that get the most attention are those that best explain data. In fact, the truth is much more "interesting" than that:

> It has long been thought that a theorist is considered great because his theories are true, but this is false. A theorist is considered great, not because his theories are true, but because they are interesting. (p. 309)

Davis's introduction is actually itself an example of a principle he explains in the article, which is that one way to catch readers' attention is to challenge what they believe to be true or what the literature believes to be true. The general form would be along the lines of, "One state of affairs *seems* to be the case, or is *believed* to be the case, but in fact *something else* is true." Much of his article involves the elaboration of that basic principle in a variety of different scenarios, e.g., what seems stable is actually changing; what seems disorganized and chaotic is actually highly structured and predictable; phenomena that seem very diverse are in fact all essentially similar. And this holds for their opposites as well, that is, something that always seems to be changing is in fact very stable, what seems structured and predictable is actually highly chaotic and disorganized, and some things that seem very similar need to be distinguished.

If there is a general message here about what makes something interesting, it is that readers are captivated when we challenge what they know, when we give information that encourages a new way of thinking about an issue, or when we inform them on a topic they know little about. The question for you as an author therefore becomes how best to present your research so that readers immediately see the value it might have for them. Some of the specific ways these justifications play out can be seen in Table 15.1.

Hooks. Remember that the primary purpose of your introduction is simply to introduce the research that you've done, but recall also how we said that part of the trick of writing well is to identify all of the pieces of the puzzle that you are trying to put together. It is for this reason that some people suggest that you should actually leave the writing of your introduction to the end. Becker (2007), for example, recalls how one of his mentors, Everett Hughes, would tell him, "Introductions are supposed to introduce. How can you introduce something you haven't written yet? You don't know what it is. Get it written and then you can introduce it" (p. 80).

While there is a lot to be said for writing the introduction last, we personally do not do it that way, preferring instead to take a shot at an introduction even though we know it is no more than a preliminary statement of what we think the paper will be about and thus knowing that one of our future editing tasks will be to figure out what parts of our first draft still belong, what in the end was irrelevant, and what is missing that needs to be included. But lying behind these statements is another lesson about writing your papers—the various parts of it must interconnect, be consistent, and lead from one to the next.

TABLE 15.1   ●   Five of the Many Ways You Can Frame Your Work to Make It "Interesting" for Readers

Making Things "Interesting"	Explanation
1. "The common wisdom says" or "everyone knows" X is true. But is it?	So much of what we "know" is based on "the common wisdom" or what "everyone knows," which often turns out not to be true at all. If your research was designed to shed light on such a state of affairs, and particularly if your findings *do* challenge people's assumptions, then inform readers of that right from the start.
2. Some people think X is true. Some people think Y. What is going on?	Controversy is interesting. If you've been doing research in an area where there has been considerable debate about what is "true" and/or where there has been disagreement over the "appropriate" thing to do, then offering your report as an effort to better understand and perhaps resolve the controversy is another way of capturing your reader's attention.
3. Our policies (and/or procedures) about X assume that Y is the case. But is it?	Policies and procedures always involve understandings or assumptions about (1) the nature of the problem the policy was designed to address, (2) the people for whom the policy is intended, (3) those who will be responsible for implementing the policy, and (4) what options led this particular policy initiative to be considered the "best" way for dealing with the situation at hand. If your research was designed to address these assumptions, then one way to frame your research is to identify the assumption and assert your interest in testing it out, for example, by seeing whether the people who apply for a program really are of a certain type or whether the treatment (or supplement or method) really is the best one available, and so on.
4. X is a phenomenon we know little about. It is interesting because …	There are many things in the world that catch our interest that we don't know much about. It may be a relatively new phenomenon or a bourgeoning phenomenon that is only now starting to appear on our radar screen, or perhaps doesn't appear at all but you would like to suggest it should. If your research pertains to such a phenomenon, then your introduction should describe what we know about it and supply any information about the pervasiveness of the phenomenon and/or the attention the issue has been receiving and/or why it deserves more attention than it has received thus far.
5. A theory suggests a certain phenomenon is interesting.	Those taking a more deductive approach may be engaged in explicit theory testing and may well have decided to investigate a particular phenomenon because it so clearly embodies the conditions addressed by the theory and, hence, is conducive to testing hypotheses derived from the theory. If that is the case, then your introduction should explain the theory and articulate the connection you see between the theory and the research setting or phenomenon.

For example, in a class that Ted taught, former graduate student Patricia Ratel completed a term project that involved interviewing single-parent mothers who were trying to balance the demands of single parenthood with those of being a student trying to complete a degree. In her introduction, Ratel (2008) cited several key findings from the literature that dealt with women who were balancing parenting with other life demands (usually work), including that (1) most single parents are women; (2) women in that situation are often in poverty and/or living on social assistance; (3) balancing the demands of single parenthood with other responsibilities has impacts for the mother such as sleeplessness, poor nutrition, high stress, and an inadequate social life; (4) social resources such as family and friends you can rely on to share the burden of responsibility are important; and (5) impacts on the children include their becoming "latchkey" children and having more than the usual level of responsibility placed on them at a young age.

We call these elements "**hooks**" because they are the themes on which the rest of the paper will hang. What you talk about in the introduction should be the variables and concepts that are integral to your research, which is what you will talk about in your results, which is what you should highlight in your conclusions. Chenail (1997) talks about this in an excellent article entitled "*Keeping things plumb.*" He talks about your area of curiosity, your research question, the data you collect, and the data analysis as four successive steps that all have to be in line, and the perils of being in the situation when you realize that you have gone off the plumb line and are effectively changing the topic. Ratel is a very positive example in that regard: After noting in her introduction that most single parents are women, we are not surprised to hear in a later section that her own research focuses on women. Of course, the same introduction could also serve the opposite purpose in order to make the paper "interesting" by saying that, while most single parents are women, very little is known about the men who find themselves in that role, and hence that is where the research will take us. Either way, the literature cited in the introduction provides the segue into the next part of the paper.

When we get to the methods section and she tells us about her interviews, we are not surprised to hear that she will ask about finances, social resources, impacts on the women, and impacts on their children. This in turn sets up the conclusion that connects back to those themes she introduced at the beginning. You should be able to see more clearly now what we mean when we say that the biggest challenge in writing a tight paper is in determining what puzzle pieces you have to work with and ensuring that you keep that consistency throughout the paper. Similarly, when we say that you should expect to do multiple drafts, it is because part of your job will be to ensure that each of the sections "speaks to" and sets up the next, which will give your paper continuity and flow. The last line of your introduction should be some statement about what you will be looking at, and the reader's response should be, "Of course. That makes perfect sense. Why would you want to do anything else?"

Middle

The middle of the paper is normally the largest part—as in any film or novel—because it is the place where the plot thickens as we articulate all the specifics of our research. This includes a *Methods* section, where you describe *what you did* (your procedures, including any research instruments) and *with whom or with what you did it* (your research sample), and a *Results* section, which outlines *what you found* (the data). Let's consider each in turn.

Methods. There are a number of elements that need to be included in any methods section. One would be to describe your sampling and solicitation procedures and the sample that resulted: who or what were your basic units of analysis? where did you find them? how did you gain access? how did you get people to participate? and what makes your research site an appropriate venue and your sample an appropriate one in/ with which to have done your research? An important point to make here will be in how your sampling is related to your research objectives. For example, were you trying to describe a particular group and sought to identify a representative sample? or were you more interested in exploring the variety of perspectives that exist within an organization on some issue and thus sought to identify more of a purposive sample? Recall that one of the main themes in the chapter on sampling (Chapter 5) is that there is no one "best" sampling technique; the appropriateness of any choice is a function of several factors, not the least of which is how well it matches your research questions and objectives. The methods section is where you explain how that connection plays out in your particular project.

It is also important in the methods section to show that you understand enough about the validity issues that will concern your reader to provide information about your sample that bears on these issues. For example, was there a prior relationship between the researcher and the participants that might have affected the completeness and authenticity of responses to interviews? In Ratel's (2008) study of single-parent mothers, for example, Ratel felt that her pre-existing knowledge of and friendship with the women, as well as the fact that she, too, was both a student and a single-parent mother, likely enhanced their trust in her and led to open reporting and valid data. In contrast, when Zellerer (1996) interviewed Inuit women in a remote northern community about their experiences with sexual violence, she believed that being a woman and a *stranger* to the community helped because the women knew they could share their stories without having to worry about the repercussions that might arise after the research ended if they were to speak with people from within their community.

At the same time, just because a researcher says everything went wonderfully does not make it so. Ideally you also will be able to point to other evidence that is consistent with the idea of full and accurate reporting. This might take the form of noting the length of time that was spent in the community or simply the length of the interviews—a 2-hour interview presumably shows greater commitment than a more superficial half-hour interview, for example. Alternatively, the kind of information that was shared might be an indication of the degree of rapport that existed; the more important, sensitive, and detailed the information, the more we are prepared to believe in its comprehensiveness and truthfulness.

Also useful in your methods section is an overall description of your participants. In Ratel's case, the emphasis was placed on showing how her small sample of single-parent mothers ($n = 9$) was nonetheless quite diverse with respect to such variables as their academic major, how many children each woman had, how long each had been a single parent, and the age(s) of their child(ren). In many survey-based studies, a portion of the survey will ask for demographic information not only because of its usefulness for analysis but also because it allows you to describe who your participants were. Also to be noted here as appropriate would be such facts as your response rate, whether any participants were excluded from the analysis and why (e.g., flippant responses; combative attitude; too much missing data).

The methods section also will describe how the data were generated and any implications of these choices on the validity of the information should be explained. Was there a structured survey or interview schedule or observational protocol or was a less-structured approach such as a guided interview taken? Why? Copies of any research instruments used would be included in an appendix to a thesis or report from a course project; journals and books rarely publish such items but they should be made available to anyone who asks for a copy. Also to be noted are how the data were recorded. For example, were the responses to a survey recorded automatically through an online form and database or with a data capture program? Or did respondents write responses down on paper, which required subsequent transcription? In the case of interviews, did they occur in a private or public location? Was confidentiality promised? In the case of interviews, did you record the conversation or take notes? In the case of observation, how were notes recorded and what procedures were implemented to ensure reliability and validity of encoding?

Generally speaking, this is the section where you outline what you did and why. The emphasis at this point should be on the positives, i.e., why you made the choices that you did and what advantages you gained by doing so. The possible limitations of your choices normally will be considered in a later section when you reflect on the strengths and limitations of what you have done in the context of that specific project.

Results. You always gather more data than you end up writing about in a report. Frequency distributions, cross-tabulations, correlations, and measures of difference in many quantitative studies can go on for dozens and dozens of pages of printout. Transcriptions of field notes and interviews from more qualitative studies can quickly run into hundreds of pages. There is no way you can report all that data. Your challenge is to prepare a summary of the data that is concise and informs your audience of the main themes or patterns that emerge from your analysis.

There are at least three basic principles that can guide the writing of a good *Results* section. First, the organization of the results section as a whole, and every table and statement within it, should be connected explicitly to whichever research question or other methodological matter the data address. Second, you should present data summaries concisely; don't use three tables if you can collapse them into one. Third, avoid redundancy. For example, if something is already in a table, then do not also describe it in the text; stick to pointing out individual highlights that speak to specific issues you want to address or patterns in the data to which you want to draw the reader's attention.

To return to Ratel's (2008) study of single-parent mothers in academe, recall how we talked about the "hooks" she included in her introduction. These included mentioning several key variables that were important in understanding the single-parenting experience, such as women's financial situation; the physical and emotional stress of trying to keep up with responsibilities by oneself in multiple, and often competing, domains; impacts on the children; the mitigating role of social support mechanisms; and the unique interest that Ratel brought forth in wanting to examine how single-parent women fared in the academic context. It thus should come as no surprise that her interviews, which she outlined in her methods section, focused on those very issues. Nor will it be surprising that the themes around which she organizes her results include headings such as "Financial Circumstances," "Physical and Emotional Stress," "The Children," "Social Support," and "Academics." By organizing her results section using themes first identified in the introduction, Ratel is making it easier for the reader to make connections with that material.

The way you present data will depend in part on the type of data you gathered. For numerical data, you should follow the principles discussed in Chapter 14 regarding the proper formatting of tables. For nonnumerical data, the presentation is handled in a somewhat different way, although once again the type of data you have and the analytical strategy you employ will make a difference. In some projects the data may involve describing how some phenomenon occurs, or how a particular organization or other group works. It will be up to you to determine how best to present that data—if it is a process you are focusing on, then the data might be presented chronologically, organized around how the process or narrative develops; if an organization, your data might be organized by the different clusters of people who work there, the various roles they fill, and how the various clusters interact with each other. In more structured interview-based studies like Ratel's, the presentation could be by theme, as we described. Whichever you choose, the basic process involved in the presentation of nonnumerical data involves going back and forth between the researcher's interpretation of what went on and the evidence that bears on that interpretation.

We see the presentation of qualitative data as very much a credibility building exercise that plays out between the researcher who writes the report and their reader. The job of the researcher is to present their interpretation of what is going on and then to present illustrative evidence that the researcher sees as supportive of that interpretation. For example, consider the following paragraph from Ratel's discussion of "Physical and Emotional Stress" as it plays out in the mothers' lives:

> All the women interviewed stated emphatically that they were physically exhausted. The multifaceted nature of their lives, the adoption of three separate and distinct roles (i.e., wage earner, student, and mother) created demands on their time and energy that were difficult to manage. Inevitably, the women sacrificed their own wellbeing to meet these demands. Collectively, they reported that they are in poor physical health and pointed to lack of sleep, lack of exercise, and inadequate diet as the key contributing factors. The women contend with some anxiety because of their financial situations, but also must face the pressures associated with the academic environment, as well as meeting the challenge of raising their children alone. There is a distinct cyclical element to this situation in which the inability to cope with the physical demands manifests itself in an inability to deal with the emotional stresses. This in turn takes a toll on their physical well-being. As Karen stated:

> I was on anti-depressants for the first year I was in school. I came very close to having a nervous breakdown, twice actually. I have a prescription for Valium but

I'm trying not to rely on the drugs any more. I live on coffee and cigarettes; I'm always exhausted. After I deal with the kids at night, cook and clean, read bedtime stories, you know … I have to work until two or three in the morning because it's the only time I have to study. I get up at 5:30 in the morning so I can have a half an hour to myself before the kids get up and I start all over again. Occasionally, I force myself to back off and get some sleep. As soon as the semester starts, I'm counting down the weeks hoping I can make it through to the break. People tell me I don't deal with the stress appropriately, that I should get some exercise and get some more sleep. I know they're right but I have to laugh. Who's got the time? They just don't have a clue what I'm dealing with here.

Note that Ratel presents data in two ways: (1) by offering her statement about one of the themes that emerged from her interviews and (2) by including a quotation from one particular interview that illustrates the theme. We can compare the two. In the first paragraph, Ratel describes how the women are exhausted, they burn the candle at both ends, they don't sleep or eat well, and it all takes a toll on their health. The quotation that follows gives the words of a particular respondent ("Karen"), and what is she saying? That she's exhausted, burns the candle at both ends, doesn't sleep much, and that it all takes a toll on her health—a perfect illustration of exactly what Ratel had said was going on. This is of course only one quote, and ideally you would have two or three brief ones to include just to show that you were not making a big deal about something that only one respondent had said, but the general form here is exactly what the reader is looking for. We get to the end of it and think, "Yup. Sounds like stress to me. And poor nutrition, lack of sleep … all those contributing things that Ratel said were there." Ratel thereby earns some credibility points and we continue on from there, and each successive round of concept/evidence establishes more and more credibility for Ratel as an insightful observer.

But now read the following example, which we made up:

The women all relied heavily on superstition and saw conspiracies everywhere. With all of life's forces beyond their control, the end result, not surprisingly, was a sense of abandonment and alienation that manifest itself in apathy toward the other women whom they previously thought of as sisters. For example, one woman stated:

My mother always told me that "what goes around comes around," so I guess I've always tried to go out of my way to treat others how I would like them to treat me. I know some of the others view it differently, and they have every right to, but that's just how I always thought of it, I suppose.

If we were to read a paper that included something like the above, our reaction would be "Huh? Are you kidding?" Is it reasonable to see a phrase such as "what goes around comes around" as evidence of "superstition"? Or to pull the phrase "I know some of the others view it differently" out of context and infer that the woman was seeing "conspiracies"? Or to see the source's acknowledgment that women all have a right to their own opinions as "apathy"? We think not. And on the assumption that the kinds of examples a researcher will give are in all likelihood the *best* examples from the interviews that *most clearly* illustrate the concept offered by the researcher, then our fictitious researcher is on truly thin ice. There are just too many other ways to look at that quotation, and we begin to have doubts about everything else the researcher claims. If we can't agree with the researcher on the matters for which evidence is put forward, how can we ever trust their claims on other summary statements where don't have direct access to the data to know what misinterpretations may be operating? We can't. Contrast this with Ratel's clear connections between conceptual assertions and data. You believe Ratel because she demonstrates to you that her observations are credible and the inferences she draws are reasonable.

Another notable aspect of Ratel's results section is the manner in which she identifies her respondents, where each quote is attributed to a particular person. The names are, of course, fictitious, as she makes clear in a footnote, consistent with her pledge to maintain confidentiality. However, use of a name does two things. First, it maintains a human touch; the respondent is "Karen" rather than "Subject 28" or "Respondent A." Second, with respect to our methodological concerns, it helps us to keep track of who is being quoted throughout the paper.

To appreciate this point, consider the presentation of results from a sampling perspective. With quantitative data presented in tabular form, the summary data that appear in the table "represent" the sample in the sense that everyone who is part of the sample is contained in the distribution and have had their data included in the computation of the mean. We paid a certain price for that. Everyone accepted that their views would only be expressed as a checkmark indicating a preference between predetermined categories, and we lost all the texture and nuance that comes when we hear people speak in their own words. What we gain in return is the ability to make charts and graphs that can easily and succinctly summarize people's views.

When we stay with qualitative data, as Ratel did, we have the advantage of getting all that texture as we read the words of the women, but, because we cannot quote everything every woman said, we present only "illustrative" quotations where Karen (in this instance) presents a view that "stands for" the sample. The thing you have to demonstrate when you present data of that sort is that you are not simply selectively presenting one individual's opinions that you happen to like and that you are sampling more than one point of view.

One way to do this is to provide a source for each quotation. Citing pseudonyms allows us to see in the paper as a whole who is being quoted at different times, without violating any confidences. Another problem with our fictitious quotation, therefore, is that we simply attributed it to "a woman" but did not attribute a particular source. How can you tell whether the next quotation comes from the same woman, who we may be quoting again and again, or someone different? In our case you can't, but you could if, like Ratel, we attributed every quote to a particular source, which would allow the reader to see that we are offering quotations from various participants and not simply quoting the same one again and again.

End

Discussion and Conclusions. The image to keep in mind as you prepare your report is of an **hourglass,** as we show in Figure 15.2. In the introduction, you start off broadly at the top end of the hourglass by connecting with the literature and noting the big social issues and concerns that got you interested in the subject matter. As the introduction proceeds, you narrow things further as you get more and more specific about your interests and gradually lay the framework for your study. You end by outlining the more concrete and specific focus of your particular research project.

The methods and results sections represent the middle portion of the hourglass, where all you're writing about is what you encountered in your research. Your challenge is to do as good a job as possible with your research participants on the topic you have chosen to study. It's not that we don't care about the bigger issues at that point; it's just not the time to be discussing them.

That time comes in the discussion and conclusion sections, which sometimes are combined, depending on the preference of the author and the dictates of the situation. You have several loose ends remaining to be tied in these sections: (1) offering a brief final statement of how your results "speak" to your research questions; (2) indicating what the implications of these results are for the bigger issues that made this research "interesting" for you in the first place; (3) tempering your inferences with critical reflection on the strengths and weaknesses of your research; and (4) any final statements you want to make about your research and its implications, which often will include suggestions for future research. All four are expected to be done in a straightforward manner with a minimum of flourish or hype.

FIGURE 15.2 ● Hourglass Shape of a Standard Written Report

ABSTRACT
- Offers an overview of the research in no more than 150 words.
- Usually written last to ensure it reflects the content of the final research report.
- Should include an overview of your study's objectives, sample, research site, method(s), main finding(s), and, if appropriate, a statement of its implications for policy or practice.
- Must stand alone sufficiently well that readers can look at it and determine whether it speaks to issues of interest to them.

INTRODUCTION
- Provides the overall context for the research and describes why it might be "interesting" to persons who engage in research and/or develop policy and/or develop theory.
- Presents a clear statement of the problem motivating the research.
- Moves from more general to more specific and provides a justification for the research.
- Includes a focused and critical review of the literature that "sets up" the research by identifying themes that will be addressed in the research and considered in the discussion/conclusion - no more and no less.
- Concludes with a specific statement of the purpose of the research and any specific research questions being posed.

METHODS
- Offers an overall description of the research procedures.
- Outlines and justifies choices made with respect to sampling of research participants and setting.
- May include copy of research instrument if a standardized protocol is being followed or may simply include it as an appendix.
- Provides a clear statement of the research question(s) that the research has been designed to answer.

RESULTS
- Clear and specific presentation of research findings, integrating the primary data collected into the analysis.
- The 'facts' demonstrated by the data are weighted and judiciously used.
- Organized thematically to reflect research question(s) and any other issues set out in the Introduction; this section anticipates the Discussion section.

DISCUSSION/CONCLUSIONS
- Begins with a summary statement of the research question or purpose of the research and gives a succinct answer to that question.
- Integrates the current study into the extant literature. Consistencies are noted and discussed in light of the generalizability of findings this reveals. Inconsistencies are also noted, and the researcher speculates on what the sources of these differences might be. Original contributions of the current research are highlighted.
- Engages in final consideration of the strengths and limitations of the research, often with an eye toward making suggestions for further research that will address any limitations/gaps that are identified.
- Concludes with general discussion of the implications of the research for other research, related policy, future research possibilities, and so on.

If the results of your research are *at odds with* the research literature, then your next task would be to consider what differences between your research/sample/context and that other research might account for any differences in findings. That will have implications for the kinds of research you might do next to see whether your speculations about the basis of those differences have any merit. However, if your research is more *consistent with* the extant literature, then your research adds evidence that speaks to the generalizability of those original findings. In that case, you might speculate on what sorts of research might be done next to further extend the generalizability of the findings, e.g., to other groups of people or perhaps to other kinds of processes or research sites. We join Becker (1998) in suggesting that the best place to go to next is to the place or group of people from whom you can learn the most, which often means looking for the situation that has the greatest potential to shoot down your developing views.

Tracking. You would be amazed at how often we go to read research reports that have been prepared by students and find that the introduction looks reasonable, and the methods section on its own sounds good, and the discussion and conclusions are alright, but where the three sections have no connection to one another! The introduction may raise some interesting issues, but if these issues do not find their way into the research, then why raise them in the first place? Most painful of all is when students seem afraid for one reason or another to bluntly ask the question they want to know the answer to and instead dance all around it and end up not being able to offer any direct answer to the question they posed! It is for this reason that we have emphasized how any research report should exhibit continuity from one section to the next:

- The introduction should lead us to the research question, lay the groundwork for the methods section, interest us in the outcomes of certain data, and provide the thematic framework that we will want to return to in the discussion and conclusion section.

- The methods section is connected to the introduction insofar as it addresses the research question(s) introduced there and tells us how they will be answered, thereby providing direction for the results and discussions sections that follow.

- The discussion and conclusions section connects back to the introduction by offering answers for the research issues introduced there, being integrated with the literature cited there, and commenting on the bigger context first considered there. It connects back to the methods and results sections because it arises from and incorporates the data and data gathering procedures outlined there.

A colleague of ours—John Lowman—uses the word "tracking" to describe this aspect of the rewriting process. He is referring to that one aspect of redrafting:

ensuring that what you have written "tracks" correctly, so that all the essential elements of your paper follow from each other and speak to each other following a logical flow. His general point is similar to the one we noted in Chenail's (1997) article about "keeping things plumb," although Chenail is using the concept more in relation to the process of doing the research, while Lowman is referring to the same type of connectedness and consistency in the various sections of the written report. No information is missing that is required to maintain the flow; nor is there any superfluous information since these are tangents and distractions.

Finish at the Beginning

We suggest the last thing you write is the element that goes first: the **Abstract**. Abstracts are brief summaries of your paper—normally no more than 150–200 words—that give an overview of your study's objectives, sample, research site, method(s), main finding(s), and, depending on your objective and the venue of publication, sometimes an implication or two of the findings for policy or practice. The reason for waiting until you finish the paper to write the abstract is that it needs to reflect what is in your paper, and since the paper itself will change to some degree as you redraft and hone its content, it's not until you've finalized the paper that you can summarize it.

There are really two main purposes an abstract serves when it's published in a journal or book. The first is that it gives readers a quick fix on the general thrust and implications of your research, which allows them to decide whether the paper is relevant to them and whether they want to spend time on the whole article. The second is that many researchers catch up on the literature by going through compendia of abstracts of recent research both to get an overall sense of recent developments and to locate those articles of special relevance and interest that they can then download or locate in the library, so your abstract should be both concise *and* self-sufficient.

CREATING EFFECTIVE PRESENTATIONS

Venues for Presentation
Conferences and Symposia

While writing is an important venue for getting the word out regarding your research, so, too, is taking advantage of whatever opportunities you have to present your work to different audiences. One such place you may do so is at conferences. We won't try and give you an exhaustive tour of the conference circuit. Suffice it to say that there are hundreds of these every year in venues around the world that tend to be organized around one of two lines.

First are disciplinary-based conferences. These can range from smaller local and regional groups of anywhere from 50 to a few hundred people, to national and international meetings where the number of people attending extends well into the thousands with numerous simultaneous sessions listed in conference programs a hundred pages long. Second are more topic-focused conferences that also come in all sizes from a couple of dozen to thousands. Discipline-based conferences bring together people who are mostly from that discipline, and sessions will typically cover a broad range of topics that reflect the diversity of the discipline. Topic-focused conferences will deal with a range of topics within that area, often bringing together people with diverse disciplinary backgrounds.

We recommend you start checking out conferences in your senior undergraduate and graduate school years and view these as part of career development. Given the sort of lag time that exists between when people finish their research and when it actually appears in print, which can often be a year or two, conferences are a great way to hear what people are doing right now, which leaves you much more current than if you rely solely on the literature. It is also a splendid opportunity to start networking with people who share your interests. In our undergraduate and graduate years, it was always a thrill to see and often to meet some famous scholar who we otherwise only knew as a name in the literature. And although every discipline has its divas and divos who are overly consumed with their own sense of self-importance, for the most part we have found academics to be very generous of their time and encouraging of new scholars who are still trying to find their way in the academic world. And it's not just the people at the front of the room who are of interest; seeing who is in the audience and hearing the questions they ask often connects you with a kindred spirit who might become a lifelong colleague. As you near the end of your studies, conferences also can be a great place to check for job opportunities as many institutions and agencies, both academic and other, see conferences as a great way to get the word out to a targeted audience and have preliminary face-to-face discussions with many people for the price of one plane ticket.

Many academics see a conference presentation as the first step in publishing their work. Disciplinary-based conferences are organized and advertised well ahead of time. There normally will be a "call for papers" 6 or 8 months before the actual conference where interested parties are invited to submit a 200-word or 300-word summary of the paper they hope to deliver. It should be pretty easy to do a summary like that as you complete a research project. The conference organizers will use these to decide who will be allowed to present (and acceptance rates for these typically are quite high) and to organize papers into thematically connected panels of three or four papers who will present in a session that might be 90 minutes long. Your paper normally will be allocated about 15–20 minutes of program time, which is enough to give the basic nuts and bolts of your work while allowing time for questions and feedback that can help you when you get back home and start writing a longer version of your work for submission to a journal.

Finally, O'Leary (2014) reminds us that yet another reason to go to conferences is to have fun. As you gain more experience, do more research, attend more conferences, and grow your research networks, conferences become a great way to make new friends and catch up with people you haven't seen in a while. It is a reminder that you are part of a broader community than just the people in your home department and provides opportunities for you to be a part of that community. Conferences also are a way to see parts of the country and the world you have never been to before and often even to have someone else pay for all or part of it! How good is that? Funding for conferences can come from a variety of sources. Sometimes these will be covered by grant funds, but even if you are not in a position to acquire such funding yourself, many universities have funds available that you can access to pay or at least subsidize your travel.

Community and Stakeholder Audiences

There are likely to be audiences other than academics who are interested in your work as well. Community groups, high school classes, and profession-based groups are often looking for speakers for their monthly or annual meetings. Alternatively, you may have done a research project in an organization you work with and have now been tasked with presenting your work to those in the company or agency who will be most interested in hearing about it, perhaps because they were the participants, or will be the ones implementing the recommendations you came up with, or will be developing new policies based on your findings, or will be managing those most affected when any changes come into effect. These can be great opportunities to talk about the implications of your work to audiences who are actually in a position to put your ideas into practice as well as to offer you constructive commentary from a more practical perspective.

Included among these groups will be the people with whom you did your research. If it was done with a community group or organization or company or agency, what better way to reconnect with those who made your research possible than to go back and share what you found? In addition to going full circle and feeding the fruits of your labor to people who helped enable it in the first place, what better place to get feedback on what you have done, to discuss implications of your work you may not have thought of, and to discuss potential opportunities for future research that would address issues there was no time to include in the previous research or that were identified in that preliminary study.

Elements of a Great Presentation
You and Your Audience

As was the case with written media, when you are presenting your work in person, a huge factor to consider is your audience because you want to "speak" to them in a manner that is meaningful to them. If you are doing a conference presentation, for example, you will want to meet the expectations of a conference audience, which will involve being explicit about your research question, how you went about answering it, your major findings, a caveat or two about the limitations of what you did and what could be done next, and how your study contributes to the literature.

If you are doing a presentation to community members who assisted in your research by providing facilities and/or access to special populations, you will probably spend less time detailing your methods other than in general descriptive terms (e.g., how many people participated and what methods you employed) and much more in detailing what you found that would be of interest to them. It might be advice about how they might better serve their community, or how the data you gathered might be instrumental in helping them acquire better financing from whoever funds them, or to recruit new members. Remember this is not about you or about trying to impress people with how much you know; they will be most impressed if you speak in a language they understand and have the flexibility to adapt what you present to what is most meaningful and helpful for them to know.

General Structure

As was the case with written reports, a great presentation will have a beginning, a middle, and an end. The beginning is when you connect with your audience and set the stage for what is to come. Your first slide will show your title and your name as well those of any co-authors. This is a good time to set the ground rules you will be operating by. Will you be giving any handouts? If so, do this before you begin the presentation, or after it is over, as doing it in the middle will be a distraction. Would you prefer for people to interrupt you if they have any questions? Or should they wait for the end?

With those details out of the way, you are ready to transition into the presentation. One good way to begin with the title slide still showing on the screen is with a story of how you became interested in the topic. Alternatively, you may have a poignant story about something you heard or saw during the research, or that might have appeared in the news recently, that highlighted for you why this was an important piece of research to do. The research has dominated your life for a while; this is where you bridge the gap to your audience's world and captivate their interest by giving an indication there was meaning in this research for them. Whichever way you go, keep this brief. Remember that a typical conference presentation is only 15–20 minutes long, and that time will fly by, so any preamble should be short because it is already eating into precious time—aim for 1 minute and never go beyond 2 unless you have a much longer time slot.

Then it's off to slide number 2 which, for many people, is the place to give a roadmap or outline of what is to come. For others, including us, it is more useful to make this the place where you begin the overall story arc of your talk by outlining the question your research was designed to address and then gives a tour of your work that emphasizes those aspects that will be of greatest interest to your audience. Depending on who you are speaking to, that might be some combination of the intricacies of the design and analysis, and/or some of the challenges you faced in completing the research, and/or the main findings, and/or the implications of what you found for members of your audience.

Gray (2014) outlines various structural templates that you can follow. The first is a more inductive approach, where you present people with a series of facts and then tell them the conclusion you derived from it. That can make for an engaging presentation because it invites readers to figure out where they see it all heading to and allows you and the audience to compare notes at the end. The second template is a more deductive one where you present the conclusion first and then outline the facts on which you based that conclusion. The more deductive approach is a "safer" route because it invites a confirmation bias; the question people ask themselves is whether the data you are presenting is consistent with the conclusion you have drawn. In contrast, we find the more inductive approach more engaging for audiences because it invites them to come up with their own conclusion, and we rather like it when we get to the end and someone inevitably starts with a comment along the lines of, "Gee, the place I thought you were going was X, but you took it to Y; have you considered this alternative way of looking at it?" Perhaps we have been around long enough and done enough presentations that we enjoy the challenge of that situation and simply enjoy having people offer alternative ways of thinking about our work; our work improves because of it. Although no one likes a hostile audience, we would rather have a thoughtful and challenging one than a complacent one.

A third presentation structure that Gray (2014) offers is a discursive structure in which you first present the two sides of an argument and then present the evidence that led you to choose one side more than the other. Sometimes a controversy in the literature may offer the opposing positions that you then made an effort to resolve through your research. Sometimes there will be two or more different policy approaches that you or your organization will need to choose between, and perhaps your study speaks to the assumptions on which the alternatives are based, or perhaps deals with evidence of the differential effectiveness of one approach over the other, or simply compares costs and benefits of each route. A fourth alternative that Gray (2014) refers to as "situation, options, and the way forward" is similar to the discursive approach. The story line here involves first presenting the audience with a dilemma that has to be resolved—the situation. Next come the alternatives to dealing with the situation that have been considered, with arguments for and against each option presented along the way. Last comes your suggestion for the way forward, where you justify your choice.

Avoiding Death by PowerPoint

What did the world do before PowerPoint? If we had a penny for every speech or presentation that was offered using PowerPoint slides, we would be rich enough to retire comfortably, but we suppose Bill Gates is the only one who gets to do so. But while PowerPoint has become ubiquitous as a backdrop for our presentations, so, too, have complaints about its use. The fact that there are now many alternatives to PowerPoint that do roughly the same thing simply means that the pain has spread more broadly, not that we have become better at presenting. The phrase "Death by PowerPoint" has become synonymous with the situation where the audience is so underwhelmed by a presentation they die from boredom, as is reflected in the cartoon in Figure 15.3. Try putting "Death by PowerPoint" in your favorite search engine and you will have enough links to keep you busy for a long time.

Although the concept is generally considered to be metaphorical, it seems there was a time that a PowerPoint presentation literally did contribute to the deaths of seven people (see Thomas, 2019). In January 2003, the space shuttle *Columbia* launched successfully and would complete 16 days worth of scientific experiments that were its primary mission. However, a day after launch, while the shuttle was still in orbit, engineers reviewing video footage of the launch saw that a piece of insulating foam had come loose and collided with one of the tiles on the shuttle's left wing. Pieces of falling foam were no big deal, but the tile this piece collided with was one that played an important role in protecting the shuttle from the heat that occurred when the shuttle re-entered earth's atmosphere. NASA managers had a choice to make: They

FIGURE 15.3 ● Scene of the Crime: Death by PowerPoint

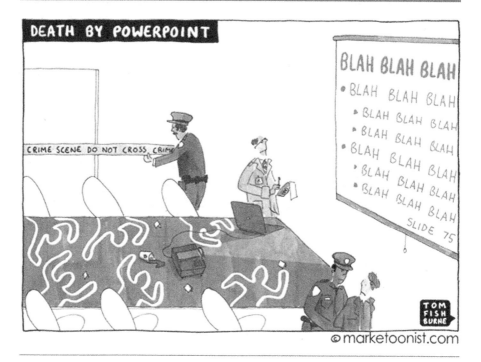

could (1) ask the astronauts to do a spacewalk to check for damage; (2) get another space shuttle to go up and bring the astronauts home; or (3) risk re-entry. As Thomas (2019) explains,

> *NASA officials sat down with Boeing Corporation engineers who took them through three reports; a total of 28 slides. The salient point was whilst there was data showing that the tiles on the shuttle wing could tolerate being hit by the foam this was based on test conditions using foam more than 600 times smaller than that that had struck* Columbia. *[The slide shown in Figure 15.4] is the slide the engineers chose to illustrate this point. … NASA managers listened to the engineers and their PowerPoint. The engineers felt they had communicated the potential risks. NASA felt the engineers didn't know what would happen but that all data pointed to there not being enough damage to put the lives of the crew in danger. They rejected the other options and pushed ahead with* Columbia *re-entering Earth's atmosphere as normal.*

FIGURE 15.4 ● A PowerPoint Slide Outlining Risks for Space Shuttle *Columbia*

Review of Test Data Indicates Conservatism for Tile Penetration

- The existing SOFI on tile test data used to create Crater was reviewed along with STS-87 Southwest Research data
  - Crater overpredicted penetration of tile coating significantly
    - Initial penetration to be described by normal velocity
      - Vaires with volume/mass of projectile (e.?g. 200ft/sec for 3cu. Ln)
    - Significant energy is required for the softer SOFI particle to penetrate the relatively hanrd tile coating
      - Test results do show that it is possible at sufficient mass and velocity
    - Conversely, once tile is penetrated SOFI can cause significant damage
      - Minor variations is total energy (above penetration level) can cause significant tile damage
  - Flight condition is significantly outside of test database
    - Volume of ramp is 1920cu in vs 3 cu in for test

Source: Thomas (2019).

All seven astronauts died when the shuttle disintegrated as it returned to earth's atmosphere on February 1, 2003.

Edward Tufte is Professor Emeritus of Political Science, Computer Science, and Statistics at Yale University. He is also an expert in "statistical evidence and scientific visualization" who did an analysis of the PowerPoint presentations on which the Columbia decision was made (see Tufte, n.d.; see also Harris, 2004). His analysis, which was incorporated into the official *Columbia* Accident Investigation Board report (CAIB, 2003, p. 191), explained how poorly the slide communicated what Boeing Engineers thought they were communicating. Among other things, he notes how packed with information the slide is, how it uses six different levels of hierarchy in its bullet structure that do not correspond with the relative importance of the information, how the space limitations of a Power-Point slide encourage cryptic phrases and abbreviations that were not necessarily understood by non-Engineers instead of full explanatory sentences, how the main heading and the first levels of information all point to there being little to be concerned about, and how the main caveat about risk—the very bottom line that conveys in cryptic fashion that the actual velocity with which the piece of foam hit the wing was more than 600 times the force of the testing they were reporting—was completely lost under the weight of the more positive information above it.

The *Columbia* tragedy and Tufte's subsequent analysis is a reminder of the costs of poor communication and also, for our purposes, shows how viewers are influenced by different aspects of a PowerPoint presentation and thereby helps us begin to generate some basic principles that will make your presentations that much better. We start by showing you the opposite in Table 15.2—20 things you can do to create a horrible presentation. Stated in a more positive way, there are several more fundamental points that characterize a great presentation. One key point several observers make is for you to understand that *you* are the presentation, not the PowerPoint slides (e.g., Gray, 2014; Harris, 2004; James, 2011; O'Leary & Hunt, 2016; Phillips, 2014). It is a subtly different way of thinking, but a profound one, because it shifts the main

---

TABLE 15.2 ● Twenty Ways to Commit Death by PowerPoint

Take a paper you have written and try and put all the same information into your slides	Use a bright background that ensures people will pay more attention to the screen than you
Include a long introduction so that you will have to rush through the rest of your presentation	Put as many points on a slide as you can to reduce the number of slides you have
Use complicated graphics because people are visual learners	Make your headline as big as possible because that's the most important part of the slide
Treat each slide as speaking notes and read them while people read along with you	Use lots of animation and sounds because twirling images and zippy sounds grab people's attention
Face the screen to read your slides because the slides are more important than you	Assume that the technology is functional and will work when you get in the room
If you are running out of time and still have lots of slides to go, speak faster	If you practice your presentation ahead of time, do so by reading it silently to yourself
Use jargon and acronyms that only some of the audience will understand	Flip back and forth between slides as you make different connections as you speak
Include information that is tangential to your topic just in case you need it	Copy and paste complex charts, graphs, and flowcharts directly into your presentation
Use up all your speaking time so that people will not have an opportunity to ask questions	Go off on tangents whenever a slide reminds you of an interesting story
Give the speech you want to give rather than the one that would be meaningful to your audience	Use fonts that look great on your monitor but are too small for people in the back to see

Source: A compilation of advice from Kapterev (2007), James (2011), Phillips (2014), and our own experience.

question for you to address from "what do I need to put in my slides to make it a good presentation?" to "what slide content will help me underline the points I am trying to make to this audience?"

With that frame in mind, Phillips (2014) offers an excellent TED talk that includes a reference to the kinds of features and phenomena that capture our brain's attention—and which thus will keep attention on the slides—and suggests these are the exact opposite of what you should do if you want to have the attention on you as presenter. Because we attend to movement, size, contrast, and signaling color, for example, he suggests we stay away from glitzy animation, finds it ironic that we make the headline of each slide the largest item on the slide when it is the content below it that is typically much more important, and dismisses the screaming attention of a default white background with black letters to a much calmer black background with white text that does not compete with you for attention.

Several of the suggestions in our antilist of Table 15.2 also refer to the amount of material on each slide. While the antilist urges you to put as much as possible on one slide, Phillips (2014) and others (e.g., Gray, 2014; James, 2011; Kapterev, 2007) urge us to keep the content to one idea per slide. Any numeric tables you include should be simplified, and the parts you want people to pay attention to should be highlighted above the rest of the table so that people are not left searching for whatever it is you are talking about. They also suggest no more than six items on a slide because our brain can capture six items at a glance, while more than that requires processing time, which takes the attention away from you. Even six items is a lot, however, such that you are advised to open them one at a time, with the appearance of each one linked to the preceding ones losing contrast and fading into the background. If you want to give people notes, the authors we cite here suggest you put it in a separate handout that gives the detail, not to put it in the slides. Generally speaking, the rule is "less is best" (Berk, 2012; O'Leary & Hunt, 2016).

Getting Ready

The key that all the authors we cite suggest that is needed for a great presentation is to practice, practice, practice, both to reduce nervousness and allow us to show up confident and minimally needing our notes. How many of us have suffered through a presentation where the speaker reads their notes in a monotone voice that bores us to tears, or worse yet, turns around, and reads their text-filled slides as if to show off their literacy skills to an illiterate audience while we get to see the backs of their heads. If you can practice in the room in which you will be delivering your talk, so much the better. Similarly, if you can practice delivering to real people—friends, family, other presenters—that will help as well.

The big thing about practicing is that it needs to be done orally, i.e., you need to speak your speech rather than just read it to yourself. There are two main reasons for this. First is that we talk differently than we write, so you need to make sure that your presentation sounds right, which you can only really do by saying it to ensure the words roll off your tongue smoothly. Second is that practicing your talk orally will give you a better sense of how much time it will take. Some of the worst presentations come from people who swear that it only took them 15 minutes to go through their presentation, but now realize after 20 minutes they still have six slides to go. This of course causes them to speak even faster in an effort to save at least some small portion of the time that was to be devoted to questions and, at worst, will lead them to commit the ultimate conference no-no, moving into the next speaker's time.

Finally, if at all possible, make sure you check out the room beforehand that you will be presenting in as well as the technology in the room. Given the size of the room, will people at the back be able to see your slides? If you wanted people to break into small groups in the middle of your presentation, does the seating allow for that to be done comfortably? Regarding the technology, there is no worse time than the beginning of your presentation to find out that you don't know how something works, or that an adapter is missing, or that you should have brought your remote control because the one you thought would be supplied wasn't. We also advise you assume that Murphy's law will prevail and come prepared for the fact the internet may be down by having all the material you need on a USB and are prepared for the room computer to malfunction by bringing your own laptop as backup.

Dealing With Questions

Some people worry most about the question period at the end of their talk, particularly over the prospect of looking foolish or ignorant if they do not have an answer. As Gray (2014) suggests, when you do get a question, step 1 is to make eye contact with the person asking it. Step 2 is to make sure you heard it correctly and understand what is being asked ... and if you don't, then to politely ask them to repeat or clarify the question. If you are speaking in a larger forum where the people asking questions are not using a microphone, you may want to repeat the question to ensure everyone in the audience has heard it as well. And finally, don't feel that the responsibility for answering every question lays with you. Although as speaker you always have the first opportunity, there are no rules that say you can't open up an interesting question to the audience, e.g., to ask whether anyone else has experienced those problems or has other interpretations to offer. People don't typically go to talks to humiliate speakers (and those few who do probably need therapy more than answers) but to hear something they are interested in and possibly join an interesting conversation about something they care about, too.

O'Leary and Hunt (2016) remind us that getting questions at the end of a talk is something you should see as a positive sign rather than a negative one. There is no way one talk is going to cover everything that can be covered about a topic. If people are asking questions, it is because you have engaged their interest and they want to know more. The worst thing to experience when you get to the end of your talk is silence.

As to the types of questions you might get, O'Leary and Hunt (2016) note that questions at a presentation tend to fall into one of the three categories:

- *Clarification* (What is that first word on slide 5? What year is that data from? Does your recommendation require any ongoing costs?)

- *Analysis* (How did you decide between the alternative recommendations? How do we know the problem of X is caused by Z? How did you estimate the cost of delaying action?)

- *Gaps* (Did you consider X? I would have considered X, you should consider X.)

The most common questions are questions of clarification. They typically can be answered in a word or two and more than likely will be something you already know and considered that might just need a reaffirmation and possibly a source to justify. The other two types of question will probably involve a lengthier response where you explain reasons for your choice. For the "have you considered…?" questions, if you have considered the alternative, then explain why you rejected it in favor of the one you chose. If you hadn't, then you could either respond with, "That's interesting, I'll look into that further when I get back home," or respond with a question to the questioner, such as, "Could you explain a bit why you see that as a more plausible (or useful or practical) alternative?"

DISSEMINATING FINDINGS THROUGH SOCIAL MEDIA

Understanding Why, Who, and How

As we have seen, most of the time social and health researchers publish or present their findings exclusively through academic channels. For these researchers, the primary vehicles for disseminating findings are dissertations, journal articles, books, or presentations at professional conferences (which are often closed to the public and require both researchers and audience members pay a fee to participate). Increasingly, funding agencies and organizations are demanding that findings from the research they fund be disseminated beyond academic circles. Researchers working outside of the academy frequently seek to influence key policy and decision-makers by disseminating their research findings through more public channels such as general reports made available through organizational websites, publishing in open access publications, issuing press releases, and participating in mainstream news or public affairs media stories, segments, or features.

Social media is comprised of a collection of information communication technologies (ICTs) and platforms built upon a web 2.0 foundation. This foundation focuses on design, functionality, and ease of use for users, where users often are active participants in the creation and/or dissemination of content. At present, some of the most popular social media platforms are Facebook; YouTube, Instagram, Tumblr, Reddit, SnapChat, Twitter, LinkedIn, and Pinterest. While still comparatively underutilized, social media platforms represent a rapidly evolving and expanding channel of public communication that can be used to disseminate and exchange knowledge generated from our research to a wide range of individuals, groups, and organizations.

Before you dive into using social media to disseminate your research findings, it is important that you take some time to understand what the different platforms do, how people use them, and to see if it makes sense for you to use them to disseminate your research findings. Next, and probably more importantly, you need to determine if you have the capacity, capability, and/or desire to take part in social media. Here you need to be realistic and honest with yourself about your knowledge, understanding, and comfort level with using ICTs. You also need to decide if you are the type of person who is willing and able to invest considerable time and energy into navigating and staying up-to-date on the emergence of different social media platforms and how to use them. Moreover, you need to decide if you are willing to put part of your life out there for public consumption, weighing out the benefits and burdens that being a public intellectual has for your privacy and even your personal safety. In the end you might decide that you are not cut out for social media, in which case you will want to consider alternative vehicles for disseminating your research findings. If, however, you do decide that social media is right for you and that it would be a valuable tool for disseminating your research findings, you will need to take steps to: identify the best platforms to connect with your audience, establish your social media presence or identity, determine how to best package information to communicate it to your target audience(s), and take the necessary steps to engage your target audience.

Identifying and Connecting to Your Audience

Perhaps one of the greatest advantages of social media for social and health researchers is that it provides a platform to reach a broader audience and potentially boost the influence of your research findings. Step 1 is to identify the audience that you feel could benefit most from your research. Make a list of these individuals, groups, and organizations who could or you feel should be interested in your work, including practitioners, community members, legislators and policy makers, key stakeholders associated with an issue, key news media outlets and reporters, government agencies, or health and support service organizations, to name a few.

Once you have identified your target audience, you need to determine which social media platform is the most appropriate to use to relay your research findings. In order to do this, you need to establish which members of your target audience use social media and what platforms they use. Failing to do so means your message may never even be received. In a recent community-based case study Chris was involved in, the government had set aside resources for the creation of information "hubs" where parents of children under 6 years old could go to access information about specific programs and services being offered in their community. The organization charged with creating one of the hubs invested significant resources into researching the community programs and services and decided that an optimal way to disseminate this information to families would be by creating a Facebook group. Unfortunately, results from the case study revealed that the majority of parents with children under 6 years old in the community did not use Facebook—they preferred Instagram—so the time and energy spent mobilizing Facebook as a vehicle for disseminating needed information to the community was wasted.

The moral of the story is that in order to identify which platforms your target audience uses, you need to spend some time researching the individuals and organizations that you're targeting. To do this you might want to start by seeing if they have a personal or organization website, and if they do, see if they provide any links to social media accounts on their site. You also could search for them using the search functions of the different social media platforms. If this doesn't work, you could run a Google search for the person or groups name along with "Facebook," "Instagram," or "Twitter." Hopefully the person or group you are searching has a unique name; a common name could leave you with hundreds or thousands of results to sort through. To narrow down the results, you could do a Google image search instead and scroll through the results looking for the person's image. Chances are you will come across their profile picture for Facebook, Twitter, Instagram, Pinterest, or another site. If their social media accounts are linked, as is the case when someone posts tweets from their Twitter account on their Facebook page, you can identify the multiple social media accounts they use. Finally, you can use search sites like PeekYou, Pipl, YoName, or Zoom Info that use web crawlers to catalog information from the public profiles of people that exist across the web.

Establishing a Social Media Presence or Identity

Social media platforms have the potential to increase the reach and impact of your research findings by getting them to the individuals or groups that can most benefit from them or who can put them to best use. If done well, health and social science researchers who use social media to disseminate their findings can raise not only the profile of the research but also their own reputation in a way that establishes them as an authority in the field.

If you are affiliated with a particular organization, company, or institution, you may be able to use their existing social media account to disseminate your findings. If not, you will have to take steps to create new social media accounts and establish your social media presence or identity. When you first create your social media account(s), your audience often has no way of knowing who you are and if the information you are sharing is worth monitoring, so you have to take steps to legitimate your social media presence. It is important to keep in mind that this process of establishing your social media identity and following takes time and effort and it can take even longer before your target audience starts seeing you as a trusted source of information. Fortunately, there are a few strategies that we have tried over the years that have proven to be quite effective in establishing a social media presence for different research projects that we have been involved in.

The first thing we have found is that it is vital that you create a fully descriptive profile on your social media accounts. This means you will need to provide a clear description of who you are and what your research is about. It is also really helpful to provide photos of you and/or your team or at the very least a logo that visually represents your research. If you opt to provide a logo, make sure that you keep the visuals associated with your account (e.g., the colors, images, and fonts) consistent as this creates an air of professionalism. In team research environments it can be beneficial for each member of your research team to create social media profiles related to the research.

Once you have created your accounts, publicize them as far and wide as you can. Make it as easy as possible for people to follow you by placing follow buttons or icons on all of your websites, email signatures, or other digital content. If you publish material in other forms such as websites or blogs, make it easy for people to share that content by including sharing buttons (e.g., Twitter and Facebook logos and Pinterest article pins) on each page, ensure that you use proper content or page titles that social media search engines like Hootsuite and Buffer can read, and provide graphics with your content so that when people post it to their social media feeds the post gets noticed. Also, include links to your social media accounts in the content title.

Next you will want to connect with the individuals and groups that are central nodes in the networks of your target audience. Here a good place to start is by following "influencers" or "thought leaders." Influencers or thought leaders are individuals or organizations that several members of the population that you are targeting follow. For example, thought leaders in Chris's area of research include the Centers for Disease Control and members of major news media outlets who produce television media segments or write feature articles on issues associated with Chris's research program. It is important to try to engage the influencers or thought leaders so that they will acknowledge your account and potentially follow you and like or forward or repost your posts. A good way to do this is to make an effort to repost or share their posts on topics or issues related to your research. It is not unusual for influencers or thought leaders to follow you back if you share their content and occasionally they will share your content as well.

Once you have established your social media presence or identity, you need to work to ensure that your target audience continues to see you (or your account) as a legitimate source of valuable information. To help you with this, we recommend setting and maintaining a consistent schedule for disseminating findings, and when you do not have specific findings to share with your growing network of followers, take time to post or repost information that you come across during your day-to-day activities that you think might be relevant or of interest to your following. It is important that your followers see your social media account as not only an important source of information about the research you are involved in but also as a good resource for more information. For example, when he is not posting quotes from his published articles or infographics summarizing a particular story that emerged from his research, Chris generally spends 30 minutes a day posting information he thinks might interest his followers. This information can include citations to recent research publications or summaries of important findings; blog posts that are relevant to his audiences' interests; links to current television or print media features or articles; or information about upcoming funding opportunities or public events.

Communicating Information to Your Audience

One of the neat features of using social media as a vehicle for sharing the findings of your research is that it offers you greater flexibility when it comes to how you can package the information you share. For example, you can employ more traditional formats such as PDF articles or graphics of tables and figures depicting results or you can provide links to more detailed content such as full publications, blog posts, or websites. Alternatively, you can develop more animated or interactive formats such as videos, podcasts, infographics, or interactive models such as the one our colleague Patrick John Burnett created depicting the network of social science faculty of major research Universities between 1977 and 2017 (see http:// www.relational-academia.ca/canada-network.html). That said, the format you choose can also limit your ability to provide the level of detail, nuance, or quality that you want to provide. For example, the 140 or 280 character limit that Twitter places on individual tweets would make it very difficult to disseminate all but the most superficial of research findings. You need to package your information in a way that is appropriate for the particular social media platform you're using. Determining which formats fit on which platform takes time to learn; get started by studying the different social media platforms and look at the types of posts that appear on each.

In addition to making sure that the format fits the platform, it is important to be creative in how you present the information that you post. Generally speaking, in the land of social media, images, and video rule. This is probably why social media sites such as Instagram are so popular right now, Facebook live videos get far more engagement than other types of content, and Twitter tweets that have graphics and videos are shared significantly more than text posts. While such graphic and video contents get more traction, it is important to keep in mind that producing more dynamic content such as videos, podcasts, and infographics often requires you to have the time and skills with video editing, podcasting, or visual information display. If you are pressed for time or you or someone on your team doesn't have the skills to produce such content you may find it beneficial to hire a graphic designer, web producer/videographer, and/or communications specialist who does—assuming you or your organization has the budget to do this.

Connecting With and Engaging Your Audience

Different social media platforms have the potential to enable a more timely and cost-effective dissemination and exchange of information. However, in order for this to occur, you need to take steps to ensure that your posts are connecting with and engaging your target audience. The ever-growing amount of information now being transmitted via social media makes it more challenging for target audiences to filter out relevant and valid content (information overload). You must be mindful that important information you want to relay may be getting lost in translation or in the technological abyss.

Again, there are several steps you can take to improve the chances that you will indeed connect with your target audience. The first and arguably most important thing you can do is stay on topic or on brand. Post information that is directly relevant or reflective of the theme of your account (i.e., if your research area is sexual health, consistently post information relevant to sexual health and avoid posting pictures of your latest family vacation). This allows your target audience to start to associate your social media account with a particular topic and facilitates "brand recognition." To enhance this "brand" connection, use tags to distinguish or high-light the theme of your posts. For example, on Twitter, the hashtag is an essential tool for people to find content on the topics that they're interested in. If you make use of hashtags, people will be able to find the content that you reference.

A key attribute of social media is that it is "social," meaning that it is not static like traditional knowledge dissemination platforms. Using it affords you the opportunity to engage in a dialogue with an audience. Whenever possible, create a feedback loop or dialogue between you and your audience so that you can assess how they are interpreting and utilizing the findings you have shared. You can do this by making sure that you like or repost the posts in which you are mentioned and if someone tags you, respond to them directly.

It is also a good idea to set and follow a posting schedule. If you're posting on a consistent basis, it is more likely that people will follow you and pay attention to your posts. Having a posting schedule will also allow you to fine-tune your posts for different platforms and maximize engagement. Use the insights and analytics each platform provides to track or gauge (using various metrics) the level of social engagement (i.e., the size of your audience and who you are reaching with your posts) over time. The analytics will tell you what days of the week and times of the day your differing posts receive the most views, likes, or reposts. This way you can determine the optimal day, time, and type of post in order to best reach your target audience.

Some Final Thoughts and Considerations

Social media offers a variety of opportunities and advantages for social and health researchers who wish to disseminate their research findings to a broader or more targeted population of knowledge consumers. Despite this, it is important to keep in mind that effectively using these platforms requires technological knowledge, skills, access, and understanding. While the gap between the technological haves and have-nots is closing, a digital divide still exists both in terms of the researchers that will have the access, knowledge, and capacity to use social media (Grande et al., 2014) and the audiences with whom we wish to share our research findings.

There are also important issues that need to be taken into consideration with respect to participant privacy and confidentiality and professional and personal vulnerability. When we are transmitting information over open networks, particularly when we are targeting particular social networks in our knowledge dissemination efforts, there is always a risk that what we say in our posts could result in individuals who participated in our research being identified, which would compromise their privacy and confidentiality. For example, if in the course of conducting an interview with a participant they mention their Twitter account and you then go and follow them, there is a chance that someone will put 2 + 2 together and infer that the person was one of your research participants. A good rule to follow when using social media is to avoid following accounts of people or groups that participated in your research and just allow them to follow you.

On a related note, the use of these platforms also poses a potential professional risk to us as researchers since it places us firmly within a public domain where we are more vulnerable to personal attacks by trolls, being doxed, having our privacy invaded, etc. This vulnerability not only has implications for our professional status and advancement, it could also have repercussions for our personal safety as well. For example, despite the fact that Chris does not post anything on his various social media accounts that advocate a particular political position with respect to his research on the sex industry, over the years he has been the target of several attacks launched by people and organizations that use social media as a platform for advocating a particular moral and political agenda with respect to the sex industry. Some of these attacks have even gone so far as to publish pictures of him that have been captured from his appearances on different televised news and public affairs segments.

Used effectively, social media can be another valuable tool in the researcher's toolbox for disseminating research findings, both within and beyond the academic community. As is the case with every other research tool we have discussed throughout the book, as a researcher you must always weigh the opportunities and advantages of any strategy or technique against its disadvantages or challenges. When it comes to disseminating research findings, social media should not be used as a replacement for more traditional forms of disseminating research findings; instead, it should be used to complement traditional ways of relaying information from our research to the audiences that will benefit most from having access to our findings.

SUMMING UP AND LOOKING AHEAD

The primary purpose of this chapter is to give you some advice on how to disseminate the results of your research to a wider audience, something many readers of this book will be doing in conjunction with a course on research methods where this book is being used. A central theme of the chapter is that although each part of the paper has a unique purpose and provides unique information, the various parts all are linked and interdependent insofar as each part sets up, anticipates, and speaks to issues that are raised in other sections.

The parts of a research paper and the roles each part fulfills were depicted in Figure 15.2. The way linkages can be accomplished between the various sections of the paper was emphasized; each should prepare the ground for the next, i.e., the introduction introduces the issues that are then taken up in the research methods and results section that provides the basis for revisiting and forming conclusions in relation to the issues that were raised in the introduction.

Publishing papers for other academics is an important part of our work, but researchers these days are often just as interested in sharing their work with those who would potentially benefit from hearing about it. Presentations—whether to academic or community audiences—are a second important way researchers disseminate their findings that offer networking opportunities as well. Although many of the principles to follow for presentations are similar to those for papers—the need to engage your audience and tell a story with a beginning, a middle, and an end—the time-limited oral setting poses unique challenges in a very different medium.

Finally, the 21st century researcher also should consider carefully developing a presence on social media both to facilitate networking with others in the field and to cultivate an audience for your work. Accordingly, we finished the chapter by explaining some of the considerations to keep in mind when deciding whether and how to use social media to both build and maintain communication with a community of interest.

Key Concepts

Abstract 642
Beginning-middle-end 628
Death by PowerPoint 647
Hooks 632

Making it "interesting" 629
Hourglass shape 639
Know your audience 626
Social media platforms 654

"Spew" draft 625
Tracking 641

STUDY QUESTIONS

1. Explain the "hourglass" form that most papers follow.

2. Explain why it is important to create "hooks" in your introduction.

3. What does Chenail mean when he says that you should keep your work "plumb"?

4. What makes a paper or presentation "interesting"?

5. Your authors say that every paper and presentation will have a beginning, a middle, and an end. Explain in your own words what goes into each section.

6. Find out about your disciplinary conferences. Look for a smaller local or regional one and another larger national or international one. Ask a professor or check them out online.

7. Check out two journals that publish articles in your area of interest. Compare and contrast them on subject area, mission, length, citation style, and focus.

8. What are some considerations to keep in mind when choosing a media platform to disseminate information?

9. What benefits arise from using social media to talk about your research? What are some potential disadvantages or problems that can arise?

APPENDIX A

CRITICAL VALUES OF CHI-SQUARE

df	Level of Significance for a Nondirectional Test				
	.10	.05	.02	.01	.001
1	2.71	3.84	5.41	6.64	10.83
2	4.60	5.99	7.82	9.21	13.82
3	6.25	7.82	9.84	11.34	16.27
4	7.78	9.49	11.67	13.28	18.46
5	9.24	11.07	13.39	15.09	20.52
6	10.64	12.59	15.03	16.81	22.46
7	12.02	14.07	16.62	18.48	24.32
8	13.36	15.51	18.17	20.09	26.12
9	14.68	1 6.92	19.68	21.67	27.88
10	15.99	18.31	21.16	23.21	29.59
11	17.28	19.68	22.62	24.72	31.26
12	18.55	21.03	24.05	26.22	32.91
13	19.81	22.36	25.47	27.69	34.53

(Continued)

df	Level of Significance for a Nondirectional Test				
	.10	.05	.02	.01	.001
14	21.06	23.68	26.87	29.14	36.12
15	22.31	25.00	28.26	30.58	37.70
16	23.54	26.30	29.63	32.00	39.29
17	24.77	27.59	31.00	33.41	40.75
18	25.99	28.87	32.35	34.80	42.31
19	27.20	30.14	33.69	36.19	43.82
20	28.41	31,41	35.02	37.57	45.32
21	29.62	32.67	36.34	38.93	46.80
22	30.81	33.92	37.66	40.29	48.27
23	32.01	35.17	38.97	41.64	49.73
24	33.20	36,42	40.27	42.98	51.18
25	34.38	37.65	41.57	44.31	52.62
26	35.56	38.88	42.86	45.64	54.05
27	36.74	40.11	44.14	46.96	55.48
28	37.92	41.34	45.42	48.28	56.89
29	39.09	42.69	46.69	49.59	58.30
30	40.26	43.77	47.96	50.89	59.70

The table lists the critical values of chi-square for the degrees of freedom shown at the left for tests corresponding to the significance levels that head the columns. If the observed value of X^2obs [the observed value of chi-square] is greater than or equal to the tabled value, reject H_0 [the null hypothesis]. All chi-squares are positive. *Source*: Sir R.A. Fisher & F. Yates (1974). *Statistical tables for biological, agricultural and medical research* (6th ed.). Harlow, UK: Addison Wesley Longman, Table IV. Reprinted by permission of Pearson Education Limited.

APPENDIX B

CRITICAL VALUES OF r

df = N−2	Level of Significance for a Nondirectional (Two-Tailed) Test				
	.10	.05	.02	.01	.001
1	0.9877	0.9969	0.9995	0.9999	10.0000
2	0.9000	0.9500	0.9800	0.9990	0.9990
3	0.8054	0.8783	0.9343	0.9587	0.9912
4	0.7293	0.8114	0.8822	0.9172	0.9741
5	0.6694	0.7545	0.8329	0.8745	0.9507
6	0.6215	0.7067	0.7887	0.8343	0.9249
7	0.5822	0.6664	0.7498	0.7977	0.8982
8	0.5494	0.6319	0.7155	0.7646	0.8721
9	0.5214	0.6021	0.6851	0.7348	0.8471
10	0.4973	0.5760	0.6581	0.7079	0.8233
11	0.4762	0.5529	0.6339	0.6935	0.8010
12	0.4575	0.5324	0.6120	0.6614	0.7800
13	0.4409	0.5139	0.5923	0.6411	0.7603
14	0.4259	0.4973	0.5742	0.6226	0.7420
15	0.4124	0.4821	0.5577	0.6055	0.7246

(*Continued*)

df = N−2	Level of Significance for a Nondirectional (Two-Tailed) Test				
	.10	.05	.02	.01	.001
16	0.4000	0.4683	0.5425	0.5897	0.7084
17	0.3887	0.4555	0.5285	0.5751	0.6932
18	0.3783	0.4438	0.5155	0.5614	0.6787
19	0.3687	0.4329	0.5034	0.5487	0.6652
20	0.3598	0.4227	0.4921	0.5368	0.6524
25	0.3233	0.3809	0.4451	0.4869	0.5974
30	0.2960	0.3494	0.4093	0.4487	0.5541
35	0.2746	0.3246	0.3810	0.4182	0.5189
40	0.2573	0.3044	0.3578	0.3932	0.4896
45	0.2428	0.2875	0.3384	0.3721	0.4648
50	0.2306	0.2732	0.3218	0.3541	0.4433
60	0.2108	0.2500	0.2948	0.3248	0.4078
70	0.1954	0.2319	0.2737	0.3017	0.3799
80	0.1829	0.2172	0.2565	0.2830	0.3568
90	0.1726	0.2050	0.2422	0.2673	0.3375
100	0.1638	0.1946	0.2301	0.2540	0.3211

If the observed value of r is greater than or equal to the tabled value for the appropriate level of significance (columns) and degrees of freedom (rows), reject H_0 [the null hypothesis]. The degrees of freedom are the number of pairs of scores minus two, or $N-2$. The critical values in the table are both + and − for nondirectional (two-tailed) tests. *Source*: Sir R.A. Fisher & F. Yates (1974). *Statistical tables for biological, agricultural and medical research* (6th ed.). Harlow, UK: Addison Wesley Longman, Table VII. Reprinted by permission of Pearson Education Limited.

APPENDIX C

CRITICAL VALUES OF *t*

df	Level of Significance for a Nondirectional (Two-Tailed) Test				
	.10	.05	.02	.01	.001
1	6.314	12.706	31.821	63.657	636.619
2	2.920	4.303	6.965	9.925	31.598
3	2.353	3.182	4.541	5.841	12.941
4	2.132	2.776	3.747	4.604	8.610
5	2.015	2.571	3.365	4.032	6.859
6	1.943	2.447	3.143	3.707	5.959
7	1.895	2.365	2.998	3.499	5.405
8	1.860	2.306	2.896	3.355	5.041
9	1.833	2.262	2.821	3.250	4.781
10	1.812	2.228	2.764	3.169	4.587
11	1.796	2.201	2.718	3.106	4.437
12	1.782	2.179	2.681	3.055	4.318
13	1.771	2.160	2.650	3.012	4.221
14	1.761	2.145	2.624	2.977	4.140
15	1.753	2.131	2.602	2.947	4.073
16	1.746	2.120	2.583	2.921	4.015

(Continued)

	Level of Significance for a Nondirectional (Two-Tailed) Test				
df	.10	.05	.02	.01	.001
17	1.740	2.110	2.567	2.898	3.965
18	1.734	2.101	2.552	2.878	3.922
19	1.729	2.093	2.539	2.861	3.883
20	1.725	2.086	2.528	2.845	3.850
21	1.721	2.080	2.518	2.831	3.819
22	1.717	2.074	2.508	2.819	3.792
23	1.714	2.069	2.500	2.807	3.767
24	1.711	2.064	2.492	2.797	3.745
25	1.706	2.060	2.485	2.787	3.725
26	1.706	2.056	2.479	2.779	3.707
27	1.703	2.052	2.473	2.771	3.690
28	1.701	2.048	2.467	2.763	3.674
29	1.699	2.045	2.462	2.756	3.659
30	1.697	2.042	2.457	2.750	3.646
40	1.684	2.021	2.423	2.704	3.551
60	1.671	2.000	2.390	2.660	3.460
120	1.658	1.980	2.358	2.617	3.373
∞	1.645	1.960	2.326	2.576	3.291

The value listed in the table is the critical value of t for the number of degrees of freedom listed in the left column for a directional (one-tailed) or nondirectional (two-tailed) test at the significance level indicated at the top of each column. If the observed t is greater than or equal to the tabled value, reject H_0 (the null hypothesis). Since the t distribution is symmetrical about $t = 0$, these critical values represent both + and − values for nondirectional tests. Source: Sir R.A. Fisher & F. Yates (1974). *Statistical tables for biological, agricultural and medical research* (6th ed.). Harlow, UK: Addison Wesley Longman, Table III. Reprinted by permission of Pearson Education Limited.

GLOSSARY

Abduction: Moving away from prediction and hypothesis testing; the idea is to consider which of various different explanations best explains the phenomenon observed. (p. 33, Chapter 2)

Abstract: A brief summary of a paper, normally no more than 150–200 words, that gives an overview of the study's objectives, sample, research site, method(s), main finding(s), and implications of the findings. (p. 642, Chapter 15)

Academic freedom: It been defined as "the right to teach, learn, study and publish free of orthodoxy or threat of reprisal and discrimination" consistent with the ethical standards of one's discipline. Free inquiry is seen as the foundation upon which innovation, creativity, and theoretical development can grow. Concern about academic freedom is growing these days as the intervention of third parties into the research process—government, corporations, special interest groups—seems to be increasingly placing constraints on what researchers can do, and universities and colleges administrations themselves seem to be engaging more frequently in micromanagement of their faculty.

Activist research: Researchers who share political values with an organized group of people they study, and serving their interest by doing research that helps advocate for their cause. (p. 479, Chapter 11)

Adaptive questioning: Where answers to specific questions influence the subsequent questions asked. For example, a question early in a survey might ask you to identify your favorite sport. If you respond that it is "hockey," then instead of subsequent questions asking you about "your favorite sport" an adaptive questioning strategy would simply refer to "hockey" given that you have already identified that as your favorite sport. (p. 340, Chapter 9)

Analytic control: Adapting to a situation by anticipating and addressing all **rival plausible explanations** in our research. Contrasts with **manipulative control**, where researchers actually intervene in a situation to create conditions that are most conducive to valid inference about internal validity. (p. 273, Chapter 7)

Analytic induction: A process of theory formulation characteristic of inductive approaches. The researcher begins by making observations and formulating a tentative explanation for those observations. Next, the researcher examines the adequacy of that explanation (does it account for all the data?) and revises the explanation until it successfully accounts for all observed data. Particular attention is paid to negative cases (observations that are inconsistent with the tentative explanatory scheme), since these will suggest revisions. Once an explanatory scheme has been devised that's consistent with all the data gathered to date, the researcher gathers more data to see whether they, too, are consistent with the explanation. If not, the process continues. (p. 302, Chapter 8)

Annotations: Memos or notes about one's thoughts or insights on a particular passage of qualitative material. In NVivo annotations are virtual sticky notes that we attach to a particular element (section of text or area of image, video, or audio) of any project document. (p. 534, Chapter 13)

Anomaly: Things that aren't supposed to happen, if indeed a theory is true. For example, early astronomers, who believed that the earth was the center of the universe, were faced with the anomaly that Mars does not follow a circular or elliptical path around us, but occasionally "wanders" back and forth across the heavens. Recognition of this anomaly was a boon to theory development in astronomy; Copernicus eventually argued for the correctness of *his* theory (that we travel around the sun) because it accounted very simply for what only appeared to be Mars's irregular path, explaining why the illusion occurred. (p. 61, Chapter 2)

Anonymity: Keeping a participants name/identity unknown, even to the researcher. (p. 120, Chapter 4)

Autoethnography: The researcher uses self-reflection to explore anecdotal and personal experience to connect to a wider cultural, political, and social meanings and understandings. (p. 469, Chapter 11)

Background/demographic questions: These are straightforward questions that are useful in describing your sample and potentially also help you make distinctions within your sample that can be useful in your analysis. (p. 400, Chapter 10). Typical demographics include variables such as age, sex, education level, race/ethnicity, a measure of social class.

Beginning-middle-end: A general structure in presenting your research. The beginning is when you connect with your audience, introduce your "characters" (which typically refers to the concepts that will be featured in your research), and set the stage for what is to come. The middle is when you present your research design and analysis, results, and main findings. The end is when you review strengths and limitations of your work and discuss its implications. (p. 628, Chapter 15)

Bernie Beck trick: A method used to identify existing literature that may be connected to what your research interest is. This is performed by asking "tell me briefly what your research is all about, but without using any of the identifying characteristics of the actual case." This will produce a general description of the research, which will open doors for relevant literature for examination. (p. 46, Chapter 2)

Blind condition: Research done in a way in which experimenters do not know what type of treatment that a participant received, thereby eliminating one source of potential experimenter bias. (p. 232, Chapter 6)

Bonferroni technique: A technique that involves splitting the adopted probability required for significance across the entire range of comparisons to be made. For example, if you're adopting a significance level of $p < .05$ and plan to undertake 10 separate t-tests (or chi-squares or Pearson correlations), the Bonferroni procedure involves spreading the .05 (known as the *experiment-wise error rate*) across the 10 comparisons, with the result that a .05/10 = .005 significance level would have to be achieved on any given comparison before you'd be prepared to consider it "reliable." (p. 614, Chapter 14)

Boolean operators: Useful when engaging searches for keywords, the Boolean operators AND, OR, and NOT can be used to modify the inclusivity or exclusiveness of your searches. The wildcard character (*) can further modify your search to allow for various forms of a word (e.g., method* will search for all words that start with method, such as methodology, methodologian, methodologist). Quotation marks can be used to delimit exact phrases. (p. 48, Chapter 2]

Bounding: A procedure used to reduce errors due to **tele-scoping** that can occur when you have vague time referents such as "in the last 6 months." Bounding is when researcher uses a more specific point of reference (e.g., since last Christmas) in questionnaires in order to assist participants recollection of valid information. (p. 524, Chapter 12)

Case: A focus of study bounded in space and time; "bounded system," sometimes described as "one of many." (p. 296, Chapter 8)

Case study analysis: Analysis of a single case. (p. 16, Chapter 1)

Categorical response item: Closed item questions with predetermined response categories. (p. 354, Chapter 9)

Categorical variables: Variables that differ in kind but have no order or magnitude underlying their differences. For example, you might be counting types of fruit and your categories might include bananas, apples, and oranges. The three are simply different types of fruit, with none of them being any more or less of a fruit than the others. (p. 566, Chapter 14)

Category system: A type of coding scheme that involves using a set of mutually exclusive and exhaustive categories to code any given behavior we observe. For example, to use a category system to code for violent content in a film, we'd typically begin by breaking the film into units (on, say, a minute-by-minute or a scene-by-scene basis) and code whether the behavior in each minute or scene is predominantly violent, nonviolent, or whatever. Category systems give a better indication of the *temporal flow* of criterion acts during the observational period than do sign systems. (p. 447, Chapter 11)

Certificates of Confidentiality: A certificate issued by the National Institutes of Health in the United States that provides statutory protection for researchers engaged in health research to ensure that they cannot be forced to disclose identifying research information about their research participants to any civil, criminal, administrative, legislative, or other proceeding. See also **Privacy certificates.** (p. 124, Chapter 4)

Ceteris paribus: A Latin phrase meaning "all else being equal." This phrase—often explicitly and always implicitly—underlies theoretical statements; that is, variables *X* and *Y* are related to each other, *ceteris paribus*. It's also the cornerstone of the experimentalist methods discussed in Chapters 6 and 7. The true experiment embodies the *ceteris paribus* assumption by testing the effects of certain variables on other variables under conditions in which, overall, all other variables are equalized. (p. 246, Chapter 6; p. 290, Chapter 8)

Chi-square: A statistical test used to assess whether two categorical variables are associated beyond what would be expected on the basis of chance variation alone. The chi-square statistic describes deviations between what we'd expect (on the basis of chance, if the two variables were indeed independent) and what we actually observe. (p. 591, Chapter 14)

Clarification probes: Asking/probing questions directed to respondents in order to clarify something that they had said previously. (p. 405, Chapter 10)

Class privilege: A relationship—such as that between a lawyer and his or her client—that is recognized and protected under law so that the normal obligation we have to testify what we know when subpoenaed is set aside. In such relationships the onus of proof is on those challenging the protected nature of the communications to demonstrate what compelling reasons exist for the privilege to be set aside. (p. 125, Chapter 4)

Closed or structured questions: Questions with limited response options, such as categorical response items and rating scales. (p. 350, Chapter 9)

Cluster analysis: A method of organizing coded material that involves placing similarly thematically coded information (e.g., people, places, events, or social artifacts that share common characteristics) into relational categories that allow the analyst to make distinctions among groupings or clusters of people, places, and so on that

are meaningful to the researcher and/or participants. (p. 535, Chapter 13)

Code: The most basic unit of coding used in the program NVivo. Codes are short labels representing ideas, themes, personas, places, interests, or concepts. In NVivo codes are used to store all of the references from the data (e.g., segments of text, image, video, or audio material) that correspond to a particular theme, topic, idea, or concept we identify. (p. 544, Chapter 13)

Coding: A method of data management whereby the analyst attempts to simplify observations by way of assigning them to conceptually or theoretically relevant categories. When an analyst codes the volumes of data they have collected they are in essence organizing and reducing the data into smaller more manageable segments that can be retrieved easily and compared with other coded segments of data. A coded segment might represent or illustrate a specific theoretical or analytic concept, or it can simply reflect elements of the data that we want to highlight or think about further. (p. 532, Chapter 13)

Coding scheme: A manual, often prepared prior to the analysis of data, that outlines the rules that will be used to structure the coding of textual, visual, or audio observations in a manner that helps to improve the **validity** and **reliability** of the coding classifications made. (p. 446, Chapter 11)

Cognitive interviewing or think-aloud interview: This involves pilot testing a survey or questionnaire by having people read through the questions aloud and to articulate their thinking process while they decide how to respond. Doing so helps highlight misunderstandings and ambiguities of wording that can be used to improve questions prior to distributing the survey. (p. 376, Chapter 9)

Common law: Law based on legal precedents as established through judicial decisions as opposed to legislative decree. (p. 125, Chapter 4)

Common Rule: The regulatory system for ethics in the United States is embodied in what is known as "The Common Rule" in the *Code of Federal Regulations*, or more specifically, 45 CFR 46.102(d) and (f). The regulations, which were initially formulated in 1991 and significantly revised in 2018, apply to all "research" that involves "human subjects" in institutions that seek federal research funding.

Compensatory equalization of treatments: One of several possible threats to **internal validity** that can emerge in field settings when the treatment or program being evaluated involves goods and/or services considered desirable and where there is a large disparity between groups. Seeing the disparity, administrators, those charged with implementing the treatment, or some of the recipients may reroute some goods or provide access to services among some or all members of the disadvantaged group in an effort to alleviate the disparity. This practice makes the groups less distinct than they would otherwise have been, potentially leading to an erroneous finding of "no difference." (p. 274, Chapter 7)

Compensatory rivalry: One of several possible threats to **internal validity** that can emerge in field settings. If it's known that an evaluation is in progress, one may see compensatory rivalry by the respondents who are receiving the less desirable treatment(s). Knowing that you are in the disadvantaged group may spur a competitive spirit to overcome adversity and perform well. This is particularly likely to be the case in situations where the group already perceives itself as a group (e.g., work teams, crews, classes) and has a lot to lose if a difference is revealed. (p. 275, Chapter 7)

Complete observer: One end of the traditional observational continuum. In this role, the researcher identifies themself to the participants as a researcher who's engaged in observational research. Once in the setting, the complete observer typically does their best to remain relatively inconspicuous, doing nothing other than observe with the full knowledge of all who are present that that's why the researcher is there. Contrasts with **complete participant** (the other extreme of the role continuum). (p. 439, Chapter 11)

Complete participant: One end of the traditional observational continuum. In this role, the observer doesn't reveal himself or herself as a researcher; from the perspective of those being observed, the researcher *is* a participant. There are two ways this might occur: (1) *post hoc* observation, where a former participant writes his or her account of a setting or event well after the fact, and (2) surreptitious observation, where the researcher

observes people without their knowing that they're being observed for the purpose of research. Contrasts with **complete observer** (the other extreme of the role continuum). (p. 439, Chapter 11)

Computer-assisted social research (CASR): Using computer technology within networked environments (e.g., the Internet or an intranet) to assist researchers in creating, editing, and finalizing the research instrument. (p. 339, Chapter 9)

Concurrent mixed data analysis: Using one data source to complement and expand on the analysis of another that is administered at about the same time. (p. 555, Chapter 13)

Concurrent validity: A type of validity that involves correlating responses on our measure to some other criterion. Suppose our measure of "romantic love" involves asking two people the question "Are you in love?" We must show that responses to that question are tied to some other independent measure of "love." For example, Zick Rubin's (1973) research on this topic shows that people who say they're "in love" tend to gaze into each other's eyes more often and for longer periods than do couples who do not say they're in love. If we take those measures at approximately the same time, we're engaging in concurrent validation. "Concurrent" means "at the same time"; temporal closeness between the two measures defines concurrent validation. Contrasts with **predictive validity.** (p. 90, Chapter 3)

Confidentiality: The ethical right of people to keep information about themselves private or to share it only with those whom they trust to safeguard it. (p. 118, Chapter 4)

Confirmation bias: A type of cognitive bias where people only pay attention to information that confirms their previously existing beliefs or biases instead of being open to negative evidence that would cause them to reconsider those beliefs. (p. 303, Chapter 8)

Conflict of interest: A situation in which the aims of two or more parties are incompatible, or working against each other. It is particularly problematic when one person has power over the other, as sometimes occurs in the research context, and can impose their will to the disadvantage of the other. (p. 143, Chapter 4)

Conflict of role: It occurs where there are contradictory and incompatible demands placed upon a person relating to their position. In the research context this can occur when people interview friends or work colleagues and occupy the dual role of "researcher" and "friend" or "colleague." (p. 144, Chapter 4)

Consensus tyranny: Pressures to require a unanimous position by a group, which may mask the diversity of the group and cause the perspectives of some members of the community to be suppressed. (p. 480, Chapter 11)

Constant: Something that does not vary. (p. 564, Chapter 14)

Constructionism: The view that we actively construct reality on the basis of our understandings, which are largely, though not completely, culturally shared. It thus becomes important to understand people's and society's constructions of things because those constructions will have implications for how we study and make sense of the world. For example, men and women have been "constructed" as active and passive, respectively, for many years. This construction has even spread to our understandings of sexual intercourse and conception. We once envisioned active spermatozoa, released when the man ejaculates, swimming to the woman's ovum, which passively awaits fertilization. As our conceptions of women have changed in recent years, so, too, has our conception of conception. Now researchers bring a more egalitarian perspective to their understanding of the fertilization process: although the spermatozoa are still characterized as swimming to the ovum, the ovum is now considered to play a more active role in "send[ing] out messages to the sperm, participating actively in the process, until sperm and egg find each other and merge" (Flint, 1995, p. D8).

Content analysis: Analyzing existing artifacts of human existence which include texts of various formats, pictures, audio, or video. (p. 489, Chapter 12)

Contingency questions: A question or a subset of questions in an interview or questionnaire that require the respondent to answer only if he or she has answered in a particular way to previously asked questions, e.g.,

"If 'no,' go to question 3; if 'yes,' go to question 4." (p. 335, Chapter 9)

Contingency table: A celled matrix that is used to display the joint (or bivariate) frequencies of the distributions of responses to two nominal or categorical variables. (p. 590, Chapter 14)

Control group (or comparison group): A group that is treated identically to the experimental group in *all* respects *except* that it does not receive the independent variable. Its purpose is to control for **rival plausible explanations.** (p. 212, Chapter 6)

Convergent mixed data analysis: Merging two forms of data into a single dataset in order to compare and contrast the results. (p. 555, Chapter 13)

Convergent validity: The degree to which your measure is related to other measures to which it is supposed to be related. For example, a measure of how "in love" people are *should* be related to other measures of affection, intimacy, and commitment. If we show that our measure is related to those other indicators, we've demonstrated convergent validity. (p. 90, Chapter 3)

Correlation ≠ causation: Just because two things regularly happen together does not mean that one is necessarily causing the other. (p. 204-205, Chapter 6)

Covert observation: Collecting information by observing participants in the field without announcing your role. (p. 441, Chapter 11)

Criterion sampling: Selecting cases that meet a specific criterion that makes them eligible for our research by virtue of belonging to some group of interest or having had some particular life experience we are interested in investigating. (p. 187, Chapter 5)

Critical case sampling: Selecting cases that are most likely to contain important information for the research. (p. 188, Chapter 5)

Critical ethnography: It focuses on the implicit values expressed within ethnographic studies, with particular attention paid to injustices created or maintained by, e.g., social structures, systems of power relationships. (p. 471, Chapter 11)

Critical realism: Critical realism, or the *critical realist perspective*, can be seen as a midway resolution that acknowledges some truth in both realist and social constructionist perspectives. Like the constructionists, critical realists acknowledge that "reality" is indeed constructed and negotiated, but they also assert that reality is not *completely* negotiable, that is, all explanations are not equally viable. In other words, we *can* be "wrong." But, if we can be "wrong," there must be a reality out there that exists independent of our opinions of it.

Cultural critique: A researcher whose main primary political allegiance is to the academy, and to the knowledge from research, not to the relationship established with the organized group of people being studied. Contrasts with a more **activist** approach (p. 479, Chapter 11)

Data analysis triangulation: The practice of employing several different methods of analyzing and interpreting data in order to improve the validity of the conclusions by ensuring the robustness of your results.

Death by PowerPoint: A situation where the audience is so underwhelmed by a presentation they die of boredom. (p. 647, Chapter 15)

Deduction: See deductive approaches. (p. 7, Chapter 1; p. 33, Chapter 2)

Deductive approaches: Research perspectives characterized by the belief that researchers should begin with theory, from which they deduce hypotheses, which they then test by gathering data. If the data support the hypothesis, the theory that gave rise to that hypothesis has gained some support, and further tests of the theory (through further hypothesizing and data gathering) are formulated. If the data do not support the hypothesis, the theory's adequacy is questioned, suggesting that the theory should be either rejected or revised. Also known as the **hypothetico-deductive method**, and sometimes as *"top-down" approaches*. Contrasts with **inductive approaches**. (p. 7, Chapter 1; p. 34, Chapter 2)

Deductive coding: Where the analyst codes audio, video, or textual data using a well-specified or predefined set of interests or concepts, generally based on prior research (and the literature) and/or theory. (p. 533, Chapter 13)

Definitional operationism: A play on the term "operational definition" that refers to a type of mono-operationism in which researchers engage in the tautology of operationally defining their variables of interest by definition. For example, a researcher may develop a measure of intelligence but, instead of showing that the measure possesses **convergent and divergent validity** with respect to other measures, may simply state that the measure is its own definition; that is, what we mean by intelligence is whatever our test measures. (p. 91, Chapter 3)

Degrees of freedom: The theoretical distribution of a given inferential statistic will vary in form depending on the number of parameters that are free to vary. (p. 593, Chapter 14)

Demographic items: See demographic variables. (p. 376, Chapter 9)

Demographic variables: Information about an individual or social group that helps contextualize the person or group, usually in relation to "social facts." It includes variables such as age, sex, race, socioeconomic status, education, and gender. (p. 88, Chapter 3)

Dependent variable: In research, the variable we measure in order to assess whether the **independent variable** exerts any effects. It gains its name because a person's status on the variable (e.g., his or her score) *depends* on whatever effects the independent variable has. Also sometimes known as the *outcome* variable. (p. 206, Chapter 6)

Descriptive statistics: Statistics that are used to summarize sample data. The major ones included in Chapter 14 are statistics that describe **central tendency** (the mean, the median, and the mode) and **variability** (the mean and the standard deviation). (p. 564, Chapter 14)

Dichotomization: See dichotomy.

Dichotomous item: A type of categorical response item that contains only two response alternatives. Any question that asks you to answer yes or no, true or false, whether you own or rent, can swim or not, have ever been to Peru or not, or whether you prefer the Democratic or Republican candidate for President, would be considered a dichotomous item. (p. 354, Chapter 9)

Dichotomy: Any division into two parts; an especially popular and appropriate term with respect to classification. A sample might be dichotomized into males and females or into an experimental and a control group. But dichotomies can also be less concrete; qualitative and quantitative approaches to science, for example, represent a dichotomy of research perspectives.

Diffusion (or imitation) of treatment: One of several possible threats to **internal validity** in field evaluations, where it's not unusual to be faced with intact groups that cannot be isolated from one another. Instead of having two (or more) comparison groups that are clearly distinct on the independent variable being considered, we may find that the boundaries between the groups are or become somewhat blurred. For example, if the groups are differentiated by their access to varying sets of information, any communication between groups about the nature of this information will make each group a little more like the other(s). This diffusion of treatment will act to minimize the groups' separation and heighten their similarity, which may result in a false negative, i.e., where you conclude there is no difference between the groups when really there is. (p. 274, Chapter 7)

Direct realism (or naïve realism): It is the epistemological position that holds that there is a (i.e., one) reality out there that exists independent of us that can be understood and awaits our discovery. An implication of this view is that, if reality involves a singular truth that exists independent of the observer, it should be able to be understood by different observers in exactly the same way.

Direct relationship: See **positive relationship**. (p. 600, Chapter 14)

Disproportional stratified random sample: A probability sampling technique that is used when the researcher is primarily interested in comparing results between strata rather than in making overall statements about the population or when one or more of the subgroups are so small that a consistent sampling ratio would leave sample sizes in some groups too small for adequate analysis. The researcher begins by stratifying the population into subgroups of interest and taking a random sample within each stratum, but a different sampling ratio is used within each stratum, so that equal numbers of units of analysis end up in each of the strata samples. (p. 173, Chapter 5)

Disprovable: Falsifiable; an important quality of any theory is that it must be able to be disproved. (p. 303, Chapter 8)

Divergent validity: It involves showing that your measure is not related to other measures to which it's not supposed to be related. For example, a measure of how "in love" people are *should not* be related to independent and different concepts like respect or tolerance (since each of these can exist without love being present). If we show that our measure is independent of (i.e., not correlated with) measures of those other indicators, we've demonstrated divergent validity. Contrasts with **convergent validity**. (p. 90, Chapter 3)

Double-barrelled items: A question that asks about two different things at the same time. For example, if we were to ask you if you thought Nashville was a great city for theatre and listening to live music, you are being asked about two different things and may feel quite differently about them. (p. 370, Chapter 9)

Echo probe: Repeating or paraphrasing the last thing the respondent said and then asking them to continue with their story. It shows that you are paying attention to and understand their response, while also inviting them to expand further. (p. 404, Chapter 10)

Ecological validity: A type of **external validity** that addresses issues of representativeness and generalizability in a slightly different way. Brunswik (1955) first used this term, which refers to how well the treatments and measures you use reflect the particular milieu to which you wish to generalize. (p. 222, Chapter 6)

Emic: Perspective of the insider, the social group being studied. Contrasts with "**etic**." (p. 450, Chapter 11)

Encryption: The encoding of messages or information so that only authorized parties can access it. (p. 121, Chapter 4)

Epistemic relationship: In research we are always going back and forth between theoretical concepts and specific real-world data that we believe reflect those concepts. The epistemic relationship refers to how well those two things coincide. (p. 87, Chapter 3)

Epistemology: It deals with the question of how we know what we know and what criteria we bring to the evaluation of whether something is "true" or not.

Ethics creep: The overextension of an ethics committee's jurisdiction into areas that are not actually part of its mandate. (p. 110, Chapter 4)

Ethnography: A method of field research used in anthropology that focuses on "culture" and involves collecting information from people in their natural setting for an extended period of time. See also **participant observation** and **field research**. (p. 464, Chapter 11)

Etic: Perspective of the outsider, the observer. Contrasts with "**emic**." (p. 450, Chapter 11)

Evaluation imperialism: The view that a better world can only be created by empirically driven evaluators. (p. 284, Chapter 7)

Evolutionary epistemology: A concept positing that scientific theories will evolve over time because constant empirical testing and revision will bring us ever closer to the truth.

Exhaustive: Covering all possible alternatives. A term often used in relation to response options provided in a questionnaire or structured interview such as a CATI. (p. 355, Chapter 9)

Experience/behavior questions: These questions ask the interviewee to describe overt actions and events that you might have seen had you been there to observe it. (p. 400, Chapter 10)

External validity: The **generalizability** of results beyond the specifics of the study, particularly to other people, situations, and times. (p. 221, Chapter 6)

Extreme or deviant case sampling: Selecting cases that are vastly different or extremely out of the ordinary for research. (p. 185, Chapter 5)

Face validity: The degree to which a set of measures appear to measure what it is intended to measure; at face value. (p. 503, Chapter 12)

Fallibilist realism: A philosophical position that maintains that human beings can be wrong about our beliefs and understandings of the world as a result we must be open to evidence that contradicts our beliefs and understandings. It is also known as **critical realism**.

Feeling questions: These questions try and get at respondents' emotional responses to events or whatever phenomenon you are asking about. (p. 401, Chapter 10)

Field research: A data collection method that aims to observe, interact, and understand people *in situ*, i.e., while they are in the environment in which the phenomenon of interest normally happens. (p. 464, Chapter 11)

Gatekeeper: A person who controls access to research participants or other research data such as archival content. Gatekeepers often hold a position of power or status relative to the researcher who seeks access to the individuals, groups, organizations, or social artifacts that the gatekeeper safeguards. (p. 143, Chapter 4)

Generalizability: The ability to extend the results or findings of the research to other people, situations, or times. (p. 153, Chapter 5)

Go native/overidentify: A term used by positivists in a pejorative way that is said to occur when a researcher takes on the values and perspectives of the group being studied and abandon the detached, analytical stance that, according to positivists, is required to effectively study the world. Positivists believe that getting too "involved" with the people we study will destroy our objectivity.

Google Scholar: A publicly accessible web search engine that indexes the full text and metadata of literature across an array of publishing formats and disciplines.

Granularity: The level of detail in the data. The greater the granularity, the deeper the level of detail. (p. 363, Chapter 9)

History: In experimental research, it is one of many threats to **internal validity**. In this context, the term refers to any specific events that occur during the course of the research in addition to the independent variable. To the extent that such other variables exist, they threaten internal validity because those other variables end up being **rival plausible explanations** for any changes we observe. One way history is effectively controlled is by including a control group, which is a group that's treated identically in all respects to the experimental group (and hence subject to all the same historical factors), except for administration/receipt of the independent variable. (p. 207, Chapter 6)

Hit-and-run research: It is done when researchers enter a community and extract data without prior permission, or due acknowledgement of local partners and collaborators, and then leave immediately after they have gotten what they want. (p. 475, Chapter 11)

Hooks: An element in your research paper where you introduce an initial theme or concept that will be picked up later in the design and analysis of you research. (p. 632, Chapter 15)

Hourglass shape: An image to keep in mind as you prepare your report: in the introduction, start off broadly at the top end of the hourglass by connecting with the literature and noting the big social issues and concerns that got you interested in the subject matter. Then you become more specific as you move into the details of your particular project, including your methods and findings, after which you broaden out again as you connect back with the literature and explore the broader implications of your work. (p. 639, Chapter 15)

Humanistic obligation: A moral responsibility to uphold values that respect human dignity in our research. (p. 112, Chapter 4)

Hypotheses: See **hypothesis**. (p. 33, Chapter 2; p. 69, Chapter 3)

Hypothesis: An unambiguous statement about the results that you expect to occur in a situation if the theory that guides your work is true. Hypotheses are generally associated with deductive inquiry, which believes that "good research" should begin with theory and should be directed toward testing theory. Stating your hypothesis before beginning your research is a bit like placing your bets ahead of time, so that you can't come back after the results are in and say, "Oh yes, I knew that was going to happen." If you knew, you should have said so. (p. 37, Chapter 2; p. 69, Chapter 3)

Hypothetico-deductive method: The long name given to the process of deduction in social and health science research. The prefix "hypothetico" points to the role that the *a priori* (before-the-fact) specification of hypotheses plays in this brand of inquiry. Contrasts with **inductive approaches**. (p. 7, Chapter 1; p. 33, Chapter 2; p. 82, Chapter 3)

Independent variable: In research, the variable whose effects we wish to identify or assess. Also sometimes known as the *treatment* variable or the *causal* variable. Contrasts with **dependent variable**. (p. 206, Chapter 6)

Induction: See **inductive approaches**. (p. 18, Chapter 1; p. 33, Chapter 2)

Inductive approaches: Research perspectives characterized by the belief that research should begin with observation, since it is only on that basis that theory grounded in the real world will arise. Thus, researchers observe, induce empirical generalizations based on their observations, and then, through analytic induction, attempt to develop a full-blown theory that adequately reflects the observed reality. Sometimes known as *"bottom-up"* approaches; contrasts with deductive (or "top-down") approaches. (p. 12, Chapter 1; p. 36, Chapter 2)

Inductive coding: A method of coding textual, audio, or visual data where the analyst either begins with the identification of general themes and ideas that emerge from a very literal reading of the data and then proceeds to either elaborate the category by making finer and finer distinctions or combines specific descriptive coding categories to create more general categories that bring disparate events or descriptions under the same conceptual umbrella. Contrasts with **deductive coding** where the researcher brings certain themes or codes into the analysis on the basis of theory, other research, even prior to seeing whatever data one has to work with. (p. 533, Chapter 13)

Inferential statistics: Statistics that are used to facilitate drawing conclusions about data concerning the extent to which variables are associated and whether differences exist among groups—on the basis of population estimates derived from sample data. The techniques included in Chapter 14 are the *t*-test, the chi-square, and Pearson's product—moment correlation coefficient. (p. 564, Chapter 14)

Information overload: When data or information are so voluminous and overwhelming that they render us unable to make sense of them. (p. 526, Chapter 12)

Information sheet: A clearly written and understandable written document that is presented to a research participant prior to their participation in a study that outlines what their participation would involve, any risks involved, and any promises and safeguards the researcher offers. (p. 115, Chapter 4)

Informed consent: An ethical principle that suggests you should not do things to people unless they consent, and that their consent is given on the basis of having been informed of all aspects of the study and its outcomes that might affect their willingness to participate. (p. 114, Chapter 4)

Instrumental case study: The study of a case (e.g., person, specific group, department, organization) to provide insight that can be generalized to a larger phenomenon. (p. 297, Chapter 8)

Instrumentation: One of many possible threats to the **internal validity** of research, in this instance arising from changes in the way data are collected or organized during the course of a study. For example, if we change the way a certain statistic is gathered, using the "old" way when collecting the pretest data and the "new" way when collecting the posttest data, we don't know whether any differences we observe between pretest and posttest are due to the independent variable or simply to the change in the way we gathered the data. Instrumentation effects also occur when data change over time because coders or raters become more practiced or fatigued or because equipment wears down. (p. 212, Chapter 6)

Internal validity: The extent to which differences observed in an experimental study can be unambiguously attributed to the **experimental treatment** itself, rather than to other factors. In other words, to what extent can you be certain that the differences we observe are caused by the independent variable per se, rather than by **rival plausible explanations?** (p. 206, Chapter 6)

Interquartile range (IQR): A measure of statistical dispersion that highlights the distance between the 25th and 75th percentile of a distribution of scores. A benefit of using this statistic is that it is not influenced by extreme scores—outliers—since only the middle 50 percent of the distribution of scores is taken into account. (p. 584, Chapter 14)

Inter-rater agreement: See **inter-rater reliability**. (p. 448, Chapter 11)

Inter-rater reliability: The degree to which two or more people, using the same coding scheme and observing the same people, events, or other units, produce essentially the same results. Inter-rater agreement must normally be higher than 80 percent in order to be considered acceptable. (p. 89, Chapter 3; p. 496, Chapter 12)

Interrupted time-series design: A time series of a particular outcome of interest that is used to establish an underlying trend, which is "interrupted" by an intervention at a known point in time. (p. 264, Chapter 7)

Interval-level measurement: A measure with no true zero point that has rank-ordered ordered attributes with a meaningful distance between them. The most commonly presented example of an interval measure is thermometer readings as the thermometer scale has no true zero point, the intervals between temperature readings go up or down in equal intervals, and the interval between 20° and 30° is equal to the interval between 10° and 20°. (p. 567, Chapter 14)

Interview schedule: A guide an interviewer uses when conducting a structured interview. (p. 402, Chapter 10)

Intrinsic case study: The study of a case wherein the subject itself is the primary interest. (p. 296, Chapter 8)

Inverse relationship: See **negative relationship**. (p. 600, Chapter 14)

Investigator triangulation: It refers to the practice of several different researchers contributing in the study to collect, analyze, and interpret data and observations. This practice is thought to improve both the credibility of the observations and the resulting interpretation of the research.

"It depends": A term that researchers should be comfortable with when it comes to evaluating the effectiveness of the types of research methods used. We suggest on several occasions in the book that "it depends" is the answer to every methodological question that asks which method or procedure is "best." It always depends on the specifics of the situation. (p. 350, Chapter 9)

Jackknifing: A technique used when you have a very large number of cases (e.g., 10 times as many cases as you have variables) and want to assess the replicability or reliability of your results. There are several ways to perform this procedure, but the simplest is to randomly split your sample of cases into *two* samples, do the analyses you want to do separately in the two samples, and then focus only on those results that emerge as statistically significant in *both* data sets. (p. 614, Chapter 14)

John Henry effect: When participants from the control group in an experimental design actively compete with the experimental group thereby changing their behavior. This threat to the **internal validity** of the study is based on an individual by the name of John Henry who, when he learned that his performance was to be compared to that of a steam drill, worked so hard that he outperformed the drill but died in the process. Also known as **compensatory rivalry**. (p. 275, Chapter 7)

Keyword search: They are terms (and their synonyms and antonyms) associated (or not associated) with the topic, problem, or question that your literature review is structured around that help you to further restrict the scope of your searches of the literature. Combining subject and keyword searches will likely yield fewer results but those you get will be more highly relevant for your literature review. Depending on how successful your keyword restricted search is on helping you retrieve literature, you may find that you have to narrow down or expand your list of terms. (p. 47, Chapter 2)

Know your audience: Keeping the type of audience in mind when presenting your work because you want to "speak" to them in a manner that is meaningful to them. (p. 626, Chapter 15)

Knowledge questions: Questions that seek to determine what a respondent knows about some person, event, or phenomenon. King, Horrocks, and Brooks (2019) point out that the distinction between these types of questions and opinion/value questions can be difficult to make, since the two often go hand in hand. (p. 400, Chapter 10)

KWIC (key-word-in-context) analyses: Allows you to do a word or phrase search, and displays the results in the context of several words before and after it. (p. 551, Chapter 13)

Likert-type items: A type of structured response item developed by Rensis Likert. Two attributes distinguish a "Likert-type" item. First, the item is an *assertion* (rather than a question). Second, the respondent's task is to indicate the extent to which s/he *agrees* or *disagrees* with the assertion. Likert-type items are distinguished from a Likert scale; the latter would involve some number of

Likert-type items that had been combined together and validated appropriately. (p. 359, Chapter 9)

Making it "interesting": You should begin the introduction to any paper or presentation by explaining why your research is important, and why your audience might find it "interesting." (p. 629, Chapter 15)

Mandatory reporting: Laws that require an individual to report when they see a criterion event occurring. For example, many states have laws that require you to report suspected/observed abuse, or threat to another person's life, to a legal authority. (p. 141, Chapter 4)

Manipulative control: Creating situations and invoking procedures such as random assignment of participants into groups in order to maximize the **internal validity** of an experiment. (p. 273, Chapter 7)

Matching: A method of intentionally *creating* **pretest equivalence**. Contrasts with **random assignment**, which allows you to *assume* pretest equivalence. To use matching, we begin by identifying pairs of individuals who are matched (i.e., as similar as possible) on some variable (e.g., pretest scores), and then randomly assigning one person from each pair to the **experimental group** and the other to the **control group**. In this way, we're guaranteed groups that are constituted equally with respect to that matching variable. Not a particularly useful procedure unless groups are quite small and you want to ensure your groups are as equal as possible. (p. 219, Chapter 6)

Maturation: In experimental research, it is one of many possible threats to **internal validity**. Defined as processes within the research participants that change as a function of time per se (not specific to particular events), such as growing older, more tired, getting hungrier, and so on. In other words, sometimes changes happen merely because of biological processes that happen over time, and we must be careful to recognize those processes and their effects when we're assessing the effects of other independent variables. (p. 207, Chapter 6)

Mean: The arithmetic average of a group of scores computed by taking the sum of the values of all scores and dividing them by the total number of scores. (p. 577, Chapter 14)

Median: The centermost score in a distribution of scores, the score that splits a distribution of scores in half such that 50 percent of the scores lie above it and 50 percent lie below it. (p. 577, Chapter 14)

Memo: A note that we write to ourselves where we elaborate upon the categories of meaning that are beginning to emerge from the research or coding process, just as we might write margin notes in a book we are reading, or include thoughts and other "notes to self" in our field notes as we think of them. (p. 534, Chapter 13)

Memory fade: When our ability to accurately recall information becomes weaker through the passage of time. (p. 523, Chapter 12)

Methodological triangulation: Employing multiple methods to study a particular phenomenon in order to overcome the deficiencies and biases that may result from employing a single method approach.

Mill's three causal criteria: John Stuart Mill's assertion that in order to show a causal effect, three criteria must hold: see **temporal precedence, association/relationship**, and **elimination of rival plausible explanation**. (p. 203, Chapter 6)

Mixed-methods perspective: Defined by Johnson, Onwuegbuzie, and Turner (2007) as "the type of research in which a researcher or team of researchers combines elements of qualitative and quantitative research approaches (e.g., use of qualitative and quantitative viewpoints, data collection, analysis, inference techniques) for the broad purposes of breadth and depth of understanding and corroboration" (p. 123).

Mode: The most typical or frequently occurring score or response in a distribution of scores or responses. (p. 576, Chapter 14)

Mono-operationism and mono-method bias: Two potential problems that can be produced when researchers become overly reliant on, respectively, a particular *measure* of a construct or a particular *way* of measuring it. *Mono-operationism* (sometimes called *mono-operation bias*) refers to the problem that develops when we use only one operational definition of a variable (e.g., if we use only IQ tests to measure intelligence, never trying to measure it any other way). *Mono-method bias* refers to reliance on only one method (e.g., self-report interviews) instead of investigating a phenomenon in a number of different ways (e.g., also incorporating

observational and/or archival research). See also **definitional operationism**. (p. 88, 91, Chapter 3)

"Monte Carlo" computer simulations: A technique that's used to address what occurs when certain assumptions that are required by probability theory are violated. Much of probability theory, on which most statistics are based, is based on "long-run" expectations, expectations about what would be true if there were an infinite number of trials. One great advantage of computers derives from the fact that they'll do the same thing over and over again—and do so incredibly quickly—until you tell them to stop. And although you cannot have them process any information an *infinite* number of times (since, by definition, the processing would never end),[1] you can nonetheless instruct a computer to process a set of instructions a *very large* number of times, where "very large" is so large a number that the observed outcomes will closely approximate what you would find if you were to repeat the instructions an infinite number of times. Monte Carlo simulations have been used in this way to evaluate such questions as (1) whether you'd get incorrect results if you violated the assumptions of the *t*-test and found that the dependent variable is not normally distributed in the population or (2) whether you'd be misled if you accidentally subjected ordinal data to a *t*-test. (p. 569, Chapter 14)

Mortality: A threat to **internal validity** that arises when some individuals drop out of the research before it's completed. Single-session, short-term laboratory experimentation virtually precludes mortality as a problem. But in the field, where time-series data and a succession of follow-ups are more likely, the mortality problem increases in relevance. Some individuals who are recorded as participants at the beginning of the study do not return to receive the dependent measure at follow-up; for example, they drop out of therapy, choose to resign from the group, move to another jurisdiction, are released on parole, join another club, get lost, or die. The problem is one of *selection bias*, since the people or units that "survive" to the posttest are no longer the same group that was measured at the pretest. (p. 276, Chapter 7)

---

[1] The one exception here would be for Chuck Norris, who is said to have counted to infinity *twice*!

Multiple or collective case study: A chosen set of cases where each case is treated as its own individual entity, to be compared or contrasted with one another. (p. 297, Chapter 8)

Multiple time-series: A quasi-experimental design where measurements are taken from two groups of test units (usually from an experimental group and a control group). The experimental group is exposed to a treatment/independent variable, and then another series of measurements is taken from both groups. (p. 270, Chapter 7)

Multiple-response item: Questions that allow the participants to choose more than one alternative. (p. 356, Chapter 9)

Multistage cluster sampling: A probability-based sampling technique that is employed when no **sampling frame** is available. This technique involves randomly sampling clusters within clusters until one reaches the desired unit of analysis. (p. 174, Chapter 5)

Mutually exclusive: The property of a questionnaire item where the categories of response provided do not overlap with one another so that a participant can realistically select only one response option. (p. 355, Chapter 9)

Negative (or inverse) relationship: It refers to a correlation in which one variable increases in value as the other variable decreases. For example, as temperature increases, the number of layers of clothing we wear decreases. (p. 600, Chapter 14)

Negative case sampling: When you keep a vigilant eye open for cases that challenge your thinking or what you know thus far about a phenomenon. (p. 189, Chapter 5)

Negative evidence: Cases or evidence that is contradictory to a working hypothesis or your current understanding. (p. 302, Chapter 8)

Nominal definition: A statement of what a concept means to the researcher; much like a dictionary definition. Expressing nominal definitions for the key concepts or variables involved in your research allows other researchers to consider whether they would agree with your definition of the term. See also **operational definition** and epistemic relationship. (p. 85, Chapter 3)

Nonequivalent controls: They are used in situations where **random assignment** of participants cannot be achieved; to make reasonable comparisons with our experimental group of interest, and to rule our **rival plausible explanations**. They are called nonequivalent because you cannot assume the groups are equal, but the ideal is to make them as similar to the experimental group as possible. (p. 268, Chapter 7)

Normal distribution: A symmetrical or bell-shaped continuous probability distribution with a single peak and whose distribution conforms to the empirical rule (e.g., where 68 percent of the distribution of scores represented fall within one standard deviation, 95 percent of scores fall within two standard deviations and 99.7 percent fall within three standard deviation points of the mean). (p. 607, Chapter 14)

Nuremberg Code: A set of research ethics principles for human experimentation created as a result of the Nuremberg trials at the end of World War II. (p. 105, Chapter 4)

NVivo: A software application mainly used for working with nonnumeric data. (p. 541, Chapter 13)

Occam's Razor: The general principle that simplicity is preferred in scientific theorizing. While the success of any theory is measured by its ability to explain the phenomena it purports to explain, if two different theories do an equally good job, then the one that does so more simply or that posits less complex mechanisms will be preferred.

Open coding: A technique for coding textual, visual, or audio content where the analyst identifies general themes and ideas as they emerge from a literal reading of the data. (p. 533, Chapter 13)

Open-ended questions: Questions that allow the respondent to answer however they wish rather than being forced to choose from among predetermined category alternatives. (p. 349, Chapter 9)

Operational definition: The way we actually define the variables of interest within the confines of the research project. Suppose you're interested in looking at romantic love. How will you determine whether any two people in your research are actually "in love"? You might decide to ask them, "Are you two in love?" If they say "yes," you will consider them "in love." Their response to the question

"Are you in love?" has become the operational definition of the concept of "love" in their research. See also **nominal definition** and **epistemic relationship**. (p. 86, Chapter 3)

Operationalizing: Explaining a phenomenon through defining variables into measureable factors. (p. 85, Chapter 3)

Opinion/values questions: These types of questions ask the respondent to reflect on the topic at hand in terms of their own values, goals, and priorities. (p. 400, Chapter 10)

Ordinal measurement: A measure that has rank-ordered attributes that have no meaningful distance between them and no meaningful zero point. An example of an ordinal measure would be when we ask people to rank order different activities in terms of how much they enjoy doing them. The ranks create a hierarchy, but the distance between 1 and 2 is not necessarily the same as between 2 and 3 and so on. (p. 566, Chapter 14)

Outliers: A data point that is significantly different from other observations; extreme scores. (p. 581, Chapter 14)

Parachute research: See **hit and run research**. (p. 475, Chapter 11)

Participant observation: A method used in sociology. Learning the activities of people in the natural setting through observing or participating in those activities. See also **ethnography** and **field research**. (p. 464, Chapter 11)

Participatory Action Research (PAR): A collaborative approach to research where a researcher and participants from a community or group work together to identify difficulties and gather information designed to promote change that benefits the community or group. (p. 473, Chapter 11)

Pearson's r: A statistical test used to represent the degree to which the values of one variable change as the values of another variable also change. This statistic, also known as Pearson's r, is used to summarize the direction (positive or negative) and degree (closeness) of the linear relationship between two variables. The Pearson's r statistic can have a value ranging from -1.0 to $+1.0$. A Pearson's r value of -1.0 represents a perfect negative association between two variables (i.e., as the value of

one variable goes up the other goes down). A value of $+1.0$ represents a perfect positive association between two variables (i.e., as the value of one variable goes up so does the value of the other). Finally, a value of 0 means that the two variables are completely unrelated (i.e., as the value of one variable changes the values of the other do not change in any systematic and linear way). (p. 598, Chapter 14)

Phenomenologism: An approach to understanding whose adherents assert that we must "get inside people's heads" to understand how they perceive and interpret the world. According to theorists such as Weber, phenomenological understanding is a virtual prerequisite for achieving **Verstehen**.

Pilot study: A study that takes place prior to the actual study where the researcher is able to test out features of their design such as sampling and recruitment strategies or research instruments. (p. 376, Chapter 9)

Population: An aggregation of all **sampling elements**, that is, the total of all the sampling units that meet the criterion (or criteria) for inclusion in a study. The **sampling frame**, if available, defines the population. (p. 160, Chapter 5)

Positive (or direct) relationship: It refers to correlations between two or more variables where, as one variable increases in value, the other increases in value as well. For example, the more one studies, the higher the grades that one receives. (p. 600, Chapter 14)

Positivism: A school of thought marked by a *realist* perspective, an emphasis on quantitative precision, the belief that effective research requires avoiding over-identification, and a search for general truths unearthed through the gathering and analysis of aggregated data. Chapter 1 focuses on "orthodox" or classic positivism, which developed in the 19th and early 20th centuries.

Practice effects: Changes or improvements that result from practice or repetition of having taken similar tests/experiments. (p. 209, Chapter 6)

Pragmatism: A philosophical tradition which emerged in the late 19th century through the works of Charles Sanders Pierce, John Dewy, and William James and played a major role in the emergence of symbolic interactionism (e.g., Mead and Cooley) that rejects the idea that there is a single view of reality. In doing this pragmatists reject traditional dualisms of realism versus constructivism, free will versus determinism, subjectivism versus objectivism, and induction versus deduction in favor of a position that emphasizes adopting the approach that works best in a particular situation.

Predictive validity: A type of validity that involves assessing the extent to which your measure does in fact predict whatever it's supposed to predict. For example, if you develop tests like the LSAT (Law School Admission Test) or GRE (Graduate Records Exam), which are supposed to predict success in law school and graduate school, respectively, then demonstrating the tests' predictive validity would require you to show that scores on the test do indeed relate to later success in law school or graduate school, respectively. Contrasts with **concurrent validity**. (p. 90, Chapter 3)

Pretest equivalence: When two (or more) groups are equal, or similar on average prior to the introduction of the independent variable. This is a very important assumption that underlies experimentalist logic. (p. 216, Chapter 6)

Pretest sensitization: See **testing**. (p. 209, Chapter 6)

Privacy certificate: A certificate issued by the National Institutes of Justice in the United States that provides legal protection for researchers to ensure that they cannot be forced to disclose identifying research information about participants to any civil, criminal, administrative, legislative, or other proceeding. Compare to **Certificates of Confidentiality**. (p. 124, Chapter 4)

Privilege: A term describing a relationship whereby the persons in that relationship are exempt from the normal requirement that all of us have to testify when asked to do so in a court of law when and if information discussed in the context of that relationship becomes of interest to the court. The lawyer–client relationship is protected by a privilege, for example, so that you can go and talk freely to your lawyer and seek legal advice without fearing that they will get subpoenaed and be on the witness stand the next day giving evidence against you. (p. 123, Chapter 4)

Probabilistic sampling: A sampling technique in which cases are selected from a population based on probabilities,

when you need to ensure the sample is representative of the population from which it was drawn. (p. 163, Chapter 5)

Probe for examples: Asking a respondent to provide a concrete example of what they are talking about. (p. 404, Chapter 10)

Project file: The name used to describe the central space in the qualitative data analysis software program NVivo that is used to store all documents (e.g., text, audio, image, or video files), links, and memos that emerge at various stages of the research process from design to reporting. (p. 542, Chapter 13)

Proportional stratified random sampling: A type of **stratified random sampling** where the number of elements sampled in each stratum are proportionate to their numbers in the wider population. For example, if women account for 65 percent of students enrolled in your research methods class and males account for 35 percent drawing a proportionate stratified random sample of students from your class would result in 65 percent of your sample being female and 35 percent male. (p. 172, Chapter 5)

Pseudonyms: A fictitious name used in order to conceal and thereby protect the real source of an interview or other research data. (p. 120, Chapter 4)

Purposive (or strategic) sampling: A general class of sampling techniques that are based on an acknowledgement that the parameters of the population are unknown. Instead of attempting to acquire a statistically representative sample, purposive samples are drawn to achieve a particular theoretical, methodological, or analytical objective. (p. 184, Chapter 5)

Qualitative approaches: Research methods characterized by an inductive perspective, a belief that theory should be grounded in the day-to-day realities of the people being studied, and a preference for applying phenomenology to the attempt to understand the many "truths" of reality. Such approaches tend to be constructionist. Qualitative researchers tend to be cautious about numbers, believing that the requirements of quantification distance us even further from phenomenological understanding we should embrace. Qualitative researchers tend to engage most commonly in case study analysis.

Qualitative data analysis (QDA) software: Computer-assisted data analysis software that assists with transcription analysis, coding, and text interpretation. (p. 538, Chapter 13)

Quantitative approaches: Research methods that emphasize numerical precision; a detached, aloof stance on the researcher's part (i.e., the avoidance of over-identification); and, often, a hypothetico-deductive approach. Quantitative researchers tend to prefer gathering similar structured data across large samples as this will facilitate their ability to engage in statistical analysis of their data to identify broader patterns across individuals.

Quasi-probabilistic sampling: Selecting cases that will offer a reasonable approximation of a truly random sample when actually getting one is not possible, typically because of the absence of a **sampling frame**. (p. 174, Chapter 5)

Quota sampling: The **quasi-probabilistic** equivalent of stratified random sample where the researcher purposively selects participants to fill a predetermined quota of substantively relevant groups. (p. 175, Chapter 5)

Random: A very special word in the methodological world that means that every unit has an equal probability of being selected (in the case of sampling) or assigned (in the experimental context). (p. 153, Chapter 5)

Random assignment: A very powerful research procedure that directly addresses the assumption of **pretest equivalence**, i.e., the crucial experimental assumption that your experimental and control groups are equal in all respects *before* the imposition or administration of your independent variable. Given that you have a group of people ready to participate in your research, random assignment is achieved by letting "chance" be the *sole* determinant of which group (i.e., experimental or control) any given person is a member of. Random assignment, coupled with adequate group sizes (i.e., at least 30 per group), allows you to assume, with a reasonable degree of confidence, that the two (or more) groups, on average, are fairly equal on all preexperimental variables. (p. 217, Chapter 6)

Random digit dialing (RDD): A technique for selecting and contacting participants for telephone survey research where the unique identifier portion of the phone number (i.e., the numbers not associated with the area code or exchange) are dialed at random. (p. 337, Chapter 9)

Random error: The vagaries of chance. Refers to errors that have no systematic biasing effect on a study's results. (p. 166, Chapter 5)

Range: A measure of dispersion representing the distance between the highest and lowest scores in a distribution. Because it can be affected by unusual outliers, the **inter-quartile range** is often thought of as a better measure. (p. 583, Chapter 14)

Rapport: The development of a bond of mutual trust between researcher and participant that is considered to be the foundation upon which access is given and valid data are built. (p. 11, Chapter 1; p. 391, Chapter 10)

Rate data: Data that are expressed as a frequency per some unit of population; for example, birth rates, crime rates, death rates, unemployment rates, and infant mortality rates. For example, Vancouver's murder rate is currently about 6 per 100,000 per year while the murder rate for Seattle, just across the border, is more than 5 times higher at 32 per 100,000 per year. Specifying rates rather than raw numbers allows researchers to compare rates in a single location over time or to compare two or more locations despite differences in their population size.

Ratio-level measurement: A measure with an absolute and meaningful zero point and rank-ordered categories of values with meaningful intervals of difference between them. Count or weight measures such as number of years in school or the number of pounds a baby weighs at birth are common examples of ratio measures. (p. 567, Chapter 14)

Reactivity (or reactive bias): The degree to which (if at all) the researcher's presence causes research participants to react by changing from their "usual" or "normal" behavior patterns because they know they're being observed. (p. 444, Chapter 11)

Real and virtual libraries: Two main sources to obtain information for any research. Buildings that house physical books and journals (real libraries), and online library catalogues (virtual libraries). (p. 41, Chapter 2)

Realism: The idea that a reality exists out there independently of what and how we think about it. Contrasts with **constructionism**.

Redact: Censor or remove part of a text, particularly names or other identifying information, for security/ confidentiality purposes. (p. 120, Chapter 4)

Reflexive: A process whereby the researcher remains consciously and critically aware of the multiple influences they have on the research process while also acknowledging how the research process also influences them. (p. 78, Chapter 3)

Regression toward the mean: One of many possible threats to **internal validity**. Unlike testing, where *real* change occurs between pretest and posttest (e.g., because of practice, sensitization to issues, or greater motivation), regression toward the mean involves changes that are more apparent than real. Regression toward the mean refers to the propensity of extreme scorers on the first testing to score closer to the mean (average) of the group on the second testing. This phenomenon arises because of the random error that is present in any measurement and occurs because chance events are unlikely ever to stack up to precisely the same degree on two successive occasions. Also known as **statistical regression**. (p. 209, Chapter 6)

Reliability: The degree to which repeated observation of a phenomenon—the same phenomenon at different times, or the same instance of the phenomenon by two different observers—yields similar results. Underlying this concept are scientific beliefs about the importance of stability and repeatability in the generation of understanding. Two types of reliability are **inter-rater reliability** and **test-retest reliability**. (p. 89, Chapter 3)

Replication: Reproducing a study that was previously done to determine if the findings of the original research can be applied to other participants and circumstances. If we get the same results, we are more confident in the robustness of the phenomenon; if we get different results, we have the challenge of figuring out why the phenomenon appears sometimes and not others. However important this is, most journals do not publish straight replications. (p. 58, Chapter 2)

Representative: Accurately mirrors or reflects. (p. 155, Chapter 5)

Research questions: An essential aspect of research; a focused question that can be addressed empirically that a research project sets out to answer. (p. 44, Chapter 2; p. 69, Chapter 3)

Resentful demoralization: One of several possible threats to **internal validity** that can emerge in field settings. Given the same situation as is described under **compensatory rivalry**—it's known that an evaluation is in progress—participants may demonstrate the opposite response to the discrepancy among groups. With compensatory rivalry, the disadvantaged group rises to the challenge. With resentful demoralization, members of that group perceive the result as adverse and inevitable; they therefore may not even try to compete, and may even intentionally reduce their performance. In this instance, the researcher may *overestimate* the actual potency of the treatment being evaluated. (p. 275, Chapter 7)

Response rates: The number of respondents who completed the survey as a proportion of those who were asked to participate; also known as completion rate, or return rate. (p. 334, Chapter 9)

Response sets: These occur when a survey or scale is set up so that agreement (or disagreement) with the items is always associated with more of the characteristic being studied. For example, in the original F-scale, which measured right-wing authoritarian tendencies, all the items were written so that agreement was the "authoritarian" response. The concern with response sets is that people start to pay less attention to the items and just keep on checking at the same end of the scale, which reduces validity. For this reason, scales normally should have about half their items written in a positive direction, and half worded in a negative direction.

Response symmetry: The response categories in a survey should have equal balance (e.g., equal number of positive and negative response categories). (p. 364, Chapter 9)

River sampling: An online sampling method that drives potential respondents to an online portal (the river) where they are screened for studies. Respondents who meet a specified criterion are invited into the study. (p. 187, Chapter 5)

Sample: A subset of the population that the researcher wishes to research. (p. 152, Chapter 5)

Sampling error: The degree to which the distribution of characteristics in a sample deviates from the distribution of those characteristics in the population from which the sample was drawn. Estimates of the sampling error can be computed only when random sampling has been done. The two types of sampling error are **systematic error** and **random error**. (p. 166, Chapter 5)

Sampling frame: A complete list of all the sampling elements of the population we wish to study. For example, if we want to sample voters in an upcoming election, the voters' lists represent a sampling frame of all eligible voters who have been enumerated. The availability of a sampling frame can influence a researcher's choice of sampling techniques because in most cases random sampling cannot be done without one. (p. 165, Chapter 5)

Sampling ratio: A way of expressing what proportion of a population is actually sampled. For example, if the population numbers 1,000 people and if you sample 200 of them, your sampling ratio is 200:1,000 (i.e., 200 out of 1,000), or 1:5 (i.e., 1 in 5). (p. 170, Chapter 5)

Scientific obligation: The obligation to do research according to the highest scientific and disciplinary-based standards [p. 112, Chapter 4].

Secondary data: Primary research data collected by another researcher for their own purposes that are subsequently made available to other members of the research community for their own purposes. (p. 117, Chapter 4; p. 488, Chapter 12)

Selection: One of many possible threats to the **internal validity** of research, particularly experimental research, because it violates the fundamental premise of pretest equivalence, that is, the assumption that all experimental and control groups are equal before the experiment begins, so that any differences we observe after administering the independent variable must have arisen during the course of the study. (p. 212, Chapter 6)

Selective deposit: A term referring to the fact that some people, groups, and processes have a higher likelihood than others of having their views, lives, and so on made a part of the historical record. Historians can study history based only on what's in the record; thus, our understanding of history is influenced by the factors that

influence selective deposit into that record. (p. 425, Chapter 10; p. 441, Chapter 11)

Self-anchoring scale: It refers to a type of scale used by Hadley Cantril (see Chapter 6) in which the end points of the scale are defined by the participant. For example, in his famous international study about people's perceptions of their quality of life, he would first ask participants to think of the worst life situation they could imagine for themselves, and to call that a "1," and then the best situation they could imagine themselves in, and to call that a "10," after which he would ask them to place themselves on the scale "as their life is now." The anchors—the end points of the scale—are self-defined. (p. 358, Chapter 9)

Semantic differential-type item: A type of rating scale questionnaire item originally developed by Osgood, Suci, and Tannenbaum (1957) to assess the meaning associated with particular attitude objects using a set of bipolar adjectives (or dimensions) upon which any given attitude object could be described (e.g., respondents are asked to rate the fairness (fair versus unfair) of being punished for a variety of different behaviors). (p. 361, Chapter 9)

Semi-structured interviewing: When the interviewer has a list of topics to cover but where the researcher adapts the specific wording, order and inventory of questions depending on the directions that the respondent takes the conversation. (p. 402, Chapter 10)

Sequential mixed data analysis: Using the results of our analysis of one type of data to inform or shape how we go about analyzing the second form of data. (p. 555, Chapter 13)

Serendipity: Discoveries that happen purely by accident, as when a prospector strikes oil while searching for gold. The searcher (whether prospector or researcher) must be sufficiently knowledgeable and aware to realize what he or she has found. Many people in history have been perturbed to discover later that a serendipitous discovery had been staring them right in the face but that they'd been too unaware to recognize it at the time. (p. 61, Chapter 2)

Shadow speaking: The interviewer transcribes the interview by repeating the participant's words onto a speech-to-word program by listening to a slowed-down recorded interview through headphones. (p. 413, Chapter 10)

Sign systems: A type of **coding scheme** in which an observer defines what is of interest to him or her (e.g., instances of violence, prosocial behavior, or a moral dilemma) and then waits and watches, noting each time one of the predetermined criterion behaviors occurs. Sign systems give a better indication of *how many* prosocial acts are witnessed than **category systems**. (p. 447, Chapter 11)

Silent probe: Remaining silent after a respondent has given a preliminary response, thereby encouraging the respondent to continue with their story. (p. 404, Chapter 10)

Simple random sampling: The **probability sampling** technique that allows a researcher to minimize sampling error and allows him or her to calculate the degree of **sampling error** that probably exists. To perform simple random sampling, in most cases you must have a **sampling** frame in which every sampling element is listed once and only once. Simple random sampling is then accomplished by merely choosing sample elements at random from the list. This can be done by putting all the names (or whatever) into a hat or drum and pulling them out at random, by numbering all elements in the sampling frame and then using a table of random numbers or random number generator to guide your selection, or using a computer program such as Microsoft Excel® or Open Office Calc® to select randomly from the sampling frame using whatever sampling ratio you specify. (p. 166, Chapter 5)

Single-response item: A survey response item format that requires the participant to indicate their response to a question in an empty space provided (e.g., In what year where you born?). (p. 353, Chapter 9)

Skew: An asymmetrical distribution. Mathematicians use the convention of describing the direction of the skew based on where the distribution's thinner end, or "tail," (i.e., positively or negatively skewed). (p. 579, Chapter 14)

Snowball sampling: Collecting samples by starting with one or two individuals, and through their connections and referrals, obtaining more cases to create a larger sample. (p. 190, Chapter 5)

Social facts: Life's "big" realities (e.g., the legal and economic system), which wield significant influences on people and are beyond people's control in any direct sense. They are important to positivists because such social realities are believed to exert their effects no matter what we think about them and thus are some of the more stable and pervasive social factors we can observe.

Social media platforms: A collection of information communication technologies (ICTs) platforms built upon a web 2.0 foundation, where users can actively participate, create, and disseminate content (e.g., Facebook, YouTube) (p. 654, Chapter 15)

Sociological imagination: Termed by C. W. Mills (1959), a practice of being able to pull away from the situation and think of your experience as one of many and part of broader social factors and forces. (p. 56, Chapter 2)

"Spew" draft: Spitting out your story on a document, saying everything you feel you want to say quickly on this first draft. A potential cure for writer's block that can help get you going. (p. 625, Chapter 15)

Stakeholder sampling: Selecting cases by identifying key stakeholders who are highly involved in the program/service that the researcher is evaluating. (p. 185, Chapter 5)

Stakeholders: Any individuals who have a direct interest or concern with a particular aspect of the design, implementation, or outcome of the research. Stakeholders can include research participants, research ethics board members, the individuals, or organizations that sponsor or fund the research, and the researchers themselves. (p. 78, Chapter 3)

Standard deviation: A measure of dispersion, expressed in the standard units, that indicates the average distance that any given score in a distribution of scores will be from the mean score in that distribution. A low standard deviation indicates that scores or observations tend to cluster close to the mean while a high standard deviation indicates that scores are spread out from the mean. Standard deviation is calculated by taking the square root of the variance. (p. 588, Chapter 14)

Starting from where you are: A method suggested by Lofland, Snow, Anderson, and Lofland (2006) to begin research with your own life situation and the concerns and issues that arise therefrom. (p. 55, Chapter 2)

Statistical conclusion validity: A measure of how reasonable a research or experimental conclusion is that takes into account whether appropriate statistical tests and reliable and valid measures have been used. (p. 221, Chapter 6)

Statistical significance: The likelihood that a relationship between two or more variables is caused by chance alone. (p. 227, Chapter 6)

Statute-based protections: Legislative protections for the confidentiality of identifiable information that ensure that research data cannot be used in any legal proceeding without the permission of the participant. In the United States, health research can be protected through **Certificates of Confidentiality** that are administered by the National Institutes of Health, while some criminological research is protected through the **Privacy certificates** administered by the National Institute of Justice. (p. 123, Chapter 4)

Stratified random sample: A probabilistic sampling technique where the researcher divides the population into groupings (or strata) of interest and then samples randomly within each stratum. This technique is used when there is some meaningful grouping variable on which the investigator wishes to make comparisons and where the probabilities of group membership are known ahead of time. (p. 170, Chapter 5)

Structured interviewing: When the interviewer prepares a set of predetermined questions for the participant to answer during an interview. (p. 402, Chapter 10)

Surveillance capitalism: This concept, put forth by Zuboff (2018), refers to the collection and accumulation of information about individuals whenever they use any digital search, app, or website, which is then used by giant corporations (primarily Google and Facebook) to sell advertising and sold to other corporations to use how they like for purposes ranging from innocuous to nefarious. (p. 527, Chapter 12)

Systematic error: One of two types of sampling error. Systematic error occurs when aspects of your sampling procedure act in a consistent, systematic way to make some sampling elements more likely to be chosen for participation than others. For example, Chapter 4 describes a 1992 call-in survey in which an American TV program's viewers expressed their opinions about a presidential speech. To participate, respondents had to,

among other things, own a touch-tone phone, be interested in and able to understand a TV show dealing with political analysis, and be motivated enough to take the time to express their opinion. These factors created a systematically biased sample: wealthier people, more educated people, and people who wanted to complain were more likely to be represented in that sample than poorer people (who might be unable to afford a touch-tone phone), less educated people (who might be less able to follow the political analysis), and apathetic, uncertain, or contented people (who might have less motivation to call). Contrasts with **random error**. (p. 166, Chapter 5)

Systematic sample with random start: A **probabilistic sampling** technique where the researcher selects a randomly determined starting point within a **sampling frame** and samples every n^{th} element (based in a sampling ratio) until the desired sample size is reached. (p. 170, Chapter 5)

Telescoping: It uses the metaphor of a telescope—something that brings distant objects closer—to refer to when survey or interview respondents perceive events as being more recent than they are. Contrast with **memory fade**; addressed by **bounding**. (p. 524, Chapter 12)

Tell-me-more probe: Simply asking the respondent to elaborate on their initial response (e.g., "can you explain a bit more about how exactly that works?"). (p. 404, Chapter 10)

Temporal precedence: One of John Stuart Mill's three criteria of causality that maintains that the cause must come before the effect. (p. 204, Chapter 6)

Testing: In experimental research, it is one of many possible threats to **internal validity**. Testing refers to the effects of taking a test on scores in the second testing. Such effects can operate in several different ways. The first, **pretest sensitization**, involves the fact that taking a test can sensitize you to issues in a way that you wouldn't have been aware of otherwise. It threatens **internal validity** because, if we observe that your attitudes have changed, we can't be sure whether the change was produced by the independent variable or by the greater sensitization to issues induced by the pretest. Another way in which testing can threaten **internal validity** is through practice effects. If we were trying to assess your abilities, for example, it would be difficult to know in the posttest situation whether you had improved purely because of the practice the pretest gave you or because of the independent variable we had imposed upon you. (p. 208, Chapter 6)

Test-retest reliability: The degree to which a measure shows reliability (i.e., consistency) by producing similar results when a test is administered on two successive occasions; that is, where the same group of people are tested and retested. If the test (or scale or other type of measure) is reliable, the two sets of scores should correlate highly: people who score high (or low) on one occasion should also score high (or low) on the second occasion. Compare **inter-rater reliability**. (p. 89, Chapter 3)

Text search query: Searches for words or phrases within the document. (p. 551, Chapter 13)

Theoretical triangulation: Employing multiple theories throughout the design, collection, and analysis process. Proceeding in this manner would involve a researcher or group of researchers developing research questions from different theoretical vantage points and thereby studying a phenomenon through multiple lenses.

Theory: A set of concepts and a description of how they're interrelated that, taken together, purport to explain a given phenomenon or set of phenomena. The word "theory" is also sometimes used more broadly to refer simply to abstractions; thus, when I look at your behavior and call you studious, we are making the jump from the concrete (your observable behavior, i.e., the number of hours per week you spend studying) to the theoretical (the concept of studiousness). (p. 8, Chapter 1; p. 33, Chapter 2; p. 69, Chapter 3)

Think-aloud Interview: See **cognitive interviewing**.

Time-series design: Research design that involves a single subject/research units that are measured repeatedly at intervals over time. (p. 273, Chapter 7)

Tracking: A process during redrafting of your research paper, where your "tracks" are written correctly to ensure that all essential elements of your paper follow from each other and speak to each other following a logical flow. (p. 641, Chapter 15)

Transcribing: The process of transferring recorded audio/video interviews to a word document. (p. 412, Chapter 10)

Tree maps: A diagram that displays the hierarchical relationships among coded contents in NVivo. (p. 553, Chapter 13)

Triangulation: A research strategy that permits us to validate our observations by drawing upon multiple theories, methods, investigators, or data analysis techniques within the same investigation in order to enhance the validity of the findings (p. 22, Chapter 1).

***t*-statistic:** A measure of whether two group means differ more than would be expected on the basis of chance variation alone. (p. 610, Chapter 14)

Typological analysis: A method of organizing coded material that involves placing similarly thematically coded information (e.g., people, places, events, or social artifacts that share common characteristics) into relational categories that allow the analyst to make distinctions among groupings or clusters of people, places, and so on that are meaningful to the researcher and/or participants. (p. 535, Chapter 13)

Typologies: Classifying and organizing similarly coded material according to a general type.

Units of analysis: The units or elements about which information will be gathered, they are the "things" you wish to study. Units of analysis can include individuals, groups, organizations, or social artifacts. (p. 164, Chapter 5)

Universe: A theoretical aggregation of all possible sampling elements. (p. 164, Chapter 5)

Unstructured interviewing: When there is no specific set of predetermined questions, although the interviewers may have certain topics in mind that they wish to cover during the interview; flows similar to an everyday conversation and tends to be more informal and open-ended. (p. 401, Chapter 10)

Validity: A term that refers, in the most general sense, to whether research measures what the researcher thinks is being measured. This text discusses many kinds of validity, including **predictive validity**, **internal validity**, **external validity**, and **ecological validity**. All relate to whether you are indeed accomplishing what you think you are. (p. 89, Chapter 3)

Variable: Stated most simply, it is anything that varies. For example, in your methods class, "sex" is probably a variable, since the students in your class (unless you go to a sex-specific university or college) probably include both males and females. Variables contrast with *constants*, which are things that do *not* vary. (p. 82, Chapter 3; p. 564, Chapter 14)

Variance: A measure of dispersion or spread of scores around the mean. It is calculated by taking the average squared difference of each score from the mean of all scores in the distribution. (p. 588, Chapter 14)

Variety: The range of information available—one of the 3 Vs used to evaluate an archival database. See also velocity and volume. (p. 525, Chapter 12)

Velocity: The speed with which the archival database is created—one of the 3 Vs used to evaluate an archival database. See also variety and volume. (p. 525, Chapter 12)

Verstehen: A German word, first used in the social sciences by Max Weber, that refers to a profound understanding evidenced by the ability to appreciate a person's behavior in terms of the interpretive (i.e., phenomenological) meaning they attach to it (p. 11, Chapter 1).

Volume: The amount of information available—one of the 3 Vs used to evaluate an archival database. See also velocity and variety. (p. 525, Chapter 12)

Waitlist controls: Potential participants who are on a waitlist for a service or treatment can be used as a control group to evaluate the effectiveness of that service or treatment. (p. 268, Chapter 7)

Wigmore criteria or Wigmore test: A set of four criteria used by Canadian and US courts to evaluate whether communications in a certain relationship (e.g., researcher–participant, doctor–patient, priest–penitent) should be considered "privileged" and exempt from the normal requirement to testify in a court of law. The criteria require that (1) there be a shared expectation of confidentiality by those in the relationship; (2) confidentiality be essential to the relationship; (3) the relation be an important and socially valued one; and (4) the damage that would be done the relationship by disclosure be greater than the damage to the case at hand by nondisclosure. (p. 128, Chapter 4)

Wildcards: See Boolean operators

Word frequency query: A search of a specific word or concept which appears the most often in any textual data. (p. 552, Chapter 13)

z-scores: A statistical measure of how far a score deviates from the mean of a group that is expressed as a number of standard deviation units. (p. 608, Chapter 14)

REFERENCES

Abramson, P. R., & Hayashi, H. (1984). Pornography in Japan: Cross-cultural and theoretical considerations. In N. M. Malamuth & E. Donnerstein (Eds.), *Pornography and sexual aggression* (pp. 173–185). Cambridge, MA: Academic Press.

Adelman, C. (1993). Kurt Lewin and the origins of action research. *Educational Action Research*, 1(1), 7–24.

Adler, P. A., & Adler, P. (1994). Observational techniques. In N. K. Denzin, & Y. S. Lincoln (Eds.), *Handbook of qualitative research* (pp. 377–392). Thousand Oaks, CA: SAGE.

Adler, P. A., & Adler, P. (2002). Do university lawyers and the police define research values? In W. C. van den Hoonaard (Ed.), *Walking the tightrope: Ethical issues for qualitative researchers* (pp. 34–42). Toronto, Canada: University of Toronto Press.

Aldridge, J., Medina, J., & Ralphs, R. (2010). The problem of proliferation: Guidelines for improving the security of qualitative data in a digital age. *Research Ethics Review*, 6(1), 3–9.

Altemeyer, R. A. (1970). Adverbs and intervals: A study of Likert scales. In *Proceedings of the 78th Annual Convention of the American Psychological Association*, 5: 397–398.

Altemeyer, R. A. (1981). *Right-wing authoritarianism*. Winnipeg, Canada: University of Manitoba Press.

American Anthropological Association. (2012). *Principles of professional responsibility*. Retrieved from http://ethics.americananthro.org/ethics-statement-0-preamble/

American Political Science Association. (2012). *A guide to professional ethics in political science* (2nd ed.). Washington, DC: Author. Retrieved from https://www.apsanet.org/portals/54/Files/Publications/APSAEthicsGuide2012.pdf

American Psychological Association. (1973). *Ethical principles in the conduct of research with human participants*. Washington, DC: Author.

American Psychological Association. (2010). *Publication manual of the American Psychological Association* (6th ed.). Washington, DC: Author.

American Sociological Association. (2018). *Code of ethics*. Retrieved from https://www.asanet.org/sites/default/files/asa_code_of_ethics-june2018.pdf

Anderson, K., & Jack, D. C. (1991). Learning to listen: Interview techniques and analyses. In S. B. Gluck & D. Patai (Eds.), *Womens words: The feminist practice of oral history* (pp. 11–26). New York, NY: Routledge.

Angrosino, M. V., & Mays de Perez, K. A. (2003). Rethinking observation: From method to context. In N. K. Denzin & Y. S. Lincoln (Eds.) *Collecting and interpreting qualitative materials* (2nd ed., pp. 107–154). Thousand Oaks, CA: SAGE.

Argyris, C. (1975). Dangers in applying results from experimental social psychology. *American Psychologist*, 30, 469–485.

Aronson, E., & Carlsmith, J. M. (1968). Experimentation in social psychology. In G. Lindsey & E. Aronson (Eds.), *The handbook of social psychology* (Vol. 2, 2nd ed., pp. 1–79). Reading, MA: Addison-Wesley.

Atchison, C. (1996). *Turning the trick: The development and partial implementation of a multi-dimensional research instrument designed for clients of sex sellers*. BA (hons.) thesis, Simon Fraser University.

Atchison, C. (1998). *Men who buy sex: A preliminary description based on the results from a survey of the Internet-using population*. M.A. thesis, Simon Fraser University.

Atchison, C. (1999). Navigating the virtual minefield: Using the Internet as a medium for conducting primary social research. In D. Currie, D. Hay, & B. MacLean (Eds.), *Exploring the social world: Social research in action*. Vancouver, BC: Collective Press.

Atchison, C., Lowman, J., & Fraser, L. (1998). Men who buy sex: Preliminary findings of an exploratory study. In J. Elias, V. L. Bullough, & V. Elias (Eds.), *Prostitution: On whores, hustlers, and Johns*. Northridge, CA: Prometheus Press.

Atkinson, P., & Hammersley, M. (1994). Ethnography and participant observation. In N. K. Denzin & Y. S. Lincoln (Eds.), *Handbook of qualitative research* (pp. 248–261). Thousand Oaks, CA: SAGE.

Atlantic Sugar v. United States. (1980). *85 Cust. Ct. 128*.

Badets, J., and Chui, T. W. L. (1994). *Canada's changing immigrant population*. Catalogue No. 96-311E. Published by Statistics Canada and Prentice-Hall Canada. Retrieved from http://publications.gc.ca/collections/collection_2012/statcan/rh-hc/CS96-311-1994-eng.pdf

Bailey, C. (2007). *A guide to qualitative field research* (2nd ed.). London: Pine Forge Press.

Baker, R., Blumberg, S. J., Brick, J. M., Couper, M. P., Courtright, M., Dennis, J. M., ... Zahs, D. (2010). Research synthesis: AAPOR report on online panels. *Public Opinion Quarterly*, 74(4), 711–781.

Barry, D. (2001). Assessing culture via the Internet: Methods and techniques for psychological research. *Cyberpsychology and Behavior*, 4(1), 17—21.

Bauman, S., Airey, J., & Atak, H. (1998). Effective use of web-based technology: Using the Internet for data collection and communication applications. Internet Survey Research White Paper.

Baumrind, D. (1964). Some thoughts on ethics of research: After reading Milgram's "Behavioral study of obedience." *American Psychologist*, 19, 421–423.

Bazeley, P. (2012). Integrative analysis strategies for mixed data sources. *American Behavioral Scientist*, 56(6), 814–828. doi:10.1177/0002764211426330

Beatty, P. C., & Willis, P. C. (2007). Research synthesis: The practice of cognitive interviewing. *Public Opinion Quarterly*, 71(2), 287–311.

Becker, H. S. (1963). *Outsiders: Studies in the sociology of deviance*. New York, NY: Free Press.

Becker, H. S. (1964). Against the code of ethics. *American Sociological Review*, 29, 409–410.

Becker, H. S. (1970). Problems of inference and proof in participant observation. In H. S. Becker, *Sociological work*. Chicago, IL: Aldine.

Becker, H. S. (1979). Do photographs tell the truth? In T. D. Cook & C. S. Reichardt (Eds.), *Qualitative and quantitative methods in evaluation research* (pp. 99–117). Thousand Oaks, CA: SAGE.

Becker, H. S. (1993). How I learned what a 'crock' was. *Journal of Contemporary Ethnography*, 22, 28–35.

Becker, H. S. (1996). The epistemology of qualitative research. In R. Jessor, A. Colby, & R. Schweder (Eds.), *Ethnography and human development: Context and meaning in social inquiry* (p. 62). Chicago, IL: University of Chicago Press. Retrievd from www.soc.ucsb.edu/faculty/hbecker/qa.html

Becker, H. S. (1998). *Tricks of the trade: How to think about your research while you're doing it*. Chicago, IL: University of Chicago Press.

Becker, H. S. (2007). *Writing for sociologists* (2nd ed.). Chicago, IL: University of Chicago Press.

Becker, H. S. (2020). *Writing for social scientists: How to start and finish your thesis, book, or article* (3rd ed.). Chicago, IL: University of Chicago Press.

Becker, H. S., & Faulkner, R. R. (2008). Studying something you are a part of: The view from the bandstand. *Ethnologie Francaise*, 38, 15–21. Retrieved from http://www.howardsbecker.com/articles/ffbparis.html

Becker, H. S., Geer, B., Hughes, E. C., & Strauss, A. L. (1961). *Boys in white: Student culture in medical school*. Chicago, IL: University of Chicago Press.

Benmayor, R. (1991). Testimony, action research, and empowerment: Puerto Rican women and popular education. In S. B. Gluck & D. Patai (Eds.), *Womens words: The feminist practice of oral history* (pp. 159–174). New York, NY: Routledge.

Berg, B. L. (2001). *Qualitative research methods for the social sciences* (4th ed.). Boston, MA: Allyn & Bacon.

Berg, B. L. (2007). *Qualitative research methods for the social sciences* (6th ed.). Boston, MA: Pearson.

Berk, R. A. (2012). How to create *"Thriller"* PowerPoints in the classroom. *Innovation in Higher Education*, 37, 141–152.

Bernard, H. R. (2013). *Social research methods: Qualitative and quantitative approaches* (2nd ed.). Thousand Oaks, CA: SAGE.

Bhaskar, R. (1986). *Scientific realism and human emancipation*. Bristol, UK: Verso (New Left Books).

Black, D. J. (1970). Production of crime rates. *American Sociological Review*, 35, 733–748.

Black, M., & Ponirakis, A. (2000). Computer-administered interviews with children about maltreatment: Methodological, developmental, and ethical issues. *Journal of Interpersonal Violence*, 15, 682–695.

Black, D. J., & Reiss, A. (1970). Police control of juveniles. *American Sociological Review*, 35, 63–77.

Blumberg, S. J., Luke, J. V., & Cynamon, M. L. (2006). Telephone coverage and health survey estimates: Evaluating the need for concern about wireless substitution. *American Journal of Public Health*, 96(5), 926–931. doi:10.2105/AJPH.2004.057885

Blumer, H. (1969). *Symbolic interactionism: Perspective and method*. Englewood Cliffs, NJ: Prentice-Hall.

Bodanis, D. (2001). $E = mc^2$: A biography of the world's most famous equation. New York, NY: Penguin.

Bogardus, E. (1925). Measuring social distance. *Journal of Applied Sociology*, 9, 299–308.

Boilevin, L., Chapman, J., Deane, L., Doerksen, C., Fresz, G., Joe, D. J., ... Winter, P. (2019). *Research 101: A manifesto for ethical research in the downtown eastside*. Retrieved from https://open.library.ubc.ca/cIRcle/collections/ubccommunityandpartnerspublicati/52387/items/1.0377565

Bollas, C., & Sundelson, D. (1995). *The new informants: The betrayal of confidentiality in psychoanalysis and psychotherapy*. Lanham, MD: Jason Aronson.

Borland, K. (1991). "That's not what I said": Interpretive conflict in oral narrative research. In S. B. Gluck & D. Patai (Eds.), *Womens words: The feminist practice of oral history* (pp. 63–76). New York, NY: Routledge.

Boruch, R. F., & Cecil, J. S. (1979). *Assuring the confidentiality of research data*. Philadelphia, PA: University of Pennsylvania Press.

Bourdieu, P. (1977). *Outline of a theory of practice*. Cambridge, UK: Cambridge University Press.

Brancati, D. (2018). *Social scientific research*. Thousand Oaks, CA: SAGE.

Brandt, L. L. (1975). Scientific psychology: What for?. *Canadian Psychological Review*, 16, 23–34.

Brantingham, P. J. (1991). Patterns in Canadian crime. In M. A. Jackson & C. T. Griffiths (Eds.), *Canadian criminology: Perspectives on crime and criminality* (pp. 371–402). Toronto, Canada: Harcourt Brace Jovanovich.

Brantingham, P. J., & Brantingham, P. L. (1984). *Patterns in crime*. New York, NY: Macmillan.

Broadhead, R. S., & Rist, R. C. (1976). Gatekeepers and the social control of social research. *Social Problems*, 23(3), 325–336.

Brock, D. R., & Kinsman, G. (1986). Patriarchal relations ignored: An analysis and critique of the Badgley report on sexual offenses against children and youths. In J. Lowman, M. A. Jackson, T. S. Palys, & S. Gavigan (Eds.), *Regulating sex: An anthology of commentaries on the findings and recommendations of the Badgley and Fraser reports* (pp. 107–126). Burnaby, BC: School of Criminology, Simon Fraser University.

Bronfenbrenner, U. (1979). *The ecology of human development*. Cambridge, MA: Harvard University Press.

Bronskill, J., & Blanchfield, M. (1998, September 20). Canadian convicts used as test subjects in experiments. *Vancouver Sun*, p. 41.

Bruner, J. (1986). *Actual minds, possible worlds*. Cambridge, MA: Harvard University Press.

Brunswik, E. (1955). Representative design and probabilistic theory in a functional psychology. *Psychological Review*, 62, 193–217.

Bryman, A. (2007). Barriers to integrating quantitative and qualitative research. *Journal of Mixed Methods Research*, 1(1), 8–22.

Bungay, V., Oliffe, J., & Atchison, C. (2016). Addressing underrepresentation in sex work research: Reflections on designing a purposeful sampling strategy. *Qualitative Health Research*, 26(7), 966–978.

Burrows, R., & Savage, M. (2014). After the crisis? Big Data and the methodological challenges of empirical sociology. *Big Data & Society*, 1(1), 205395171454028. doi:10.1177/2053951714540280

Butler-Kisber, L. (2018). *Qualitative inquiry: Thematic, narrative and arts-based perspectives* (2nd ed.). Thousand Oaks, CA: SAGE.

Byrne, D., & Kelley, K. (1989). Basing legislative action on research data: Prejudice, prudence, and empirical limitations. In D. Zillmann & J. Bryant (Eds.), *Pornography: Research advances and policy considerations* (pp. 363–385). Hillsdale, NJ: Erlbaum.

Cadwalladr, C., & Graham-Harrison, E. (2018, March 17). Revealed: 50 million Facebook profiles harvested for Cambridge Analytica in major data breach. *The Guardian*. Retrieved from https://www.theguardian.com/news/2018/mar/17/cambridge-analytica-facebook-influence-us-election

Campbell, D. T. (1957). Factors relevant to the validity of experiments in social settings. *Psychological Bulletin*, 54, 297–312.

Campbell, D. T. (1963). Social attitudes and other acquired behavioural dispositions. In S. Koch (Ed.), *Psychology: A study of a science* (Vol. 6, pp. 94–172). New York, NY: McGraw-Hill.

Campbell, D. T. (1969a). Definitional versus multiple operationism. *Et al*, 2(1), 14–17.

Campbell, D. T. (1969b). Reforms as experiments. *American Psychologist*, 24, 409–429.

Campbell, D. T. (1969c). Ethnocentrism of disciplines and the fish-scale model of omniscience. In M. Sherif & C. W. Sherif (Eds.), *Interdisciplinary relationships in the social sciences* (pp. 328–348). Chicago, IL: Aldine.

Campbell, D. T. (1974). Evolutionary epistemology. In P. A. Schlipp (Ed.), *The philosophy of Karl Popper* (pp. 413–463). LaSalle, IL: Open Court.

Campbell, D. T. (1978). Qualitative knowing in action research. In M. Brenner, P. Marsh, & M. Brenner (Eds.), *The social contexts of methods* (pp. 184–209). London: Breem Helm.

Campbell, D. T. (1979a). "Degrees of freedom" and the case study. In T. D. Cook & C. S. Reichardt (Eds.), *Qualitative and quantitative methods in evaluation research* (pp. 49–67). Thousand Oaks, CA: SAGE.

Campbell, D. T. (1979b). A tribal model of the social system vehicle carrying scientific knowledge. *Knowledge: Creation, Diffusion, Utilization*, 1, 181–201.

Campbell, D. T. (1984). Can we be scientific in applied social science? In R. F. Connor, D. G. Altman, & C. Jackson (Eds.), *Evaluation studies review annual* (Vol. 9, pp. 26–48). Thousand Oaks, CA: SAGE.

Campbell, D. T. (1986). Science's social system of validity-enhancing collective belief change and the problems of the social sciences. In D. W. Fiske and R. A. Schweder (Eds.) *Metatheory in social science: Pluralisms and subjectivities* (pp.108–148). Chicago, IL: University of Chicago Press.

Campbell, D. T. (1991). Methods for the experimenting society. *American Journal of Evaluation Research*, 12(3), 223–260.

Campbell, D. T., & Ross, L. H. (1968). The Connecticut crackdown on speeding: Time-series data in quasi-experimental analysis. *Law and Society*, 3, 33–53.

Campbell, D. T., & Stanley, J. C. (1963). *Experimental and quasi-experimental designs for research*. Chicago, IL: Rand McNally.

Cantril, H. (1965). *The pattern of human concerns*. New Brunswick, NJ: Rutgers University Press.

Caporaso, J. A. (1973). Quasi-experimental approaches to social science: Perspectives and problems. In J. A. Caporaso & L. L. Roos Jr. (Eds.), *Quasi-experimental approaches: Testing theory and evaluating policy*. Chicago, IL: Northwestern University Press.

Carspecken, P. F. (1996). *Critical ethnography in educational research: A theoretical and practical guide*. New York, NY; London, UK: Routledge.

Cecil, J. S., & Wetherington, G. T. (Eds.). (1996). Court-ordered disclosure of academic research: A clash of values of science and law. *Law and Contemporary Problems (Special Issue)*, 59(3), 1–191.

Chakravartty, A. (2011). Scientific Realism. In E. N. Zalta (Ed.), *The Stanford encyclopedia of philosophy*. Retrieved from http://plato.stanford.edu/archives/sum2011/entries/scientific-realism/. Last checked 7 November 2011.

Chenail, R. J. (1997). Keeping things plumb in qualitative research. *The Qualitative Report*, 3(3), 1–10.

Christians, C. (2000). Ethics and politics in qualitative research. In N. K. Denzin & Y. S. Lincoln (Eds.), *Handbook of qualitative research* (2nd ed., pp. 133–155). Thousand Oaks, CA: SAGE.

Cicourel, A. V. (1964). *Method and measurement in sociology*. New York, NY: Free Press.

Clifford, J. (1986). Introduction: Partial truths. In J. Clifford & G. E. Marcus (Eds.), *Writing culture: The poetics and politics of ethnography* (pp. 1–26). Berkeley, CA: University of California Press.

Cohen, S. (1985). *Visions of social control: Crime, punishment and classification*. Cambridge, UK: Polity.

Collins, A. (1988). *The sleep room*. Toronto, Canada: Lester & Orpen Dennys.

Collins, P. H. (1991). Learning from the outsider within: The sociological significance of black feminist thought. In M. M. Fonow & J. A. Cook (Eds.), *Beyond methodology: Feminist scholarship as lived research* (pp. 35–59). Bloomington, IN: Indiana University Press.

Columbia Accident Investigation Board. (2003). *Report* (Vol. 1). Washington, DC: Government Printing Office. Retrieved from https://www.nasa.gov/columbia/home/CAIB_Vol1.html

Confessore, N., & Kang, C. (2018, December 30). Facebook data scandals stoke criticism that a privacy watchdog too rarely bites. *New York Times*. Retrieved from https://www.nytimes.com/2018/12/30/technology/facebook-data-privacy-ftc.html

Cook, K. E. (2008). Critical ethnography. In L. Givens (Ed.), *The SAGE encyclopedia of qualitative research methods* (Vol. 1, pp. 148–151). Thousand Oaks, CA: SAGE.

Cook, T. D. (2000). Toward a practical theory of external validity. In L. Bickman (Ed.), *Validity and social experimentation: Donald Campbell's legacy* (pp. 3–43). Thousand Oaks, CA: SAGE.

Cook, T. D., & Campbell, D. T. (1979). *Quasiexperimentation*. Boston, MA: Houghton Mifflin.

Cooley, C. H. (1902). *Human nature and the social order*, New York, NY: Charles Scribner's Sons.

Cope, B., & Kalantzis, M. (2015). Sources of evidence-of-learning: Learning and assessment in the era of big data. *Open Review of Educational Research*, 2(1), 194–217.

Cote, D. (2012, February 15). Researchers weigh in on Belfast Project legal drama. *The Heights*. Retrieved from http://bcheights.com/2012/02/15/researchers-weigh-in-on-belfast-project-legal-drama/

Cowles, M., & Davis, C. (1982). On the origins of the .05 level of statistical significance. *American Psychologist*, 37, 553–558.

Crabb, B. B. (1996). Judicially compelled disclosure of researchers' data: A judge's view. *Law and Contemporary Problems*, 59, 9–34.

Crawford, S., Couper, M. P., & Lamias, M. J. (2001). Web surveys: Perceptions of burden. *Social Science Computer Review*, 19, 146–162.

Cressey, D. R. (1953). *Other people' money: A study in the social psychology of embezzlement*. New York, NY: Free Press.

Cresswell, J. W. (2016). *30 essential skills for the qualitative researcher*. Thousand Oaks, CA: SAGE.

Crowne, D. P., & Marlowe, D. A. (1960). A new scale of social desirability independent of pathology. *Journal of Consulting Psychology*, 24, 351.

Cusumano, M. A., & Yoffie, D. B. (1998). *Competing on internet time: Lessons from Netscape and its battle with Microsoft*. New York, NY: The Free Press.

Dahlen, M. (2002). Learning the web: Internet user experience and response to web marketing in Sweden. *Journal of Interactive Advertising*, 3(1), 25–33.

Daisley, B. (1994, December 28). Clear evidence needed to invoke Wigmore rules. *The Lawyer's Weekly*.

Darwin, C. (1859). *On the origin of species*. London: John Murray.

Davis, M. (1971). That's interesting! Towards a phenomenology of sociology and a sociology of *phenomenology*. *Philosophy of the Social Sciences*, 1, 309–344.

Davis, S. (1990). Men as success objects and women as sex objects: A study of personal advertisements. *Sex Roles: A Journal of Research*, 23, 43–50.

Dawes, R. M. (1972). *Fundamentals of attitude measurement*. Hoboken, NJ: Wiley.

de Vaus, D. (2002). *Surveys in social research* (5th ed.). London: Routledge.

Deloria, V., Jr. (1991). Commentary: Research, redskins, and reality. *American Indian Quarterly*, 15(4), 457–468.

Denzin, N. K. (1970). *The research act: A theoretical introduction to sociological methods*. Chicago, IL: Aldine.

Denzin, N. K. (1978). The logic of naturalistic inquiry. In N. K. Denzin (Ed.), *Sociological methods: A sourcebook*. New York, NY: McGraw-Hill.

Denzin, N. K. (1989). *The research act: A theoretical introduction to sociological methods* (3rd ed.). Englewood Cliffs, NJ: Prentice-Hall.

Denzin, N. K., & Lincoln, Y. S. (1994). Introduction: Entering the field of qualitative research. In N. K. Denzin & Y. S. Lincoln (Eds.), *Handbook of qualitative research* (pp. 1–18). Thousand Oaks, CA: SAGE.

Denzin, N. K., & Lincoln, Y. S. (2003). Introduction: The discipline and practice of qualitative research. In N. K. Denzin & Y. S. Lincoln (Eds.) *The landscape of qualitative research: Theories and issues* (2nd ed., pp. 1–46). Thousand Oaks, CA: SAGE.

Devlin, A. S. (2018). *The research experience: Planning, conducting and reporting research*. Thousand Oaks, CA: SAGE.

Dillman, D. A. (2009). Some consequences of survey mode changes in longitudinal surveys. In P. Lynn (Ed.), *Methodology of longitudinal surveys* (pp. 127–140). Chichester, UK: Wiley. doi:10.1002/9780470743874.ch8

Dillman, D. A., Smyth, J. D., & Christian, L. M. (2009). *Internet, mail, and mixed-mode surveys: The tailored design method* (3rd ed.). Hoboken, NJ: Wiley.

Dillman, D. A., Smyth, J. D., & Christian, L. M. (2014). *Internet, phone, mail, and mixed-mode surveys: The tailored design method* (4th ed.). Hoboken, NJ: Wiley.

Dingwall, R. (2008). The ethical case against ethical regulation in humanities and social science research. *Twenty-First Century Society*, 3(1), 1–12.

Ditton, J. (1979). *Contrology: Beyond criminology*. London: Macmillan Press.

Donnerstein, E., & Berkowitz, L. (1981). Victim reactions in aggressive erotic films as a factor in violence against women. *Journal of Personality and Social Psychology*, 41, 710–724.

Doob, L. W. (1959). Review of "*Propaganda analysis: A study of inferences made from Nazi propaganda in World War II* by Alexander L. George." *American Journal of Sociology*, 65(3), 318–319.

Dotinga, A., Van Den Eijnden, R. J. J. M., Bosveld, W., & Garretsen, H. F. L. (2005). The effect of data collection mode and ethnicity of interviewer on response rates and self-reported alcohol use among Turks and Moroccans in The Netherlands: An experimental study. *Alcohol and Alcoholism*, 40(3), 242–248. doi:10.1093/alcalc/agh144

Douven, I. (2017). Abduction. In E. N. Zalta (Ed.), *The Stanford encyclopedia of philosophy*. Retrieved from https://plato.stanford.edu/archives/sum2017/entries/abduction/

Dow Chemical Co. v. Allen. 672 F.2d 1262, 1274-77 (7th Cir. 1982).

Doyle, A. C. (1986). The adventure of Silver Blaze. In A. C. Doyle (Ed.), *The original illustrated Sherlock Holmes* (pp. 185–200). Secaucus, NJ: Castle Books. (Originally published 1892.).

Draper, H., Wilson, S., Flanagan, S., & Ives, J. (2009). Offering payments, reimbursements and incentives to patients and family doctors to encourage participation in research. *Family Practice*, 26(3), 231–238.

Duneier, M. (1999). *Sidewalk*. New York, NY: Farrar, Straus & Giroux.

Duran, B., & Duran, E. (2000). Applied postcolonial clinical and research strategies. In M. Battiste (Ed.), *Reclaiming indigenous voice and vision* (pp. 86–100). Vancouver, BC: UBC Press.

Durkheim, E. (1951). *Suicide: A study in sociology* (J. Spaulding & G. Simpson, Trans.). New York, NY: Free Press.

Durkheim, E. (1968). Social facts. In M. Brodbeck (Ed.), *Readings in the philosophy of the social sciences* (pp. 245–254). New York, NY: Macmillan. (Reprinted from E. Durkheim, 1938, *The rules of sociological method*, New York: Free Press.)

Dutton, D. G., Boyanowsky, E. O., Palys, T. S., & Heywood, R. (1982). *Community policing: Preliminary results from a national study of the RCMP*. Research report prepared for the Research Division of the Solicitor General Canada.

Ellis, C., Adams, T. E., and Bochner, A. P. (2011). Autoethnography: An overview. *Forum Qualitative Sozialforschung/ Forum: Qualitative Social Research*, 12(1), Art. 10, http://nbn-resolving.de/urn:nbn:de:0114-fqs1101108

Epstein, J., & Klinkenberg, W. D. (2001). From Eliza to Internet: A brief history of computerized assessment. *Computers in Human Behavior*, 17, 295–314.

Epstein, J., Klinkenberg, W. D., Wiley, D., & Mckinley, L. (2001). Insuring sample equivalence across Internet and paper-and-pencil assessments. *Computers in Human Behavior*, 17, 339–346.

Etter-Lewis, G. (1991). Black women's life stories: Reclaiming self in narrative texts. In S. B. Gluck & D. Patai (Eds.), *Womens words: The feminist practice of oral history* (pp. 43–58). New York, NY: Routledge.

Farris, G. F. (1969). The drunkard's search in behavioral science. *Compensation and Benefits Review*, 1(2), 29–33.

Faulconer, J. E., & Williams, R. N. (1985). Temporality in human action: An alternative to positivism and historicism. *American Psychologist*, 40, 1179–1188.

Faulkner, R. R., & Becker, H. S. (2008). Studying something you are a part of: The view from the bandstand. *Ethnologie Française*, 38(1), 15–21. Retrieved from http://home.earthlink.net/~hsbecker/articles/ffbparis.html

Federal Communications Commission. (2011). *Telephone subscribership in the United States*. Washington, DC: FCC Reference Information Center. Retrieved from https://www.fcc.gov/general/telephone-subscribership-report

Festinger, L. (1953). Laboratory experiments. In L. Festinger & D. Katz (Eds.), *Research methods in the behavioral sciences* (pp. 136–172). New York, NY: Holt, Rinehart and Winston.

Festinger, L. (1957). *A theory of cognitive dissonance*. Evanston, IL: Row, Peterson.

Festinger, L., & Katz, D. (Eds.). (1953). *Research methods in the behavioral sciences*. New York, NY: Holt, Rinehart and Winston.

Festinger, L., Riecken, H. W., & Schachter, S. (1956). *When prophecy fails*. Minneapolis, MN: University of Minnesota Press.

Filstead, W. J. (1979). Qualitative methods: A needed perspective in evaluation research. In T. D. Cook & C. S. Reichardt (Eds.), *Qualitative and quantitative methods in evaluation research* (pp. 33–48). Thousand Oaks, CA: SAGE.

Fine, M., Weis, L., Weseen, S., & Wong, L. (2003). For whom? Qualitative research, representations, and social responsibilities. In N. K. Denzin & Y. S. Lincoln (Eds.), *The landscape of qualitative research: Theories and issues* (2nd ed., pp. 167–207). Thousand Oaks, CA: SAGE.

Fishbein, M. (Ed.). (1967). *Readings in attitude theory and measurement*. Hoboken, NJ: Wiley.

Fishbein, M., & Azjen, I. (1975). *Belief, attitude, intention, and behavior: An introduction to theory and research*. Reading, MA: Addison-Wesley.

Fisher, R. A. (1925). *Statistical methods for research workers*. Edinburgh, Scotland: Oliver & Boyd.

Fisher, W. A. (1986). The emperor has no clothes: On the Badgley and Fraser Committees' rejection of social science research on pornography. In J. Lowman, M. A. Jackson, T. S. Palys, & S. Gavigan (Eds.), *Regulating sex: An anthology of commentaries on the findings and recommendations of the Badgley and Fraser Reports* (pp. 159–176). Burnaby, BC: School of Criminology, Simon Fraser University.

Fisher, W. A., & Grenier, G. (1994). Violent pornography, anti-woman thoughts, and antiwoman acts: In search of reliable effects. *The Journal of Sex Research*, 31, 23–38.

Fitzgerald, M. H. (2004). Punctuated equilibrium, moral panics and the ethics review process. *Journal of Academic Ethics*, 2, 315–338.

Flint, A. (1995, June 3). The scientists and the radicals square off. *The Globe & Mail*, D8.

Foley, D., & Valenzuela, A. (2005). Critical ethnography: The politics of collaboration. In N. K.Denzin and Y. S. Lincoln (Eds.), *Handbook of qualitative research* (pp. 217–234). Thousand Oaks, CA: SAGE.

Fontana, A., & Frey, J. H. (2003). The interview: From structured questions to negotiated text. In N. K. Denzin & Y. S. Lincoln (Eds.), *Collecting and interpreting qualitative materials.* (2nd ed., pp. 61–106). Thousand Oaks, CA: SAGE.

Fox, J., Murray, C., & Warm, A. (2003). Conducting research using web-based questionnaires: Practical, methodological and ethical considerations. *Social Research Methodology*, 6, 167–180.

Fox, N., & Roberts, C. (1999). GPs in cyberspace: The sociology of a 'virtual community'. *Sociological Review*, 47(4), 643–671.

Freidson, E. (1964). Against the code of ethics. *American Sociological Review*, 29(3), 410.

French, D. P., Cooke, R., McLean, N., Williams, M., & Sutton, S. (2007). What do people think about when they answer theory of planned behaviour questionnaires? *Journal of Health Psychology*, 12(4), 672–687.

Fricker, R., & Rand, M. S. (2002). Advantages and disadvantages of Internet research surveys: Evidence from the literature. *Field Methods*, 14, 347–367.

Friere, P. (1982). Creating alternative research methods: Learning to do by doing it. In B. Hall, A. Gillette, & R. Tandon (Eds.), *Creating knowledge: A monopoly? Participatory research in development* (pp. 29–37). New Delhi, India: Participatory Research Network Series.

Fry, C. L., Hall, W., Ritter, A., & Jenkinson, R. (2006). The ethics of paying drug users who participate in research: A review and practical recommendations. *Journal of Empirical Research on Human Research Ethics*, 1(4), 21–35.

Galliher, J. (1973). The protection of human subjects: A reexamination of the professional code of ethics. *The American Sociologist*, 8(3), 93–100. Retrieved October 24, 2020, from http://www.jstor.org/stable/27702088

George, A. A. (1959). *Propaganda analysis: A study of inferences made from Nazi propaganda in World War II*. Evanston, IL: Row, Peterson.

Gluck, S. B. (1984). What's so special about women: Women's oral history. In D. Dunaway & W. K. Baum (Eds.), *Oral history: An interdisciplinary anthology* (pp. 221–237). Nashville, TN: American Association for State and Local History.

Gluck, S. B. (1991). Advocacy oral history: Palestinian women in resistance. In S. B. Gluck & D. Patai (Eds.), *Womens words: The feminist practice of oral history* (pp. 205–220). New York, NY: Routledge.

Gluck, S. B., & Patai, D. (Eds.). (1991). *Womens words: The feminist practice of oral history*. New York, NY: Routledge.

Gold, R. L. (1958). Roles in sociological field investigation. *Social Forces*, 36, 217–223.

Golder, S. A., & Macy, M. W. (2014). Digital footprints: Opportunities and challenges for online social research. *Annual Review of Sociology*, 40, 129–152.

Gorden, R. L. (1980). *Interviewing: Strategy, techniques and tactics* (3rd ed.). Homewood, IL: Dorsey Press.

Gosling, S., Vazire, S., Srivastava, S., & John, O. P. (2004). Should we trust web-based studies? A comparative analysis of six preconceptions about Internet questionnaires. *American Psychologist*, 59(2), 93–104.

Grande, D., Gollust, S. E., Pany, M., Seymour, J., Goss, A., Kilaru, A., & Meisel, Z. (2014). Translating research for health policy: Researchers' perceptions and use of social media. *Health Affairs*, 33(7), 1278–1285.

Gravlee, C. (2002). Mobile computer-assisted personal interviewing with handheld computers: The Entryware System 3.0. *Field Methods*, 14, 322–336.

Gray, D. E. (2014). *Doing research in the real world* (3rd ed.). Thousand Oaks, CA: SAGE.

Gray, G., & Guppy, N. (1994). *Successful surveys: Research methods and practice*. Toronto, Canada: Thomson Nelson.

Greenwald, G. (2014). *No place to hide: Edward Snowden, the NSA, and the US surveillance state*. New York, NY: Picador.

Greschner, D. (1992). Aboriginal women, the constitution and criminal justice. *University of British Columbia Law Review (special edition)*, 26, 338–359.

Groopman, J. (2008). *How doctors think*. New York, NY: Houghton Mifflin Harcourt.

Hagan, F. E. (1989). *Research methods in criminal justice and criminology* (2nd ed.). New York, NY: Macmillan.

Hagey, R. S. (1997). The use and abuse of participatory action research. *Chronic Diseases in Canada*, 18(1), 1–4.

Haggerty, K. D. (2004). Ethics creep: Governing social science research in the name of ethics. *Qualitative Sociology*, 27(4), 391–414.

Hale, S. (1991). Feminist method, process, and self-criticism: Interviewing Sudanese women. In S. B. Gluck & D. Patai (Eds.), *Womens words: The feminist practice of oral history* (pp. 121–136). New York, NY: Routledge.

Hale, C. R. (2006). Activist research v. Cultural critique: Indigenous land rights and the contradictions of politically engaged anthropology. *Cultural Anthrology*, 21(1), 96–120.

Hamburger, P. (2005). The new censorship: Institutional review boards. *Supreme Court Review*, 2004, 271–354.

Hampton, K., & Wellman, B. (1999). Netville online and offline: Observing and surveying a wired suburb. *The American Behavioral Scientist*, 43, 475–493.

Harris, S. (2004). Missing the point. Is PowerPoint the enemy of thought? *Government Executive*, 36(15), 48–56.

Hart, P. (1991). Irving L. Janis's Victims of Groupthink. *Political Psychology*, 12(2), 247–278.

Harvey, L. (2012–2019). Social research glossary. *Quality Research International*. Retrieved from http://www.qualityresearchinternational.com/socialresearch/

Henry, S (1987). The construction and deconstruction of social control: Thoughts on the discursive production of state law and private justice. In J. Lowman, R. J. Menzies, & T. S. Palys (Eds.), *Transcarceration: Essays in the sociology of social control* (pp. 89–108). Aldershot, UK: Gower.

Herbert, P. B., and Young, K. A. (2002). Tarasoff at Twenty-Five. *Journal of the American Academy of Psychiatry and Law*, 30, 275–281.

Hill, K. (2014, June 28). Facebook maniulated 689,003 users' emotions for science. *Forbes Magazine*. Retrieved from https://www.forbes.com/sites/deloitte/2018/12/14/the-march-toward-equality-and-inclusion-must-become-a-sprint/#717be0994b65

Hoare, T., Levy, C., & Robinson, M. P. (1993). Participatory action research in Native communities: Cultural opportunities and legal implications. *The Canadian Journal of Native Studies*, 13, 43–68.

Hoffman, J. E. (1980). Problems of access in the study of social elites and boards of directors. In W. B. Shaffir, R. A. Stebbins, & A. Turowetz (Eds.), *Fieldwork experience: Qualitative approaches to social research* (pp. 45–56). New York, NY: St. Martin's Press.

Hooks, B. (1989). *Talking back: Thinking feminist, thinking black.* Boston, MA: South End.

Horowitz, I. (1967). *The rise and fall of Project Camelot: Studies in the relationship between social science and practical politics.* Cambridge, MA: MIT Press.

Horowitz, R. (1983). *Honor and the American dream.* New Brunswick, NJ: Rutgers University Press.

House, E. R. (1976). Justice in evaluation. In G. V. Glass (Ed.), *Evaluation studies review annual* (Vol. 1, pp. 75–100). Thousand Oaks, CA: SAGE.

Huberman, A. M., & Miles, M. B. (1994). Data management and analysis methods. In N. K. Denzin & Y. S. Lincoln (Eds.), *Handbook of qualitative research* (pp. 428–444). Thousand Oaks, CA: SAGE.

Huff, D. (1954). *How to lie with statistics.* New York, NY: Norton (reissued in 1982 and 1993).

Humphreys, L. (1970). *Tearoom trade: Impersonal sex in public places.* Chicago, IL: Aldine.

In re Grand Jury Proceedings: James Richard Scarce. 53d 397 (9th Cir. 09/17/1993).

In re Michael A. Cusumano and David B. Yoffie [United States of America v. Microsoft Corporation], No. 98-2133, United States Court of Appeals for the First Circuit]. (1998). Retrieved August 20, 2002, from http://www.law.emory.edu/1circuit/dec98/98-2133.01a.html

Inquest of Unknown Female. (1994, October 20). Oral reasons for judgement of the Honourable L.W. Campbell, 91-240-0838. Burnaby, BC.

Irwin, J. (1970). *The felon.* Englewood Cliffs, NJ: Prentice-Hall.

Irwin, J. (1980). *Prisons in turmoil.* Boston, MA: Little, Brown.

Irwin, J. (1985). *The jail: Managing the underclass in American society.* Berkeley, CA: University of California Press.

Israel, M. (2004a). *Ethics and the governance of criminological research in Australia.* Report for the New South Wales Bureau of Crime Statistics and Research. Retrieved from http://www.lawlink.nsw.gov.au/bocsar1. nsf/files/r55.pdf/$file/r55.pdf

Israel, M. (2004b). Strictly confidential? Integrity and the disclosure of criminological and socio-legal research. *British Journal of Criminology*, 44, 715–740.

Israel, M. (2015). *Research ethics and integrity for social scientists: Beyond regulatory compliance* (2nd ed.). Thousand Oaks, CA: SAGE.

Israel, J., & Tajfel, H. (Eds.). (1972). *The context of social psychology: A critical assessment.* Cambridge, MA: Academic Press.

Jackson, K., & Bazeley, P. (2019). *Qualitative data analysis with Nvivo* (3rd ed.). Thousand Oaks, CA: SAGE.

Jackson, M., & MacCrimmon, M. (1999). *Research confidentiality and academic privilege: A legal opinion.* Submission prepared for the Simon Fraser University Ethics policy Review Task Force. Retrieved August 21, 2002, from http://www.sfu.ca/~palys/JackMac Opinion.pdf

Jaffee v. Redmond (95-266). 518 U.S. 1 (1996).

James, G. (2011, September 30). Top 20 reasons presentations suck and how to fix them. *CBS News.* Retrieved from https://www.cbsnews.com/media/top-20-reasons-presentations-suck-and-how-to-fix-them/

Janis, I. L. (1972). *Victims of groupthink.* Boston, MA: Houghton Mifflin.

Johnson, R., & Onwuegbuzie, A. (2004). Mixed methods research: A research paradigm whose time has come. *Educational Researcher,* 33(7), 14–26.

Johnson, R., Onwuegbuzie, A., & Turner, L. (2007). Toward a definition of mixed methods research. *Journal of Mixed Methods Research,* 1(2), 112–133.

Jordan, S. (2003). Who stole my methodology? Co-opting PAR. *Globalisation, Societies and Education,* 1(2), 185–200.

Kahneman, D., Slovic, P., & Tversky, A. (1982). *Judgment under uncertainty: Heuristics and biases.* Cambridge, UK: Cambridge University Press.

Kapterev, A. (2007) *Death by PowerPoint.* Retrieved from https://www.slideshare.net/thecroaker/death-by-powerpoint/2-There_are_300_million_PowerPoint_users_in_the_world

Karr, L. (2000). New horizons in cross-national experimentation. *Current Research in Social Psychology,* 5(13), 190–205.

Katz, J. (2007). Towards a natural history of ethical censorship. *Law & Society Review,* 41(4), 797–810.

Katz, D., & Braly, K. (1933). Racial stereotypes of one hundred college students. *Journal of Abnormal and Social Psychology,* 28, 280–290.

Kaye, B., & Johnson, T. J. (1999). Research methodology: Taming the cyber frontier: Techniques for Improving online surveys. *Social Science Computer Review,* 17, 323–337.

Kelly, G. A. (1955). *The psychology of personal constructs (2 vols.).* New York, NY: Norton.

Kelly, P. J. (2005). Practical suggestions for community interventions using participatory action research. *Public Health Nursing,* 22(1), 65–73.

Kelly, C. D. (2006). Replicating empirical research in behavioral ecology: How and why it should be done but rarely ever is. *Quarterly Review of Biology,* 81(3), 221–236.

Kemmis, S., & McTaggart, R. (2007). Participatory action research: Communicative action and the public sphere. In N. K. Denzin & Y. S. Lincoln (Eds)., *Strategies of qualitative inquiry* (3rd ed., pp.271–330). Thousand Oaks, CA: SAGE.

Kerlinger, F. N. (1973). *Foundations of behavioral research* (2nd ed.). New York, NY: Holt, Rinehart and Winston.

Kidd, S. A., & Kral, M. J. (2005). Practicing participatory action research. *Journal of Counseling Psychology,* 52(2), 187–195. doi: 10.1037/0022-0167.52.2.187

Kidder, L. H. (1981). Qualitative research and quasi-experimental frameworks. In M. B. Brewer & B. E. Collins (Eds.), *Scientific inquiry and the social sciences: A volume in honor of Donald T. Campbell* (pp. 226–256). San Francisco, CA: Jossey-Bass.

Kidder, L. H., & Campbell, D. T. (1970). The indirect testing of social attitudes. In G. F. Summers (Ed.), *Attitude measurement* (pp. 333–385). Chicago, IL: Rand McNally.

Kiesler, S., & Sproull, L. S. (1986). Response effects in the electronic survey. *Public Opinion Quarterly,* 50, 402–413.

King, N., Horrocks, C., & Brooks, J. (2019). *Interviews in qualitative research* (2nd ed.). Thousand Oaks, CA: SAGE.

Kinsey, A., & Mart, C. E. (1948). *Sexual behavior in the human male.* Bloomington, IN: Indiana University Press.

Kirby, J., & Marsden, P. (2006). *Connected marketing: The viral, buzz and word-of-mouth revolution* (1st ed.). Oxford, UK: Butterworth-Heinemann.

Kirk, R. E. (1968). *Experimental design: Procedures for the behavioral sciences.* Pacific Grove, CA: Brooks/Cole.

Kitchin, H. (2002). The tri-council on cyberspace: Insights, oversights, and extrapolations. In W. C. van den Hoonaard (Ed.), *Walking the tightrope: Ethical issues for qualitative researchers* (pp. 160–174). Toronto, Canada: University of Toronto Press.

Knox, R. E., & Inkster, J. A. (1968). Postdecision dissonance at post time. *Journal of Personality and Social Psychology,* 8, 319–323.

Kolar, K., & Atchison, C. (2013). Recruitment of sex buyers: A comparison of the efficacy of conventional and computer network-based approaches. *Social Science Computer Review,* 31(2), 178–190. doi:10.1177/0894439312453001

Kramer, A. D. I., Guillory, J. E., & Hancock, J. T. (2014, June 17). Experimental evidence of massive scale emotional contagion through social networks. *Proceedings of the National Academy of Sciences of the United States of America,* 111(24), 8788–8790. Retrieved from https://www.pnas.org/content/111/24/8788

Krippendorff, K. (2019). *Content analysis: An introduction to its methodology* (4th ed.). Thousand Oaks, CA: SAGE.

Krueger, R. A. (2015). *Focus groups: A practical guide for applied research* (5th ed.). Thousand Oaks, CA: SAGE.

Kuhn, T. S. (1970). *The structure of scientific revolutions* (2nd ed.). Chicago, IL: University of Chicago Press.

Kuhn, T. S. (2012). *The structure of scientific revolutions. 50th anniversary* (4th ed.). Chicago, IL: University of Chicago Press.

Kyle, J., & Gultchin, L. (2018). *Populists in power around the world*. London: Tony Blair Institute for Global Change. Retrieved from https://institute.global/insight/renewing-centre/populists-power-around-world

Lahman, M. E. (2018). *Ethics in social science research: Becoming culturally responsive*. Thousand Oaks, CA: SAGE.

Lakoff, G. (1987). *Women, fire, and dangerous things: What categories reveal about the mind*. Chicago, IL: University of Chicago Press.

LaPiere, R. T. (1934). Attitudes versus actions. *Social Forces, 13*, 230–237.

Latour, B. (1987). *Science in action*. Cambridge, MA: Harvard University Press.

Leavy, P. (2011). *Essentials of transdisciplinary research: Using problem-centered methodologies*. Walnut Creek, CA: Left Coast Press.

Levitin, D. J. (2017). *Weaponized lies: How to think critically in the post-truth era*. Toronto, Canada: Penguin.

Lewis, P., Barr, C., Clarke, S., Voce, A., Levett, C., & Gutiérrez, P. (2019, March 6). Revealed: The rise and rise of populist rhetoric. *The Guardian*. Retrieved from https://www.theguardian.com/world/ng-interactive/2019/mar/06/revealed-the-rise-and-rise-of-populist-rhetoric

Lewis, P., Clarke, S., & Barr, C. (2019, March 6). How we combed leaders' speeches to guage populist rise. *The Guardian*. Retrieved from https://www.theguardian.com/world/2019/mar/06/how-we-combed-leaders-speeches-to-gauge-populist-rise

Likert, R. (1932). A technique for the measurement of attitudes. *Archives of Psychology, 140*, 44–53.

Lindesmith, A. (1952). Comment on W. S. Robinson's the logical structure of analytic induction. *American Sociological Review, 17*, 492–493.

Liu, M., Papathanasiou, E., & Hao, Y.-W. (2001). Exploring the use of multimedia examination formats in undergraduate teaching:

Results from the fielding testing. *Computers in Human Behavior, 17*, 225–248.

Lofland, J. (1971). *Analyzing social settings: A guide to qualitative observation and analysis*. Belmont, CA: Wadsworth.

Lofland, L. H. (1973). *A world of strangers: Order and action in urban public space*. New York, NY: Basic Books.

Lofland, J., & Lejeune, R. A. (1960). Initial interaction of newcomers in Alcoholics Anonymous. *Social Problems, 8*, 102–111.

Lofland, J., & Lofland, L. H. (1984). *Analyzing social settings: A guide to qualitative observation and analysis* (2nd ed.). Belmont, CA: Wadsworth.

Lofland, J., Snow, D., Anderson, L., & Lofland, L. H. (2006). *Analyzing social settings: A guide to qualitative observation and analysis* (4th ed.). Belmont, CA: Wadsworth.

Lombroso, C. (1911). *Crime: Its causes and remedies*. Boston, MA: Little, Brown.

Lord, F. M. (1953). On the statistical treatment of football numbers. *American Psychologist, 8*, 750–751.

Lowman, J. (1989). *Street prostitution: Assessing the impact of the law (Vancouver)*. Ottawa, ON: Ministry of Supply and Services.

Lowman, J. (2014). *In the eye of the storm: The (ab)use of research in the Canadian prostitution law reform debate*. Paper presented at a conference on "Sex Work and Human Rights: Lessons from Canada for the UK" held at Durham Law School, Durham University, September 18–19. Excerpt online at https://www.sfu.ca/~palys/Lowman-2016-ExpertTestimonyInBedford&McPherson.pdf

Lowman, J., & Palys, T. S. (2000). Ethics and institutional conflict of interest: The research confidentiality controversy at Simon Fraser University. *Sociological Practice: A Journal of Clinical and Applied Sociology, 2*, 245–255.

Lowman, J., & Palys, T. S. (2001a). The ethics and law of confidentiality in criminological research. *International Journal of Criminal Justice, 11*, 1–33.

Lowman, J., & Palys, T. S. (2001b). Limited confidentiality, academic freedom, and matters of conscience: Where does CPA stand?. *Canadian Journal of Criminology, 43*, 497–508.

MacDonald, C. (2012). Understanding participatory action research: A qualitative research methodology option. *Canadian Journal of Action Research, 13*(2), 34–50.

MacFarlane, Br., & Cordner, S. M. (2008). *Wrongful convictions: The effect of tunnel vision and predisposing circumstances in the criminal justice system*. Toronto, Canada: Government of Ontario. Retrieved from https://www.attorneygeneral.jus.gov.on.ca/

inquiries/goudge/policy_research/pdf/Macfarlane_Wrongful-Convictions.pdf

Madison, D. S. (2005). *Critical ethnography: Method, ethics and performance*. Thousand Oaks, CA: SAGE.

Malamuth, N. M. (1978). Erotica, aggression and perceived appropriateness. Paper presented at the 86th annual convention of the American Psychological Association, Toronto, ON. (Cited in Malamuth 1984.)

Malamuth, N. M. (1989). Sexually violent media, thought patterns, and antisocial behavior. In G. Comstock (Ed.), *Public communication and behaviour* (Vol. 2, pp. 159–204). New York, NY: Academic Press.

Malinowski, B. (1922). *Argonauts of the western Pacific*. London: Routledge & Kegan Paul.

Malinowski, B. (1967). *A diary in the strict sense of the term*. New York, NY: Harcourt Brace Jovanovich.

Malka, A., & Chatman, J. A. (2003). Intrinsic and extrinsic work orientations as moderators of the effect of annual income on subjective well-being: A longitudinal study. *Personality and Social Psychology Bulletin*, 29(6), 737–746.

Manicas, P. T., & Secord, P. F. (1983). Implications for psychology of the new philosophy of science. *American Psychologist*, 38, 399–413.

Manning, P. K. (1991). Analytic induction. In K. Plummer (Ed.), *Symbolic interactionism: Contemporary issues* (Vol. 2, pp. 401–430). Brookfield, VT: Edward Elgar. (Reprinted from R. Smith & P. K. Manning (Eds.), 1982, *Qualitative methods*. Cambridge, MA: Ballinger.)

Manz, W., & Lueck, H. E. (1968). Influence of wearing glasses on personality ratings: Cross-cultural validation of an old experiment. *Perceptual and Motor Skills*, 27, 704.

Margolis, E. (1994). Video ethnography: Toward a reflexive paradigm for documentary. *Jump Cut*, 39, 122–131.

Marquart, J. W. (2001). Doing research in prison: The strengths and weaknesses of full participation as a guard. In J. M. Miller & R. Tewksbury (Eds.), *Extreme methods: Innovative approaches to social science research* (pp. 35–47). Boston, MA: Allyn & Bacon.

Maxcy, S. (2003). Pragmatic threads in mixed methods research in the social sciences: The search for multiple modes of inquiry and the end of the philosophy of formalism." In A.Tashakkori & C.Teddlie (Eds.), *Handbook of mixed methods in social and behavioral research*. Thousand Oaks, CA: SAGE.

Maxwell, J., & Loomis, D. (2003) Mixed methods design: An alternative approach. In A. Tashakkori & C. Teddlie (Eds.), *Handbook of mixed methods in social and behavioral research*. Thousand Oaks, CA: SAGE.

McFarland, D. A., Lewis, K., & Goldberg, A. (2016). Sociology in the era of big data: The ascent of forensic social science. *The American Sociologist*, 47(1), 12–35.

McGhee, J. W. (1985). *Introductory statistics*. Los Angeles, CA: West Publishing.

McGuire, W. J. (1973). The yin and yang of progress in social psychology: Seven koan. *Journal of Personality and Social Psychology*, 26, 446–456.

McNamee, R. (2019). *Zucked: Waking up the Facebook catastrophe*. New York, NY: Penguin.

McNeeley, S., & Warner, J. J. (2015). Replication in criminology: A necessary practice. *European Journal of Criminology*, 12(5), 581–597.

McTaggart, R. (1991). Principles for participatory action research. *Adult Education Quarterly*, 41(3), 168–187. doi:10.1177/0001848191041003003

Mead, G. H. (1934). *Mind, self, and society: From the standpoint of a social behaviorist*. Chicago, IL: University of Chicago Press.

Mead, M. (1960). *Coming of age in Samoa: A psychological study of primitive youth for Western civilization*. New York, NY: Mentor. (Originally published 1928.)

Menikoff, J., Kaneshiro, J., & Pritchard, I. (2017). The common rule, updated. *New England Journal of Medicine*, 376(7), 613–615.

Merton, R. K. (1987). The focussed interview and focus groups: Continuities and discontinuities. *Public Opinion Quarterly*, 51(4), 550–566.

Meyer, R. (2014, June 28). Everything we know about Facebook's secret mood manipulation experiment. It was probably legal. But was it ethical? *The Atlantic*. Retrieved October 24, 2020, from https://www.theatlantic.com/technology/archive/2014/06/everything-we-know-about-facebooks-secret-mood-manipulation-experiment/373648/

Miles, M., & Huberman, M. (1994). *Qualitative data analysis* (2nd ed.). Thousand Oaks, CA: SAGE.

Milgram, S. (1963). Behavioral study of obedience. *Journal of Abnormal and Social Psychology*, 67, 371–378.

Milgram, S. (1974). *Obedience to authority: An experimental view*. New York, NY: Harper & Row.

Mill, J. S. (1965). *A system of logic*. London: Longman's, Green. (Reprint of 8th edition, originally published 1881; 1st edition published 1843.)

Miller, J. M., & Tewksbury, R. (Eds.). (2001). *Extreme methods: Innovative approaches to social science research.* Boston, MA: Allyn & Bacon.

Mills, C. W. (1959). *The sociological imagination.* New York, NY: Oxford University Press.

Mindell, J. S., Giampaoli, S., Goesswald, A., Kamtsiuris, P., Mann, C., Männistö, S., … Tolonen, H. (2015). Sample selection, recruitment and participation rates in health examination surveys in Europe – experience from seven national surveys. *BMC Medical Research Methodology, 15*(1), 78. doi:10.1186/s12874-015-0072-4

Miner, H. (1956). Body ritual among the Nacirema. *American Anthropologist, 58,* 503–507.

Mitchell, A. (1994, July 13). Study debunks immigration myths: Harder working, better educated than Canadian-born, Statscan says. Globe and Mail, pp. A1, A2.

Mlodinow, L. (2008). *The drunkard's walk: How randomness rules our lives.* New York, NY: Random House.

Moloney, M. (2010). *Voices from the grave.* London: Faber & Faber.

Monette, D. R., Sullivan, T. J., & DeJong, C. R. (1994). *Applied social research: Tool for the human services.* Fort Worth, TX: Harcourt Brace.

Monture-Okanee, P. A. (1993). Reclaiming justice: Aboriginal women and justice initiatives in the 1990s. In Royal Commission on Aboriginal Peoples (Eds.), *Aboriginal peoples and the justice system* (pp. 105–132). Ottawa, Canada: Canada Communication Group Publishing.

Mook, D. G. (1983). In defence of external invalidity. *American Psychologist, 38,* 379–387.

Morden, H. K., & Palys, T. (2019). Measuring crime. In N. Boyd (Ed.), *Understanding crime in Canada: An introduction to criminology* (2nd ed.). Toronto, Canada: Edmond Montgomery.

Morgan, G. (1983). Research as engagement: A personal view. In G. Morgan (Ed.), *Beyond method: Strategies for social research* (pp. 383–391). Thousand Oaks, CA: SAGE.

Morgan, D. L. (1988). *Focus groups as qualitative research.* Thousand Oaks, CA: SAGE.

Morgan, D. L. (2008). Sampling. In L. Givens (Ed.), *The Sage encyclopedia of qualitative research methods* (Vol. 2, pp. 799–800). Thousand Oaks, CA: SAGE.

Morgan, D. L. (2019). *Basic and advanced focus groups.* Thousand Oaks, CA: SAGE.

Morse, J. M. (1994). Designing funded qualitative research. In N. K. Denzin & Y. S. Lincoln (Eds.), *Handbook of qualitative research* (pp. 220–235). Thousand Oaks, CA: SAGE.

Mudde, C. (2004). The populist zeitgeist. *Government and Opposition, 39*(4), 541–563.

Mudde, C. (2015, February 17). The problem with populism. *The Guardian.* Retrieved from https://www.theguardian.com/commentisfree/2015/feb/17/problem-populism-syriza-podemos-dark-side-europe

National Center for Health Statistics. (2017). *National health interview survey early release program.* Retrieved from https://www.cdc.gov/nchs/data/nhis/earlyrelease/Wireless_state_201903.pdf

Native kids used for experiments. (2000, April 26). *Vancouver Sun,* p. A12.

Neuendorf, K., Gore, T., Dalessandro, A., Janstova, P., & Snyder-Suhy, S. (2010). Shaken and stirred: A content analysis of women's portrayals in James Bond films. *Sex Roles, 62*(11-12), 747–761.

Olesen, V. (1994). Feminisms and models of qualitative research. In N. K. Denzin & Y. S. Lincoln (Eds.), *Handbook of qualitative research* (pp. 158–174). Thousand Oaks, CA: SAGE.

Olson, K., & Shopes, L. (1991). Crossing boundaries, building bridges: Doing oral history among working-class men and women. In S. B. Gluck & D.Patai (Eds.), *Womens words: The feminist practice of oral history* (pp. 189–204). New York, NY: Routledge.

Osgood, C. E., Suci, G. J., & Tannenbaum, P. H. (1957). *The measurement of meaning.* Urbana, IL: University of Illinois.

Oskamp, S. (1977). *Attitudes and opinions.* Englewood Cliffs, NJ: Prentice-Hall.

O'Doherty, T. (2011a). Criminalization and off-street sex work in Canada. *Canadian Journal of Criminology and Criminal Justice, 53*(2), 217–245.

O'Doherty, T. (2011b). Victimization in off-street sex industry work. *Violence Against Women, 17*(7), 944–963.

O'Leary, Z. (2014). *The essential guide to doing your research project* (2nd ed.). Thousand Oaks, CA: SAGE.

O'Leary, Z., & Hunt, J. S. (2016). *Workplace research: Conducting small scale research in organizations.* Thousand Oaks, CA: SAGE.

O'Neil, R. M. (1996). A researcher's privilege: Does any hope remain? *Law and Contemporary Problems, 59,* 35–50.

Palys, T. (1978). Simulation methods and social psychology. *Journal for the Theory of Social Behavior*, 8, 343–368.

Palys, T. (1986). Testing the common wisdom: The social content of video pornography. *Canadian Psychology*, 27, 22–35.

Palys, T. (1989). Addressing the "third criterion" in experimentalist research: Towards a balance of manipulative and analytic control. In I. Benbasat (Ed.), *The information systems research challenge: Experimental research methods*. Boston, MA: Harvard Business School. (Vol. 2 of the Harvard Business School Research Colloquium Series, J. I. Cash, Jr., & J. F. Nunamaker, Jr. [Eds.].) Retrieved from http://www.sfu.ca/~palys/Palys1989-Addressing TheThirdCriterion.pdf

Palys, T. (1990). Ideology, epistemology, and modes of inquiry: Aboriginal issues, trajectories of truth, and the criteria of evaluation research. Paper presented at a meeting of the West Coast Law and Society Group, Vancouver, BC. Retrieved from https://www.sfu.ca/~palys/ideology.htm

Palys, T. (1994). *Statement of Dr. Ted S. Palys: Comments on the statement by Dr. Neil Malamuth*. Report prepared for Arvay Findlay, solicitors for Little Sister's Book and Art Emponum, for the case of Little Sister's v. The Queen. Last Retrieved December 23, 2011, from http://www.sfu.ca/~palys/court.htm

Palys, T. (1999). Vancouver's Aboriginal Restorative Justice Programme: The challenges ahead. *Aboriginal Justice Bulletin*, 3(1), 2–3.

Palys, T. (2003). Histories of convenience: Images of Aboriginal peoples in film, policy and research. In H. N. Nicholson (Ed.), *Screening culture: Constructing Image and Identity* (pp. 19–34). Lanham, MD: Lexington Books.

Palys, T. (2008). Purposive sampling. In L. Givens (Ed.), *The Sage encyclopedia of qualitative research methods* (Vol. 2, pp. 697–698). Thousand Oaks, CA: SAGE.

Palys, T. (2016). The cost of free: Implications of contemporary internet governance for the future of criminological research. Paper presented at the annual meetings of the Western Society of Criminology, Vancouver, BC. Speaking notes online at https://www.sfu.ca/~palys/WSC-2016-TheCostOfFree.pdf

Palys, T., & Atchison, C. (2012). Obstacles and opportunities: Qualitative research in the digital age. *International Journal for Qualitative Methods*, 11(4), 352–367.

Palys, T., & Atchison, C. (2014). *Research decisions: Quantitative, qualitative and mixed methods approaches* (5th ed.). Toronto, Canada: Thomson Nelson.

Palys, T., Boyanowsky, E. O., & Dutton, D. G. (1984). Mobile data access terminals and their implications for policing. *Journal of Social Issues*, 40(3), 113–127.

Palys, T., Olver, J. O., and Banks, L. K. (1983). Social definitions of pornography. Paper presented to the annual meetings of the Canadian Psychological Association, Winnipeg, MN.

Palys, T., & Lowman, J. (1984). Methodological meta-issues in pornography research: Ecological representativeness and contextual integrity. Paper presented at the annual meetings of the Canadian Psychological Association, Ottawa, ON.

Palys, T., & Lowman, J. (2000). Ethical and legal strategies for protecting confidential research information. *Canadian Journal of Law and Society*, 15(1), 39–80.

Palys, T., & Lowman, J. (2001). Social research with eyes wide shut: The limited confidentiality dilemma. *Canadian Journal of Criminology*, 43, 255–267.

Palys, T., & Lowman, J. (2002). Anticipating law: Research methods, ethics and the common law of privilege. *Sociological Methodology*, 32, 1–17.

Palys, T., & Lowman, J. (2012). Defending research confidentiality "to the extent the law allows": Lessons from the Boston College subpoenas. *Journal of Academic Ethics*, 10(4), 271–297.

Palys, T., & Lowman, J. (2014). *Protecting research confidentiality: What happens when law and ethics collide*. Toronto, Canada: Lorimer.

Palys, T., and Lowman, J. (2015). A Belfast Project Autopsy: Who can you trust? In M. Tolich (Ed.), *Qualitative ethics in practice* (109–119). Walnut Creek, CA: Left Coast Press.

Palys, T., & MacAlister, D. (2016). Protecting research confidentiality via the wigmore criteria: Some implications of *parent and bruckert v The Queen and Luka Rocco Magnotta*. *Canadian Journal of Law and Society*, 31(3), 473–493.

Palys, T., Schaefer, R., & Nuszdorfer, Y. (2014). Lessons from a case study of Aboriginal and Canadian justice coexistence in Vancouver. *Justice as Healing*, 19(4), 1–8.

Palys, T., Turk, J., & Lowman, J. (2018). Statute-based protections for research participant confidentiality: Implications of the US experience for Canada. *Canadian Journal of Law and Society*, 33(3), 381–400.

Palys, T. S., & Williams, D. W. (1983). Attitudes regarding capital punishment: On the assessment of false dichotomies. Paper presented at the annual meetings of the Canadian Psychological Association, Winnipeg, MN.

Park, R. E. (1952). *The collected papers of Robert Ezra Park, Vol. 2: Human communities: The city and human ecology.* Glencoe, IL: Free Press.

Parsons, T. (1959). Some problems confronting sociology as a profession. *American Sociological Review, 24,* 547–559.

Patai, D. (1991). US academics and Third World women: Is ethical research possible? In S. B. Gluck & D. Patai (Eds.), *Womens words: The feminist practice of oral history* (pp. 137–154). New York, NY: Routledge.

Patton, M. (1990). *Qualitative evaluation and research methods* (pp. 169–186). Thousand Oaks, CA: SAGE.

Pearce, M. (2002). Challenging the system: Rethinking ethics review of social research in Britain's National Health Service. In W. C. van den Hoonaard (Ed.), *Walking the tightrope: Ethical issues for qualitative researchers* (pp. 43–58). Toronto, Canada: University of Toronto Press.

Pedhazur, E. J. (1982). *Multiple regression in behavioral research: Explanation and prediction* (2nd ed.). New York, NY: Holt, Rinehart and Winston.

Peiris, D. R., Gregor, P., & Alm, N. (2000). The effects of simulating human conversational style in a computer-based interview. *Interacting With Computers, 12,* 635–650.

Pepinsky, H. (1987). Justice as information sharing. In J. Lowman, R. J. Menzies, & T. S. Palys (Eds.), *Transcarceration: Essays in the sociology of social control* (pp. 76–88). Aldershot, UK: Gower.

Petersen, A. M. (1994). *Waltzing with an elephant: First Nations womens experience in creating a shelter for women in crisis.* Unpublished master's thesis, Simon Fraser University, Burnaby, BC.

Pettit, F. (2002). A comparison of World-Wide Web and paper-and-pencil personality questionnaires. *Behavior Research Methods, Instruments, and Computers, 34,* 50–54.

Pew Research Centre. (2010). State of the news media 2010: Declines in news audience, revenue, reporting – And a grim picture for economic models for online news. Retrieved October 24, 2020, from https://www.pewresearch.org/internet/2010/03/15/state-of-the-news-media-2010/

Phillips, D. J. P. (2014). *How to avoid death by PowerPoint. TEDx-StockholmSalon talk.* Retrieved from https://www.youtube.com/watch?v=Iwpi1Lm6dFo

Popkin, S. (2001). Interview with Samuel Popkin. In B. Schultz & R.Schultz (Eds.), *The price of dissent: Testimonies to political repression in America* (pp. 339–347). Berkeley, CA: University of California Press.

Popper, K. R. (1959). *The logic of scientific discovery.* New York, NY: Basic Books.

Preissle, J. (2008). Analytic induction. In L. Givens (Ed.), *The Sage encyclopedia of qualitative research methods* (Vol.1, pp. 15–16). Thousand Oaks, CA: SAGE.

Punch, M. (1994). Politics and ethics in qualitative research. In N. K. Denzin & Y. S. Lincoln (Eds.), *Handbook of qualitative research* (pp. 83–97). Thousand Oaks, CA: SAGE.

Ragin, C. (1987). *The comparative method.* Berkley, CA: University of California Press.

Ragin, C. C. (1992). Introduction: Cases of "What is a case?" In C. C. Ragin & H. S. Becker (Eds.), *What is a case: Exploring the foundations of social inquiry* (pp. 1–18). New York, NY: Cambridge University Press.

Ragin, C. C., & Amoroso, L. M. (2018). *Constructing social research: The unity and diversity of method* (3rd ed.). Thousand Oaks, CA: SAGE.

Ratel, P. (2008). One day at a time: Single parent mothers in academe. In T. Palys & C. Atchison, *Research decisions: Quantitative and qualitative perspectives.* (4th ed., pp. 404–414). Toronto, Canada: Thomson Nelson. Retrieved from http://www.sfu.ca/~palys/Ratel.pdf

Rawls, J. (1971). *A theory of justice.* Cambridge, MA: Harvard University Press.

Redelmeier, D. A. (2005). The cognitive psychology of missed diagnoses. *Annals of Internal Medicine, 142,* 115–120.

Reeve, B. B., Willis, G., Shariff-Marco, S. N., Breen, N., Williams, D. R., Gee, G. C., … Levin, K. Y. (2011). Comparing cognitive interviewing and psychometric methods to evaluate a racial/ethnic discrimination scale. *Field Methods, 23*(4), 397–419.

Reinharz, S. (1992). *Feminist methods in social research.* New York, NY: Oxford University Press.

Reverby, S. M. (2012). Ethical failures and history lessons: The US Public Health Service Research Studies in Tusekegee and Guatemala. *Public Health Reviews, 34*(1), 1–19.

Rice, S. A. (Ed.). (1931). *Methods in social science.* Chicago, IL: University of Chicago Press.

Richards of Rockford Inc. v. Pacific Gas and Electric Co. 71 F.R.D. 388 (N.D. Cal, 1976).

Richards, L. (1999). *Using NVivo in qualitative research.* London: SAGE.

Richardson, L. (1994). Writing: A method of inquiry. In N. K. Denzin & Y. S. Lincoln (Eds.), *Handbook of qualitative research* (pp. 516–529). Thousand Oaks, CA: SAGE.

Richardson, L. (2003). Writing: A method of inquiry. In N. K. Denzin & Y. S. Lincoln (Eds.), *Collecting and interpreting qualitative materials* (2nd ed., pp. 499–541). Thousand Oaks, CA: Sage.

Riecken, H. W. (1969). The unidentified interviewer. In G. J. McCall & J. L. Simmons (Eds.), *Issues in participant observation* (pp. 39–43). Reading, MA: Addison-Wesley.

Rigakos, G. (1995). Constructing the symbolic complainant: Police subculture and the non-enforcement of protection orders for battered women. *Violence and Victims*, 10(3), 127–147.

Ripley, E. B. D. (2006). A review of paying research participants: It's time to move beyond the ethical debate. *Journal of Empirical Research on Human Research Ethics*, 1(4), 9–19.

Robinson, S. B., & Leonard, K. F. (2019). *Designing quality survey questions*. Thousand Oaks, CA: SAGE.

Rosenhan, D. L. (1973). On being sane in insane places. *Science*, 179, 250–258.

Rosenstock, I. (1974). Historical origins of the health belief model. *Health Education Monographs*, 2(4), 328–335.

Rosenthal, R., & Rosnow, R. L. (1969). *Artifact in behavioral research*. New York, NY: Academic Press.

Rosenthal, R., & Rosnow, R. L. (1984). *Essentials of behavioral research: Methods and data analysis*. New York, NY: McGraw-Hill.

Roth, J. A. (1969). A codification of current prejudices. *American Sociologist*, 4, 159.

Rubenstein, S. M. (1995). *Surveying public opinion*. Belmont, NY: Wadsworth.

Rubin, Z. (1973). *Liking and loving*. New York, NY: Holt, Rinehart and Winston.

Rubington, E., & Weinberg, M. S. (Eds.). (1968). *Deviance: The interactionist perspective*. New York, NY: Macmillan.

Rubin, H. J., & Rubin, I. S. (2012). *Qualitative interviewing: The art of hearing data* (3rd ed.). Thousand Oaks, CA: SAGE.

Rugg, D. (1941). Experiments in wording questions: II. *Public Opinion Quarterly*, 5(1), 91–92.

Ryan, C. (2017). Computer and internet use in the United States: 2016. American Community Survey Reports, ACS-39, U.S. Census Bureau, Washington, DC.

Saari, L. M., & Judge, T. A. (2004). Employee attitudes and job satisfaction. *Human Resource Management*, 43(4), 395–407.

Salamon, E. (1984). *The kept woman: Mistresses in the 80s*. London: Orbis.

Salazar, C. (1991). A Third World woman's text: Between the politics of criticism and cultural politics. In S. B. Gluck & D. Patai (Eds.), *Womens words: The feminist practice of oral history* (pp. 93–106). New York, NY: Routledge.

Samuels, M., & Ryan, K. (2011). Grounding evaluations in culture. *American Journal of Evaluation*, 32(2), 183–198.

Sanders, J., & Patterson, D. (2018, December 11). Facebook data privacy scandal: A cheat sheet. *Tech Republic*. Retrieved from https://www.techrepublic.com/article/facebook-data-privacy-scandal-a-cheat-sheet/

Santos, D. (2013). (Participatory) action research and the political realm. *Counterpoints*, 354, 492–513.

Scarce, R. (1990). *Eco-warriors: Understanding the radical environmental movement*. Chicago, IL: The Noble Press. Updated editions published in 2006 (Left Coast Press) and 2016 (Routledge).

Scarce, R. (1994). (No) trial (but) tribulations: When courts and ethnography conflict. *Journal of Contemporary Ethnography*, 23, 123–149.

Scarce, R. (1999). Good faith, bad ethics: When scholars go the distance and scholarly associations do not. *Law and Social Inquiry*, 24, 977–986.

Scarce, R. (2005). *Contempt of court: A scholar's battle for free speech from behind bars*. Oxford, UK: Altamira Press.

Schatzman, L., & Strauss, A. L. (1973). *Field research: Strategies for a natural sociology*. Englewood Cliffs, NJ: Prentice-Hall.

Schmidt, W. C. (2002). A server-side program for delivering experiments with animations. *Behavior Research Methods, Instruments, and Computers*, 34, 208–217.

Schrag, Z. (2017). *Ethical imperialism: Institutional review boards and the social sciences, 1965-2009*. Baltimore, MD: Johns Hopkins University Press.

Schuler, E. A. (1967). Report of the Committee on Professional Ethics. *American Sociologist*, 2, 242–244.

Schuman, H., & Presser, S. (1981). *Questions and answers in attitude surveys: Experiments on question form, wording and context*. New York, NY: Academic Press.

Schutz, A. (1970). Interpretive sociology. In H. R. Wagner (Ed.), *Alfred Schutz: On phenomenology and social relations* (pp. 265–293). Chicago, IL: University of Chicago Press.

Schwandt, T. A. (1994). Constructivist, interpretivist approaches to human inquiry. In N. K. Denzin & Y. S. Lincoln (Eds.), *Handbook of qualitative research* (pp. 118–137). Thousand Oaks, CA: SAGE.

Scriven, M. (1976). Maximizing the power of causal investigations: The modus operandi method. In F. V. Glass (Ed.), *Evaluation studies review annual* (Vol. 1, pp. 101–118). Thousand Oaks, CA: SAGE.

Seidman, D., & Couzens, M. (1974). Getting the crime rate down: Political pressure and crime reporting. *Law and Society Review*, 8, 457–493.

Shadish, W. R., Cook, T. D., & Campbell, D. T. (2001). *Experimental and quasi-experimental designs for generalized causal inference.* New York, NY: Houghton Mifflin.

Shank, G. (2008a). Deduction. In L. M. Given (Ed.), *The Sage encyclopedia of qualitative research methods* (Vol. 1, pp. 207–208). Thousand Oaks, CA: SAGE.

Shank, G. (2008b). Abduction. In L. M. Given (Ed.), *The Sage encyclopedia of qualitative research methods* (Vol. 1, pp. 1–2). Thousand Oaks, CA: SAGE.

Shea, C. (2000). Don't talk to the humans: The crackdown on social science research. *Linguafranca*, 10(6), 1–17.

Sheehan, K. B., & Hoy, M. G. (1999). Using e-mail to survey Internet users in the United States: Methodology and assessment. *Journal of Computer Mediated Communication*, 4(3), JCMC435. Retrieved from http://www.ascusc.org/jcmc/vol4/issue3/sheehan.html

Sherif, M., Harvey, O. J., White, B. J., Hood, W. E., & Sherif, C. W. (1961). *Intergroup conflict and cooperation: The Robber's Cave experiment.* Norman, OK: University of Oklahoma Book Exchange.

Silverman, D. (1985). *Qualitative methodology and sociology.* Brookfield, VT: Gower.

Skogan, W. G. (1975). Measurement problems in official and survey crime rates. *Journal of Criminal Justice*, 3, 17–32.

Smith, L. T. (2001). *Decolonizing methodologies: Research and indigenous peoples.* London: Zed Books.

Social Sciences and Humanities Research Ethics Special Working Committee (SSHWC). (2004). *Giving voice to the spectrum: Report of the Social Sciences and Humanities Research Ethics Special Working Committee.* Report prepared for the federal Interagency Advisory Panel on Research Ethics. Retrieved from http://www.re.ethics.gc.ca/english/workgroups/sshwc/SSHW-CVoiceReportJune2004.pdf

Social Sciences and Humanities Research Ethics Special Working Committee (SSHWC). (2008). SSHWC recommendations regarding privacy and confidentiality. Report prepared for the Interagency Advisory Panel on Research Ethics. Retrieved from https://www.sfu.ca/~palys/SSHWC-RecommendationsRePrivacyAndConfidentiality2008.pdf

Soothill, K., & Sanders, T. (2005). The geographical mobility, preferences and pleasures of prolific punters: A demonstration study of the activities of prostitutes' clients. *Sociological Research Online*, 10(1), 17–30. Retrieved from http://socresonline.org.uk/10/1/soothill.html

Stake, R. E. (2003). Case studies. In N. K. Denzin & Y. S. Lincoln (Eds.), *Strategies of qualitative inquiry* (pp. 134–164). Thousand Oaks, CA: SAGE.

Starr, L. (1984). Oral history. In D. Dunaway & W. K. Baum (Eds.), *Oral history: An interdisciplinary anthology* (pp. 3–26). Nashville, TN: American Association for State and Local History.

Stevens, S. S. (1951). Mathematics, measurement, and psychophysics. In S. S. Stevens (Ed.), *Handbook of experimental psychology* (pp. 1–49). Hoboken, NJ: Wiley.

Stinchcombe, A. (1968). *Constructing social theories.* New York, NY: Harcourt Brace Jovanovich.

Stones, M., & McMillan, J. (2010). Payment for participation in research: A pursuit for the poor?. *Journal of Medical Ethics*, 36(1), 34–36.

Strauss, A. L. (1987). *Qualitative analysis for social scientists.* New York, NY: Cambridge University Press.

Strunk, W., Jr. (1999). *The elements of style.* New York, NY: Bartleby. (Originally published 1918). Retrieved from www.bartleby.com/141

Sudman, S., & Bradburn, N. M. (1982). *Asking questions.* San Francisco, CA: Jossey-Bass.

Tajfel, H. (1972). Experiments in a vacuum. In J. Israel & H. Tajfel (Eds.), *The context of social psychology* (pp. 69–119). London: Academic Press.

Team Populism & The Guardian. (2019, March 5). *Coding rubric and anchor texts for the global populism database.* Retrieved from https://populism.byu.edu/App_Data/Publications/Populism%20codebook_The%20New%20Populism%20201903%20(2).pdf

Teddlie, C. & Tashakkori, A. (2003). Major issues and controversies in the use of mixed methods in the social and behavioural sciences. In Tashakkori, A. & Teddlie, C. (Eds.), *Handbook of mixed methods in social and behavioral research.* Thousand Oaks, CA: SAGE.

Temple, E. C., & Brown, R. F. (2011). A comparison of Internet-based participant recruitment methods: Engaging the hidden population of cannabis users in research. *Journal of Research Practice*, 7(2), Article D2. Retrieved January 15, 2020, from http://jrp.icaap.org/index.php/jrp/article/view/288/247

Terkel, S. (1975). *Working*. New York, NY: Avon.

Terry, W. (1984). *Bloods: An oral history of the Vietnam War by black veterans*. New York, NY: Random House.

Thomas, W. I. (1928). *The child in America: Behavior problems and programs*. New York, NY: Knopf.

Thomas, J. (1993). *Doing ethnography*. Thousand Oaks, CA: SAGE.

Thomas, G. (2016). *How to do your case study* (2nd ed.). Thousand Oaks, CA: SAGE.

Thomas, J. (2019). *Death by PowerPoint: The slide that killed seven people*. Online at McDdreemie's Meducational & Medhistorical Musings blog. See https://mcdreeamiemusings.com/new-blog/2019/4/13/gsux1h6bnt8lqjd7w2t2mtvfg81uhx

Thornton, G. R. (1943). The effect upon judgments of personality traits of varying a single factor in a photograph. *Journal of Social Psychology*, 18, 127–148.

Thornton, G. R. (1944). The effects of wearing glasses upon judgments of personality traits of persons seen briefly. *Journal of Applied Psychology*, 18, 203–207.

Tinati, R., Halford, S., Carr, L., & Pope, C. (2014). Big data: Methodological challenges and approaches for sociological analysis. *Sociology*, 48(4), 663–681.

Traynor, M. (1996). Countering the excessive subpoena for scholarly research. *Law and Contemporary Problems*, 59, 119–148.

Trigger, B. G. (1988). The historians' Indian: Native Americans in Canadian historical writing from Charlevoix to the present. In R. Fisher & K. Coates (Eds.), *Out of the background: Readings on Canadian Native history* (pp. 19–44). Toronto, Canada: Copp Clark Pitman.

Tuckel, P., & O'Neill, H. (2002). The vanishing respondent in telephone surveys. *Journal of Advertising Research*, 42, 26–48.

Tufte, E. (n.d.). *PowerPoint does rocket science: Assessing the quality and credibility of technical reports*. Retrieved from https://www.edwardtufte.com/bboard/q-and-a-fetch-msg?msg_id=0001yB&topic_id=1&topic=Ask+E%2eT%2e

United Nations. (2004). *Information and communications technology (ICT): Vital statistics*. Retrieved September 2004, from http://cyberschoolbus.un.org/Cyberschoolbus/Briefing/Technology/Index.htm

United States Census Bureau. (2017). *Voting and registration in the election of November 2016*. Retrieved from https://www.census.gov/data/tables/time-series/demo/voting-and-registration/p20-580.html

van den Hoonaard, W. C. (2001). *Walking the tightrope: Ethical issues for qualitative researchers*. Toronto, Canada: University of Toronto Press.

Verma, I. M. (2014, July 22). Editorial expression of concern and correction. *Proceedings of the National Academy of Sciences of the United States of America*, 111(29), 10779.

Vidich, A. J., and Lyman, S. M. (1994). Qualitative methods: Their history in sociology and anthropology. In N. K. Denzin & Y. S. Lincoln (Eds.), *Handbook of qualitative research* (pp. 23–59). Thousand Oaks, CA: SAGE.

Vidich, A. J., and Lyman, S. M. (2003). Qualitative methods: Their history in sociology and anthropology. In N. K. Denzin & Y. S. Lincoln (Eds.), *The landscape of qualitative research: Theories and issues* (2nd ed., pp. 55–130). Thousand Oaks, CA: SAGE.

Wagner, D. G. (1984). *The growth of sociological theories*. Thousand Oaks, CA: SAGE.

Warwick, D. P., & Lininger, C. A. (1975). *The sample survey: Theory and practice*. New York, NY: McGraw-Hill.

Watson, J. B. (1913). Psychology as the behaviorist views it. *Psychological Review*, 20, 158–177.

Webb, E. T., Campbell, D. T., Schwartz, R. D., & Sechrest, L. (1966). *Unobtrusive measures: Nonreactive research in the social sciences*. Skokie, IL: Rand McNally.

Weber, M. (1968). Objectivity in social science. In M. Brodbeck (Ed.), *Readings in the philosophy of the social sciences* (pp. 85–97). New York, NY: Macmillan. (Reprinted from M. Weber, 1949, *The methodology of the social sciences*, New York: The Free Press.)

Weick, K. E. (1968). Systematic observational methods. In E. Aronson & G. Lindzey (Eds.), *The handbook of social psychology* (Vol. 2). Boston, MA: Addison-Wesley.

Weiss, C. H. (1975). Evaluation research in the political context. In E. L. Streuning & M. Guttentag (Eds.), *Handbook of evaluation research* (Vol. 1, pp. 13–26). Thousand Oaks, CA: SAGE.

Weiss, C. H. (1993). Politics and evaluation: A reprise with mellower overtones. *American Journal of Evaluation Research*, 14(1), 107–109.

Weiss, C. H. (2000). The experimenting society in a political world. In L. Bickman (Ed.), *Validity and social experimentation: Donald Campbell's legacy* (pp. 283–302). Thousand Oaks, CA: SAGE.

Whyte, W. F. (1943). *Street corner society: The social structure of an Italian slum*. Chicago, IL: University of Chicago Press.

Whyte, W. F. (1993). *Street corner society: The social structure of an Italian slum* (4th ed.). Chicago, IL: University of Chicago Press.

Wiggins, E. C., & McKenna, J. A. (1996). Researchers' reactions to compelled disclosure of scientific information. In J. S. Cecil & G. T. Wetherington (Eds.), *Court-ordered disclosure of academic research: A clash of values of science and law.* Law and contemporary problems (special issue) (Vol. 59(3), pp. 67–94). Durham, NC: Duke University School of Law.

Wigmore, J. H. (1905). *A treatise on the system of evidence in trials at common law, including the statutes and judicial decisions of all jurisdictions of the United States, England, and Canada.* Boston, MA: Little, Brown.

Willis, G. B., & Miller, K. (2011). Cross-cultural cognitive interviewing: Seeking comparability and enhancing understanding. *Field Methods, 23*(4), 331–341.

Wilson, S. (2008). *Research is ceremony: Indigenous research methods.* Black Point, NS: Fernwood Publishing.

Wolcott, H. F. (2009). *Writing up qualitative research* (3rd ed.). Thousand Oaks, CA: SAGE.

Wolf, M. (1992). *A thrice-told tale: Feminism, postmodernism, and ethnographic responsibility.* Stanford, CA: Stanford University Press.

Wolf, L. E., Patel, M. J., Williams, B. A., Austin, J. L., & Dame, L. A. (2013). Certificates of confidentiality: Protecting human research subject research data in law and practice. *Minnesota Journal of Law, Science & Technology, 14*(1), 11–87.

Woodward, J. L. (1934). Quantitative newspaper analysis as a technique of opinion research. *Social Forces, 12*(4), 526–537.

Woong Yun, W., & Trumbo, C. W. (2000). Comparative response to a survey executed by post, e-mail, and web form. *Journal of Computer Mediated Communication, 6*(1), JCMC613.

Wright, R. (1992). *Stolen continents: The "New World" through Indian eyes since 1492.* Toronto, Canada: Penguin.

Yerkes, R. M., & Dodson, J. D. (1908). The relation of strength of stimulus to rapidity of habit-formation. *Journal of Comparative Neurology and Psychology, 18,* 459–482.

Yin, R. K. (2018). *Case study research and applications: Design and methods* (6th ed.). Thousand Oaks, CA: SAGE.

Zellerer, E. (1996). Community-based justice and violence against women: Issues of gender and race. *International Journal of Comparative and Applied Criminal Justice, 20*(2), 233–244.

Zimbardo, P. G., Ebbesen, E. B., & Maslach, C. (1977). *Influencing attitudes and changing behavior: An introduction to method, theory, and applications of social control and personal power* (2nd ed.). Boston, MA: Addison-Wesley.

Zinger, I. (1999). *The psychological effects of 60 days in administrative segregation.* Doctoral dissertation. Department of Psychology, Carleton University.

Zinger, I., Wichmann, C., & Andrews, D. A. (2001). The effects of administrative segregation. *Canadian Journal of Criminology, 43,* 47–83.

Znaniecki, F. (1934). Analytic induction. In F. Znaniecki (Ed.), *The method of sociology* (pp. 249–331). New York, NY: Farrar & Rinehart.

Zuboff, S. (2015). Big other: Surveillance capitalism and the prospects of an information civilization. *Journal of Information Technology, 30,* 75–89.

Zuboff, S. (2019). *The age of surveillance capitalism: The fight for a human future at the new frontier of power.* New York, NY: Hachette Book Group.

INDEX

Made in the USA
Las Vegas, NV
10 August 2023

75892171R00413